Social and Community Psychiatry

Stelios Stylianidis
Editor

Social and Community Psychiatry

Towards a Critical, Patient-Oriented Approach

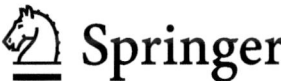

Editor
Stelios Stylianidis
Department of Psychology
Panteion University
Athens
Greece

The Work was first published in 2014 by TOPOS BOOKS/MOTIBO PUBLISHING SA with the following title: Σύγχρονα θέματα κοινωνικής και κοινοτικής ψυχιατρικής: Για μια κριτική ανθρωποκεντρική ψυχιατρική

ISBN 978-3-319-28614-3   ISBN 978-3-319-28616-7 (eBook)
DOI 10.1007/978-3-319-28616-7

Library of Congress Control Number: 2016936100

© Springer International Publishing Switzerland 2016
This work is subject to copyright. All rights are reserved by the Publisher, whether the whole or part of the material is concerned, specifically the rights of translation, reprinting, reuse of illustrations, recitation, broadcasting, reproduction on microfilms or in any other physical way, and transmission or information storage and retrieval, electronic adaptation, computer software, or by similar or dissimilar methodology now known or hereafter developed.
The use of general descriptive names, registered names, trademarks, service marks, etc. in this publication does not imply, even in the absence of a specific statement, that such names are exempt from the relevant protective laws and regulations and therefore free for general use.
The publisher, the authors and the editors are safe to assume that the advice and information in this book are believed to be true and accurate at the date of publication. Neither the publisher nor the authors or the editors give a warranty, express or implied, with respect to the material contained herein or for any errors or omissions that may have been made.

Printed on acid-free paper

This Springer imprint is published by Springer Nature
The registered company is Springer International Publishing AG Switzerland

Foreword

Social psychiatry deals with the context that shapes mental health and mental illness. This is done on a macro level as exemplified by the work on how mental health and mental health problems are framed within the value system of a society with the core topic of discrimination and stigma as well as by epidemiological data like those currently widely debated on inequality and health and mental health. The meso-level concerns key institutions in our societies such as schools, health and social services, housing, employment and legal situations and essentially how help for dealing with mental health problems and disabilities is organised and delivered in a community. The micro-level is dominated essentially by what happens between people with core topics such as therapeutic as well as family and peer communication and support.

All these and more of our field's fundamental issues will be dealt with in this book. As a textbook of social psychiatry, it provides insight into its scientific and political foundations, its core policies and practices and their evolvement to date. All along it also addresses current dynamics and future developments of social psychiatry.

"The future of academic psychiatry may be social" is a convincing 2013 editorial statement in the *British Journal of Psychiatry* by eminent social psychiatrists and researchers Stefan Priebe, Tom Burns and Tom Craig.

Let me take this opportunity to state my conviction that the future of all psychiatry will be social. And let us acknowledge that much of its presence is.

While the great reforms in psychiatric services and treatment of the past decades are far from completed, community-based, integrated service models have by and large replaced the institutional psychiatry that had been dominant in earlier years, at least in the Western industrial nations. Psychiatric inpatient treatment increasingly takes place in general hospital units and is essentially restricted to the provision of crisis intervention over a few days or weeks. While the 1960s were still dominated by the aim of avoiding "institutionalism", i.e. the negative consequences of long institutional stays, nowadays these concerns are confounded by economical considerations calling for ever shorter inpatient stays.

What shape acute services should ideally take and what role hospital beds and their location might play are questions that remain at the forefront of service planners' concerns. Nowadays, in mental health emergency situations, brief inpatient treatment in general hospitals is considered a significant alternative, as well as models of acute mental health home treatment, a form of community-integrated crisis intervention. From a scientific perspective, the minimal number of hospital beds needed remains undetermined as are questions about effectiveness, suitability and possible adverse effects of different community-integrated acute interventions as well as the "dosage", i.e. the intensity of the required community-integrated services that are capable of preventing hospitalisations. This book describes various specific developments for specific situation in different parts of Greece, such as day centres, mobile health teams, ACT and home care.

Fact is, hospital stays take up only a fraction of time in patients' lives. Psychiatric treatment occurs essentially in the community. In the community, that is where mental health and social care workers are busy every day to help other people – in times of crisis as well as in situations of long-term needs for different types of assistance for their life in the community in various roles.

All these activities and interactions in the community together constitute social psychiatry: prevention, treatment, rehabilitation, the provision of assistance in everyday real-life situations, healing and empowering people and communities towards inclusive community life. However, there is a mismatch between the real-life everyday efforts and the conceptual formulations of this kind of essential work. Consequently, textbooks on social psychiatry are rare. This one is a great step. With its comprehensive range of information, it will reach, educate and motivate different professional groups as well as policymakers, but hopefully also activists and various stakeholders including prominently users of services and their families and friends. It will be welcomed as a state-of-the art textbook as well as an orientation and inspiration for further developments.

Professor Stelios Stylianidis is held in highest regard in the international research, policy as well as the mental health practice community. His experience covers essential working fields from grassroot developments to leadership positions in global organisations, clinical practice in different contexts as well as organisational and policy activities on the local, national and international arena over quite some time – times that have seen and brought on tremendous changes.

He and his co-authors address the specific situation in Greece on several levels with relevant historical and conceptual assumptions and a variety of practice examples in different locations and situations. They also introduce topical international developments and their implications for Greece, importantly recovery-orientation and the actual patient and human rights situation, especially with regard to persons with psychosocial disabilities.

Current government policies of recovery-orientation in traditionally influential English-speaking countries follow important changes in mental healthcare over the last decades. Deinstitutionalisation and the community support movement have been accompanied and are intertwined with a strong family movement and a politically influential voice of users of services.

People with a lived experience of mental health problems and treatments have been an essential force among the pioneers of the recovery movement, who have created the concepts and a language for recovery. As authors of the groundwork for the movement, they have developed and impacted not only alternatives but also international mental health system transformation efforts and specific models of recovery-oriented practice.

From their work we know that much of recovery is lived outside clinical settings, but also that important challenges concern the roles and responsibilities of mental health professionals in supporting and assisting people with mental health problems in their efforts towards making full use of their health and resilience and achieving their goals in life. Self-determination and individual choice of flexible support and opportunities, promoting empowerment and hope and assistance in situations of calculated risk are the new indicators of the quality of services. In contrast to a deficit model of mental illness, recovery-orientation includes a focus on health promotion, individual strengths and resilience. A shift from demoralising prognostic scepticism towards a rational and optimistic attitude towards recovery and broadening treatment goals beyond symptom reduction and stabilisation require specific skills and new forms of cooperation between practitioners and service users, between mental health workers of different backgrounds and between psychiatry and the public. New rules for services, for example, user involvement on all levels and person-centred organisation of care, as well as new tools for clinical collaborations, for example, shared decision-making and psychiatric advance directives, are being complemented by new proposals regarding more ethically consistent anti-discrimination and involuntary treatment legislation, as well as participatory approaches to evidence-based medicine and policy.

Recovery demands all our best efforts in terms of human rights, patients' rights, scientific and clinical responsibility and service, in the interest of those of us who might become patients and those who have. We learn from those who are using services, those who have used services (ex-users) and those who define themselves through overcoming harmful experiences in the support system (survivors).

One prominent example of successful engagement of activists with a lived experience is the explicit inclusion of persons with psychosocial disabilities in the recently widely ratified UN Convention on the Rights of Persons with Disabilities (CRPD). The CRPD puts the force of law behind rights to non-discrimination in key areas, including health, housing, education and employment as well as standards of living and social, political and cultural participation (Bartlett 2012). Community-based services are central to the implementation of the treaty's provisions.

In many ways the first human rights treaty of the twenty-first century epitomises the essentials of recovery. Forged between diplomats and a throng of civil society representatives – many of them persons with disabilities as experts in their own right, including those with psychosocial disabilities (Sabatello and Schulze 2013) – the treaty is the product of a truly participatory process. In a corresponding logic, it makes the consultation of its constituency – persons with disabilities and their representative organisations, respectively – an obligation.

The reality of "nothing about us without us" seems to have arrived and is irreversibly here to stay: no policy development and no amendment of legislation or elaboration of new regulations shall be undertaken without including experts in their own right – persons with a lived experience of mental health problems and services. The Mental Health Action Plan for Europe, the WHO Global Mental

Health Action Plan, the recommendations of the first trialogic task force of the World Psychiatric Association (WPA) providing for a partnership with users of services and their families and friends (Wallcraft et al. 2011) and the call for "user involvement", a "partnership approach" or participatory approach are evidences that henceforth no significant development can be advanced without the meaningful involvement of experts in their own right.

It is against these historic developments and future perspectives that this book presents the breadth and depth of social psychiatric thinking and doing. The reader will be able to understand and roam with pleasure and urgency the landscape opened up by this essential way of looking at reality and knowing how to play a significant role in shaping it. Readers will be motivated and ready for the promotion and implementation of social psychiatric concepts and practice for the good of psychiatry, for medicine and for society.

Wien, Austria   Michaela Amering

Bibliography

Amering M, Schmolke M (2009) Recovery in mental health. Reshaping scientific and clinical responsibilities. Wiley-Blackwell, London

Bartlett P (2012) The United Nations convention on the rights of persons with disabilities and mental health law. Mod Law Rev 75(5):752–778

Priebe S, Burns T, Craig TK (2013) The future of academic psychiatry may be social. Br J Psychiatry, 202(5):319–320

Sabatello M, Schulze M (Eds) (2013) Human rights and disability advocacy. University of Pennsylvania Press

Schulze M (2010) Understanding the convention on the rights of persons with disabilities. Handicap International, New York. Retrieved from: http://hiproweb.org/uploads/tx_hidrtdocs/HICRPDManual2010.pdf

Wallcraft J, Amering M, Freidin J, Davar B, Froggatt D, Jafri H, … Herrman H (2011) Partnerships for better mental health worldwide: WPA recommendations on best practices in working with service users and family carers. World Psychiatry 10(3):229–236

About the Book

Dr. Stylianidis and his colleagues have produced a comprehensive marriage of theoretical social psychiatry and current practice. Their analysis of the historical and conceptual assumptions prevalent in the Greek situation and their impact on attempts to overcome and/or make use of recent chaotic opportunities for change, carry lessons relevant for many other parts of the world wishing to transform mental health services.

Dr. Marianne Farkas
Center for Psychiatric Rehabilitation
Boston University, USA

This book about social psychiatry and public mental health in Greece represents a unique effort to bridge social psychiatry as a theory and as a set of applied strategies. Its middle-income country perspective provides a rather innovative insight

Prof. Benedetto Saraceno,
School of Medical Sciences,
Nova University of Lisbon, Portugal

This book deals with principles of social psychiatry as applied in the current environment that is especially critical for mental health. While awareness on mental health has increased substantially, there are new threats to essential services due to lack of adequate resources. The lessons of this book will be important to keep in mind as countries and communities discuss their plan for mental health.

Dr. Shekhar Saxena
Department of Mental Health and Substance Abuse
World Health Organization, Geneva, Switzerland

This is a book that has much to offer to readers interested in psychiatry and mental health. It includes a comprehensive and original overview of the historical, conceptual, and operational aspects of social psychiatry. It critically discusses the process of mental health reform in Greece, showing the impact of the economic crisis on the mental health of the population in one the most affected countries in Europe. Finally, it introduces the reader to the most recent contributions of psychiatric epidemiology, of the recovery approach, and of global health and mental health promotion, helping to understand why these contributions have radically changed mental health across the world.

Dr. José Miguel Caldas de Almeida
Department of Mental Health
NOVA University of Lisbon, Portugal

Introduction

Social and community psychiatry cover wide, complex fields. Our contemporary world requires that we re-examine those fields both from an interdisciplinary and public health perspective.

The scope of social psychiatry ranges from understanding the impact of social structures and experiences on the appearance, course and outcome of mental disorders, through the development and evaluation of complex social interventions and services, right up to the impact of society on the construction of mental disorders and the responses it provides to them (Morgan and Bhugra 2010). From that viewpoint we can argue that social psychiatry interacts with intercultural and community psychiatry, taking a philosophical approach about the emergency and aetiology of mental disorders, and intersects with a series of other scientific disciplines including clinical psychiatry, various schools of individual and group psychotherapy, social epidemiology, public health, sociology and anthropology. By formulating the basic hypothesis that mental disorders like all mental phenomena cannot be seen outside of the historical, socio-cultural and economic environment in which they emerge, social psychiatry occupies an interim position between biomedicine, genetics, the neurosciences, psychology and the social disciplines.

Social psychiatry has changed over time as it followed wider scientific, cultural and policy developments in community psychiatry. According to Thornicroft and Tansella (2001, 2010), community-based mental health services are those which provide a full range of effective mental healthcare to a specific population and which, in cooperation with other local bodies, train and help people with mental disorders, so as to relieve their stress and pain.

Our key argument is that despite fears over the disappearance of both social psychiatry and the special nature of psychiatry overall as a discipline for studying, understanding and treating psychopathological phenomena, social psychiatry can only be theorised about and implemented in practice through constant interaction between genetics, biology, psychology and the social sciences. These disciplines should not compete against each other or vie for importance with each other, but ought to be factors in a common effort to understand the psychopathology of the complex living being that is man, by taking a holistic approach to his existence.

The proclamations made by the world psychiatric community about the biopsychosocial model of mental illness remain a lot of hot air in day-to-day clinical practice, to the extent that emphasis is only placed on one of those aspects (such as biological treatments to ease symptoms, or psychotherapy or psychosocial interventions).

In conclusion, social psychiatry deals with the impact of the social environment on an individual's mental health and with how individuals facing mental problems interact with their social environment.

Social Psychiatry and the Situation in European Countries

First, some specific data: one in four European citizens will have some sort of mental health problem over the course of their lifetime (Herman et al. 2005). It's estimated that more than 27 % of adult European citizens will experience a mental disorder every year, the most frequently occurring being stress-related disorders and depression (Fryers et al. 2003; WHO 2010). In Europe, mental disorders are estimated at 20 % of all disability, and according to the WHO by 2020 depression will be the main cause of disability and disability-adjusted life years (DALYS) in the developed world (WHO 2008). Despite governments, international organisations, health policymakers, international research centres and universities having jointly realised that the extent and scale of the mental health problem is immense, the way in which mental health services are organised and funded in Europe varies wildly and is far from being considered satisfactory. Given the current socioeconomic crisis, which by the look of things will be long-lasting, the massive increase in social inequalities and the increase in the vicious cycle of poverty, social exclusion, stigmatism, self-stigmatism and the major increase in mental disorders, mental health as a major public health problem continues to be very low on the political agenda of EU countries, save for very few exceptions.

Implementing the WHO guidelines (2001, 2003) calling for a series of real actions to promote and improve public mental health and defend the basic constitutional rights of European citizens suffering from a serious mental disorder remains, to a large degree, mere statements of principle that are far from offering the possibility of comprehensive psychosocial interventions that meet the population's real needs.

In addition, given the diverse economic, social and institutional crisis which is shaking the very European venture to its core, and calling into question the viability of the welfare state, the problem of limited resources, means and targets for psychiatric care systems has been raised and strongly reiterated by all stakeholders: politicians, mental health professionals, family associations, users of mental health services, local communities and local governments.

However, we find ourselves faced with a major paradox, at both global and European levels: the few resources available for mental health are unevenly distributed, without any real evaluation and monitoring of the quality of care or the outcome of all services provided. For example, the WHO's *Mental Health Atlas* (2005) states that Europe has the largest number of psychiatric clinics per capita in the general population (8/10,000 residents) while 70 % of resources for mental health are still being invested in old-style psychiatric hospitals or asylums – new community-based institutions. Even though the differences in GDP between various

European states are not large, it is clear that mental health policy and the psychiatric care models and culture which prevail are determined by a series of factors such as the number of psychiatric clinics, the number of psychiatrists compared to other mental health professionals, the number of hospitalisations on orders from the Public Prosecutor, the *revolving door* phenomenon, the operation of social networks to provide social care, the real involvement and participation of families and users in the design and running of mental health services, and so on.

Consequently, a key issue in the current debate about mental health resources, and about harmonising in- and outpatient models for providing psychiatric care (what one might call a balanced care model approach), clearly highlights the importance of social and community psychiatry for the contemporary socioeconomic situation (Thornicroft and Tansella 2013). As Thornicroft and Tansella (2001) so aptly point out, "Social care … is a vehicle for providing services. It can allow treatment to be provided to a patient, but is not treatment in itself". As part of this work, by exploring different scientific and social approaches, we will attempt to show that even today the key elements of treatments and the outcomes of different models and schools are being inadequately monitored, assessed and evaluated.

Relatively recent European naturalistic studies such as the *EPSILON* Study, *ODIN Study* and *EuroSC* and experimental studies (*EQOLISE, EDEN Study, Quatro Study*) (Ruggeri and Bertani 2010) are very important pilot research attempts which are sadly an exception despite the need to understand what is really going on, both from the viewpoint of professionals and from the perspective of users of services and their families.

One also needs to add to all these aforementioned problems and impasses in older models of how services were organised, the problems of new objects of psychopathology and current clinical practice, which derive from conditions of extreme social exclusion, social insecurity, social inequalities and new forms of social pain and day-to-day life of European citizens. The complexity of these new needs requires innovative, inventive answers from interdisciplinary mental health teams, which the simplistic reductionism of both the hospital-centred and biomedical models cannot provide. On the other hand, the social mandate given to mental health professionals by the State, which is unable to support its welfare aspect, is to provide social control of those fluid, new forms of social pathologies via the systematic logic of psychiatrising them (via changes in DSM-5) (Karavatos 2014; Kleinman 2012; Parker 2014).

Psychiatric and Mental Health: Conceptual Clarifications

It is commonly accepted both in the field of mental health and in related scientific disciplines (philosophy, sociology, social anthropology) that there is conceptual ambiguity, even confusion one might say, between the concepts of mental health and psychiatry. That confusion, and the inability to demarcate the two disciplines, has frequently affected theory and practice in social and community psychiatry and also therapeutic work in clinical psychiatry.

Let's take a more systematic look at the reasons for this confusion, by going on a brief historical journey. Over the last 30 years at European and global level, an extension and impressive transformation in the role of the initial mission and objectives of public psychiatry (namely, prognosis, treatment and rehabilitation of mental illnesses) have been observed. This expansion has benefited general mental health policy aimed at preventing and treating all forms of psychological pain, including non-pathological forms, while it has also attempted to modify social representations of the general public using mental health promotion and education methods.

Thanks to that development, the initially "closed" discourse of clinical psychiatry began to spread to all levels of social organisation (social work, education, the workplace, trade union, associations, civic organisations, even lifestyle magazines), but there had not been any real debate about what the boundaries, objectives and nature of its clinical and therapeutic work were. One visible consequence of this dissemination of "psy" discourse through all levels and networks of day-to-day life (Stylianidis 2008), among others, was an immense mushrooming in the "psy" market through the unthinking, unsubstantiated multiplication of hundreds of psychotherapeutic schools that sought to "treat the normal" and "develop everyone's personal skills and potential".

In the 1880s American psychiatrists were already using the expression "mental health" in reference to preventative actions in the urban environment, to avoid behavioural disorders emerging in children (Ehrenberg and Lovell 2001). Thirty years later the psychiatrist Adolf Meyer founded the American "mental health" movement, whose key aim was to prevent psychiatric illnesses through research and psychiatric care for mental disorders in the community.

In 1922 the French psychiatrist Edouard Toulouse (1865–1947) took the initiative to set up a "mental disease prevention" clinic in Paris which combined open structures and social services, making it the forerunner of the French psychiatric sector, which only crystallised in the form we know it today in 1960 (Lovell, op. cit.). Toulouse believed then that synergies between the American and French mental health movement could trigger a radical transformation of traditional psychiatry on a global scale (Ahrenfeld 1958). One can clearly understand that that so-ambitious forecast came to naught.

There are various definitions of mental health, none of which is really satisfactory. The most comprehensive definition is given by the WHO, which defines mental health as "a state of well-being in which every individual realises his or her own potential, can cope with the normal stresses of life, can work productively and fruitfully, and is able to make a contribution to her or his community". The positive dimension of mental health is stressed in WHO's definition of health which states that "health is a state of complete physical, mental and social well-being and not merely the absence of disease or infirmity".

The inadequacy of the definition derives from the fact that the concept of mental health necessarily requires a value judgement: mental health means nothing except in the context of a socio-cultural system which dominates in a given historical period. This relativisation makes it difficult to recognise objective elements in the definition which are universally acceptable. A brief analysis of some of the prevailing definitions shows that the same criteria systematically crop up again and again: there are definitions based on the absence of mental illness, on identifying mental health with normalcy, or even vague states of "well-being" deriving from a balanced personality or from problem-free adjustment and integration to the social world. Psychiatry is a scientific discipline dealing with the treatment of mental disorders, but mental health is a discipline relating to the psychosocial well-being of individuals and communities. Consequently, the twin ideas of illness/treatment are not sufficient for or capable of incorporating the aspect of social pain, exclusion and vulnerability which are characteristic of millions of individuals on the planet, irrespective of the presence or absence of specific mental disorders.

Consequently, such a reading raises major epistemological difficulties. The first difficulty is associated with the nature of psychopathology, since the term "disease" on its own is a source of confusion about the special nature of psychiatry to the extent that it applies too across the rest of medicine. The second difficulty is that the field of psychopathology, and the wider field of mental disorders, has become exceptionally complicated, as evidenced by the successive, constantly expanding classification systems that encompass the ever-increasing number of new pathologies, which are published by the WHO (ICD) and IPA (DSM). The third difficulty derives from the diversity and relativity of mental illnesses, which are widely known thanks to the contribution of phenomenology, psychoanalysis and ethnopsychiatry. Thus, defining mental health by reference to normalcy and problem-free adjustment criteria remains exceptionally fluid and fragile. Besides, the well-documented concerns expressed by Georges Canguilhem (*Le normal et le pathologique* 1972) and a series of other philosophers have made it legitimate for us to ask the question "what is normal?" To render the definition clear, do we need to adapt ourselves to a statistical model or a simplifying model? Both one and the other conflict with ordinary observation and the logic of a "neutral" evaluator.

In contrast to these approaches, references to purely subjective criteria, i.e. the subjective condition and experience of "well-being", the way in which we perceive our self image personal balance and happiness, quite self-evidently are not firm scientific criteria, especially if one espouses Popperian logic.

In the context of this book, it is necessary to examine this paradoxical condition about the fluidity of definitions of mental health from three viewpoints. Firstly, as a field of special activities for promoting mental health and educating others about it, which is something constantly evolving and developing. Secondly, as a body of new knowledge, especially in relation to new forms of social pain and new social pathologies (new forms of depression, new forms of addiction, new forms of grief, new forms of "antisocial" behaviour) (Ehrenberg 2008, 2010). Thirdly, mental health can be understood as a set of historically defined ways in which psychological pain can be expressed. By examining these three viewpoints together, we can better formulate a definition for mental health, both from the results of new practices (deinstitutionalisation and care in the community, the recovery movement, the movement of users of mental health services and their families, new forms of empowerment and advocacy) and from a fresh reading of its dynamic representations.

In conclusion one might say that this brief overview of mental health definitions has revealed that these three perspectives refer to three intervention rationales. First, mental health can be viewed as a part of what it means to be human and the need to promote health. Second, mental health can be viewed a forum within which pain is expressed, whose social and cultural elements must be integrated. Third, mental health can be viewed as a way for individuals to address diversity, life events and different social, environmental and individual factors (Patel et al. 2006) utilising a dynamic life plan and searching for a new equilibrium.

As Benedetto Saraceno so succinctly puts it (2014, p. 181), "being involved in mental health means being involved with situations of pain which frequently include diagnosed illnesses, which in most cases, are characterised by physical and mental vulnerability, humiliation, poverty, social marginalisation, and exclusion from access to basic rights. Being involved in mental health also means being involved with pain and illness, with individuals and groups, with psychological, physical and social aspects, not only with human bodies but also with emotions and feelings, resources, opportunities and violations of rights".

Maroussi, Greece   Stelios Stylianidis

Bibliography

Ahrenfeld RH (1958) Psychiatry in the British Army in the second world war. Routledge & K. Paul.
Becker T, Knapp M, Knudsen HC, Schene A, Tansella M, Thornicroft G (1999) The EPSILON study of schizophrenia in five European countries. Design and methodology for standardising outcome measures and comparing patterns of care and service costs. Br J Psychiatry 175(6):514–521
Canguilhem G (1972) Le normal et le pathologique. Presses Universitaires de France
Ehrenberg A (2008) La fatigue d'être soi: dépression et société. Odile Jacob, Paris
Ehrenberg A (2010) La Société du malaise. Odile Jacob, Paris
Ehrenberg A, Lovell A (2001) Maladie mentale en mutation (La): Psychiatrie et société. Odile Jacob, Paris
Fryers T, Melzer D, Jenkins R (2003) Social inequalities and the common mental disorders. Soc Psychiatry Psychiatr Epidemiol 38(5):229–237
Herrman H, Saxena S, Moodie R (2005) Promoting mental health: concepts, emerging evidence, practice: a report of the World Health Organization, Department of Mental Health and Substance Abuse in collaboration with the Victorian Health Promotion Foundation and the University of Melbourne. World Health Organization.
Kleinman A (2012) Culture, bereavement and psychiatry. Lancet 379:608–609
Morgan C, Bhugra D (2010) Principles of social psychiatry. Wiley-Blackwell
Parker G (2014) The DSM-5 classifications of mood disorders: same fallacies and fault lines. Acta Psychiatr Scand 24 Feb. [early view] doi:10.1111/acps.12253
Patel V, Saraceno B, Kleinman A (2006) Beyond evidence: the moral case for international mental health. Am J Psychiatry 163(8):1312–1315
Ruggeri M, Elena Bertani M (2010) Mental Health in Europe: learning from differences. In: Principles of social psychiatry, 2nd edn., pp 499–516
Saraceno B (2014) Discorso globale, sofferenze locali. Analisi critica del Movimento di salute mental globale. Il Saggiatore, Milano
Tansella M, Thornicroft G (2001) The principles underlying community care. In: Textbook of community psychiatry. Oxford University Press, Oxford, pp 155–165

Thornicroft G, Tansella M (2009) Better mental health care. Cambridge University Press, Cambridge, pp 1–184

Thornicroft G, Tansella M (2013) The balanced care model for global mental health. Psychol Med 43(04):849–863

World Health Organization (WHO) (2005) Mental health atlas: 2005, http://www.who.int/mental_health/evidence/atlas/global_results.pdf. Accessed on 7 Jul 2014

World Health Organization (WHO) (2008) The global burden of disease 2004 update. http://www.who.int/healthinfo/global_burden_disease/GBD_report_2004update_full.pdf. Accessed 7 Jul 2014

World Health Organization (WHO) (2010) mhGAP intervention guide for mental, neurological and substance use disorders in non-specialised health settings: mental health Gap Action Programme (mhGAP)

World Health Organization (WHO) (2013) Mental health action plan 2013–2020. http://apps.who.int/iris/bitstream/10665/89966/1/9789241506021_eng.pdf Accessed 7 Jul 2014

Karavatos T (2014) Acceptance of DSM-5: "The problem with DSM-5 isn't in the 5 but in the DSM". (in Greek) Synapsis J 32(10):4–8

World Health Organization (2001) The World Health report 2001: mental health: new understanding, new hope. World Health Organization

Stylianidis S (2008) Transformations in psychiatry: in search of new examples for a new mental health policy (in Greek). In: Stylianidis S, Stylianoudi MGL (ed.) Community and psychiatric reform: The experience of Evia, 1988–2008. Topos Press, Athens, pp 443–477

Contents

Part I Social Psychiatry

1 A Brief Historical Overview of Madness
   in Social Psychiatry.. 3
   Stelios Stylianidis

2 Philosophical and Sociological Foundations
   of Social Psychiatry.. 17
   Stelios Stylianidis

3 Psychiatric Epidemiology and Its Applications
   in Social Psychiatry.. 41
   Lily Evangelia Peppou and Stelios Stylianidis

4 Global Mental Health... 59
   Michail Lavdas, Stelios Stylianidis,
   and Christina Mamaloudi

5 Psychiatric Reform in Greece 77
   Panagiotis Chondros and Stelios Stylianidis

6 The Contribution of Psychoanalytical Thinking
   and Practice to Social Community Psychiatry.................. 93
   Michael A. Petrou

Part II Applications of Social Psychiatry

7 Promoting Mental Health: From Theory
   To Best Practice... 117
   Stelios Stylianidis, Pepi Belekou,
   Lily Evangelia Peppou, and Athina Vakalopoulou

8 Social Suffering and Mental Health in Metropolitan
   Athens: A Qualitative Approach 133
   Stelios Stylianidis, Athina Vakalopoulou,
   and Lily Evangelia Peppou

9 **The Recovery Model and Modern Psychiatric Care: Conceptual Perspective, Critical Approach and Practical Application**.................................... 145
Stelios Stylianidis, Michail Lavdas, Kalomira Markou, and Pepi Belekou

10 **Mobile Mental Health Units on the Islands: The Experience of Cyclades**................................. 167
Stelios Stylianidis, Stella Pantelidou, Antonios Poulios, Michail Lavdas, and Nikos Lamnidis

11 **Community Child Psychiatry: The Example of Mobile Mental Health Units in the NE and Western Cyclades**.. 193
Stella Pantelidou, Vicky Antonopoulou, Antonios Poulios, Jenny Soumaki, and Stelios Stylianidis

12 **A Modern-Day Community Daycare Centre in Operation**... 215
Stelios Stylianidis and Dimitris Trivellas

13 **Assertive Community Treatment: Home Intervention for People with Severe and Enduring Mental Health Problems: Designing the Greek Model**.................................. 249
Alex Krokidas, Xenia Varvaressou, and Stelios Stylianidis

14 **Brief Psychotherapy in a Community Framework**............... 277
Marina Skourteli and Stelios Stylianidis

15 **Community Mental Healthcare for Migrants**.................. 309
Nikos Gionakis and Stelios Stylianidis

16 **Modern Technologies and Applications and Community Psychiatry**.................................. 331
Orestis Giotakos

17 **Assessment and Management of Domestic Violence Cases Within a Community Mental Health Services Framework**... 343
Stella Pantelidou, Athina Vakalopoulou, and Stelios Stylianidis

18 **Sexuality of Patients with Serious Psychiatric Disorders in Psychosocial Rehabilitation Units**......................... 365
Stelios Stylianidis, Pepi Belecou, and Stelios Farsaliotis

Part III Evaluation

19 **Evaluation of Social Psychiatry Services**..................... 389
Stelios Stylianidis, Petros Skapinakis, Venetsanos Mavreas, and Michael Lavdas

20	**Implications of the Socioeconomic Crisis for Staff in Community PSR Units: The Case of an NGO** .... Stelios Stylianidis, Klimis Navridis, and Anna Christopoulou	405
21	**Staff Evaluation and Presentation of Organisational Culture in Mental Health Structures** .... Stelios Stylianidis, Meni Koutsosimou, Nikos Symeonidis, Panagiotis Chondros, and Giorgos Chadoulis	419

Part IV Empowering and Rights in Mental Health

22	**User and Family Participation in Mental Health Services** .... Panagiotis Chondros, Stelios Stylianidis, and Michael Lavdas	437
23	**Involuntary Hospitalisation: Legislative Framework, Epidemiology and Outcome**................................. Stelios Stylianidis, Lily Evangelia Peppou, Nektarios Drakonakis, and Emilia Panagou	451
24	**The Impact of the Economic Crisis in Greece: Epidemiological Perspective and Community Implications** .... Marina Economou, Lily Evangelia Peppou, Kyriakos Souliotis, and Stelios Stylianidis	469
25	**Afterword: The Economic Crisis and Mental Health** .... Stelios Stylianidis, Panagiotis Chondros, and Michael Lavdas	485
Index...		509

Part I
Social Psychiatry

A Brief Historical Overview of Madness in Social Psychiatry

Stelios Stylianidis

Abstract

The definition of madness and how it has been dealt with in different historical periods establish the social, cultural and institutional foundations for the emergence of psychiatry as a separate scientific discipline and the development and establishment of the schools of social and community psychiatry. This chapter examines the historical background of psychiatry and mental health from the viewpoint of the change in the social and scientific handling of madness and the interplay of wider cultural and social processes. This historical development begins in antiquity, continues with the emergence of asylums and the examination of "nervous disorders" in the Victorian age through the development of measures to promote mental health taken between WWI and WWII and the wider mental health movements which emerged in both Europe and the USA and came to fruition in the modern age and concludes with us highlighting contemporary issues, conflicts and concerns.

1.1 Introduction

This chapter focuses our attention on the development of the discipline of psychiatry and of mental health from the age of asylums (1800–1900) to the modern day.

Tomorrow, during the visit, when you try to communicate with those people without any dictionary, remember and realise that you are superior is only one regard: Strength.
F. Basaglia (1963)
(From the Manifesto of the French Surrealist painters to the Asylum Directors, 1923)

S. Stylianidis
Department of Psychology, Panteion University, Athens, Greece
e-mail: stylianidis.st@gmail.com

By examining its historical development from the vantage point of a twenty-first-century observer, it is impressive to see how the field of mental health has developed via institutions, new psychiatric care structures, professionals and users of services. For example, in 1890, only a very small number of professionals could call themselves psychotherapists in the USA (VandenBos et al. 1992). Today, even applying stricter criteria and in the same country, a minimum of 100,000 professionals are now considered to be highly specialised psychotherapists, and using wider criteria, more than 250,000 psychotherapists and mental health counsellors meet the needs of the US population.

In addition, the mental health sector has improved in terms of quality: the range of treatment options has expanded impressively from institution- and asylum-based care to the "traitement moral" of the nineteenth century to a wide diversity of psychological and pharmacological interventions which have become available over the last decade. Likewise, the number of related scientific disciplines has grown too at a rapid pace, frequently via harsh struggles with one school of psychotherapy vying for pole position against another. Today, the field of mental health does not only include psychiatrists, psychologists and psychoanalysts but also psychotherapists from various schools and creeds, nurses, social workers, speech therapists, logopedists, mental health counsellors, as well as priests, and GPs with special training in psychosomatic conditions.

The growth of the mental health sector is also tied – in a quite complex way – with cultural and social mechanisms and with the development of the scientific disciplines of psychiatry and psychology. On the one hand, it reflects wider cultural processes at play such as individualisation, the appearance of social management and the psychiatrisation of social phenomena.

Via the general, brief historical overview we provide, we attempt to show the turning points in the social and scientific handling of madness and how this ties into wider mental health movements which emerged in both Europe and the USA. This historical development commences with the emergence of asylums and an examination of "nervous disorders" in the Victorian age, goes on to examine the growth in measures to promote mental health between WWI and WWI and ends with a short analysis of contemporary tensions in the field of psychiatry.

1.2 From Antiquity to the Emergence of Asylums (Fifth Century BC to 1800)

Deviant forms of behaviour, which we nowadays associate with mental disorders, were examined in detail by Hippocrates (460–377 BC), Asclepius, Galen (130–200 BC) and Aristotle (384–322 BC) in antiquity. Findings brought to light during archaeological excavations provide firm evidence of this: skulls with holes drilled into them, clearly in an attempt to free the diseased person of the spirit which possessed him (Kaprinis et al. 2009).

Later when the Byzantine Empire was at its peak, under the influence of Arabic culture, methods for dealing with mental disorders which were more humane came to the fore, involving protecting the rights of the mentally disturbed and avoiding non-beneficial forced periods of hospitalisation; in fact the ways in which health and mental health services were organised could be characterised as forerunners of current mobile mental health units (Stylianidis et al. 2007). Reliable historical sources note that medicine in Byzantium was strongly influenced by the advances made in the Classical period and the Hippocratic approach. Byzantine doctors, many of whom were also men of the cloth (bishops, metropolitans, etc.), studied in Athens, and their medical practice placed particular emphasis on caring for the mentally disturbed. It is worth noting that closed care facilities in Byzantium (poorhouses) had features of modern-day milieu therapy and included industrial therapy as well. In contrast to the medieval West, the "psychiatric culture" of Byzantium drew a clear distinction between perceptions and practices of demonic possession and mental illness.

Under the Ottoman Empire, various foundations were set up which served more as places for treatment and rehabilitation and less so as places of imprisonment (Ploumpidis and Evans 1993).

1.3 The Emergence of Asylums and the "Traitement Moral" (1800–1900)

Before asylums were set up, there was no organised system for treating deviant behaviour. In the Middle Ages in the West, people considered to be mentally ill who exhibited strange or dangerous forms of behaviour were cared for by their families or the community, and only rarely were they locked up in special, separate homes like the "dolhuysjes" of Holland (Abma 2004).

The first known asylum for the chronically ill was founded in Valencia in 1409. Asylums then spread rapidly through Spain and other European countries. The vast majority of these institutions were under the aegis of the Catholic Church and only provided asylum-style care (Foucault 1961a).

Then in the mid-seventeenth century, as more people began moving to cities and farmers began abandoning the countryside *en masse* for large European urban centres, city authorities had to urgently impose rules for preserving social order and cohesion. The monumental work of the philosopher Michel Foucault and his general contribution to our understanding of the "great confinement" has been a guiding force in tracing instances of social exclusion of diversity throughout that historical period, which is a matter explored in more detail in the next chapter.

The Hôpital Général was founded in Paris in 1656, designed to lock up the unemployed, the poor and anyone who deviated from the model of productivity and rationalism and constituted a threat to the preservation of the social order. The shared dogma of that time in Western Europe was that "normal" people act rationally, respect social order and accept the economic ideal of productivity. Those who did not comply were deemed "mad" and "affected" (aliénés) and had to be locked up in major institutions. The goal of locking them up was to educate these individuals through forced labour and religious practices, in the belief that these "immoral" individuals would be able to internalise the moral rules being forced on them.

During the eighteenth century, doctors in various European countries, influenced by the ideas of the Enlightenment, confirmed that as a disease "madness" could be treated. In England, William Battie published the *Treaties of Madness* in 1758, thereby announcing that psychiatry was both a science and a form of treatment. Some decades later, doctors like William Tuke in England, Philippe Pinel in France, Johann Reil in Germany and Vincenzo Chiarugi in Italy developed theories and hypotheses about the organic aetiology of madness. In the same vein, the American doctor Benjamin Rush wrote in 1812: "The cause of madness is seated primarily in the blood vessels of the brain, and it depends upon the same kind of morbid and irregular actions that constitute other arterial diseases". These biological views about the causes of madness had almost no therapeutic value. It is no coincidence that the first treatment methods were based on social and psychosocial principles rather than medical ones. The forms of treatment/care which developed consisted of an intensive, detailed system of discipline aimed at "reinstilling" morality into the mental life of patients. For that reason, the mentally ill were confined to separate institutions in their countries, which were specialised in the "traitement moral". The first of these was the Retreat Institution in York, founded in 1796 by William Tuke. In France, Philippe Pinel in his work *Traité médico-philosophique sur l'aliénation mentale, ou la manie* (translated under the English title of the Treatise on Insanity) focused on the psychological core of the "traitement moral". The patient had to place himself under the imposing prestige of an individual "who through his physical and moral properties is able to exert an invincible impact on the patient and change his perverse chain of ideas". In other words, by "liberating" the mad from their chains, the "traitement moral" was imposed on them as a mixed system of persuasion and effect, focused on the moral prestige of the doctor, all of which took place within a well-organised institution.

However, because the "traitement moral" was not medically substantiated, it was also invested in by other professionals. For example, philosophers, judges, priests and even "charitable volunteers" preached that they too could do just as well and be as effective in implementing the "traitement moral". In the end, the "traitement moral" was considered to be an ineffective method, as had initially been suspected, and in 1880, it was abandoned as a form of treatment.

As far as the development of psychiatry itself is concerned, in the first half of the nineteenth century, psychological interpretations dominated the understanding of mental phenomena, especially in Germany, where two schools of thought, the Psychiker and the Somatiker schools, were in conflict. However from 1850 onwards, an organic approach to the pathogenesis of mental illnesses began to prevail. One example of this is the German professor Wilhelm Griesinger, who argued in one of his works in 1845 in a quite dogmatic manner that "mental illnesses are diseases of the brain", a view supported by the boost given to medical research by the discovery of the syphilis bacteria at that time. Likewise the work of Morel in France and Maudsley in England contributed to the purely biological orientation of research into psychiatry (Abma 2004, p. 98).

However, at the end of the nineteenth century, both the psychological and biological approach experienced a crisis, to the extent that no theory could adequately explain the pathogenesis of mental illnesses. However, the immense contribution of the German psychiatrist, Emil Kraepelin (1856–1926), appeared to show a way out of the crisis. Successive editions of his work on dementia praecox, as schizophrenia used to be called, and his important development of a system for classifying mental illnesses, based on tens of clinical observations of patients in psychiatric institutions, meant that Kraepelin exerted a major influence on the shape of psychiatric nosography and therapeutic practice.

In short, through the culture of "curability" which prevailed in the nineteenth century in Western countries, asylums which had been used to lock up the insane gradually began to transform into treatment institutions, hosting an increasingly growing number of patients. However, treatment in the context of an asylum did not also go hand in hand with corresponding developments in psychiatric theory. Theoretically speaking, the focus was on rational and scientific explanations of mental phenomena, but the dominant theoretical references and forms of treatment still derived from the Enlightenment tradition. Towards the end of the nineteenth century, the golden age of psychiatry appeared to be reaching the end of its own delusion. At a therapeutic level, the "traitement moral" was considered a failed method to the extent that those few patients who were able to abandon the asylum returned to it, thereby bolstering the "revolving door" phenomenon so well known to us all today.

1.4 Nervous System Diseases and Victorian Era Illnesses (1870–1920)

In addition to the emergence of large institutions, treatments and theories concerning serious psychiatric disorders (madness) at the end of the nineteenth century, another form of mental illness also emerged, milder forms of mental disorders, more paroxysmal and not so chronic, with symptoms and vexations such as fatigue, a general sense of weakness, mental instability and a feeling of impending collapse. These "nervous disorders" were introduced, along with madness, as a new class of mental problems. This development not only defined the expansion of the field of psychiatry into what we nowadays call mental health but also highlighted a new professional group within that discipline, called neurologists.

Victorian era illnesses, primarily characterised by symptoms of fatigue and weakness, without any determinate organic foundation, had already been described in various forms in the seventeenth and eighteenth centuries. During those periods, these illnesses were dealt with using a variety of treatments, including mesmerism and "animal magnetism". The fluidity of these symptoms led to them being lumped together in as "neurasthenias", meaning weaknesses of the nerves. For example, one can mention the American doctor, George M. Beard, who described the illness in depth in his book entitled *American Nervousness* (1881). Neurasthenia was a "useful" diagnostic term, because it medicalised a series of mental symptoms while also releasing mental illnesses from the stigma of madness.

In that way, from the mid-1800s to the historically recent full segregation of the disciplines of psychiatry and neurology (which took place in the 1970s and 1980s in Europe), neurology developed as a new medical specialisation which backed up its therapeutic approach in medical terms, generating remarkable results both concerning conditions of the nervous system and mental disorders in general. In addition to criticising the asylum system as anti-therapeutic and ineffective, neurologists also proposed that Victorian era illnesses be treated in private clinics and university clinics using treatment methods which included everything from hypnosis and suggestion to exhortations towards moral improvement, travel and rest at specially designed sanatoria.

The underlying theory on which these practices rested was the belief that conditions of the nervous system could be treated through some form of physical treatment. With that in mind, S. Weir Mitchell, a famous neurologist of the period, stated that *You treat the body and in some way you find that the mind is also treated* (Zakzanis et al. 1998).

The counterweight to the causes of neurasthenia and hysteria, which date from the eighteenth century, focuses not on the nervous system but on mental functions. In Europe, the roots of these diseases were thought to rest in the individual unconscious, in the form of unchecked base urges: it was therefore thought that these urges could be suppressed through hypnosis or free association. Hypnotism was used and developed by the famous French neurologist Jean-Martin Charcot at Paris' Pitié-Salpêtrière Hospital, where Freud (1856–1939) himself studied, and was an important turning point in the process of discovering unconscious functions and the role of sexual drives in the emergence of neuroses and more generally in establishing psychoanalytic theory and practice.

The introduction of the concept of neurasthenia, which we examined above, made a decisive contribution to a clear dividing line between the two types of mental disorders, madness and nervousness, and a dividing line between psychiatrists on the one hand and neurologists and all other types of psychotherapists on the other, as professionals.

However, because psychiatrists believed they were losing ground and their clinical practice would be limited to work in large institutions, they attempted to bridge the gap between madness and neurasthenia by introducing the concept of prevention. This concept brought major changes to the world of mental health, based as it was on the assumption that the failure of the traitement moral for madness was due to the fact that serious psychiatric disorders had already become chronic as a development of non-treatable forms of neurosis.

So, in the name of prevention, a methodology for timely diagnosis and treatment of neuroses in the community could be applied. Through this development, the boundaries between academic discipline and the practice of psychiatry and neurology became blurred and fluid. The emergence of psychiatrists from asylums also contributed to a new area of specialisation developing, that of psychiatric social work, which in effect, if practised by a psychiatrist, was the forerunner of professional social psychiatry. The psychiatrist, Adolf Meyer, who studied medicine in Switzerland, migrated to the USA in 1892, where he played a leading role in setting up the movement for community mental healthcare, as part of his work at the New York State Psychiatric Institute. His working hypothesis was that psychiatric disorders were a manifestation of an unhealthy life and ineffectual adjustment by the individual to his social environment. However, we need to take a critical stance towards that innovation for its time, to the extent that it proposed not just individual treatment but a complex web of precautionary mental health and social control measures for all forms of deviant behaviour, such as sexual perversions, rape and violent criminal behaviour.

On the initiative of a former patient, Clifford Whittingham Beers, who suffered from bipolar disorder, the first social mental health association was set up on the advice of Meyer in 1908, and the national mental health committee followed in 1909 (Reisman 1991). However, what is of interest is the different types of interventions that fell under the "mental health" umbrella. The prevention principle expanded the field of mental health, to incorporate not just patients with mental and nervous conditions but also all persons who were at risk. What Meyer wrote in 1930 is illustrative indeed of this point: *mental health as a prevention philosophy is an ideal, and a guiding principle in work, in the context of daily life, where possible, before the 'normal' and pathological diverge*. It is worth noting at this point that the conflict between treatment/prevention and social control which runs through the field of psychiatry to this day was already present in a movement which was progressive for its time in the USA, the social mental health movement (Castel 1981). From that point in history on, the path opened up for full medicalisation of social deviance, as shown by the works of Foucault and Basaglia (Foucault 1961b; Basaglia 1963). In the USA in particular, we can see a synergy between psychiatrists, churches and social workers, to expand the role of the discipline of psychiatry, to include not just treatment of serious psychiatric disorders and also to promote "proper" adjustment and mental care for "normality".

1.5 The Mental Health Movement (1914–1960)

Both the therapeutic impulse and the wish to more effectively manage mental disorders led to a truly impressive growth in the field of mental health, in the interwar years and especially so after WWII. The painful experiences of WWI played a decisive role in this change. For the first time in the history of psychiatry, psychiatrists were directly involved in military activities. Their efforts were complemented by clinical psychologists who developed a new diagnostic tool, which was more objective and rational compared to the past: psychological tests. For the general public, during the 1920s and 1930s, any basic knowledge about psychology had to do with psychoanalysis. At the same time, social policymakers viewed both psychoanalysis and its main competitor at that time, behaviourialism, as important pillars in their attempt to regulate normal and deviant behaviour.

With the outbreak of WWI in 1914, new destructive technologies emerged on the battle field (Binneveld 1997). These new technologies also led to the emergence of new mental disorders, such as hysterical blindness, paralytic crises, terrors, exhaustion and total disorientation. In 1916, the British psychiatrist Myers coined the phrase "shell shock" to describe persistent symptoms which were initially attributed to shell explosions. Those symptoms (inability to reason, disturbed sleep patterns, hyperactivity, verbal diarrhoea, loss of self-control) were initially attributed to physical causes (the explosions) affecting soldiers serving in the artillery and if they emerged in other soldiers were thought to be neurotic reactions of individuals exposed to traumatic situations.

New clinical data forced traditional military psychiatrists to move beyond classic treatment methods being used at that time (military drills, electroshock treatment, isolation, cold showers, imaginary surgical procedures, "drowning" treatment) and to implement new psychiatric and psychotherapeutic methods. Military neuroses offered new material for observation and stressed the already well-known relationship between mental disorders and everyday living conditions.

From the 1920s onwards, psychological interpretations of human behaviour attracted increasingly more popular attention (Burnham 1988). The populist new psychology manuals which began to be published, A. G. Tansley's *The New Psychology and Its Relation to Life* (1920), exerted a particular influence, while a series of articles in the press made the key elements of Freudian theory widely known, and to a large extent it was adopted by the general public as a new cultural phenomenon. With the rise of Nazism in Germany in the 1930s, in particular, a whole generation of European psychoanalysts migrated to the USA resulting in psychoanalysis becoming the dominant theoretical orientation of psychiatry up until the end of the 1960s.

WWII marked the emergence of a large range of innovations and the development of the field of mental health, due to the fact that the war embroiled a large number of healthcare professionals in various ways of diagnosing and treating military men. At the same time, the social reorientation of psychiatry, both in terms of its theoretical prospects and preventative and therapeutic interventions, led to the creation of social structures providing psychiatric care. It is worth pointing out that the war made it easier for a large number of clinical psychologists to actively participate in various mental health activities. Moreover, the psychological needs of the military and the rest of the population during WWII meant that not only were then-current psychiatric and psychological treatments more widely disseminated, but so too did psychological ideas and techniques between common currencies among military personnel. The mass production of self-help books relating to self-management of one's emotions in times of crisis allows us to better understand the current massive growth (especially in the English language literature) of populist self-help for specific psychiatric disorders and the multiplication of the number of manuals available on personal growth and how healthy individuals can improve their skills. Effective adaptation to the environment and the ability to manage difficult social and psychological techniques became the new goal for clinicians in the field. For example, we can cite Carl Rogers, who was the clinical psychologist who exerted a decisive influence on counselling for mental health issues in America and who defined clinical psychology as the technique and the art of applying psychological principles to the individual's problems to achieve a more satisfactory degree of adjustment.

Against this backdrop of an expanding mental health sector, it should be noted that the National Committee for Mental Health in the USA adopted an action plan in the 1960s. It foresaw the establishment of numerous mental health centres in all States, to bolster social cohesion and stability. That plan was given legal substance under the presidency of John F. Kennedy when the Mental Health Act was enacted in 1963.

While psychotherapists from various schools and trends were constantly expanding their activities in the provision of mental health services in the community, psychiatrists in psychiatric hospitals were attempting to find therapeutically effective approaches to the psychosocial rehabilitation of serious psychiatric disorders, and in particular schizophrenia. The majority of psychiatrists relying on their belief that the fits in grand mal epileptic crises were biological competitors of schizophrenia attempted to apply that principle to the treatment of schizophrenic patients using artificially induced insulin comas and electroconvulsive therapy (ECB). These shock treatments appeared to suppress certain symptoms, but no one – not even at that time – could ignore the serious and sometimes long-term side effects they caused.

At the same time, a more extreme and irreversible form of medical intervention entered the psychiatric realm: prefrontal lobotomies. This method was developed in 1935 by the Portuguese neurosurgeon, Egas Moniz, who won the 1949 Nobel Prize for Medicine for inventing it. These developments were complemented by the discovery of chlorpromazine in 1952, by the Frenchmen Delay and Deniker, at Paris' Sainte-Anne Hospital, which was a historical turning point as the first effective antipsychotic treatment. Despite the fact that neuroleptics were discovered by accident (chlorpromazine was initially used as an anaesthetic) and at that time there was no scientific evidence to support the precise biological action of psychoactive substances, this discovery caught the interest of both medical research and the pharmaceutical industry. These changes, plus the publication of the first edition of the DSM by the American Psychiatric Association, radically altered the general public's image of psychiatry, calling into doubt phenomenology and psychodynamic practice in clinical treatment which had dominated up until that point.

However, it is worth noting that both psychoanalysts and the representatives of other psychotherapeutic schools at that time (person-centred treatment and the counselling of C. Rogers, all post-psychoanalytic therapies, such as behaviourialism) supported the importance of the psychological pathogenesis of mental disorders, compared to the biological reductionism of emerging biological psychiatry, and that psychotherapies should be provided in a social context and ought to be scientifically backed up and should not be based on moral and philosophical approaches.

1.6   Radicalism: From Psychiatry to the Deinstitutionalism Movement (1960–1980)

The 1960s and 1970s were a period of radical upheavals both in sociopolitical terms and in the mental health sector. On the one hand, Western societies gradually showed an increasing interest in mental health and improving care for sufferers, which was accompanied by the "personal growth" movement as we already mentioned. On the other hand, influenced by radical ideologies (Marxist ideology, demands for social and political liberation, the emergence of the concept of the subjective and social integration of diversity, social liberation movements like feminism, the gay movement, etc.), various social collectives transformed the basic assumptions of traditional psychiatry and psychology into a key question. Institutional/asylum-based psychiatry and culture underwent intense, subversive criticism because of the social control they exerted and because of the suppression and stigmatism of mental patients, who were now viewed as the victims of a social injustice. From this ideological viewpoint, mental illnesses were considered by certain authors and mental health professionals to be a myth which disguised social deviance and gave a pseudoscientific legitimacy to the suppressive power and violence of asylums. As a result, alternative theories and interpretations of mental illness were developed, such as antipsychiatry and the Italian deinstitutionalisation movement (these two ought not to be confused though) which formed a mass social movement which contested the institutional and neo-institutional culture and the dominance of the biomedical model's culture. The theoretical views of these movements which contested traditional approaches, and their practical consequences on changing traditional psychiatric care, will be explored in more detail in Chap. 3 of this book. Here we will limit ourselves to pointing out certain illustrative views from the protagonists of this theoretical and social challenge to the role of psychiatry.

First, Thomas Szasz (1976) published *The Myth of Mental Illness* where he argued that most mental disorders are an expression of problems, exclusions and conflicts in social life and are not due to a chemical imbalance in the brain or some other type or organic aetiology. Consequently, biological, surgical or pharmaceutical treatments were a fraud, and covered over the real problem, both for mental health professionals and the general public. While Szasz was developing his theoretical views in the USA, in Europe, alternative therapies were being developed for psychotic and neurotic patients, such as group therapy, systemic family psychotherapy and a myriad of other psychotherapeutic techniques which, although lacking in serious scientific documentation, created an anti-culture which competed against traditional psychiatry. In Great Britain, for example, R. Laing, inspired by existentialism, phenomenology and social analyses conducted by the American sociologist E. Goffman into "total institutions" (1963) and the unjustified power of psychiatrists, experimented with new forms of group and family psychotherapy for schizophrenic patients. At around the same time, David Cooper coined the term antipsychiatry in his well-known book *Psychiatry and Anti-psychiatry* (Cooper 1967).

At the same time, leading intellectuals from other countries like the French philosopher Michel Foucault, in his monumental work *The History of Madness* (1961a) and the social psychiatrists Dorner (1969) in Germany, in his work *Citizens and Madness* (*Burger und Irre*), and Foudraine (1974) in Holland, in his well-known work *Not Made of Wood*, enriched the literature of critical psychiatry. All these intellectuals, with the assistance of Franco Basaglia, who set himself apart from antipsychiatry by calling himself and his approach anti-institutional (Basaglia and

Tranchina 1979; Stylianidis et al. 2010; Tzanakis 2008; Louzoun and Stylianidis 1987), agreed that instead of performing the humanitarian and scientific role which they professed in treating mental disorders, traditional psychiatrists were in effect merely servants of a repressive, alienating power which aimed to ensure social control over socially and politically deviant citizens.

The impact of these antipsychiatry and deinstitutionalisation movements, despite their occasionally simplistic formulations about understanding the complexity of mental illness, made a decisive contribution to the development of social mental health structures, fully replacing psychiatric asylums with best psychiatric reform practices and improving the exploration, acceptance and destigmatisation of mental illness.

1.7 "Rationalism" (1980 to the Present Day)

In the age of humanitarian psychotherapies and the antipsychiatry and anti-institutionalist movement, social care and psychotherapy reached their apogee. All these changes are consistent with the accelerating rise in requests from the public for social mental health services including counselling services and treatment for "normal" people. In many Western countries, psychotherapeutic practice was an integral part of public mental health and the increase in requests for psychotherapy made the cost of these services skyrocket. The gradual rolling back of the welfare state and its collapse at the present time in quite a few European countries, and the dominance of the neoliberal dogma and the culture of financial capital and the markets, resulted in all public mental health services being "rationalised". The now urgent strategic goal in mental health policies inspired by liberal models was to introduce the concept of "managed care" from the USA to Europe and to measure cost-effectiveness of the system's benefits using new diagnostic and treatment tools.

DSM-III (Gonon 2013) released in 1987 was now thoroughly "atheoretical" in character, free of any psychodynamic or phenomenological approach (by abolishing neuroses, personality structure and defence mechanisms in the new classification) and formulated a purely neutral descriptive terminology which is supposed to improve the credibility of psychiatry and put it on a par with other medical specialisations.

The discovery of neurotransmitters, genetics, neurophysiology and psychoneuroimmunology, pharmaceutical research and new imaging methods (MRI, PET) that allow us to see how the central nervous system works have generated significant evidence that anomalies in brain function correspond to specific mental disorders. Consequently, from the 1990s to the present day, the new treatment culture is based purely on the biomedical model, to the extent that the interests of both mental health policymakers and the pharmaceutical industry and the large majority of the psychiatric community "converge" about the adoption of low-cost, rapid, easy treatment solutions for all forms of psychological functions. Whatever is not evidence-based psychiatry and cost-effective and does not involve a standardised approach to the treatment of mental disorders no longer has any place in the psychiatric landscape.

Measurable effectiveness of behavioural/cognitive psychotherapies and an extension of the indications for using psychotropic drugs on "new pathologies" and on younger ages (e.g. hyperactivity disorder in children, antisocial behaviour in adolescents) require *manu militari* the dominance of biological psychiatry and short-term psychotherapeutic interventions compared to any long-term, financially costly forms of psychoanalytical approach or any holistic handling of complex biopsychosocial and spiritual-cultural needs of the patient, compared to any long-term individualised care and psychosocial rehabilitation plan for serious psychiatric disorders (Stylianidis and Lavras 2012; Dimitriadis 2013; Stylianidis and Ploumpidi 2014). However, new and constantly expanding complex needs for psychiatric care and mental health in the general population and new vulnerable social groups afflicted by globalisation and the economic crisis (Patel and Prince 2010) have necessarily raised new challenges for psychiatry, governments and groups of users of services as well as their families.

In order to rise to those challenges, a change in psychiatric culture and ways of thinking is needed, and new practices and innovations via a new form of scientific documentation must be promoted. In other words, a fourth psychiatric revolution is needed which will promote a new scientific and social culture for psychiatry, mental health, education and research focused on understanding and treating subjective and social pain and diversity.

Bibliography

Abma R (2004) Madness and mental health. In: Jansz J, Van Drunen P (eds) A social history of psychology. Blackwell, Malden, pp 93–128

Basaglia F (1963) Le istituzioni della violenza. In: Basaglia F (ed) Basaglia Scritti I 1953–1968. Einaudi Paperbacks, Torino, pp 471–505

Basaglia F, Tranchina P (1979) Autobiografia di un movimento-1961–1979: dal manicomio alla riforma sanitária. Unione Province Italiane, Regione Toscana, Amministrazione Provinciale di Arezzo

Beard GM (1881) American nervousness, its causes and consequences: a supplement to nervous exhaustion (neurasthenia). Putnam, New York

Binneveld H (1997) From shell shock to combat stress: a comparative history of military psychiatry. Amsterdam University Press, Amsterdam

Burnham JC (1988) Paths into American culture: psychology, medicine, and morals. Temple University Press, Philadelphia

Castel R (1981) Le Psychanalysme: L'ordre psychanalytique et le pouvon. Flammarion, Paris

Cooper D (1967) Psychiatry and anti-psychiatry. Tavistock Publications, London

Dimitriadis G (2013) Special file: psychopathology (in Greek). Synapsis J 29(9):46–47

Dorner K (1969) Burger und Irre. Zur Sozialgeschichte der Wissenschaftssoziologie der Psychiatrie. Europaische Verlagsanstalt, Frankfurt a. Main

Foucault M (1961a) Folie et déraison: histoire de la folie à l'âge classique, vol 169. Plon, Paris

Foucault M (1961b) Histoire de la folie à l' âge classique. Gallimard, Paris

Foudraine J (1974) Not made of wood. Quartet Books, London

Goffman E (1963) Asylums: essays on the social situation of mental patients and other inmates Penguin. Anchor, Asylums, New York

Gonon F (2013) Quel avenir pour les classifications des maladies mentales? Une synthèse des critiques anglo-saxonnes les plus récentes. Inf Psychiatr 89(4):285–294

Kaprinis G, Giozepas I, Iakovidis A, Kandylis D, Fokas K (2009) Clinical psychiatry, vol I. Parisianou Scientific Publications S.A, Athens (in Greek)

Louzoun C, Stylianidis S (1987) La nouvelle psychiatrie italienne. Mission interministérielle recherche-expérimentation, Paris

Patel V, Prince M (2010) Global mental health: a new global health field comes of age. JAMA 303(19):1976–1977

Ploumpidis D, Evans NJR (1993) An outline of the development of psychiatry in Greece. Hist Psychiatry 4(14):239–244

Reisman JM (1991) A history of clinical psychology. Taylor & Francis, New York

Stylianidis S, Lavdas M (2012) Comments on trauma and social exclusion: is psychiatrification the answer to the complexity of social pain? Synapsis J 26(8):16–19 (in Greek)

Stylianidis S, Theoharakis N, Chondros P (2007) The suspended step of psychiatric reform in Greece: a timeless approach featuring topical questions. Archaeol Arts 105:45–54 (in Greek)

Stylianidis S, Ghionakis N, Chondros P (2010) La riforma psichiatrica greca attraverso lo spettro dell'esperienza della riforma italiana. Psichiatr di Comunità 1:93–106

Szasz T (1976) Involuntary Psychiatry. U Cin L Rev 45, 347

Tzanakis M (2008) Beyond the asylum, Social psychiatry and the issue of the subject (Synapses Series). Exantas Press, Athens (in Greek)

VandenBos GR, Cummings NA, DeLeon PH (1992) A century of psychotherapy: economic and environmental influences. In: Freedheim DK, Freudenberger HJ, Kessler JW, Messer SB, Peterson DR, Strupp HH, Wachtel PL (eds) History of psychotherapy: a century of change. American Psychological Association, Washington, DC, pp 65–102

Zakzanis K, Leach L, Kaplan E (1998) On the nature and pattern of neurocognitive function in major depressive disorder. Cogn Behav Neurol 11(3):111–119

Philosophical and Sociological Foundations of Social Psychiatry

2

Stelios Stylianidis

Abstract

We will deal in this chapter some aspects of the work of Michel Foucault and some of the major figures of existentialism, a work that laid the sociological and philosophical foundations for the formation of the critical psychiatry and deinstitutionalisation movement. We will also explore the subject formation problematic, by looking into the contribution of phenomenological psychoanalysis and the connection between the phenomenological approach to philosophy and Franco Basaglia's thought, which constitutes the essential challenge to the psychiatric implementation of the biomedical model. In the same perspective, we will finally analyse some of the transformations that contemporary psychiatry underwent in the age of the ideological domination of neoliberalism in the domain of mental health as well.

2.1 The Sociological Foundations of Social Psychiatry

Psychiatry and the Enlightenment, namely, the Age of Reason, diverge from one another on two principal lines of thought. There is, on the one hand, the importance attributed to the notion of reason, which, by promoting order in society and technical solutions to human problems, leads to the event of the "great confinement", as Foucault (1972) put it. In its scientific, technical, and technological expression, this tendency results in the creation of psychiatry, whereas another line of Enlightenment thought focuses on the individual, the exploration of subjectivity and the Cartesian forms of phenomenology and psychoanalysis. Scientific reductionism, i.e. the oversimplification by academic and traditional psychiatry of complex psychopathological

S. Stylianidis
Department of Psychology, Panteion University, Athens, Greece
e-mail: stylianidis.st@gmail.com

phenomena or phenomena expressing the human psychic and mental function, is formed at the end of nineteenth century. Reductionism is a one-dimensional attempt to explain aspects of a multileveled individual and collective sensegiving (psychic, social, mental, anthropological, political, historical) by means of scientific entities, such as genes and neurotransmitters. The tradition of reductionism in psychiatry places great emphasis on the role of experts, namely, those who have the privilege to be the narrators in what happens during the technological framing of problems and, therefore, in identifying and establishing the causal processes that can be scientifically manipulated. Put schematically, there is no scientific knowledge if there is no documentation.

This viewpoint establishes a methodological individualism; it focuses, in other words, on aspects of human behaviour, such as the symptoms, independently of the context within which the latter are observed. Therefore, when referring to the sociological foundations of traditional psychiatry and to the criticism it underwent by community psychiatry in order to transform itself into a new body of knowledge and a novel social practice, it is important to remark that its primordial interest lies in an understanding founded solely on science and in the promotion of therapeutic approaches based on technology. Traditional psychiatry is interested in notions like sense, values or relations only marginally, secondarily and in an attempt perhaps to find a democratic alibi for its practice. In contrast to this epistemological, ethical and philosophical approach, critical psychiatry, from whose current stems social psychiatry, focuses primarily on the ethics and hermeneutics of madness, on social malaise, social suffering and alienation. Its interest in the development and analysis of special technologies is only secondary. In the first of the following figures, one can discern the dissociation between biology, psychology and culture pertaining to the viewpoint of the "hard" biomedical paradigm; the perspective changes radically in the second figure, whereby the suffering subject and its lived experience is placed in the centre of the intersecting domains. In this chapter, the ontology of mental suffering, along with the soul-body dualism, will be studied in more depth within the context of phenomenological psychiatry.

The hard biomedical model (Fig. 2.1) has biology, psychology and culture at its centre, whereas the soft biomedical model (Fig. 2.2), the model on which social and community psychiatry is based, has at its centre the experience forming the point of intersection between psychology, biology and culture. There is no actual separation between the biological, the psychological and the cultural outside of a unitary, complex and historically determined human experience.

2.2 Existentialism and Social Psychiatry

We know that the fathers of existentialism are Søren Kierkegaard and, through his philosophical individualism, Friedrich Nietzsche. With his notion of the free organic individual opposing the uniformity imposed by contemporary society and by promoting existential individuality (born biological beings, we have to become existential individuals assuming the responsibility of our actions), the French existentialist

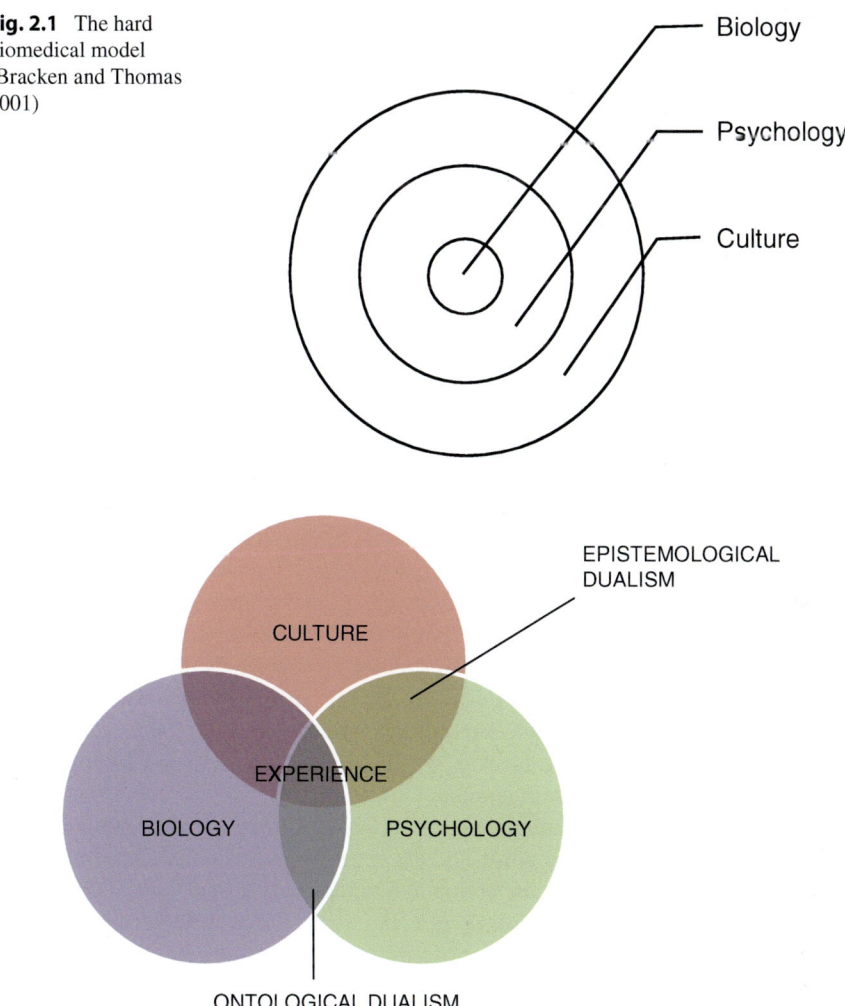

Fig. 2.1 The hard biomedical model (Bracken and Thomas 2001)

Fig. 2.2 The soft biomedical model (Bracken and Thomas 2001)

Jean-Paul Sartre is at the basis of the problematic and constitution of the concept of subject in the area of critical psychiatry. Authenticity, i.e. the state of recognition of the Other's distinct liberty, must be the dominant virtue of the individual. While referring to absolute freedom and the sense of responsibility, Sartre (1962) maintained that "people exist, objects just are". According to Sartre, the concept of existence is particularly related with transience and the responsibility of the individual before his/her freedom. Sartre claimed that a human being is nothing other than "his life project".

Following this line of thought, critical psychiatry promotes a genuinely democratic hermeneutical approach to understanding psychopathological phenomena, an approach acknowledging the possibility of autonomy and different perspectives for a subject and emphasising its value as a citizen that can eventually manifest a psychiatric or psychological problem. Critical psychiatry focuses, therefore, on the value of the suffering subject, symbolically and effectively placed in the position of active citizen. Moreover, critical psychiatry's hermeneutics stresses the role of meaning as a primordial concept referring to a complex human reality irreducible to causal explanation and gives priority to ethics over technology or the discovery of new therapeutic approaches.

Before proceeding to examine hermeneutics and phenomenology as philosophical approaches which influenced decisively the critical psychiatry movement, especially in its beginnings, we would like to mention first some basic points of convergence between the two, points that will be analysed more thoroughly subsequently:

1. Critical psychiatry's approach to knowledge aims at turning it into an instrument for a democratic debate; in other words, it puts the emphasis on the framework determining the understanding of individual reality. Consequently, the understanding of the social, cultural, temporal or bodily framework comes first, followed by the meaning of the subject's problems and symptoms.
2. According to critical psychiatry, the hermeneutical interrogation of the meaning, importance, significance and value of a suffering subject should always precede causal explication, namely, the linear connection between cause and effect in the understanding and description of psychopathology.
3. For critical psychiatry, diagnosis is not the opinion of an expert disconnected from the life context of an individual. On the contrary, it is a process of shared understanding and explanation, namely, a joint construction between the expert, the intersecting therapeutic group and the suffering individual.
4. Critical psychiatry opposes the notion of temporality to that of chronicity. There is no static phenomenology: nobody is a chronic patient or suffers from a chronic disease. On the contrary, mental suffering is structured during observation by past experiences and future possibilities. We probably have here a precursor of the notion of recovery, which is developed in other chapters of this book. Admitting "being towards death" into theory means bringing together our otherwise scattered hypotheses in the realisation of the importance of the subject's being.
5. The attempt to a comprehensive interrogation into the role of science and expertise in the field of mental health occupies an important place in critical psychiatry. Understanding science as something originating with human experience and interests is different from the "neutral, out of nowhere viewpoint", namely, the scientific demonstration of a phenomenon without an examination of the context within which the latter arises. The problem of ethics and social priorities in clinical practice is therefore primordial and cannot be merely reduced to a simply demonstrative practice, namely, a kind of medicine and psychiatry based solely on proof. Psychiatry has been the meeting point of multiple references and scientific domains: medicine, law or philosophy (romanticism in the nineteenth

century, positivism in the twentieth century). As maintained at the end of this chapter, twenty-first-century psychiatry largely disinvests and, by means of the reductionism it promotes and the biomedical model upon which it is based, obscures its own complexity. By contrast to a multileveled approach to subjectivity, this biomedical model is founded on two constitutive ideas:
(A) Mental illness is a disease commensurable to bodily diseases and, therefore, potentially curable.
(B) The mentally suffering subject is never completely destroyed and may, as a subject, actively contribute to his/her cure.

A madness-object and a partial, occasional madness of the subject constitute two different approaches. In any case, subjectivity, in its relationship both to praxis and to suffering, lies at the centre of clinical practice. The contradictions of traditional psychiatry, which critical psychiatry tries to resolve through its theory and practice, lie in the opposition between confinement and a humanist or therapeutic function of psychiatry, between a therapeutic approach and the demand for social control and management of every psychic deviation and between subjectivism and objectivism.

In this perspective, the appearance of the asylum had a double function. As thoroughly described by Foucault in his *The History of Madness*, the asylum constituted throughout the fifteenth century a space for the protection of society against troublesome individuals or outsiders; on the other hand, it was also a refuge for the insane against the damaging effects of society. Therefore, while providing a space of control for outsiders or all those tearing at the fabric of society, the asylum offers at the same time a real refuge for the mentally ill, who, as a result of the clinic's creation within the space of the asylum, become for the first time recognised as a distinct medical and psychiatric entity. All of this means that the birth and constitution of psychiatry as a distinct scientific realm take place within the asylum (Abatzoglou 1991). In 1793, at the asylum of Bicêtre, Pinel will propose a new kind of treatment for the mentally ill named **moral treatment**. The latter is opposed to natural treatment, namely, the therapeutic approaches used at that time, like bloodletting, enema, various drugs or hydrotherapy. By contrast, moral treatment proposes methods and rules aiming at the direct engagement of the mind and feelings and can, in a sense, be considered the predecessor of institutional psychotherapy (psychothérapie institutionnelle), a school that dominated France's mental institutions after 1948. Within the institutions, however, the concentration camp living conditions, violence and abandonment contrast with the implementation of a personalised care project and the investment in the personal relationship between doctor and patient, aspects that formed the basis for the realisation of Pinel's proposal for moral treatment.

Owing to the ineffectiveness of moral treatment, a biological orientation dominated psychiatry since the second half of the nineteenth century, while the asylum remained the site of treatment. Throughout his innovative and challenging work on knowledge, power, institutions, subject and psychiatry, Foucault describes with great precision both the role of the asylum and the social mechanisms that brought it about. Foucault adopts a critical stance, situating himself between Marxism, existentialism and phenomenology. His fundamental thesis is that "what matters most is to point out the historical dimension of mental illness". The latter can be totally distinguished from normality only to the extent that society rejects and excludes it. Until the eighteenth century, the mentally ill are considered demon ridden and appear as a symbol of moral decay. On the contrary, the consideration of madness as alienation, a consideration based on modern humanist and medical approaches, leads to its exclusion. As Foucault characteristically writes, "the language of psychiatry, which is a monologue of reason about madness, has been established only on the basis of such a[n imposed] silence. In our age, madness is muzzled within the beatitude of a scientific knowledge, which analyzes it so much that in the end forgets it. Exclusion and treatment thus coincide". The intention of treating and the intention of confining the suffering subject meet and go hand in hand. Despite Renaissance's wishful thinking, madness is identified with unreason, as a result of the general confinement. Because of this identification, madness acquires a moral dimension, turning into a scandal and a threat for public order. Medicine then places a mirror in front of the patient for the latter to acknowledge in it that he/she is objectively insane. According to Foucault, madness wasn't liberated but medicalised, i.e. objectivised as mental illness. It is important here to determine and come to terms with the philosophical concept of the subject. Foucault's book *Folie et déraison: Histoire de la folie à l'âge classique* (1961), originally his doctoral thesis, poses at first as an anti-history of psychiatry and, more recently, in the 1970s, as a classic of antipsychiatry. For Foucault, fear, surveillance, humiliation and censure within the asylum constitute the four active dimensions of Pinel's moral treatment. These four dimensions produce the alienated man under the conditions of the asylum.

One can observe here an analogy with Burton's notion of institutional neurosis (1959) and Basaglia's notion of double alienation, namely, the alienation produced by the asylum, the violence and the abandonment, along with the alienation stemming from mental illness. Which is the subject of madness, finally? As Tzanakis (2008) characteristically mentions, Foucault (1963) raises the question of when madness acquires the meaning of mental illness. In *The Birth of the Clinic* (1963), Foucault analyses the procedures giving birth to the clinical gaze, the one which observes the interior of the body: "This formation depends both on the space of implementation of clinical practice and on the invention of a language by means of which the point of view of death is shifted". Within the asylums, "the gaze of the doctor observes the pathological landscape giving birth to a new language. Progressively, the gaze and the discourse representing what it saw, namely, pain in its multiplicity, coincide with one another" (Tzanakis, op. cit., p. 51).

In his reading of Foucault's work, Marcel Gauchet (1997) mentions that "the insane is insane but, at the same time, alike. And since he/she is alike, the truth of madness is the truth of subjectivity itself".

Along with the antipsychiatry current of his time (Cooper 1970; Laing 1965), Thomas Szasz (1982), professor of psychiatry at Syracuse University, New York, rejected mental illness as an object. We know that, in its beginnings, antipsychiatry was an Anglo-Saxon movement that called into question classical psychiatry by presenting psychosis not only as an existential reaction to a sclerosed and alienated family environment but also as a response to traditional medicine, accused of reproducing the so-called patient's confinement in his/her solitude and social isolation by means of scientific data and proof. As Meyers (2005) remarks, English antipsychiatry tries to situate itself between the social and the medical. From a social and political point of view, psychiatry has been subjected to denunciation and condemnation by the radical European movements, because of the violent and oppressive conditions of treatment and hospitalisation of the mentally ill.

For Cooper and Laing (1970), "talking about violence in psychiatry, the violence which blinds the eyes, screams its name and declares itself as such, means talking about the subtle and disguised violence that the others, the normal people, exert upon those who call insane". Inasmuch as psychiatry represents the interests of normal people, it can be claimed that the violence exerted in the context of psychiatric practice is principally the violence of psychiatry.

The particular intrapsychic functioning of people suffering from schizophrenia or other psychoses is completely obscured by Cooper (1970). According to the antipsychiatry movement, what determines the generation of a psychopathology are the "micro-social crises, in whose context the actions and experience of a singular person are handicapped by the others for cultural or microcultural (often family) reasons". "The individual is highhandedly labelled schizophrenic by medical or quasi-medical entities".

Psychopathology is not a natural object but "a myth constructed by man". As Szasz explains, "psychiatry is conventionally defined as a medical specialty referring to the diagnosis and treatment of mental disorders. […] I would like to suggest that such a widely accepted definition places psychiatry at the same level with alchemy and astrology, making it a part of the pseudo-sciences" (Szasz 1982). For Szasz, who has been defending these views for the past 40 years, mental disorder is not an illness whose nature could be elucidated and explored by science. It is rather a myth constructed by psychiatrists in order for them to achieve professional recognition and social acceptance and to provide easy solutions to the problems of social deviation and control.

Szasz wasn't alone during that period. As Porter (2003) mentions, Foucault was arguing in *The History of Madness* along the same lines: mental disorder should be understood not as a natural event but as a cultural construction founded on a nexus of administrative and medico-psychiatric practices. To write the history of madness means to narrate not the disorder and its treatment but the problems of freedom, control, knowledge and power it entails. After the great confinement described by Foucault, a series of humanist efforts attempted to limit the power abuses within the framework of the asylum. Pinel in France, Chiarugi in Italy and Tuke in England inaugurated a period of humanisation of medical care, a period that paved the way for a more rational and humanist approach to mental illness. By the nineteenth century, the first steps were made into the study of the pathology of madness, the description and classification of its clinical types and the acknowledging of the differences between bodily disease and mental neurosis. Treatment became a subject of preoccupation within university hospitals and extra-hospital structures, while the social dimensions of psychopathology began to draw the attention of researchers. By the end of the nineteenth century, the road to the new ideas of Kraepelin (father of the psychiatric nosography), Freud (father of psychoanalysis) and Charcot and Janet (followers of the footsteps of Kahlbaum, Griesinger, Conolly and Maudsley) was already open (Porter 2003, p. 5). Revolutionary changes took place in connection with the natural treatments of illnesses, the alienating conditions in psychiatric hospitals underwent some kind of humanisation and the various therapeutic approaches began to be connected with each other, thus achieving a more personalised form and becoming organised according to a more continuous therapeutic process – what we would nowadays call the continuum of psychiatric care.

The biomedical model of mental illness starts dominating within the context of positivism's epistemological primacy. This paradigm establishes itself more widely in the field of health and illness by placing at the centre of medical interest the detection of pathogenic and pathological phenomena within the human organism or the tracking of malfunctions in the anatomy of the organs. Canguilhem's philosophical and historical understanding of the birth of medical thought in his monumental work *The Normal and the Pathological* (1972) sheds light on the double conception of illness: there is, on the one hand, the ontological representation of illness corresponding to the Pasteurian doctrines and the microbiological theory of transmissible diseases and infection and, on the other, the poetic conception of illness, identified with ancient Greek medicine and departing from the local effects of the anatomo-pathological substrate while defining illness as a disorder in the harmony and equilibrium between man and his/her environment.

As Anastasia Zisi (2013) mentions, "the starting point of the biomedical paradigm is the negative definition of health and the concomitant focusing on the different types of pathology and the biological factors generating it, leading to the patient's extraction from his/her natural and social environment". It is from this biomedical health paradigm that traditional clinical psychiatry draws its principal arguments, in order to define mental illness as a result of changes in the organism's physiology, in the brain's biochemistry and in the central nervous system's functioning. The outcome of the clinical psychiatric assessment, often completed by neuropsychological tests of memory and other cognitive functions, is the psychiatric diagnosis suggesting the type of medicinal treatment for the relief from and the suppression of psychiatric symptomatology. Despite its interest in the patient's medical history and biography, the biomedical model imposes its biological ontology pertaining to the nature of mental illness, leading to the suppression of the patient as a social subject and of his/her symptoms as forms of experience and modes of existence (Zisi, op. cit., p. 27).

Foucault's work refers critically to Pinel's contribution and realisation that by the end of the nineteenth century, the insane – until then considered criminals or demon-ridden people – are subjected, chained and confined to the most downgrading and humiliating treatments. Pinel demonstrated that these people were ill and needed to be treated humanely and kindly.

After the breakthrough of this understanding and compassionate outlook on madness, psychiatry marched from conquest to conquest, establishing definitive and concrete clinical pictures, constituting the first psychiatric classifications and trying to describe scientifically the forms, types and evolutions of mental disorders.

However, Foucault reacts to and rejects this "expansionist" mission of psychiatry for several reasons. The first one is that madness "does not constitute from the outset a medical object". Madness is first and foremost a massive cultural construction, a way of defining man as rational, normal being, thus excluding and rejecting the mentally ill. This means that the attempt to grasp madness is founded precisely on such a gesture of exclusion, a gesture reproduced for years to come. We therefore find ourselves at the very opposite of the traditional history of psychiatry, which refers to medical objectification as a liberating process for the mentally ill. Foucault's approach isn't a romantically motivated endeavour to undermine the attempts towards a scientific understanding of madness but an effort to reposition the latter and grasp the risks and consequences of such a process on the modern identity. The history Foucault writes does not follow the traditional lines of the history of science (a history of monumental errors and great discoveries) in order to make a choice between those promoting obscurantism and those favouring scientific truth. His history is archaeological; it is about excavating and bringing to light the deeper layers lying beneath the surface of declarations and institutions. Foucault studies the experience of madness, taking into account not only the social practices and medical knowledge but also the literary and artistic production referring to it. The Renaissance treated madness as a form of wandering. The insane circulate from town to town, boarded on ships, forced to live on cities' gates and to undergo social exclusion. The experience of madness brought to light by the Renaissance could be described as "secular". A very powerful problematic concerning the menace of world destruction, the menace of something absurd capable of disturbing social order and generating chaos underpins this condition of constant and structural wandering. After his brief analysis of the Renaissance, Foucault devotes many pages to the description of the experience of madness in the classical age. This description became the target of many critics, philosophers and historians who called into question the very idea of a great confinement of the insane during the seventeenth century.

Foucault highlights audaciously the historical moment of the great confinement. The insane that had been living until then in a state of constant wandering were confined behind the tall walls of the general hospital, along with those living on charity and the homeless. Such a confinement presupposes a new experience and, above all, a specific image of the mentally ill, which from now on will lie at the centre of social problems (e.g. the disorder caused by marginal population groups wandering from town to town) and political practices (like the institution of police measures detaching themselves from or bypassing the judicial realm).

The mentally ill is no more a person carrying the mystical, superstitious and disturbing aura conveyed by the absurd. He/she becomes a problem, with which society is summoned to deal. In this perspective, the role of psychiatry is called into question. Foucault manages to show that the distance between scientific objectivity and what the subject experiences as suffering and, therefore, as psychopathology is due to two factors: on the one hand, the police practices of confining the marginal population and, on the other, the moral denunciation of the absurd, inasmuch as madness constitutes a figure of alienation similar to the categories of moral deviation such as the homosexuals, the poor, the bandits or the common criminals. The idea according to which scientific objectivity is impossible outside the framework of police practices and moral condemnation will be considered a real provocation both for the science of psychiatry and the social sciences trying to establish themselves as neutral and free of prejudice. Finally, madness becomes modern when appearing not as a symptom of differentiation between truth and error but rather as a revelator of the split between a pure conscience and a mystical, obscure nature. This is what Foucault calls "the anthropological experience of madness". Madness becomes a mental illness defined as the alienation of the regular and normal mental traits of an individual and based on a cerebral malfunction. Thus, it marks the distinction not between day and night – as in the Renaissance – but between the normal and the pathological in human nature. In this way, madness becomes both very distant and very close to us (Tsalikoglou 1987, 2007): subjected to confinement through the domination and legitimisation of medical discourse, captive to its medical definition, madness nevertheless "comes closer" to us precisely because we unconsciously recognise a part of our unfamiliar self in its representation. Madness, therefore, becomes extremely human. The medical construction and the biomedical model of madness are at the very opposite of such an existential experience praised to such an extent by the Renaissance, literature and the arts and liberated by the antipsychiatry movement. In conclusion, Pinel according to Foucault didn't liberate the mentally ill by breaking their chains and instituting a medical entity, namely, mental disorder, but rather subjected them to a new form of power, namely, the power of medicine. Consequently and according to the Foucauldian analysis, the hospital appears as a field of forces of power and madness as a pole of resistance. To treat or to be treated doesn't mean to rehabilitate the truth but rather to subject or be subjected to identities imposed by power mechanisms, which, by means of medical discourse, rationalise the social exclusion of the Other.

2.3 The Subject and Phenomenology

Lived Experience and Self

The concept of the subject occupies a central place in the constitution of the theory or rather the panorama of theoretical approaches articulating the clinic of the subject, lived experiences and mental phenomena with the tradition of the German (mostly) phenomenological psychiatry and the theory and practice of understanding and emancipating the mentally ill as a suffering subject.

The way Professor Tatossian (2002) formulated the necessity of reintegrating the phenomenological approach in today's clinical practice is characteristic: "Psychiatry is in danger when, on the grounds of objectivity and positivism, it ignores its multiple origins situated in everyday experience and the living world".

Let's examine schematically the basic notions structuring phenomenological knowledge in philosophy and in connection to psychiatry. Phenomenology is the knowledge "we gain in the first person" through our everyday experience, by observing nature and its qualities within a naturalistic framework. By the latter we designate the studies compatible with the methodology of the natural sciences. Phenomenological knowledge cannot be reduced to a third person; it is the conscious knowledge one has of his/her personal lived experiences. We should, however, distinguish between experience per se (e.g. the experience of pain) and knowledge of this experience and of its qualities (e.g. the knowledge of the nature and qualities of my toothache).

There are sensory, perceptive, emotional and affective subjective experiences (like mental distress, sorrow). Living a conscious experience along with its set of distinctive qualities cannot be reduced to the state of consciousness of experience as such. The awareness of the qualities of an experience presupposes having a certain knowledge, a certain set of concepts. For example, the awareness that an irritation turns into pain or that nervousness turns into anger presupposes the "reflexive" knowledge of the notions of pain and anger.

Founding the "reflexive" nature of knowledge presupposes distinguishing between appearance and knowledge of appearance. As an example we will mention Wittgenstein (1966) who, in his notes on psychology, remarks that a person expressing pain does not necessarily have some overall knowledge as to the nature of this pain. In other words, the expression of pain is not the expression of some knowledge pertaining to pain.

While this is a controversial topic among philosophers, it is less so among clinicians, given that every subject has a certain capacity to grasp his/her own lived experiences. For example, a patient is justified and authorised to express the mental or physical pain that discomforts him/her and that he/she wishes to avoid – a point that medicine should take into account and trust.

Which is the source, however, of such a lived experience? Put schematically, one philosophical conception considers that the description of a phenomenon is based on a series of inferences having, directly or indirectly, a causal relation with the phenomenon. According to a second, epistemologically distinct, philosophical conception, there is some kind of possibility to observe, internally or externally, the phenomenon. There is for instance a connection between the various mental disorders and behaviours, as can be established through the different facial mimics corresponding to different mental states (a point made since the age of Darwin). It is clear that we do not behave in the same manner when we experience an intense pain or an intense orgasm.

At this point, phenomenologists could ask the following crucial question: can we extract safe general conclusions about complex phenomena observed in others by observing our own reactions and behaviours through a process of "neutral introspection"? As we will try to show with the following remarks, this is a key controversial point between the biomedical model, which unswervingly proceeds to classify psychiatric symptoms in every detail, and the phenomenological approach to subjective otherness within the framework of a unique encounter between two individuals (Krauss 2003; Jaspers 1963; Minkowski 1927, 1948, 1966; Lanteri-Laura 1957; Blankenburg 1982, 1991). We can argue, however, that introspection may lead us to false conclusions, even in connection with our own personal experiences and mental phenomena. Nevertheless, it is sure that, despite the limitations of "observational neutrality", by using introspection we gain privileged access to the content of such experiences, even if we commit mistakes in the description of some of their aspects.

The example of jealousy is interesting both philosophically and in terms of psychopathology. I can refer to the phenomenon of jealousy I experience in an objective and external manner, attempting to interpret it and extract some conclusions from it, even if such a process is open to interrogation and doubt. This fact does not in any way deprive me of my capacity to have access to what I experience in a more specific way, namely, by means of the lived experience I feel when I am jealous. This first person lived experience contains a quality auto-observation that does not leave room for doubt. If we transpose such a reasoning to contemporary social psychiatry – which, as we will see in the following chapters, considers the place of the first person narrator-subject crucial (Jackson 1982), as a means of empowerment and active participation in the process of recovery – it is easy to understand the philosophical basis underpinning the co-construction of a new narration by the analyst and the analysand, aiming at the process of recovery-as-healing.

Jackson's principal thesis can be formulated as follows: "Introspection can help us learn something from this specific character of our first person experiences: we can learn that this knowledge cannot be reduced and limited to an objective, scientific approach". In conclusion, the relationship between the experience of a phenomenon and the knowledge deriving from the introspection of such an experience constitutes a central problem with which every philosophical theory of introspection must come to terms. In other words, "the subject (S) cannot have access to a phenomenological type of experience (E) unless it (S) has already experienced such an experience (E)" (Stoljar 2009).

By contrast to the phenomenological approach, the alternative Cartesian one is considered the most dominant among the philosophical community since the age of Descartes. The basic idea of this "introspective approach" is the following: "the spirit is penetrable as such, meaning that it disposes of a special access to the content of its various states".

It is interesting that Freud (1957) was already interrogating the fact that "philosophers frequently define mental states as being *directly present* and perceptible to consciousness". By "mental states" we can distinguish two types of states: (1) attitudes like intentions, desires, wishes or choices and (2) occasional states like sensations, emotions, perceptions, decisions, judgements and mental "acts" in general.

The second type of states is the one to which we have privileged introspective access, according to the Cartesian approach. More specifically, an individual can gain knowledge of his/her feelings and perceptions without having previously observed his/her behaviour: the recourse to introspection bypasses the observation of the outside world. Consequently and independently of all doubts about the validity of such an approach, the fact that it is not based on external data provides it with a strong epistemological privilege (Ludwig and Kabat-Zinn 2008).

According to the Cartesian approach, we become directly aware of the content of a conscious experience the moment we experience it. This entails that our introspective judgement (what philosophers called "inner meaning") is not affected by what is considered fundamental. I do not need to think about my behaviour or the state of my teeth when I have a toothache.

Subject, Psychiatry, Phenomenology and Philosophy of Mind

The bibliography and genealogy of psychiatric phenomenology is huge. We will present here abstractly some points and historical references. It is necessary to make a preliminary remark: phenomenology is not psychopathology, despite the fact that it is precisely the ambiguous relationship between them which could probably explain not only the special importance of the phenomenological approach in the various psychological analyses (as in Jaspers and Bleuler) but also the value of a psychology transformed, through phenomenology, into an existential psychology (Tatossian, p. 13).

In this psychopathological context, *phenomenology* is defined as a *change of attitude* (Broekman 1965) consisting in bracketing the natural or "naïve" attitude according to which all of us psychiatrists and other mental health professionals evaluate complex mental, social or material situations as an objective reality existing independently of us. Such complex clinical situations place us in front of epistemological dilemmas of interpretation and understanding (Tzavaras 2002).

Phenomenology is not interested in reality itself but in the conditions rendering this reality possible. Therefore, phenomenology is practised only when it puts in motion some form of *abstraction*. This abstractive process considers that all convictions pertaining to natural reality along with the direct or indirect explanatory stances regarding reality's perception are "suspended". This abstraction, reduction or *epokhe* is the fundamental act of Husserlian phenomenology, something which immediately raises the question of the relations between phenomenological philosophy and psychiatric phenomenology (Husserl 1969). The psychiatrist may be attracted to psychiatric phenomenology and seek, in the context of psychopathological observation, some kind of application of the "results and theories" which supposedly belong to the body of phenomenological philosophy.

Binswanger (1958, 1971) compares the role played by physiology in understanding bodily illness to the role played by Husserl's transcendental phenomenology in understanding psychopathology as "a cross section of consciousness". Nothing is more erroneous than the view that psychiatric phenomenology or Daseinsanalyse "adheres" beforehand to some kind of "theory" or "systematic phenomenological psychology", which simply does not exist (Spiegelberg 1972).

Phenomenology rejects all preconceptions. The danger with a "preconstructed" theory lies in the fact that the use of notions like corporeality, interpersonal communication, and consciousness can vary from one philosophy to another. If the phenomenologist-psychiatrist were to choose one or more among various existing theoretical approaches before beginning with his clinical practice, he should not be considered a genuine phenomenologist. Psychiatric phenomenology is not grounded on some king of initial "doctrine" (Blankenburg 1982, 1991): it is rather a "fluid" way of working, aiming not so much at the simple application as to the integration of philosophical principles into the clinical outlook of the psychiatrist.

Returning to E. Husserl and his notion of "epokhe" appearing for the first time in his work in 1913, we can formulate five principal points concerning it:

1. The elimination of all latent or silent theoretical preconceptions by means of which a psychiatrist accesses (or not) experience: the psychiatrist adopts an attitude that "brackets" theoretical terms and nosographic classifications, which could hinder any possible encounter with the patient's lived experience.
2. The suspension of the positing of reality: the possibility of grasping the Other is kept open by bracketing, instantaneously "deleting" what he/she says in order to come back to it at a later stage. For example, the psychiatrist avoids saying that he/she is in front of an "auditive illusion", a perception without object or a delirium and tries to listen carefully to what the subject he/she encounters is experiencing.
3. The reflexive transformation, namely, the attempt to understand the way in which the individual's perceptions and his/her relations with life objects are situated: it is necessary to grasp that these elements exist not only for the patient but also for the psychiatrist. How are we to understand, for example, the place of kitchen knives within the patient's construction of a delirium of persecution, and what is their place in his/her narration and in the attitude we adopt? (Eidetic insight)
4. Imaginative variation is an attempt to modify the act of consciousness within imagination. Up to what point can we push variation without altering the real event, the nature of experience? The act of recollecting an ordinary experience by acknowledging the different versions given by two individuals (e.g. the analyst and the analysand) allows us to realise if we are really referring to what Husserl designated as the *essence* of experience (e.g. not only the narrated fact but also the sentimental state in which the narrator found himself/herself).
5. Phenomenology is interested not in the reproduction of external reality within the subject's consciousness but in the meaningful constitution of objects by consciousness. In other words, it is interested not in facts but in the conditions that render possible the constitution of meaning by transcendental thought. Binswanger, for example, refers to a fact not as fact but as something that can freeze or oppress the consciousness of an individual.

The above aspects of "epokhe" do not form a theoretical construction but a viewpoint or an attitude adopted by the subject in view of the constitution of any theoretical construction.

Psychiatric phenomenology is also indissolubly connected with the notion of intersubjectivity, which appears for the first time in Husserl's *Cartesian Meditations* (1929). One of Husserl's principal theses, namely, nonrepresentation, could be explained as follows: "Even if the face of my interlocutor cannot be considered the same with mine, I can nevertheless relate them as if they were the same". My body and the Other's body are the "same" in the sense that I perceive some of the traits of the Other's face as if they were mine (i.e. mimics of sorrow, joy, anger, etc.).

I perceive what I experience without seeing in the Other (i.e. a feeling) as something that I myself can experience. In other words, every expression I perceive on the face of the Other refers me to a common lived experience. In his attempt to understand mental phenomena, Husserl himself makes use of terms like ego, ground, intention, psychologism, passive synthesis and genesis, terms that cannot be analysed in the context of this chapter.

Our peregrination in the field of psychiatric phenomenology brings us to Husserl's famous pupil, Martin Heidegger. In his monumental work *Being and Time* (Heidegger and Vezin 1964; Corvez 1965), Heidegger uses for the first time the notion of Dasein, which we could reductively render by "existence". In the framework of a clinical psychiatric interview, for example, there are two people in a room. Both of them share a series of characteristics pertaining to this encounter, characteristics that the chair found within the same framework cannot experience. Heidegger suggests an abstract construct, namely, Dasein, aimed against common sense and having the following characteristics: being in the world, surrounding space, understanding, being affected by the other, being towards death, being with and temporalisation. All of these fundamental elements, which L. Binswanger (1958) included in his work, constitute the "body" of Daseinsanalyse, namely, existential analysis. Through his own special way of analysing clinical cases (cf. the case of Suzanne Urban in particular), Binswanger (1960) demonstrated that, with the exception of her delirium's or mania's theme, the patient's specific way of being excludes every other presence. Binswanger founded and developed Daseinsanalyse, a particular mode of psychiatric phenomenological approach to the "analysis of existence", between 1933 and 1958.

Daseinsanalyse is not a therapeutic technique but a mode of approaching, diagnosing and understanding different from what traditional psychiatry proposes, though not contrary to it. For example, despite the different kind of analysis to which it resorts, Daseinsanalyse does not call into question the diagnosis of psychosis operated on the basis of traditional nosography.

As semiotic basis for phenomenological psychiatry, the space of representation constitutes for Binswanger "a rich ensemble structured by millions of fragments sustained through the singularity of a personal trajectory". In order for a space of representation to be constituted, the conditions of the analogic and symbolic components have to be satisfied. The analogic components form the structured development of a set of elements allowing a better perceptive rendering of what an individual is experiencing. The symbolic components of representation are the abstract systematic codifications (linguistic type of representations) based on the analogic components through a process of linguistic mediation (i.e. a publicly articulated speech without some specific content) or attached to intuition by means of an analogic representation (cf. the recent studies of experimental psychology on embodied cognitions).

"Psychiatry as science must take into account the ontological foundations supporting its discourse: the attitudes, the mental peculiarities, the psyche in the sense of psychology and psychopathology, the character, the personality, the instinct and the symptoms. All these notions lack ontological foundation". "We came across such a foundation in Heidegger and his Existential Analysis: psychiatry as a phenomenological science of lived experience is based upon such an Analysis" (Binswanger).

Psychiatric phenomenology is an attempt to comprehend the symptoms of schizophrenic psychoses in particular and psychopathology in general. Put schematically, Binswanger returns at the end of his life to Husserlian notions like transcendence, intentionality and genesis of mental phenomena (Husserl et al. 1938), without however calling into question the framework of Daseinsanalyse. "It is about a change in perspective and not about some kind of recantation", he observes. It is interesting to stress at this point the substantial influence exercised on F. Basaglia's clinical, theoretical and political attitude by the German phenomenological psychiatric tradition and by E. Husserl's philosophical thought (Basaglia 1976; Stylianidis 1985; Louzoun and Stylianidis 1987). Basaglia's work hypothesis concerning the formation of an anti-institutional approach was based on Husserl's notion of "epokhe", a notion that allowed him to formulate the position according to which "illness is bracketed" (and not negated in its existence), in order for the effects of institutionalism (violence, abandonment, impersonal treatment of the mentally ill) covering up the authentic expression of the subject's psychopathology to be called into question.

Besides the substantial use of Husserl's notion of "epokhe", Basaglia's epistemological stance adopted phenomenological psychiatry's refusal to allow any preconstructed theory and conception into psychopathology, aiming at an authentic and free encounter with the otherness of the suffering subject, without the distorting glass of "objectifying" positivist psychiatry. Consequently, Basaglia's theoretical reference to Husserl's philosophy and to the German phenomenological psychiatric school is at the very opposite of antipsychiatry's initial attitude of calling mental illness into question. His dialogue with Laing, Cooper and Foucault was fertile and important, inasmuch as it converged around the analysis of social mechanisms of control and of the alienating role of capitalist society's institutions. However, they diverged radically from one another in questioning the biomedical model "from the inside", namely, through political change and the transformation of the violent institutions of traditional public psychiatry. Binswanger's and other important German phenomenologists' (Tatossian 2002; Minkowski 1927, 1948, 1966; Blankenburg 1982, 1991) contribution in putting forward another approach of human existence, namely, a description of the subject's being in the world and of its pathological tonality, constituted the favourable philosophical and ideological background against which flourished the most radical attempts to challenge traditional psychiatry and to put forward a new form of organisation for mental health services (deinstitutionalisation, community services, etc.), aiming at a real encounter with the suffering subject.

2.4 Observations on the Transformations of Modern Psychiatry

In *The Power of Psychiatry* (1986), Peter Miller and Nikolas Rose managed to put together a series of stories and testimonies regarding psychiatry's exercise of power. To the observation that by the end of the twentieth century psychiatric practice would not be using mechanical and chemical means of immobilisation against patients' will, Miller pointedly remarks in his own perspective as user of mental health services: "… psychiatry is not something homogeneous but a loosely structured set of practices starting from the 'hard' core represented by the asylum and electroshocks, passing through the recent creation of Mental Health Centers, and extending to the 'soft' core of various psychotherapeutic approaches. The history of psychiatry is the history of the 'system's' reorganisations and transformations".

In Goffman's classic work (1961), the critique against the alienating conditions of the asylums was aiming at the analysis of the profanation and deconstruction of the confined patient's subjective identity. Laing (1965) focused his study on the subjective-existential experience of mental illness, whereas Szasz (1982) carried out an overall critique against the detrimental effects of institutional psychiatry and the incapacity of the mentally ill to have, as subjects-citizens, any negotiating power within the psychiatric system. Put schematically, we could say that all three approaches are inspired by an a priori philosophical position emphasising the primacy of subjectivity and perhaps obscuring other aspects in the way modern psychiatry is exercised at the age of postmodernity.

As Miller (op. cit., p. 29) pointedly remarks, "the promotion of subjectivity to such a degree by traditional antipsychiatry not only fails to grasp the ways in which power is exercised and operates within modern societies, but is also in no position to understand the subtle mechanisms by means of which power invests (to the direction it wishes) subjectivity rather than crushing it".

Globalisation and the ceaseless transformations of capitalism, the contemporary domination of the market culture and the promotion of subjectivity through consumption constitute problems that should be addressed in the perspective of psychiatry's contemporary transformations as well (Stylianidis 2011). The latter reproduces old and new forms of stigmatisation and auto-stigmatisation, social exclusion, extensive medicalisation and psychiatrisation of social distress and social problems and domination of the DSM as an instrument of an expanding codification of all forms of symptoms and deviations.

Such a novel understanding of these complex phenomena could be based on Porter's (2003), Doerner's (1981), Foucault's (1972), Basaglia's (1975) and Scull's (1979) theoretical and historical contributions, on the one hand, and on contemporary sociological approaches to modernity, postmodernity and the deconstruction of the welfare state, on the other, approaches like Bauman's (2013a, b), Castel's (1981), Beck's (1992, 2002), Bracken and Thomas' (2001), Rose's (1989) or Habermas' (1994, 2000).

In his major book *Governing the Soul*, Nikolas Rose (1989) describes to the point how "the management of the self" becomes a key element to contemporary societies' governmentality. Whereas notions like "the self" or identity issues were always historically related to a fundamental political questioning, this perspective is nowadays completely obscured. Psychiatry's transformations and the contemporary boom in new psychotherapeutic approaches or new "psy" professions fall within this emerging "expertise in subjectivity".

Every human problem – not only relationship problems but diagnosed mental disorders as well – becomes the object of investment by new therapeutic techniques literally invading every space in their "lighter" version: from human resource management within corporations or organisms to the settlement of social or racial conflicts, the strengthening of the police in enforcing social control and the imposition of cognitive-behavioural approaches within mental health services, the new techniques proliferate, inasmuch as they are supposed to be efficient and measurable in solving problems "here and now".

Globalised capitalism can survive and thrive insofar as it manages to persuade every citizen that he/she is a (potential) consumer not only of material goods and products of a distinctive brand bearing a positive "narcissistic" sign and status symbol but also of new techniques of promoting self-image and bringing about the much-coveted self-realisation and social recognition.

As Hardt and Negri (2000) correctly remark: "The big industries and economic powers produce not only the instruments for an easy living but also the subjectivities. They produce "agentic" subjectivities within the given bio-political framework: they produce needs, social relations, bodies and minds".

In the age and culture of postmodernism, the self-image provided by capitalism is able to make a subject change his/her mood, to constantly adapt without the slightest questioning or mental elaboration and to settle his/her accounts with the past without the slightest guilt or reflection, since these processes are "evaluated" as anti-productive.

"Narratives are no longer long and complicated. Our personal stories and grieves must be brief. Our identities must be the product of our "lifestyle" choices, instead of being the result of a personal struggle", as Bracken and Thomas (2001, p. 97) pointedly remark.

The new technology for diagnoses, the new indications for the use of psychotropic drugs, the new psychotherapeutic techniques, all this "biochemical revolution disconnects and liberates our self from depressing narratives", as Bullard (2002, p. 269) suggests.

Besides, despite the predominance of the biomedical model in clinical practice and of treatment criteria and protocols in the operating mode of medicine and psychiatry, there is substantial proof to the fact that the new classification systems are shaped by the interests of the multinational pharmaceutical giants (Kutchins and Kirk 1999).

The new marketing tendency and technique is to provide increasingly long indications for the use of psychotropic drugs: this "scientifically unbiased" and ethically neutral procedure aims to achieve the constant expansion of the market available for these drugs.

Our basic argument could be summarised as follows: contemporary psychiatric treatments and interventions are not in fact based on scientifically neutral indications and assumptions. Contemporary psychiatric technologies are determined by the points of view, priorities, meanings and values of the market. In fact, contemporary psychiatric interventions are based on the systematic manipulation of the hopes for a rapid and efficient treatment of the population as well as on the internalised expectations of postmodern man for self-realisation and evolution ("The sky is the limit").

2.5 The Psychiatrisation of the Defeated of Neoliberalism

The crisis of postmodern individualism has been a subject of study by important contemporary philosophers and sociologists (Habermas 1975, 1994, 2000; Beck 1992, 2002; Morin 1987, 2008; Castel 1981, 1995, 2013; Balandie 1967; Lasch 1991; Laplantine and Nouss 1997; Lanteri-Laura 1957; Vattimo 1991, 1992, etc.). The various approaches converge to the realisation that this new type of individualism is culturally and historically determined.

This complex and paradoxical process is characterised by the retreat into a "hedonist" ideal, by means of which the individual overinvests his/her body and imaginary life, and by a tendency to realise all immediate desires pertaining to the confirmation of every type of performance (athletic, professional, educational), the overconsumption of new goods, the immediate and constant availability for endless communication via the new technologies and the use-consumption of new psychological and psychotherapeutic techniques aiming at self-realisation and continuous social upgrading.

This tendency to an "individualised socialisation" (Lacrosse 2007) allows us to determine more accurately some aspects of the generalised phenomenon of "internal exile" touching both the individual and the "old collectivities".

To begin with, we will briefly refer to the confusion brought about to traditional symbolic points of reference with the fragmentation of nuclear family, the disparaging of the paternal function and the zero tolerance to frustration and lack. These profound changes result, among other things, in "the escalation of phenomena of violence among children and adolescents" (Corcos 2011; Lazartigues et al. 2003), within a context of "exile of the paternal figure", economic and social crisis and growing social precariousness and uncertainty.

Secondly, the predominance of a passive attitude leads to the withdrawal of large parts of the population from participation in political, social or ecological collectivities, to the refusal to grasp the systemic cause of the crisis of globalised markets and, even worse, to the identification of an important part of the socially excluded groups with totalitarian, racist, anti-Semitic and neo-Nazi ideologies hailing a nationalist type of return to an all-powerful, unadulterated by foreign mixtures, state. In return, despair, fear and lack of hope for the future push to passivity and retreat into oneself.

In the third place, the strong and all-powerful presence of the mass media and advertising imposes artificial identification models implying the possibility for everyone to have access to an immediate and limitless satisfaction "here and now".

Despite the numerous studies proving that the continuous exposition of children to television favours the development of aggressiveness, individualism and attention deficit hyperactivity disorder (ADHD) (Christakis et al. 2004; Barkley 2004), the "society of the spectacle" (Debord 1967) persists unfailingly in exerting its mass influence. The society of the spectacle and of the simulacra is not only a factor of retreat into extreme individualism. Paradoxically, it constitutes a very efficient factor of homogenisation of people's thought, by assembling a "machine of acceptance" through the brainwashing it performs (Chomsky 2007). Along the same line of thought, Bourdieu (1996) and Ramonet (1999) uncovered the mechanisms by which television, by entirely obeying to the laws of the free market and the maximisation of profit, performs the manipulation of thought.

The society of the spectacle and consumption creates a constant confusion as to the moral bearings of one's existence: "a set of values loses its meaning: values like trust, faith in the Other, in ideas, in ourselves" (Bénilde 2007).

Furthermore, the mass media contribute to the growing influence of a psychological and medical "scientific" discourse preaching a healthier way of life or the need for a "well-being" movement able to manage the "health capital" of every citizen. This widely spread culture is founded on the mass incrimination of individuals failing to abide by specific standards of beauty, appearance, weight or lifestyle and on the exacerbation of a narcissistic ideal hugely exceeding the real potential and psychic economy of the average individual. Personal lacks are being psychologised and psychiatrised, while every deviation from the rules and norms of social and professional demand for efficiency and beauty seems to be "symbolically" penalised. In addition to the reproduction of social inequalities and social exclusion, the power of the neoliberal model consists precisely in the diffusion of this culture and its reproduction as something "natural" for society's cohesion.

Finally, the individualisation of the social bond is a process closely connected with the extreme competition in work relations aiming at an immediate and ever-growing profit. This process pushes the individual to an over-adaptation to the unequal and inhumane work relations by means of a constant internalisation of what is transient and impersonal in social relations.

Through his documented study on work relations in France, Christophe Dejours (1998) unveiled the mechanisms by means of which the individual expresses his/her fear and submission to the work atmosphere of fluidity and transience and which lead to the retreat into oneself and the rejection of social and individual suffering.

As a result of the growing social insecurity (Castel 2013) and the deregulation of work relations, the individual's professional life is tightly connected with sentiments of fear, panic, despair and doubt whether he/she will manage to stay at work. Caught up in such a vicious circle, the individual starts calling into question the core of his/her own identity.

Neoliberalism is not only an economic conception and ideology; it seems to dismantle all spheres of individual, psychic and social life.

The new narcissistic individualism is produced through a process of dehumanisation and social disintegration calling into doubt not only the state of law and welfare but also the very foundations of democracy (Le Goff 2003).

While the social bond "is emptied" of its essence, the market steps up to fill the gap and pose as the "solid" foundation of a reality that has to be modernised at all costs by a constant headlong rush.

"Social disaffiliation" (Castel 2013) leads to an individualism of "disconnection" and a refusal to commit to any objective or vision. Ehrenberg (1991, 2000) has demonstrated in his work how economic competition generates a competitive individualism channelled into an entrepreneurial activity and aiming at the recovery of an individual identity and a professional and social success posing as "the natural moral bearings which structure today's world".

The opposition between market laws, the reproduction of social inequalities and the "relaxation" of moral standards in order to achieve ever-growing profits seems to be efficiently absorbed by the magma of neoliberal ideology, which transposes or transforms every political and social problem in terms of market, performance and efficiency.

Psychiatry based on the biomedical model contributes in its turn to this process of radical depoliticisation of problems and oppositions: the new classifications of the DSM-5 (Corcos 2011; Caravatos 2014) offer answers to symptoms (i.e. worldwide expansion of the antidepressants market) closely related to social and economic problems (poverty, social exclusion, lack of investment in the future) through the expansion of the indications for the use of psychotropic drugs.

The work of Gonon (2013), neurobiologist at the CNRS in France, is highly interesting. Gonon deconstructed in an extremely documented way the pseudoscientific ideology of the new psychiatric classification systems (DSM-5) while uncovering at the same time the multiplication of brain dysfunctions and deficiencies provoked by the use of the new psychotropic drugs, even among children. For example, the DSM-5 "allows", by means of a purely abstract biomedical approach, to connect behaviour, social disorder and biological deficiency, thus expanding the indications and, at the same time, the profits for the pharmaceutical companies.

At this point, social psychiatry encounters new challenges: the need to revitalise critical thought and to promote the complexity of subjective suffering not only in terms of diagnosis but also in terms of the social, economic and cultural framework within which psychopathology is applied. This "new clinical approach" should become the new field of theoretical and practical investment by critical social psychiatry.

Bibliography

Balandier G (1967) Anthropologie politique. PUF, Paris, pp 212–214
Barkley RA (2004) ADHD and television exposure: correlation as cause. ADHD Rep 12(4):1–4
Basaglia F (1975) Il concetto di salute e malattia. Relazione al Convegno "Les ambiguïtés du concept de santé dans les sociétés industrialisées". Organisation de cooperation et de développement économiques, Paris
Basaglia F (1976) *Crimini di pace* (con Foucault, Goffman, Laing, Chomsky). Einaudi, Torino
Bauman Z (2013a) Liquid love: on the frailty of human bonds. Wiley, New York
Bauman Z (2013b) Liquid modernity. Wiley, New York

Beck U (1992) Risk society: towards a new modernity, vol 17. Sage, London
Beck U (2002) The terrorist threat world risk society revisited. Theory Cult Soc 19(4):39–55
Bénilde M (2007) On achète bien des cerveaux. La publicité et les medias. Raisons d'agir, Paris
Binswanger L (1958) Daseinanalyse, Psychiatrie, Schizophrenie. Schweiz Arch Neurol Psychiatr 81:1–8
Binswanger L (1960) Melancholie und Manie. Phanomenologische Studien. Neske, Pfullingen
Binswanger L (1971) Introduction a l'analyse existentielle (Trad. franc. de J. Vereaux et R., Kuhn). Minuit, Paris
Blankenburg W (1982) A dialectical conception of anthropological proportion. In: De Koning AJJ, Jenner FA (eds) Phenomenology and psychiatry. Academic, London, pp 35–50
Blankenburg W (1991) Der Verlust der naturlichen Selbstverstanedlichkeit. Ein Beitrag zur Psychopathologie symptomarmer Schizophrenijen. (Trad. franc., Azorin, Totoyan, PUF, 1991) Enke, Stuttgart
Bourdieu P (1996) Sur la télévision. Liber, Paris
Bracken P, Thomas P (2001) Postpsychiatry: a new direction for mental health. Br Med J 322(7288):724
Broekman JM (1965) Phanomenologisches Denken in Philosophie und Psychiatrie. Confinia Psychiatr 8:165–188
Bullard A (2002) From vastation to Prozac nation. Transcult Psychiatry 39(3):267–294
Burton R (1959) Institutional Neurosis. Ed. John Wright, Bristol
Canguilhem G (1972) Le normal et le pathologique. PUF, Paris
Castel R (1981) La gestion des risques. Ed. de Minuit, Paris
Castel R (1995) Les métamorphoses de la question sociale: une chronique du salariat. Fayard, Paris
Castel R (2013) L'insécurité sociale: Qu'est-ce qu'être protégé? Seuil, Paris
Chomsky N (2007) Democracy's invisible line. Le monde diplomatique. Available at: http://mondediplo.com/2007/08/02democracy. Accessed 30.7.2014
Christakis DA, Zimmerman FJ, DiGiuseppe DL, McCarty CA (2004) Early television exposure and subsequent attentional problems in children. Pediatrics 113(4):708–713
Cooper D (1970) Psychiatrie et antipsychiatrie. Le Seuil, Paris
Cooper D, Laing R (1970) Raison et violence. Le Seuil, Paris
Corcos M (2011) L'homme selon le DSM. Le nouvel ordre psychiatrique. Albin Michel, Paris
Corvez M (1965) L'Être et l'étant dans la philosophie de Martin Heidegger. Rev Philos Louvain 63(78):257–279
Debord G (1967) The society of the spectacle. Zone Books, New York
Dejours C (1998) Souffrance en France. La banalisation de l'injustice sociale. Seuil, Paris
Doerner K (1981) Madness and the Bourgeoisie: a social history of insanity and psychiatry. Basil Blackwell, Oxford
Ehrenberg A (1991) Le Culte de la performance. Calmann-Lévy, Paris
Ehrenberg A (2000) La fatigue d'être soi: dépression et societé. Odile Jacob, Paris
Foucault M (1961) Folie et déraison: histoire de la folie à l'âge classique, vol 169. Plon, Paris
Foucault M (1963) Naissance de la Clinique. Une archéologie du regard médical. PUF, Paris
Foucault M (1972) Histoire de la folie à l'âge classique. Gallimard, Paris
Freud S (1957) Instincts and their vicissitudes. In: The standard edition of the complete psychological works of Sigmund Freud, volume XIV (1914–1916): on the history of the psychoanalytic movement, papers on metapsychology and other works, London, pp 109–140
Gauchet M (1997) De Pinel à Freud. In: Swain G (ed) Le sujet de la folie. Calmann-Lévy, Paris
Goffman E (1961) Asylums: essays on the social situation of mental patients and other inmates. Penguin, New York
Gonon F (2013) Quel avenir pour les classifications des maladies mentales? Une synthèse des critiques anglo-saxonnes les plus récentes. Inf Psychiatry 89(4):285–294
Habermas J (1975) Legitimation crisis, vol 519. Beacon Press, Boston
Habermas J (1994) Three normative models of democracy. Constellations 1(1):1–10

Habermas J (2000) The inclusion of the other: studies in political theory. The MIT Press, Cambridge, MA
Hardt M, Negri A (2000) Empire. Harvard University Press, Cambridge MA
Heidegger M, Vezin F (1964) L'être et le temps. Gallimard, Paris, p 233
Husserl E (1969) Formal and transcendental logic. Springer, New York
Husserl E. Erfahrung und Urteil (1938).Claassen, Hambourg, 1964 (Trad. franc. par D. Souche: Expérience et jugement, PUF, Paris 1970)
Husserl E (1929) Méditations cartésiennes (Trad. franç. G. Peiffer et E. Levinas, Paris, Vrin, 1969)
Jackson F (1982) Epiphenomenal qualia. Philos Q 32(127):127–136
Jaspers K (1963) General psychopathology (Trans. J. Hoenig and M.W. Hamilton). Manchester University Press, Manchester
Krauss A (2003) How can the phenomenological-anthropological approach contribute to diagnosis and classification in psychiatry? In: Fulford B, Morris K, Sadler J, Stanghellini G (eds) Nature and narrative: an introduction to the new philosophy of psychiatry. Oxford University Press, New York
Kutchins H, Kirk S (1999) Making Us crazy. DSM: the psychiatric bible and the creation of mental disorders. Constable, London
Lacrosse JM (2007) Sujet politique, sujet psychique. En marge d'un séminaire de psychopathologie historique. PSN 5(1):83–89
Laing RD (1965) The divided self. Pelican Books, London
Lanteri – Laura G (1957) La psychiatrie phénoménologique. PUF, Paris
Laplantine F, Nouss A (1997) Le métissage. Flammarion, Paris
Lasch C (1991) The culture of narcissism: American life in an age of diminishing expectations. WW Norton & Company, New York
Lazartigues A, Doukouré M, Saint-André S, Lemonnier E (2003) Certaines caractéristiques des nouvelles parentalités favorisent-elles la violence des enfants? In: Annales Médico-psychologiques, revue psychiatrique 161(4): 265–271). Elsevier Masson, Paris
Le Goff JP (2003) La démocratie post-totalitaire. La Découverte, Paris
Louzoun C, Stylianidis S (1987) La Nouvelle psychiatrie italienne. la Documentation française, Paris
Ludwig DS, Kabat-Zinn J (2008) Mindfulness in medicine. JAMA 300(11):1350–1352
Meyers C (2005) Les lieux de la folie: d'hier à demain dans l'espace européen. Erès, Paris
Miller P, Rose N (1986) The power of psychiatry. Polity Press, Cambridge
Minkowski E (1927) La schizophrénie. Psychopathologie des schizoides et des schizophrènes, Nouvelle édition revue et augmentée. Desclée de Brouwer, Paris, 1953
Minkowski E (1948) Phénoménologie et analyse existentielle en psychopathologie. Evol Psychiatrique 13:137–185
Minkowski E (1966) Traité de psychopathologie. PUF, Paris
Morin E (1987) Penser l'Europe, vol 1990. Gallimard, Paris
Morin E (2008) On complexity. Hampton Press, Creskil, NJ
Porter R (2003) Madness: a brief history. Oxford University Press, New York
Ramonet I (1999) La tyrannie de la communication. Galilee, Paris
Rose N (1989) Governing the soul. Routledge, London
Sartre JP (1962) Literary and philosophical essays. Collier Books, New York
Scull AT (1979) Museums of madness: the social organization of insanity in nineteenth-century England. Allen Lane, London, pp 18–48
Spiegelberg H (1972) Phenomenology in psychology and psychiatry: a historical introduction. Northwestern University Press, Evanston
Stoljar D (2009) Ignorance and imagination: the epistemic origin of the problem of consciousness. Oxford University Press, New York
Szasz T (1982) The psychiatric will: a new mechanism for protecting persons against "psychosis" and psychiatry. Am Psychol 37:762–770
Tatossian A (2002) La phénoménologie des psychoses. Le Cercle Herméneutique, Paris

Vattimo G (1991) The end of modernity: Nihilism and hermeneutics in post-modern culture. Johns Hopkins University Press, Baltimore

Vattimo G (1992) The transparent society. Polity Press, Cambridge, pp 68-69

Wittgenstein L (1966) Lectures & conversations on aesthetics, psychology, and religious belief. California University Press, California

Αμπατζόγλου Γ (1991) *Ψυχιατρική και Ιατρική: Τα όρια, οι ταυτότητες και οι σχέσεις*. Αθήνα: Οδυσσέας

Ζήση Α (2013) *Κοινωνία, κοινότητα και ψυχική υγεία*. Αθήνα: Εκδόσεις Δάρδανος.

Καράβατος Θ (2014) Η υποδοχή του DSM-5: «Το πρόβλημα του DSM-5 δεν βρίσκεται στο 5 αλλά στο DSM». *Σύναψις*, 32(10), 4-8

Στυλιανίδης Σ (1985) Εισαγωγή στη σκέψη του Franco Basaglia (1924-1980), *Τετράδια Ψυχιατρικής*, 7, 46-57

Στυλιανίδης Σ (2011) Η κλινική του εφήμερου. Όψεις της ατομικής και κοινωνικής οδύνης. Κλινικά και κοινωνικά ερωτήματα μέσα από μία ψυχαναλυτική οπτική, *Οιδίπους, 5*, 229-249

Τζαβάρας, Ν (2002) Ερμηνευτική και κατανόηση. Στο: Βαρτζόπουλος και συν. (Επιμ.) Σχιζοφρένεια: Φαινομενολογική και ψυχαναλυτική προσέγγιση. Αθήνα: Εκδόσεις Καστανιώτη, 47-64

Τζανάκης Μ (2008) Πέραν του Ασύλου: Η κοινοτική ψυχιατρική και το ζήτημα του υποκειμένου (Συνάψεις, τ. 6). Αθήνα: Κοινός Τόπος Ψυχιατρικής, Νευροεπιστημών & Επιστημών του Ανθρώπου

Τσαλίκογλου Φ (1987) *Ο μύθος του επικίνδυνου ψυχασθενή*. Αθήνα: Εκδόσεις Παπαζήση

Τσαλίκογλου Φ (2007) *Σχιζοφρένεια και φόνος*. Αθήνα: Εκδόσεις Λιβάνη

Psychiatric Epidemiology and Its Applications in Social Psychiatry

Lily Evangelia Peppou and Stelios Stylianidis

Abstract

Epidemiology explores the distribution and key factors of an illness or other health-related situations so as to apply those findings to the management and treatment of the illness. In that sense, it is an essential framework for identifying healthcare policy and service provision priorities and is also a vehicle that helps to design effective and feasible prevention interventions. From that perspective, it is – in some way – in the service of public health. While drawing conclusions and extrapolate findings to the population from the sample, epidemiologists frequently take into account the role of chance, bias, confounding and the direction of causality on the association observed between the exposure and the outcome/illness. Depending on the research questions posed and the availability of materials and human resources, they select epidemiological designs that will make it easier to achieve the goals of a study. The main research designs are ecological studies, cross-sectional studies, case control studies, longitudinal cohort studies and randomised controlled trials. They also make every effort to minimise the occurrence of bias and to control for confounding. Despite the importance of epidemiology worldwide with regard to its contribution to evidence-based medicine and the provision of quality services, Greece has failed to establish an epidemiology-based psychiatry culture. Nationwide studies are scarce, and links between epidemiological findings and mental health policies have not been

---

L.E. Peppou (✉)
Association for Regional Development and Mental Health (EPAPSY), Athens, Greece
e-mail: lilly.peppou@gmail.com

S. Stylianidis
Department of Psychology, Panteion University, Athens, Greece
e-mail: stylianidis.st@gmail.com

made. To date, policies appear to be based on intuition, extreme empiricism, sloppy approaches, the "guild mentality", political interests or individual beliefs; and while there may be some examples of best practice in terms of the services provided, overall services are not imbued with and integrated into a central, national strategic plan for mental health. Under pressure from the global mental health movement, the development of psychiatric epidemiology in Greece is not only a vital necessity but also a major challenge.

3.1 Introduction: Defining Epidemiology

The term epidemiology has been defined as "The study of the distribution and determinants of health-related states or events in specified populations, and the application of this study to the control of health problems" (Last 1995). Epidemiologists firstly describe a health problem and its extent: who gets ill, when and where. They then attempt to explain those observations: why do people get ill? The description of illnesses offers signs about potential risk factors, leading to the formulation of hypotheses that can be tested in the context of well-designed studies. Studies targeting specific risk factors can also provide additional evidence about the presence of aetiological relationships. Consequently, epidemiology is above all a practical branch of science and includes systematic exploration of health, illness and human behaviour in the natural environment. It is, therefore, the main scientific tool in public health medicine.

Any descriptive endeavour must set out the necessary framework for setting priorities in healthcare policy planning and service provision, while any explanatory endeavour must lead to effective and feasible primary and secondary prevention interventions. Consequently, epidemiology and public health are complementary – if not interdependent – disciplines.

Psychiatric epidemiology lags behind as compared to other branches of epidemiology, primarily because of difficulties in homogenising and measuring mental disorders. As a result, the majority of contemporary psychiatric epidemiology studies remain descriptive and focus on calculating the prevalence of disorders and their various subtypes (Robins and Regier 1991); while other branches of epidemiology have made progress in identifying risk factors and developing protective interventions (Elwood et al. 1992). Psychiatric epidemiology studies which capture risk factors tend to focus on broad categories of factors, such as gender or socio-economic standing, rather than on modifiable factors, which could be used as specific targets in an intervention.

3.2 Causality Relations

The drawing of conclusions in epidemiology (the so-called inferences) always entails a shift from research observations to generalisations. However, the presence of an association between two variables (i.e. between an exposure and an illness/outcome) does not equate to there being a causal relationship between them. In epidemiology, before exploring the degree to which causality criteria are met between two variables, one ought to take into account the role of chance, bias, confounding and the direction of causality in relation to them.

Chance

The role of chance in explaining the observed association between two variables is addressed in the statistical analysis of the results. More specifically, the p-value (significance testing) and the confidence interval are used to demonstrate the likelihood that chance explains the observed relationship. In the case of a hypothetical association between an exposure and an illness/outcome, one can estimate the likelihood that an association exists in the data, if the zero hypothesis is true (in other words that in reality there's no association between the two variables, but the relationship observed in the data is exclusively the product of chance). Conventionally, the widely agreed scientific limit for that probability is 0.05. In other words, the results are considered real (meaning that they also occur outside of experimental conditions) if the probability that they have occurred by chance is less than 5 %. Concomitantly, 95 % confidence intervals give a range of values within which the true value will lie on 95 % of occasions. However, it is worth noting that confidence intervals do not reflect probability. For example, in 2005 the annual prevalence of serious depression in Europe (meaning the percentage of people who were found to meet the diagnostic criteria for major depression during the year before clinical evaluation) was found to be 6.9 % with a 95 % confidence interval of 4.8–8.0 (Wittchen and Jacobi 2005). Congruent with this, if the study was to be repeated 100 times by following the same methodology, but by drawing different samples from the same population, 95 out of 100 of those times the prevalence-estimate would lie somewhere in the range 4.8–8.

Of those two methods for tapping the role of chance in the association observed between two variables (significance testing and confidence interval), the problem with significance testing is that it indicates only a probability (as already mentioned the probability that the association observed can be explained solely by chance and does not exist in reality). The size of p-value does not inform about the strength of the association: a weak association of low clinical significance could be identified with a very high statistically significant result, especially if the study sample is large. On the contrary, the confidence interval can provide information about the strength of association and its statistical significance. For example, in a randomised controlled clinical trial investigating the efficacy of two methods of psychotherapy in alleviating depressive symptoms (as measured by a relevant scale), the p-value at the end of the trial merely provides information about which of the two groups performed better and whether the difference between them is statistically significant or not (if it is real or it is caused by chance). The confidence interval on the contrary will provide information about (i) the size effect (ii) whether the difference is statistically significant or not – in the case where the confidence interval includes the value 0, then the difference is statistically non-significant, and (iii) the accuracy of the measurement (a large confidence interval is associated with less accuracy). Consequently, in modern epidemiology, confidence intervals are generally preferred to significance testing methods.

Bias

Bias is systematic error arising either during the design or implementation of a study. It is always unwelcome and cannot be corrected for during statistical processing of the results, as it is frequently the case with confounders. The only way to minimise it is by carefully designing and implementing a study carefully in a targeted manner.

Bias can be divided into two main types: bias arising when the investigator selects his sample or two comparable groups in population (selection bias) and bias arising when measuring variables (information bias). Specific epidemiological designs are more vulnerable to certain types of bias than others.

Information bias emerges during the process of measuring the variables of interest. All measurements entail some degree of bias, even those relating to measurement of bodily functions such as arterial pressure. When measurements relate to categories of variables, such as diagnosing major depression, error in these cases is called misclassification. Misclassification error becomes bias when it is systematic and differential, i.e. when knowledge of other variables in the design systematically leads to misclassification error of the independent or dependent variable. An illustration of this point is when the classification of participants as depressed or non depressed (outcome variable) is influenced by knowing whether they are employed of unemployed.

Recall bias is another form of information bias and has to do with the participant's ability to recall specific past information. For example, in a case-control study exploring the association between perinatal abnormalities and the presence of schizophrenia, participants are recruited based on the outcome (schizophrenia) and divided into two groups: patients with schizophrenia and members of the general population (the control group). To explore the existence of perinatal abnormalities in the two groups, the investigator conducts interviews with the mothers (mothers of patients with schizophrenia and mothers of people from the general population). If some of the mothers in both groups do not have good memory, there is some error, but it is non-differential and non-systematic. However, if mothers in one group systematically recall the desired information better or worse and in a way which significantly differentiates them from the mothers in the other group, then there is recall bias. Note that mothers of patients with schizophrenia may be more prone to recall perinatal abnormalities – and may even confabulate in an attempt to attribute their child's illness somewhere or to cast off any tellings. That could differentiate them in a systematic manner from the mothers of healthy members of the control group, who have no reason to remember the birth process. In general terms, the presence of an illness is frequently accompanied by efforts to attach to it, which in epidemiology is known as "effort after meaning". One way to address the specific bias is by cross-checking information from different sources or by adopting a cohort design.

The third well-known type of information bias is investigator bias. In the example above concerning the association between perinatal abnormalities and schizophrenia, an investigator who believes that perinatal abnormalities cause schizophrenia may attempt to elicit that information from the mothers of individuals with schizophrenia more strongly e.g. by being more pressing than the mothers of the control group. One way to address this type of bias is to "blind" the investigator, so that he does not know the participants' group allocation or the research hypothesis or the hypothesis in the study.

Selection bias primarily relates to the comparability of two groups in the study design and usually emerges when the control group is not the most suitable. This bias primarily occurs in case-control studies when the choice of an individual for the patient group or the control group is related in some way to an exposure. For example, in a case-control study on the association between arthritis (an independent variable – exposure) and Alzheimer's disease (a dependent variable – outcome), it was found that arthritis is more frequent in the control group than in the Alzheimer's group implying therefore that arthritis is a protective factor against the onset of Alzheimer's disease. However, Alzheimer's disease patients were recruited from a specialized outpatient clinic, while the individuals from the control group were drawn from a primary care setting. In primary care, visits pertaining to arthritis are quite frequent and therefore probability of someone suffering from arthritis in this population group (individuals who visit primary care facilities) is disproportionately high as compared to the general population. Consequently, the lower frequency of arthritis among patients with Alzheimer's disease does not reflect a protect effect, but it is related to the emergence of bias during the recruitment. In this rationale, in order to reduce the probability of selection bias to occur, members of the patient and control group should be drawn from the same population (base population). One way to check for this is to think of the following question: "if the individual of the control group manifested the illness of interest, would he/she be in the patient group?" and vice versa, "if the patient did not manifest the illness would he be in the control group? he/she be found in the control group?".

In cross-sectional studies and cohort surveys, a major source of selection bias emanates from non-participation. It is widely accepted that people who agree to participate in studies differ in a systematic manner from people who refuse. Refusers are usually men, people with low educational attainment and unemployed individuals. However, for bias to occur, the difference between participants and non participants should be related to both the exposure (the independent variable) and the outcome (the dependent variable). Consequently, seldom is non-participation translated to the occurrence of bias; however, it often limits the generalisation ability of the study findings.

Likewise, attrition bias can occur as a result of loss to follow up in cohort studies. As in non-participation bias, the two groups should consistently differ in terms of their characteristics or reasons they were lost and these differences should be related to both the exposure and the outcome of interest. For example, in a study exploring the association between perinatal abnormalities and schizophrenia, bias will occur if all those who have both perinatal abnormalities and schizophrenia are lost at follow-up to a significantly greater degree than those with just schizophrenia (but not perinatal abnormalities) and/or those with perinatal abnormalities but not schizophrenia. Similarly to non-participation, bias is rarely observed in cohort studies; however, due to loss to follow-up, there may be restrictions on the generalisation of study findings.

Confounding

Confounding expresses the situation where the measured effect of an exposure is altered because the exposure is concomitantly associated with other factors, which also exert an impact on the illness/outcome of the study. Confounding can cause of prevent the outcome of a study, is not a mediating factor and is independently associated with the exposure of interest. In other words, the confounding variable provides an alternative explanation for the observed association between the exposure and the outcome. For example, in a study an association documented between grey hair and mortality. The study is very well designed, no bias has emerged, the sample is representative of the population and statistical testing substantiates a strong association. In this reasoning, the association between grey hair and mortality can be extrapolated to the population. Nonetheless, such a claim fails to take into consideration the role of confounding. In particular, in the above mentioned example, age constitutes a confounder variable.

The effect of confounding can be addressed either during the design of the study or during its statistical analysis. With regard to the former, the two basic strategies are restriction and matching. As far as restriction is concerned, the sample is limited to one confounding category. For example, if gender is a confounding variable, only men will be recruited in the study. It is worth noting that in this way limitations emerge concerning the generalisability of the results, since in this example, they cannot be applied to women. On the contrary, the method of matching groups to specific confounding factors requires careful selection of participants for the control group in order for the two groups to be as similar as possible. For example, if gender is a confounder variable and the patient group consists of 60 % of men, then the control group should include a similar percentage of male participants. Although this method is helpful, it can become tricky when trying to address several confounding variables simultaneously. Arguably, it is difficult for the groups to be similar in terms of gender, age, marital status, educational level, socio-economic background, etc. The most effective way tackle confounding variables is randomisation. The process of randomisation ensures random (and by extension non-differential) distribution of confounding variables to the two groups. It is noteworthy, that this concerns both known confounding variables (which have been measured in the study) and unknown (which are not taken into consideration during the design of the study and hence they have not been measured). However, in observational studies where randomisation is not feasible, the most common way to deal with confounding is through statistical analysis, using stratification or multivariate models.

It merits noting, that sometimes it is hard for researchers to disentangle confounders from mediator or moderator variables. However, the decision about the nature of the variable is usually subjective.

Direction of Causality

It is also important to determine the direction of causality when drawing conclusions about the causal relationship between two variables. In other words, it is essential to be able to demonstrate that the exposure causes the outcome and not vice versa. For example, in a cross-sectional survey indicating an association between unemployment and major depression, it is not clear from the nature of the study's design, if the individuals who are unemployed have a higher probability of becoming depressed or if the individuals who are depressed – due to the illness and the stigma associated with it – have a higher probability of being unemployed. As cross-sectional studies collect information about the exposure and the outcome simultaneously and case-control studies recruit on the grounds of the outcome, both designs cannot determine the direction of causality.

On the contrary, in cohort studies, where participants are recruited based on the presence/absence of an exposure while being free of disease, the temporal sequence of events can be observed and thus, direction of causality can be substantiated.

3.3 Epidemiology Research Design

Epidemiologists are have a good knowledge and understanding of the principles of research design. Ethical issues do not allow the random allocation of participants into adverse conditions or the experimental distribution of harmful exposures. For example, if one wants to investigate the effectiveness of involuntary hospitalisation in patients with psychosis, he/ she cannot randomly allocate patients into two groups: the involuntary hospitalisation group and the voluntary hospitalisation group, due to ethical constraints. On the contrary, observational studies are less susceptible to these issues but more prone to bias and confounding.

The design and analysis of a study seeks to maximise the accuracy and validity of its results. The accuracy of a measurement (such as the prevalence of depression in the general population) can be compromised due to error in sampling or measurement process. However, errors of this type are random (in other words they are not systematic, as in the case of bias) congruent with this, accuracy can be improved by using larger samples and better measurement tools. On the contrary, bias and confounding are non-random and systematic errors that impinge on the validity of the results. Therefore, the selection of a research design and the methods employed are crucial for reducing bias and maximizing the study' s validity.

The main types of research designs used in epidemiology can be divided into three broad categories: (i) observational studies (ecological studies, cross-sectional studies, case control studies, and cohort studies), (ii) experimental studies (randomised controlled trials) or (iii) systematic review (and meta-analyses).

Experimental studies are used to evaluate interventions, such as the effectiveness of Cognitive Behavioural Therapy (CBT) in treating depression. In observational studies, epidemiologists endeavour to draw inferences about diseases through natural observation of people, who have been previously classified as having/ not having the exposure or outcome of interest. In this rationale, the researcher has no control over the events under investigation.

Observational studies can either be descriptive or analytical. A descriptive study elaborates on a specific disease (like depression) or an exposure (like unemployment) with respect to the characteristics of individuals affected by it in a specific place at a specific point in time. On the contrary, analytical studies explore the strength of association between exposures and outcomes. It is noteworthy noting that this distinction is largely theoretical, since practice studies frequently entail both descriptive and analytical elements.

Moreover studies can also aggregate used data, for example, the unemployment rate in Greece, and data gleaned from individuals. The advantages and disadvantages of these research designs are summarised in Table 3.1, and a brief outline of each research design is given below.

Ecological Studies

Ecological studies explore associations between exposures and outcomes, based on populations defined either geographically, or temporally. Consistent with this, the unit of analysis is populations or groups of people, rather than individuals. For example, an ecological study has substantiated a significant correlation between unemployment and suicide rates in Greece during the recession (Branas et al. 2015). In the aforementioned example, the association found between unemployment rates and suicide should not be interpreted as indicating that the vast majority of individuals who committed suicide in Greece was unemployed. Erroneous application of conclusions drawn from the aggregate level to the individual level is termed " ecological fallacy". Another shortcoming with ecological studies is that data are not usually collected for research purposes and therefore information on potential confounder variables is not available. Lastly, as information about the exposure and outcome is gleaned simultaneously, direction of causality cannot be determined.

One of the most popular ecological studies in psychiatric epidemiology is that conducted by Emile Durkheim (1858–1917), who explored regional, national and temporal variations in suicide rates in Europe. He recorded a significant association between the suicide rates in 13 Prussian provinces and the number of residents who were Protestants (Durkheim 1951).

Synchronic/Cross-Sectional Studies

Cross-sectional studies record information from a sample of people who have been drawn from a base population defined by area (such as children aged under 16 in

3 Psychiatric Epidemiology and Its Applications in Social Psychiatry

Table 3.1 Advantages and disadvantages of different types of epidemiological study

	Cross sectional survey	Case-control studies	Cohort studies	Ecological studies	Clinical trials
Subject selection	Defined population	Caseness	Exposure	Aggregated data	Caseness
Source of bias	Selection	Selection Information (recall and observer)	Information (observer only)	Selection if population	Selection information (reduced by blinding)
	Non response information	Recall and investigator bias	Loss to follow-up (selection)	Ecological fallacy	Investigator bias, reduced considerably if blinding methods are used
	Recall and observer				
Probability of confounding	Medium	Medium	Low	High	Very low if randomised
Resources	Quick and cheap	Relatively quick and cheap	Lengthy and expensive	Relatively quick and cheap	Relatively expensive
Applications	Planning services	Rare outcomes	Rare exposure	Rare outcomes	Efficacy of new interventions
	Mapping secular and geographical trends	Single outcomes	Single exposure	Rare exposures	Effectiveness of new interventions
	Identifying correlates	Multiple exposures	Multiple outcomes	Multiple exposures	Hypothesis testing
				Population exposures such as air pollution	Mechanisms
Measurement of effect	Prevalence	Odds ratio	Relative risk	Correlation/regression coefficient	Relative risk/odds ratio/ difference between means

Adapted from: Ford, T. (2007). Introduction to epidemiological study designs. In M. Prince, R. Stewart, T. Ford & M. Hotopf, (2003). Practical psychiatric epidemiology. New York: Oxford.

Greece) or some specific characteristics (such as patients who are voluntarily admitted to psychiatric hospitals) in order to calculate the prevalence of an outcome as well as to explore potential risk factors. They are inexpensive and easy to conduct, while they are more frequently used for estimating the extent of a disease, to plan services an to identify potential risk factors that can be explored in depth in analytical studies. Since the information about exposures and outcomes is collected at the same time, cross-sectional studies cannot shed light on the temporal sequence of events and thus, they cannot indicate the direction of causality.

Low response rates in cross-sectional studies (r.e. that is below 80 %) may reduce the validity of the results, since it is likely that individuals who refused to participate differ in a consistent manner from those who participated. Recruitment strategy and the mode of data collection (phone, on-site survey, post) are important in ensuring a high response rate. The way in which participants are approached and the hassle associated with participating ought to be taken into account in the design process in order to ensure a high response rate.

Another aspect that necessitates consideration in the design of a study pertains to the careful selection of tools that are valid (i.e. they study what they are intended to study) and reliable (i.e. they are consistent over time or among different investigators). It is note worthy that tools should be valid for the population for which they are intended to be used. For example, a tool which has been validated in a clinical population is not necessarily be valid for the general population. Moreover, a tool's validity in one culture/ country is not tantamount to being valid in another culture/ country.

Cross-sectional studies frequently involve a large of participants and therefore, they can become particularly expensive if the presence of mental disorders is assessed with clinical instruments employed by psychiatrists. In this reasoning, structured diagnostic interviews made by lay people are usually preferred over clinical assessment made by psychiatrists. The structured content of the instruments, good training of interviewers and continuous supervision throughout the study design contribute to the validity and reliability of the assessment. Among the most widely used structured diagnostic instruments employed by lay interviewers are the Composite International Diagnostic Interview (CIDI) and the Revised Clinical Interview Schedule (CIS-R).

It is noteworthy that cross-sectional studies are not the appropriate design for investigating outcomes with low prevalence rate such as schizophrenia or autism. In these cases, one needs to recruit a large number of participants to be able to explore the outcome with adequate precision. Alternatively, oversampling of specific population subgroups may occur.

Case-Control Studies

Case-control studies are primarily retrospective research designs. The aim is to recruit a random sample of patients and non-patients from the same designated population and then to explore their post exposure to possible risk factors. The odds of being exposed are compared between the patients and their controls, resulting in the computation of odds ratio, which is the most frequent measure of effect size in this design.

Case-control studies are quick and inexpensive to carry out, while they are suitable for an initial exploration of rare diseases. Nonetheless, they are prone to selection bias, investigator bias and recall bias. Furthermore, as the information about the exposure is collected after the disease manifestation, the direction of causality cannot be determined.

Cohort Studies

Cohort studies have two key features:

(i) Participants are recruited on the grounds of exposure rather than disease, in contrast to case control-studies.
(ii) They are longitudinal designs: The exposure is measured prior to the onset of the disease.

Classical cohort-studies involve following-up a group of people who have been recruited based on their exposure status (presence vs, absence of the exposure) in order to record the incidence of the disease, hence the direction of causality can be establish. However, due to the large number of participants often required and the long duration of follow up periods, cohort studies are usually very expensive to conduct. For example, if one would want to study the association between perinatal abnormalities and schizophrenia by conduction a cohort-study, he/she would have to follow up participants for roughly 20 years (from birth to the onset of the disease) and he/she should recruit a large number of participants, as schizophrenia has low prevalence. In this rationale, a cohort study would be time-consuming and very expensive.

The two main sources of bias in cohort studies are non-participation bias and attrition bias (loss of follow-up).

Randomised Controlled Trials

In experimental studies, the investigator allocates the intervention (exposure) to certain individuals or communities and compares the outcome of interest among them. When the allocation of participants to intervention and control groups is randomised, the investigator endeavours to create similar groups with respect to confounding variables, whether they are known or unknown. Random allocation is usually ensured by using a statistical package such as SPSS; however, very often it is not achieved if the study has a small sample size. One can test for this by statistically comparing the characteristics if the two groups prior to the outset of the intervention phase. Moreover, randomization itself cannot guarantee that the methodology in a controlled trial is perfect, since it cannot deal with bias. Congruent with this, efforts should be made to minimize its occurrence. Specifically, it is important to employ blinding techniques for both the participants and the researchers (i.e. "double-blinding" and in the case where the statistician does not know the hypothesis of the study and the allocation of participants, it is called "triple blinding") so as to prevent the occurrence of information bias. Although many studies start by successfully "blinding" participants and researches, during the study period. Very often patients and/or investigators are able to determine to which group they belong, resulting in unsuccessful "blinding". A well-designed controlled trial should incorporate a questionnaire to measure the degree to which "blinding" of participants and investigators was successful at the end of the study (e.g.. how many participants can accurately recognize the group to which they belonged). It is noteworthy that in randomized control trials, the selection of a control group necessitates careful consideration. For example, in RCTs measuring psychotherapy effectiveness it is hard to create a placebo intervention; while ethical issues prevent researchers from depriving participants of an intervention with established effectiveness for their condition. Moreover, a waiting-list control is often inadequate, as individuals know their group allocation an hence have different expectations from participating into the study as compared to individuals receiving an intervention. In this reasoning, the difference between the two groups cannot be attributed exclusively to the intervention but to different expectations held by the participants. Randomised controlled tests are currently considered to be the *gold standard* in epidemiology. However, as they can also be pone to bias, efforts should be made to minimize its occurrence.

When the intervention group is not comprised of individual but of groups of individuals such as a community or a class in a school, the design is known as a community trial or a cluster randomised trial. In these cases, both upon designing the trial as well as when analysing its results, the researchers should take into account that there two sources of variation in them: i) between individuals in a group and ii) between different groups. For example, in a school intervention about bullying, the pupils in one school (the intervention group) will have similar characteristics setting them apart from pupils at another school (the control group).

In clinical routine settings, when randomisation is not always feasible to occur, quasi-experimental designs are frequently adopted.

3.4 Epidemiology and Evidence-Based Medicine

There is frequently an overlap between the methods employed in epidemiology and in health services. Research aims pertaining to clinical effectiveness of interventions, are usually explored by using epidemiological methods. Evidence-based medicine was developed in an attempt to substantiate clinical decisions on epidemiological and statistical groups. The implementation of systematic literature reviews so as to generate sufficient evidence that would inform routine clinical practice, is base on epidemiological principles and statistical approaches, known to epidemiologists.

However, as a corollary of this, the movement for active involvement, empowerment and advocacy for the rights of service users and their caregivers, modern trends in the fields of social psychiatry and psychosocial rehabilitation laid the foundations for new scientific, ethical and institutional arguments for applying and documenting psychiatric epidemiology in assessing and evaluating mental health services (Rogers and Pilgrim 1993; Thornicroft and Tansella 2005).

Despite the fact that there are different perspectives among service users, their families and mental health professionals (Mason et al. 2004), it has been documented in the research that user and caregiver movement in the research process of evaluating quality of care, has a positive effect on therapeutic alliance as well as treatment and case management outcomes (Roth and Crane-Ross 2002).

Conducted a study on quality of care from the standpoint of people with serious mental illness in community mental health services in 3 regions of Italy. A total of 204 service users were involved and 8 different realms of care provision were explored: the choice of therapist and patients stuff relationship, treatment effectiveness, the natural setting; the availability of different treatment modes and the configuration of services; the provision of information about diagnosis; the existence of an individualize care play; the degree of patient participation in treatment decision making; the length of a waiting list and the incorporation of home visits in services provided.

Among the above mentioned domains, the three that emerged as being of out-most importance-and in fact were significantly associated with users' satisfaction - were: the choice of professionals, the length of a waiting list and the provision of sufficient information bout treatment and their overall care plan.

Furthermore, service users and mental health professionals held different views with regard to patients' autonomy as well as the need for empowering and respecting them and their choices.

Therefore, the study demonstrates that service users can provide useful and reliable designs of care into aspects of care delivered and the responsiveness on the pt of mental health professionals contributes substantially in improving the quality of care and changing the culture of mental health services. Change cannot occure about without utilising epidemiological principles and techniques.

3.5 Epidemiological Findings in Greece

At the international level, the most widely known cross-sectional studies are the National Comorbidity Survey in the USA (Blazer et al. 1994; Kendler et al. 1996; Kessler et al. 1997), the National Psychiatric Morbidity Survey in the UK (Jenkins et al. 1997) and the WHO's World Mental Health Study, 2000 (Kessler 1999). Elaboration on these studies is beyond the scope of this chapter; however, readers are encouraged to refer to these publications to gain a complete picture of the points discussed.

At the national level psychiatric epidemiology firstly appeared in Greece when two nationwide studies were conducted by the Professors Emeritus of Psychiatry,

Kostas Stefanis and Michael Madianos, in 1978 and 1984 (Madianos and Stefanis as well as one study by Mavreas and colleagues in the Athens area (Mavreas et al. 1986). Those studies provided evidence about the general levels psychiatric morbidity, while Madianos' nationwide studies also addressed the epidemiology of major depression in particular.

Over the last decade, and under the increasing pressure exerted from the economic crisis afflicting the country, the University of Ioannina funded by the Hellenic Ministry of Health designed and implemented a cross-sectional study ("2009–2010 Psychiatric Morbidity Study") on a random, representative sample of households in Greece (Crete region was excluded due to financial constraints), so as to estimate the prevalence of common mental disorders in the country (Skapinakis et al. 2013). Psychiatric morbidity was assessment with the Revised Clinical Interview Schedule (CIS-R), which had been employed in a similar UK nationwide study, and data were collected during the period September 2009–February 2010. Although the response rate was low (54 %) and the study had certain limitations (e.g. the tool is validated for the adolescent – population, only the presence of psychotic symptoms was not assessed, 35 % of the sample used a computer to enter the answers, whereas 65 % needed the investigator's assistance), it constitutes the first attempt to generate epidemiological evidence and to explore specific diagnoses in a nationwide sample. The results indicate that one week prevalence of psychiatric morbidity (i.e. the number of people meeting diagnostic criteria the week before the interview) in Greece was found to be 14 %, which is similar to estimate by Mavreas and colleagues several decades ago (Mavreas et al. 1986). The most mental disease was found to be generalized anxiety disorder (4.1 %), followed by major depression (2.9 %), phobias (2.79 %), mixed symptoms of anxiety-depression (2.67 %), panic disorder (1.88 %) and Obsessive Compulsive disorder (OCD) (1.69 %). Futhermore, being female, divorced or widowed, having a low level of education and being unemployed were found to constitute risk factors for psychiatric morbidity.

At the same time, the University Mental Health Research Institute (UMHRI) in a series of cross-sectional nationwide studies a steady rise in one-month prevalence of major depression in the general population during the economic crisis from 3.3 % in 2008 to 6.8 % in 2009 and 8.2 % in 2011 (Economou et al. 2013; Madianos et al. 2011). Conflicting findings between the two studies concerning major depression can attribute to the different methodologies adopted: one-week vs one-month prevalence estimate, household vs, telephone survey, different tools for assessing major depression and different response rates among others.

At the local level in 2005 and 2008, the Association for Regional Development and Mental Health (EPAPSY) carried out epidemiological studies on the prevalence of common mental disorders in the areas of Evia and Paros-Antiparos, respectively. The studies were carried out in areas where EPAPSY provided services in order to assess the population's needs and to improve the design and implementation of mental health promotion activities. The Evia study was carried out as part of an international collaboration between EPAPSY and the World Health Organisation Collaborative Centre of Lille, France, and involved an assessment of psychiatric morbidity in a representative sample of the local population (Stylianidis et al. 2014). The Mini International Neuropsychiatric Interview (MINI) tool was used to capture mental health problems, along with a form for recording socio-demographic data. The study demonstrated that 29 % of the island population suffered from at least one mental health disorder at some point in their lifetime. Additionally, women displayed higher prevalence rates of mood and anxiety disorders as compared to their male participants, with the exception of dysthymia, social anxiety and Post Traumatic Stress Disorder (PTSD). On the contrary in the Paros-Antiparos study, the methodology employed was similar to the 2009–2010 Psychiatric Morbidity Study already mentioned. The results showed that the prevalence of psychiatric morbidity on both islands was around 22 % with women, the unmarried individuals and the unemployed displaying elevated odds of manifesting psychiatric morbidity; whereas participants with higher education level and with higher income levels displayed lower odds of suffering from mental disorders (Stylianidis et al. 2010).

3.6 Discussion: Conclusions

This chapter endeavored to briefly present the key principles of epidemiology and the main research designs that are used. This information is of paramount importance upon designing, implementing and critically appraising a study. It also delineated the main cross-sectional studies which have been carried out in Greece the past decades. Greek studies adopting a different research design (i.e. Other than a cross-sectional survey) were not included, primarily because epidemiology starts off with describing a health outcome and providing clues for its understanding. On these grounds, it informs interventions and policies for tackling it and subsequently assesses their impact.

In other words, if large scale epidemiological studies that explore mental health outcomes and their correlates re missing, how can we proceed into developing tailored interventions for offsetting their effect?

As already mentioned, descriptive epidemiology seeks to assist in setting priorities in was hardly based on epidemiological evidence, either local or national, or on applied epidemiological studies centered on how mental health services operate (quality of care, profile of the service, clinical outcomes, etc.). As a corollary of this, the necessary complementary and dialectical relationship between psychiatric care,psychiatric epidemiology and mental health is scarce in Greece. Policies seem to be based on intuition,personal beliefs, improvisation and sketchy planning, while they often promote political interests or those of trade unions.

At the same time, good practices have been recorded in the delivery of mental health services (e.g. Evaluation of th Psychiatric reform, see the relevant chapter of this book); however, they are not widely disseminated and they are not incorporated in a national strategic plan for mental health.

Reports by foreign experts (EU, WHO, Institute of Psychiatry, readers can find more information about them in the germane chapters of this book) appear to act primarily as a political alibi for the leadership of the Ministry of Health and Social

Insurance rather than as a valuable tool that can guide the implementation and monitoring of the psychiatric reform in the country. Consequently, in the absence of a strong political will,epidemiology – which constitutes a tool of public health – remains underutilized, at least in the mental health sector in Greece.

Psychiatric epidemiology should formulate insightful hypothesis and research aims prior to the design of study, so that it can generate evidence that would contribute substantially at the individual level, improving the quality of care; to changes in monitoring of the national operational plan.

In this reasoning, psychiatric epidemiology should not become an end in itself, a self-referred and "fetishistic" object of public health. In other words, epidemiological studies should not be conducted just for promoting epidemiology an for the production of scientific publication.

Taking into consideration the special characteristics of Greece,public health and epidemiology should meet in an organized and cohesive manner,so as to provide solutions to the dead-end of the mental health care system in the country. This change in mentality and practice – i.e. that public mental health priorities should be based in epidemiological evidence –, must occur rapidly, given the growing dissemination of the global mental health movement,which in turn exerts pressures for the homogenization and adaptation to a specific model of epidemiology worldwide (Pearce 2004, see pertinent chapter of this book).

Soon, research areas will extend from the individual, community and national level to the international. Congruent with this, there is a risk that conclusions emanating from countries with advanced psychiatric epidemiology and evidence-based mental health care, will be applied to countries that cannot generate their own evidence base; ignoring, therefore, their cultural, institutional and social characteristics.

In conclusion, psychiatric epidemiology is still on its infancy in Greece and thus its development remains challenging. Psychiatric epidemiology should be closely tied to public health and to the development and improvement of services. It should also substantiate the integration of innovations into the system (e.g. patient an caregivers' participation in research and service delivery, implementation of the recovery model, cost-effective interventions, among others) in parallel with international findings. Good knowledge of international scientific standards s well as examples of good practice can provide framework fro developing our own national approach.

Bibliography

Barbato A, D'Avanzo B, D'Anza V, Montorfano E, Savio M, Corbascio CG (2014a) Involvement of users and relatives in mental health service evaluation. J Nerv Mental Dis 202:479–486

Barbato A, Rapissarda F, D'Anza V, De Luca F, Inglese C, Iapichino S, Mauriello F, D'Avanzo B (2014b) Quality assessment of mental health care by people with severe mental disorders: a participatory research project. Community Ment Health J 50:402–408

Blazer DG, Kessler RC, McGonagle KA, Swartz MS (1994) The prevalence and distribution of major depression in a national community sample: the National Comorbidity Survey. Am J Psychiatry 151:979–986

Branas C, Kastanaki A, Michalodimitrakis M, Tzougas J, Kranioti E, Theodorakis P et al (2015) The impact of economic austerity and prosperity events on suicide in Greece: a 30-year interrupted time-series analysis. BMJ Open 5(1):e005619–e005619

Durkheim E (1951) Suicide: a study in sociology. Free Press, Illinois

Economou M, Madianos M, Peppou LE, Patelakis A, Stefanis CN (2013) Major depression in the era of economic crisis: a replication of a cross-sectional study across Greece. J Affect Disord 145:308–314

Elwood MJ, Little J, Elwood JH (1992) Epidemiology and control of neural tube defects. Oxford University Press, Oxford

Jenkins R, Lewis G, Bebbington P, Brugha T, Farrell M, Gill B, Meltzer H (1997) The national psychiatric morbidity surveys of Great Britain–initial findings from the household survey. Psychol Med 27(04):775–789

Kendler KS, Gallagher TJ, Abelson JM, Kessler RC (1996) Lifetime prevalence, demographic risk factors, and diagnostic validity of nonaffective psychosis as assessed in a US community sample: the National Comorbidity Survey. Arch Gen Psychiatry 53:1022–1031

Kessler RC (1999) The World Health Organization International Consortium in Psychiatric Epidemiology (ICPE): initial work and future directions the NAPE lecture 1998a. Acta Psychiatr Scand 99(1):2–9

Kessler RC, Zhao S, Blazer DG, Swartz M (1997) Prevalence, correlates and course of minor depression and major depression in the National Comorbidity Survey. J Affect Disord 45:19–30

Last JM (1995) A dictionary of epidemiology, 3rd edn. Oxford University Press, Oxford

Madianos MG, Stefanis CN (1992) Changes in the prevalence of symptoms of depression and depression across Greece. Soc Psychiatry Psychiatr Epidemiol 27:211–219

Madianos MG, Economou M, Alexiou T, Stefanis CN (2011) Depression and economic hardship across Greece in 2008 and 2009: two cross-sectional surveys nationwide. Soc Psychiatry Psychiatr Epidemiol 46:943–952

Mason K, Olmos-Gallo AO, Bacon D, McQuilken M, Henley A, Fisher S (2004) Exploring the consumers' and providers' perspective on service quality in community mental health care. Community Ment Health J 40:33–46

Mavreas VG, Beis A, Mouyias A, Rigoni F, Lyketsos GC (1986) Prevalence of psychiatric disorders in Athens. A community study. Soc Psychiatry 21:172–181

Pearce N (2004) The globalization of epidemiology: introductory remarks. Int J Epidemiol 33:1127–1133

Robins LN, Regier DA (1991) Psychiatric disorders in America: the epidemiologic catchment area study. Free Press, New York

Rogers A, Pilgrim D (1993) Service users' views of psychiatric treatments. Sociol Health Illn 15:612–631

Roth D, Crane-Ross D (2002) Impact of services met needs, and service empowerment on consumer outcomes. Ment Health Serv Res 4:43–56

Skapinakis P, Bellos S, Koupidis S, Grammatikopoulos I, Theodorakis PN, Mavreas V (2013) Prevalence and sociodemographic associations of common mental disorders in a nationally representative sample of the general population. BMC Psychiatry 13:163–176

Stylianidis S, Skapianakis P, Pantelidou S, Chondros P, Avgoustakis A, Ziakoulis M (2010) Prevalence of common mental disorders in an island area: needs assessment and planning of mental health actions. Greek Med Arch 27:675–683 (in Greek)

Stylianidis S, Pantelidou S, Chondros P, Roelandt JL, Barbato A (2014) Prevalence of mental disorders in the Greek island of Evia. Psychiatriki 25:19–26

Thornicroft G, Tansella M (2005) Growing recognition of the importance of service user involvement in mental health service planning and evaluation. Epidemiol Psichiatr Soc 14:1–3

Wittchen HU, Jacobi F (2005) Size and burden of mental disorders in Europe- a critical review and appraisal of 27 studies. Eur Neuropsychopharmacol 15:357–376

Global Mental Health

4

Michail Lavdas, Stelios Stylianidis, and Christina Mamaloudi

Abstract

The emergence of the term "global mental health" has been driven by the multifactorial aetiology of the onset of mental disorders, the need for equal access to mental health services and the long-standing finding of inequalities in healthcare and mental healthcare which prevail not just at international level but also at national and local levels. As the human rights movement has promoted a form of globalisation of rights, a more comprehensive view of mental health has gradually emerged, meaning it is now possible to perceive the data which affect it depending on age, gender, geographical location, socioeconomic status, as well as cultural factors that vary from location to location. This chapter seeks to outline the emergence of global mental health and explain the complex terminology so characteristic of it, in an attempt to create a shared vocabulary for mental health which allows one to recognise inequalities and engage in comprehensive prevention and intervention for mental disorders.

4.1 Introduction

Global health has been defined as "the area of study, research and practice that places a priority on improving health and achieving equity in health for all people worldwide". Global mental health is the application of those principles to the area of mental health.

M. Lavdas • C. Mamaloudi
Association for Regional Development and Mental Health (EPAPSY), Athens, Greece
e-mail: ml@epapsy.gr

S. Stylianidis (✉)
Department of Psychology, Panteion University, Athens, Greece
e-mail: stylianidis.st@gmail.com

© Springer International Publishing Switzerland 2016
S. Stylianidis (ed.), *Social and Community Psychiatry: Towards a Critical, Patient-Oriented Approach*, DOI 10.1007/978-3-319-28616-7_4

Table 4.1 Frequency (%) of individuals with physical and mental disorders treated in low-, middle- and high-income settings

	High-income settings	Low- and middle-income settings)
Physical disorders		
Diabetes	94	77
Heart disease	78	51
Asthma	65	44
Mental disorders		
Depression	29	8
Bipolar disorder	29	13
Panic disorder	33	9

Adapted from Ormel et al. (2008)

Respecting the rights of individuals with mental problems and equity in access to mental health services is a central issue addressed in international treaties and conventions, the most recent being the UN's Convention of the Rights of Persons with Disabilities (CPRD). However, despite the importance given to this topic, inequalities in the protection of rights remain; inequalities that emerge on numerous levels, the main one being segregation based on income bracket. The different levels have been set by the World Bank (World Bank 2010) which divides countries into four categories depending on per capita income: (a) low income (£US$995), low middle income (US$996–3.945), high middle income (US$3.946–12.195) and high income (^{3}US$12.196). Below we will adopt the Thornicroft and Tansella (2013) distinction who have joined the two intermediate categories into one (middle income), thereby giving three categories.

The main inequality lies in the fact that while low- and middle-income countries are home to more than 80 % of the world's population, they control just 20 % of the mental health resources. Inequalities also exist in terms of available human resources. In low-income countries, there are on average 0.05 psychiatrists and 0.16 psychiatric nurses per 100,000 residents, but those numbers of 200 times lower than in high-income countries (WHO 2005). Countries in sub-Saharan Africa have less than one psychiatrist per one million people, compared to 137 psychiatrists per one million in the USA (Ndyanabangi et al. 2004). Likewise, training courses and infrastructure for mental health professionals are extremely inadequate (Saxena et al. 2007), while there are numerous violations of rights, which are particularly serious when it comes to individuals with mental disorders. As far as the right to equal access to health and mental health services is concerned, international literature has devised the term "treatment gap" to determine the number of individuals suffering but not receiving treatment. It is a fact that more than 75 % of those diagnosed with severe anxiety and emotional disorders, impulse control disorders and addiction disorders do not receive any treatment in the countries they live in (low- and middle-income countries).

However, that problem remains on a smaller but equally serious scale in countries which are better off. In Greece, the rate of use of mental health services does not exceed one third of the population of individuals suffering from some mental disorder (Skapinakis et al. 2013). The treatment gap rate for mental disorders compared to physical diseases is indicative, as we can see from Table 4.1 which helps us better understand the discrimination against mental health within the range of diseases and disabilities:

Patel and Prince (2010) have said that the failure to meet basic needs such as food, clothing, housing, comfort and privacy is a failure of mankind and also adds incarceration without control and monitoring mechanisms, as well as recorded cases of abuse and torture, restraints, etc. Documenting effective treatments and respect for human rights are two fundamental principles on which the global mental health movement, which took form on 10 October 2008, is based (Patel et al. 2011). The movement developed as a synergy between individuals and institutions committed to collective action, which seeks to address the treatment gap for individuals suffering from mental disorders irrespective of where they live. Inequalities are not limited only to uneven deployment of services but also resources invested in investigative and research activities. Less than 1 % of resources for health research have been given for low- and middle-income countries, even though 90 % of the world population lives in those countries, while the average allocation of resources for mental health in low-income countries does not exceed 0.5 % of the total health budget. In short, there is a robust body of evidence and documentation concerning the disastrous effects of mental disorder on a personal and social level. Among those unfortunate effects, it is important to single out the fact that mental disorders are a major risk factor in suicide, since 90 % of persons who commit suicide suffer from some mental disorder and in particular mood disorders dominated by major depression and bipolar disorder, which have been associated with 60 % of suicides (Mann et al. 2005). On an economic level, the impacts do not only relate to the cost of treatment in the event of potential relapse or mental disorder episodes but the cost of lost productivity which translates into an economic cost that globally exceeded $2.5 trillion in 2010 and is expected to rise to $6 trillion in 2013 (Bloom et al. 2012). However, the strongest incentive for action is none other than the violation of the rights of individuals with mental disorders who frequently have to endure unusual forms of restraint, isolation in psychiatric institutions, being locked up in penitentiaries, being restrained and chained up in their own home, being excluded from society and treatment and frequent abuse from traditional treatment methods (Patel et al. 2012).

The aims of the global mental health movement have been summarised by MGMH as follows:

Promoting the protection of human rights and prevention of discrimination and prejudice against people with mental disorders and psychosocial disabilities
Strengthening the full implementation of the International Convention on the Rights of Persons with Disabilities (CRPD) and the mechanisms for human rights protection
Enabling people with mental disorder and psychosocial disabilities to make decisions about their own lives and actively participate in issues that affect them
Ensuring equal access to people with mental disorder and psychosocial disabilities in health, education, life and other activities in order not to leave "anyone behind"

Bridging the large and increasing treatment gap in mental health and improving access to health and social support
Integrating mental health into development activities

Likewise Patel (2014) supplemented those objectives, stating in a more practical manner the importance of empowering individuals with mental disorders and their families to provide mutual support. He also added that the creation of a diverse workforce in mental health is important in provide psychosocial interventions, be they suitably trained or supervised non-specialised healthcare professionals. Taking into account the constantly growing technology sector, he proposed the use of technology to improve access to mental healthcare by using computers, for example, in self-directed psychological treatment exercises. He also stressed the critical importance of early identification and treatment of mental disorders, such as interventions in schools or other areas where children and infants are kept busy, and he considered it equally important to reduce premature death rates by improving care for physical health problems among those with mental disorders.

4.2 Historical Background

The scale of the mental health problem worldwide involves 450 million people suffering from mental or behavioural disorder, while almost 1 million people attempt suicide every year. One key indicator in epidemiology is mortality, with mental and behavioural disorders occupying a low position. However the size of their impact is demonstrated by the global burden of disorder since depression (unipolar depression) ranks in third place worldwide and is expected to climb to the first cause of global burden by 2030. Moreover, four of the six main causes of years lived with disability (YLD) are mental and behavioural disorders (depression, alcohol abuse disorders, schizophrenia and bipolar disorder). More specifically, 33 % of YLD are due to depression. While mental disorders have a relatively low mortality rate, depression and substance abuse are associated with more than 90 % of suicide cases. Moreover, higher mortality rates not associated with suicide have been found in individuals who live with schizophrenic, bipolar disorder and dementia. Serious mental disorders increase the probability of a stroke or heart disease in individuals before the age of 55 and of living less than 5 years after the episode. The reasons for this are that individuals with serious mental disorders frequently live in social isolation and healthcare services are prejudiced against the health problems those individuals face. Moreover, they are less likely to have a checkup and receive preventative care. Lastly, psychotropic drugs also contribute to premature death. The impact of mental disorders such as depression, for example, has been shown to directly affect the outcome of a chronic disease.

It is particularly important to look at the key papers and scientific studies which have shown the importance of mental disorders and the need to prioritise them when planning policies worldwide. In 1993 the University of Harvard's School of Public Health working with the World Bank and the WHO assessed the burden of disorder worldwide for the first time in a study which had been launched in 1988 to quantify the burden of disease and trauma on the population and identify global health challenges. The objectives of the study into the Global Burden of Disease (GBD) were as follows:

1. To facilitate the integration of nonfatal health effects in the international debate on health policies that too often focused on mortality.
2. To disconnect the epidemiological assessment of the pressure for changes in policy and to calculate the mortality and disability caused by a disease as objectively as possible. At national and international level, individuals taking decisions (decision-makers) often accepted estimates of the burden of a disorder or injury that makes a group of people who are seeking a specific change in policy.
3. To quantify the burden of disease using a tool that can also be used in cost-effectiveness analysis.

The DALY (disability-adjusted life years) unit was designed to meet the above objectives by measuring the treatment gap in health and combining the lifetimes lost due to premature mortality and those of "healthy life" lost due to disability. The formula for calculating DALY is set out below:

$$DALY = (Years\,Life\,Lost - YLL) + (Years\,lived\,with\,disability - YLD)$$

Desjarlais et al. (1995) then went on to draft the first global report on mental health (the World Mental Health Report) recognising problems and priorities in low-income countries and providing documentation of the consequences of the health burden worldwide in terms of epidemiology, anthropology and mental health and behavioural problems. Mental health disorders are responsible for 8.1 % of lost years of quality life.

The next turning point for global health and mental health was 2001 when the WHO published its 2001 World Health Report (WHO 2001) which referred to the burden of mental and behavioural disorders and estimated (Tables 4.2 and 4.3) that they relate to more than 25 % of people at some point in their life. At the same time, it stressed the global impact of disorders on individuals irrespective of country, society, age, gender, economic status or urban or agricultural environment. The common disorders which normally cause severe disability include depressive disorders, substance abuse disorders, schizophrenia and epilepsy. Alzheimer's disease, mental retardation and childhood and adolescence disorders were also studied. The factors related to the prevalence, onset and course of mental and behavioural disorders include poverty, age, conflict and disasters, major physical diseases and the family and social environment. The relationships between mental health and primary healthcare which had already been stressed in the Caracas Convention of 1990 were also studied.

In 2004 the WHO extended and bolstered the GBD study, which was updated in 2008 (WHO 2008a).

Table 4.2 Wider economic burden of mental disorders (WHO 2003)

	Cost of care	Productivity cost	Other costs
Sufferers	Treatment and cost of services	Inability to work, lost earnings	Pain, side effects of treatment, suicide
Family and friends	Informal care	Time off work	Pain, isolation, stigma
Employers	Contribution to care and treatment	Reduced productivity	–
Society	Mental healthcare and general healthcare (taxation/insurance funds)	Reduced productivity	Lives of people lost, untreated diseases (needs not addressed), social isolation

Table 4.3 Type of estimate cost (WHO 2003)

	Core cost	Other costs unrelated to health
Direct cost	Treatment and payment for services	Management of social welfare
		Burden on judicial system
		Transportation
Indirect cost	Cost of lost productivity	Value of time of caregivers in the family
	Cost due to mortality	

In 2005 in the spirit of ensuring social justice, the WHO set up a Commission on Social Determinants of Health which undertook to collect documentation on the promotion of equity in health, to bolster the steps needed to be taken as part of a global movement to address inequalities. The Commission completed its report in 2007 setting out key social determinants of health (Solar and Irwin 2007).

The 2008 World Health Report made health equity a priority, requiring a renewal of primary healthcare with an emphasis on integrating mental health into it. The factors identified relate directly to mental health since a multifactorial aetiology in mental disorders has already been documented (Patel and Kleinman 2003; Susser et al. 2006; Goldberg and Huxley 1992). There are multiple social determinants of mental disorders which impact directly or indirectly on the emergence of a mental disorder.

Those determinants require comprehensive prevention and intervention to improve mental health, using strategies that improve the conditions in which individuals are born, raised, work and grow. Inequalities at the socioeconomic level, for example, directly affect the rate of onset for mental disorders. For example, depression and anxiety disorders do not appear with the same frequency in all social groups. Individuals who experience inequality and financial difficulties more intensely have those mental disorders more frequently. Documentation of the link between financial debt and an increased probability of the onset of a mental disorder is important and appears in the WHO's recent report on the social determinants of mental health (WHO 2014). To be able to understand how socioeconomic status is associated with the onset of mental disorder, one merely needs to realise that the frequency, intensity and duration of "stressful" experiences coupled with skills and defences at individual and collective levels that an individual or society has make someone more or less vulnerable to mental disorder. Individuals who lower down the social ladder are more likely to experience financial difficulties as well as tougher social and environmental living conditions and to have reduced access to support and care mechanisms. Those inequalities begin even before the individual is born and normally accumulate over the course of his life, but we should not forget that no individual, even if he shares certain common "burden factors", who does not react to his vulnerability in the same way. Below is a summary of the areas of intervention that could reduce the risk of mental disorder or provide a chance for intervention:

- *Life expectancy*: Prenatal period, pregnancy and perinatal period, early childhood, adolescence, working life and development of family and older age – all in relation to gender
- *Parents, families and households*: Parental behaviour, material conditions (income, resources, food, water, hygiene, accommodation, work), working conditions and unemployment, parents' physical and mental health, pregnancy and maternal care and social support
- *Community*: Trust and security in the neighbourhood, involvement in local community life, violence/crime and isolation
- *Local services*: Early childhood and education, schools, services for adolescents and youth, health services, social services and services ensuring local hygiene conditions such as fresh water
- *National level*: Reduction in poverty, inequality, discrimination, "prudent" government, human rights, military conflict and national policies relating to access to education, work, health, housing and social policies

Returning to the key aspects of global mental health, it is essential to cite the 2007 edition of the scientific journal *The Lancet* which brought together the work of many experts in the field. Researchers who participated in writing the articles demonstrated the high burden generated by mental disorders, which account for 14 % of the global burden (Prince et al. 2007), the connections and interconnections between mental disorders and other health disorders and the relationship between mental health and the achievement of the Millennium Development Goals. They presented the needs of mankind in general and compared these with the scarcity of resources for mental health and the unequal distribution and ineffectual use of resources (Saxena et al. 2007). They recorded the documented efficacy of interventions to treat and prevent mental disorders in low-resource conditions and showed the inadequate infrastructure which existed for mental healthcare (Patel et al. 2007; Saraceno et al. 2007). The evidence collectively gathered has been used to formulate a call for improvements in mental health services in all countries, especially those with low and middle incomes (Jacob et al. 2007). Estimates about the financial cost have also been made since $2 per person per year in low-income countries and $3–$4 per person in middle-income countries are sufficient to improve mental healthcare

(Patel et al. 2007). They also gathered together indicators which could be used to map developments and research priorities. Chisholm et al. (2007) also stressed the need for political will, for collective action by all stakeholders in global health and for resources to implement solutions to address the mental health burden worldwide. In 2008 the WHO's Department of Mental Health and Addiction recognised the importance of the call for global mental health and launched the Mental Health Global Action Programme (mhGAP) (WHO 2008b). The programme's aim was to improve mental health services in low- and middle-income countries. The programme's main product, the mhGAP educational guide (WHO 2010), provides treatment guidelines for nine basic categories of mental and neurological disorders to increase the potential for recognising them in primary healthcare. It includes depression, psychosis, epilepsy, developmental disorders, behavioural disorders, dementia, alcohol dependence, addiction, self-harm and suicidality (Barbui et al. 2010).

A major turning point in the historical development of global mental health was 2013, when 194 ministers of health were adopted by the WHO's comprehensive mental health action plan. In doing so they recognised mental health as a global priority in the health sector which requires immediate action.

The action plan's vision is to help create a world where mental health is appreciated, promoted and protected, while bad mental health is prevented and individuals affected by it are able to fully exercise their rights and have access to high-quality services that are culturally and socially sensitive to their requirements, with priority being attached to recovery and ensuring the best possible health and involvement in the community and working environment without stigmatism and discrimination.

The comprehensive mental health action plan (WHO 2013) will help the growing endeavours of members of the global mental health movement and will increase access to health services, improve reporting of human rights violations and promote the social integration of individuals with mental disorders worldwide.

Mental health at global level now occupies a place on the global health agenda, with robust documentation of the treatments available and best practices to be used.

4.3 Web Platforms and Global Mental Health

It is worthwhile referring to online databases and platforms which record these best practices. The WHO has set up the WHO Mindu Bank (http://www.mindbank.info), which is a web platform that contains basic sources of information about mental health, substance abuse, disability, general health, human rights and development. The Mental Health Innovation Network online database was also developed for the World Innovation Summit for Health containing best practices for research and clinical practice (http://www.mhinnovation.net). The Calouste Gulbenkian Foundation has developed the Gulbenkian Global Mental Health Platform, which includes best practices from the international arena to promote mental health and provide continuing documentation of interventions which are taking place.

The dissemination of best practices using means such as the internet allows national sources of information and best practices to be exchanged between countries, while efforts like those listed above reduce the fragmentary nature of record-keeping and overlap in research documentation and applied practices. It also bolsters advocacy and helps promote rights at a global level.

4.4 Mental Health Priorities Based on Needs and Resource Availability

It is particularly important not to ignore the fact that resource availability not only determines the ability to intervene but also affects the very form of psychiatric prevalence in an area. Documenting mental disorders does not end solely with looking at their biological basis (which has been an area of particular focus over recent years) but also extends to psychosocial factors which play a definitive role in the onset of mental disorders. Reference was made above to the social determinants of mental health, and now we will look at the difference in prevalence based on the income ranking of countries. It can be seen in Table 4.4 below (WHO 2008a), which presents the ten main causes of burden (DALYS) based on the income ranking of various countries. For example, while dementia is the fourth most burdensome disease in high-income countries, it does not appear at all in countries with a lower income. That can be explained in part by life expectancy which is clearly higher in the former, and therefore, the probability of someone becoming ill with Alzheimer's disease is higher. Another important observation is that the top place is occupied by unipolar depression in middle- and high-income countries, while it occupies eighth place in low-income countries. High rates of depression are associated with psychosocial factors which are not dependent on the economic situation of each country, since the economic crisis has generated secondary unfavourable impacts on mental health, which in turn may be contributing to phenomena such as a rise in suicides, alcohol abuse and alcohol-related deaths (Skapinakis et al. 2013; WHO 2011).

The interventions possible based on resource availability conditions can be divided into three categories: (1) low resource availability, (2) middle resource availability and (3) high resource availability. One needs to bear in mind that resource availability conditions do not only relate to countries but also to their official categorisation based on income and on other issues. It is a fact that major differences and inequalities have been noted in resource availability not just among various cities but also between areas within the same large city.

Low Resource Availability Conditions

Emphasis needs to be placed on workers in primary healthcare and the community who will take up roles to be shared out based on needs assessments, the identification of mental disorders, the provision of short-term psychosocial interventions and medicated treatments (Beaglehole and Bonita 2008; Eaton 2008). The limited

Table 4.4 Main causes for burden of disease (DALYs), countries per income group, 2004

	Disease or injury World	DALYs (in millions)	% of overall DALYs		Disease or injury Low-income countries	DALYs (in millions)	% of overall DALYs
1	Lower respiratory tract infections	94.5	6.2	1	Lower respiratory tract infections	76.9	9.3
2	Diarrhoeal diseases	72.8	4.8	2	Diarrhoeal diseases	59.2	7.2
3	Unipolar depression	65.5	4.3	3	HIV/AIDS	42.9	5.2
4	Ischemic heart disease	62.6	4.1	4	Malaria	32.8	4.0
5	HIV/AIDS	58.5	3.8	5	Premature childbirth and low birth weight	32.1	3.9
6	Cerebral vascular disease	46.6	3.1	6	Neonatal infections and other	31.4	3.8
7	Premature childbirth and low birth weight	44.3	2.9	7	Perinatal asphyxia and trauma	29.8	3.6
8	Perinatal asphyxia and trauma	41.7	2.7	8	Unipolar depression	26.5	3.2
9	Road traffic accidents	41.2	2.7	9	Ischemic heart disease	26.0	3.1
10	Neonatal infections and other	40.4	2.7	10	Tuberculosis	22.4	2.7
	Middle-income countries				High-income countries		
1	Unipolar depression	29.0	5.1	1	Unipolar depression	10.0	8.2
2	Ischemic heart disease	28.9	5.0	2	Ischemic heart disease	7.7	6.3
3	Cerebral vascular Disease	27.5	4.8	3	Cerebral vascular disease	4.8	3.9
4	Road traffic accidents	21.4	3.7	4	Alzheimer's disease and other dementing disorders	4.4	3.6
5	Lower respiratory tract infections	16.3	2.8	5	Alcohol use disorders	4.2	3.4
6	Chronic pulmonary disease	16.1	2.8	6	Adult onset loss of hearing	4.2	3.4
7	HIV/AIDS	15.0	2.6	7	Chronic pulmonary disease	3.7	3.0
8	Alcohol use disorders	14.9	2.6	8	Diabetes	3.6	3.0
9	Eye diseases	13.7	2.4	9	Cancer (throat, lungs)	3.6	3.0
10	Diarrhoeal diseases	13.1	2.3	10	Road traffic accidents	3.1	2.6

number of mental health experts, who are normally to be found in the capital of the country, can only offer (a) training and supervision to professions in primary healthcare, (b) advice and feedback in difficult cases and (c) outpatient and inpatient assessments and treatment in cases which primary healthcare cannot handle (Mubbashar 1999; Alem 2002; Njega 2002; Saxena and Maulik 2003; Lund et al. 2011). The limited availability of human resources led Patel (2014) to propose task shifting in mental health. He proposes utilising aware citizens in the mental health sector after they receive special training, so be able to provide basic interventions to treat mental health cases and to interface with any available services whenever needed. To be able to achieve task sharing, Patel proposes that complex mental healthcare tasks be broken down into individual elements, some of which can be allocated to less-specialised staff or even to sensitive, capable individuals who have received the right training. Shifting and sharing tasks are vital, according to Patel, in the context of a team which will be coordinated by a mental health professional. The individual elements listed by Patel are (a) managing care in each case, (b) supporting the family, (c) social support and supervision of individuals trained to provide basic mental healthcare and (d) the prescription and administration of medication, which must remain with medical staff. However, it should be stressed in relation to these points that medication on its own is of limited efficacy, but if coupled with task sharing and overall care offered by training members of the community, it can have a high effectiveness rating (Buttorff et al. 2012).

Middle Resource Availability Conditions

Under these conditions, it is important to appreciate that there is still a need for a robust primary healthcare in order to provide care to high prevalence, common mental disorders in the general population (in some countries the annual prevalence of diseases in primary healthcare is as high as 20–30 %). In addition to the emphasis on primary healthcare, which must cover needs identification, the recognition of mental disorders, psychosocial interventions and feedback – as in the previous category – it is also essential to develop outpatient care services and short-term hospitalisation units, social mental health groups, acute case units, long-term sheltered care units in the community and opportunities for employment for the mentally disabled. Of these, major resources are used up by acute care units (Knapp et al. 1997); so in order to be able to stay open and intervene in crisis situations, it is essential to keep the length of hospitalisation down, so that resources can be used for supplementary services in the community (Lasalvia and Tansella 2010; Lelliott and Bleksley 2010; Sederer 2010; Totman et al. 2010).

High Resource Availability Conditions

Having ensured primary healthcare and the integration of mental health into it, one needs to put in place general psychiatry services for children and adults focused on the community and to deploy specialised services based on resource availability.

Specialised mental health services can provide care for eating disorders, resilient psychiatric disorders, substance dependence or mothers suffering from mental disorder. Having carried out a needs investigation in each area in which action is to be taken, one needs to develop services that meet the population's needs. With the right resources, community mental health groups could integrate Assertive Community Treatment (ACT) groups which visit anyone in need at home (Deci et al. 1995; Teague et al. 1998; Killaspy and Rosen 2011) and develop early intervention units for psychotic or other mental disorders (Power and McGorry 2011). Moreover, alternative methods for intervening in crisis situations would allow for better management while significantly protecting the rights of individuals with mental disorders which are frequently violated via procedures such as involuntary hospitalisation (Stylianidis et al. 2014; The Ombudsman 2007). Alternative crisis models are acute day hospitals which offer daycare for individuals with acute and severe psychiatric problems as an alternative to a stay in inpatient units, but their effectiveness in treating acute problems compared to inpatient units has not yet been documented (Marshall et al. 2001, 2011). Thornicroft and Tansella (2013) have also examined crisis houses, which are staffed by mental health professionals, which accept individuals who would otherwise have to be admitted for treatment to the psychiatric ward. Limited research so far shows that they can offer an alternative to treatment in the psychiatric ward or hospital, offering significantly better cost effectiveness compared to hospitalisation (Sledge et al. 1996a, b· Mosher 1999). Another alternative option is home treatment/crisis resolution teams which are mobile units that offer an assessment to patients in psychiatric crisis and offer intensive home care (Johnson and Thornicroft 2008). A recent Cochrane systematic study (Murphy et al. 2012) indicates that crisis resolution care is a viable solution in treating individuals with severe mental disorder, while studies by McCrone et al. (2009) show that it is the most cost-effective solution than hospitalisation, both in terms of cost and efficacy. Other specialised interventions are alternative forms of sheltered care in the community (sheltered apartments, daycare, etc.) and interventions involving supporting employment such as Individual Placement and Support which has been effective to a significant degree (Priebe et al. 1998; Drake et al. 1999; Crowther et al. 2001; Marshall et al. 2001; Lehman et al. 2002; Rinaldi and Perkins 2007; Bond et al. 2008).

4.5 Barriers and Challenges to Applying the Global Mental Health Principles

Ranking global mental health priorities is a particularly important objective. To that end, Collins et al. (2011) carried out a large-scale qualitative survey using the Delphi method which involved representatives from more than 60 countries, in order to set targets and identify the most important barriers to implementing global mental health principles.

We will attempt to present every objective and the challenges identified, starting from the first which relates to recognising the causes of mental and neurological disorders and risk and protective factors. For this target, barriers were identified such as recognition of an addressable social and biological risk factor during an individual's life. Moreover, the need to understand the impact of poverty, violence, war, migration and natural disasters was recorded and the need for research into the biomarkers of disorders was stressed. At this point we should stress that there is risk to global mental health from "psychiatrification" of the approach, impelled by the concern to show that illness has a biological basis. However in his attempt to document mental disorder and the struggle to identify its causes, Clark (2014) stresses that there is a risk of neglecting the psychosocial side of things and ignoring the different ways in which disorders manifest depending on the cultural context. Another risk identified by the investigator relates to limiting interventions to individual level without also bolstering community participation. That would result in what are best practices in global mental health benefiting "privileged individuals" and not communities.

The second objective relates to preventing and implementing early interventions, in an attempt to support communities, promote physical and mental well-being and reduce the duration of untreatable illnesses by developing cultural aware methods of early intervention under different conditions. Cultural data and cultures vary considerably from area to area and from country to country, and if we aim for efficient practices, we need to design interventions to adjust to local social, economic and cultural circumstances and to take into account the availability of human resources (Patel and Saxena 2014). The need to develop a set of well-documented primary prevention interventions for mental disorders has also been stressed, as has the need to drawn up local, appropriate strategies to eliminate child abuse and improve protection for children.

The third objective relates to improving treatment interventions and disseminating them throughout the entire spectrum of care provided. Here research is still needed into how to identify mental disorders and to integrate them into primary healthcare. It is also important to reduce cost, to increase and safeguard the stocks of effective medical supplies and to develop effective treatments for use by non-experts, including healthcare professionals with minimal training in these matters. Integrating a disability functionality assessment is also important, as is providing efficient, cost-effective social care and rehabilitation. Improving child access to well-documented forms of care provided by trained health providers in low- and medium-income countries is one of the challenges that many countries have yet to address. Using new technologies such as telemedicine could also make a real contribution to access to well-documented forms of care.

The fourth objective is to raise public awareness about the global burden. Here we face challenges relating to the development of cultural up-to-date methods for addressing stigma, prejudice and social despair among patients and families in different cultural conditions. Another major challenge is to establish a common international "documentation database" to record cultural and socioeconomic factors that cultivate inequalities in the prevalence, diagnosis, treatment and outcome of neuropsychiatric disorders. An equally important challenge is to develop valid, reliable definitions, models and measuring tools for quantitative assessment of the burden at individual level, as well as at overall population level, for use in different cultures and conditions. Lastly, this objective also includes establishing shared, weighted databases to collect data to monitor the predominance of treatment methods and the availability of human resources and services.

The next objective relates to developing the production capacity of human resources. This includes developing the production capacity in low- and medium-income countries by creating regional centres for mental health research and training and practice for staff in light of local conditions and needs. Another challenge that still needs to be overcome is to develop viable models to train and increase the number of non-experts and specialised professionals of different cultures and backgrounds in providing well-documented forms of services. To move towards that, training received by all healthcare professionals needs to change to include the mental health factors to a more satisfactory degree.

The last objective outlined by the experts in this study relates to transforming the health system and policy-level responses. Here it is vital to enact and implement key minimum standards/principles to deal with neuropsychiatric disorders worldwide. In making this shift, health systems need to be redesigned to integrate neuropsychiatric disorders into the care of chronic diseases and to create conditions for equality between mental and physical diseases. This means that resources need to be invested equally into research, training, treatment and prevention, while mental health needs to be integrated – both at national and international level – into international aid and development programmes, for example.

4.6 Comments: Conclusions

As we move further towards a global mental health movement as we have been doing over recent years, one ought not to let one's attention slip from the barriers still to be faced. While primary healthcare is a key pillar in improving mental health, both in high- and low-cost conditions, Stewart et al. (2010) have recorded the reasons for the "historical", proverbial failure of primary healthcare models in attempts to integrate mental health in developing countries. The reasons for failure can be summarised as follows: (1) the fragmentation of primary healthcare programmes which focus on special diagnostic categories (such as tuberculosis, HIV), (2) the prevalence of the traditional model for checking for diseases which ignores the cultural context and social determinants and (3) the serious inequalities in access to the health system for the population. Quite often, one or more of these factors are present in global mental health programmes, which partially explain their failure.

At the same time, as the global mental health movement has grown, we have seen the simultaneous dissemination of a phenomenon of the globalisation of the biomedical model of psychiatry. As Bracken and Thomas (2005) has succinctly pointed out, "we see the globalisation of biomedical psychiatry as a non-democratic, non-sustainable phenomenon without any clear ethical focus". It is also a fact that in the view of Chowdhury and Bhuiya (2001), most intervention models in global mental health are documented using the example of Western biomedical psychiatry. The systematic obfuscation of diversity, the prevalence of mental disorders, their prognosis and outcome and classification differ significantly in different cultural and social contexts. One must ask how it is possible for the global mental health movement to place emphasis on the global reach of Western diagnostic and treatment systems and minimise or ignore the differences; this approach is standard strategy for it.

As far as implementation of the above objectives is concerned, there is a lack of programmes to reduce the negative effects of social determinants (Saraceno 2014). In other words, interventions that are organised seek to relieve the symptoms of the affected population and not to eliminate the factors that negatively impact on and burden both the onset and outcome of mental disorders.

In the example of how depression and suicidality are dealt with, the approach could focus not just on pharmacological treatment of the symptoms but also on creating conditions that reduce the onset rate for depression, such as unemployment, unequal access to opportunities for economic growth and social inequalities more broadly speaking. Interventions to combat poverty, such as micro-loans provided in areas with high levels of poverty, have generated important results (Bruno 2012; Khandker and Samad 2013).

The restrictive responses that traditional psychiatry gives do not cover the constantly expanding mental health needs of the population. Consequently, an approach which does not take into account the social determinants that affect mental health is inadequate. Let us paraphrase Saraceno (2014) who described the vicious circle thus: we get depressed because we are poor and get poor because we are schizophrenic.

Bibliography

Alem A (2002) Community-based vs. hospital-based mental health care: the case of Africa. World Psychiatry 1:99–100

Barbui C, Dua T, van Ommeren M, Yasamy M, Fleischmann A, Clark N, Thornicroft G, Hill S, Saxena S (2010) Challenges in developing evidence-based recommendations using the GRADE approach: the case of mental, neurological, and substance use disorders. PLoS Med 7:e1000322

Beaglehole R, Bonita R (2008) Global public health: a scorecard. Lancet 372:1988–1996

Bloom DE, Cafiero E, Jané-Llopis E, Abrahams-Gessel S, Bloom LR, Fathima S, ... & Weiss J (2012) The global economic burden of noncommunicable diseases (No. 8712). Program on the Global Demography of Aging

Bond GR, Drake RE, Becker DR (2008) An update on randomized controlled trials of evidence-based supported employment. Psychiatr Rehabil J 31(4):280

Bracken P, Thomas P (2005) Postpsychiatry: mental health in a postmodern world. Oxford University Press, Oxford

Bruno J (2012) Microfinance or micro-commercial banking: the Great Recession's impact on women's access to microcredit in the United States. Womens Rts L Rep 34:1

Buttorff C, Hock RS, Weiss HA, Naik S, Araya R, Kirkwood BR, Patel V (2012) Economic evaluation of a task-shifting intervention for common mental disorders in India. Bull World Health Organ 90(11):813–821

Chisholm D, Flisher AJ, Lund C, Patel V, Saxena S, Thornicroft G, Tomlinson M (2007) Scale up services for mental disorders: a call for action. Lancet 370(9594):1241–1252

Chowdhury AM, Bhuiya A (2001) Do poverty alleviation programmes reduce inequities in health? The Bangladesh experience. In: Leon DA, Walt G (eds) Poverty, inequality, and health: an international perspective. Oxford University Press, Oxford, pp 312–332

Clark J (2014) Medicalization of global health 2: the medicalization of global mental health. Glob Health Action 77:24000, http://dx.doi.org/10.3402/gha.v7.24000

Collins PY, Patel V, Joestl SS, March D, Insel TR, Daar AS, Walport M (2011) Grand challenges in global mental health. Nature 475(7354):27–30

Crowther RE, Marshall M, Bond GR, Huxley P (2001) Helping people with severe mental illness to obtain work: systematic review. Br Med J 322(7280):204–208

Deci PA, Santos AB, Hiott DW, Schoenwald S, Dias JK (1995) Dissemination of assertive community treatment programs. Psychiatr Serv 46:676–678

Desjarlais R, Eisenberg L, Good B, Kleinman A (1995) World mental health: problems and priorities in developing countries. Oxford University Press, Oxford

Drake RE, McHugo GJ, Bebout RR, Becker DR, Harris M, Bond GR, Quimby E (1999) A randomized clinical trial of supported employment for inner-city patients with severe mental disorders. Arch Gen Psychiatry 56(7):627–633

Eaton J (2008) Ensuring access to psychotropic medication in sub-Saharan Africa. Afr J Psychiatry 11:179–181

Goldberg DP, Huxley P (1992) Common mental disorders: a bio-social model. Tavistock/Routledge, London

Jacob KS, Sharan P, Mirza I, Garrido-Cumbrera M, Seedat S, Mari JJ, Saxena S (2007) Mental health systems in countries: where are we now? Lancet 370(9592):1061–1077

Johnson S, Thornicroft G (2008) The classic home treatment studies. In: Johnson S, Needle J, Bindman J, Thornicroft G (eds) Crisis resolution and home treatment in mental health. Cambridge University Press, Cambridge, pp 37–50

Khandker S, Samad H (2013) Microfinance growth and poverty reduction in Bangladesh: what does the longitudinal data say? Working Paper 16. Institute of Microfinance. Available http://inm.org.bd/publication/workingpaper/workingpaper16.pdf. Accessed 24 July 2014

Killaspy H, Rosen A (2011) Case management and assertive community treatment. In: Thornicroft G, Szmukler GI, Mueser KT, Drake RE (eds) Oxford textbook of community mental health. Oxford University Press, Oxford, pp 171–184

Knapp M, Chisholm D, Astin J, Lelliott P, Audini B (1997) The cost consequences of changing the hospital–community balance: the mental health residential care study. Psychol Med 27(03):681–692

Lasalvia A, Tansella M (2010) Acute in-patient care in modern, community-based mental health services. Where and how? Epidemiol Psichiatr Soc 19:275–281

Lehman AF, Goldberg R, Dixon LB, McNary S, Postrado L, Hackman A, McDonnell K (2002) Improving employment outcomes for persons with severe mental illnesses. Arch Gen Psychiatry 59(2):165–172

Lelliott P, Bleksley S (2010) Improving the quality of acute inpatient care. Epidemiol Psichiatr Soc 19(04):287–290

Lund C, De Silva M, Plagerson S, Cooper S, Chisholm D, Das J, Patel V (2011) Poverty and mental disorders: breaking the cycle in low-income and middle-income countries. Lancet 378(9801):1502–1514

Mann JJ, Apter A, Bertolote J, Beautrais A, Currier D, Haas A et al. (2005) Suicide prevention strategies: a systematic review. Jama, 294(16):2064–2074

Marshall M, Crowther R, Almaraz-Serrano A, Creed F, Sledge W, Kluiter H, Tyrer P (2001) Systematic reviews of the effectiveness of day care for people with severe mental disorders: (1) acute day hospital versus admission;(2) vocational rehabilitation;(3) day hospital versus outpatient care. Health Technol Assess (Winchester, England) 5(21):1–75

Marshall M, Crowther R, Sledge WH, Rathbone J, Soares-Weiser K (2011) Day hospital versus admission for acute psychiatric disorders. Cochrane Database Syst Rev 12:CD004026

McCrone P, Killaspy H, Bebbington P, Johnson S, Nolan F, Pilling S, King M (2009) The REAct study: cost-effectiveness analysis of assertive community treatment in north London. Psychiatr Serv 60(7):908–913

Mosher LR (1999) Soteria and other alternatives to acute psychiatric hospitalization: a personal and professional review. J Nerv Ment Dis 187(3):142–149

Mubbashar M (1999) Mental health services in mental Pakistan. In: Tansella M, Thornicroft G (eds) Common mental disorders in primary carem. Routledge, London, pp 67–80

Murphy S, Irving CB, Adams CE, Driver R (2012) Crisis intervention for people with severe mental illnesses. Cochrane Database Syst Rev 5:CD001087

Ndyanabangi S, Basangwa D, Lutakome J, Mubiru C (2004) Uganda mental health country profile. Int Rev Psychiatry 16(1–2):54–62

Njega F (2002) Challenges of balanced care in Africa. World Psychiatry 1:96–98

Ormel J, Petukhova M, Chatterji S, Aguilar-Gaxiola S, Alonso J, Angermeyer MC, Kessler RC (2008) Disability and treatment of specific mental and physical disorders across the world. Br J Psychiatry 192(5):368–375

Patel V (2014) Vikram Patel talks with Denise Winn about practical ways to work towards mental health for all – and how the west can learn from developing countries. Hum Givens J 21(1): 28–33, Available at http://www.globalmentalhealth.org/sites/default/files/uploads/docs/Human%20Givens%20interview.pdf. Accessed 29 July 2014

Patel V, Kleinman A (2003) Poverty and common mental disorders in developing countries. Bull World Health Organ 81(8):609–615

Patel V, Prince M (2010) Global mental health: a new global health field comes of age. JAMA 303(19):1976–1977

Patel V, Saxena S (2014) Transforming lives, enhancing communities – innovations in global mental health. N Engl J Med 370(6):498–501

Patel V, Araya R, Chatterjee S, Chisholm D, Cohen A, De Silva M, van Ommeren M (2007) Treatment and prevention of mental disorders in low-income and middle-income countries. Lancet 370(9591):991–1005

Patel V, Boyce N, Collins PY, Saxena S, Horton R (2011) A renewed agenda for global mental health. Lancet 378(9801):1441–1442

Patel V, Kleinman A, Saraceno B (2012) Protecting the human rights of people with mental illnesses: a call to action for global mental health. In: Dudley M, Silove D, Gale F (eds) Mental health and human rights: vision, praxis, and courage. Oxford University Press, Oxford, pp 362–375

Power P, McGorry P (2011) Early interventions for people with psychotic disorders. In: Thornicroft G, Szmukler GI, Mueser KT, Drake RE (eds) Oxford textbook of community mental health. Oxford University Press, Oxford, pp 159–160

Priebe S, Warner R, Hubschmid T, Eckle I (1998) Employment, attitudes toward work, and quality of life among people with schizophrenia in three countries. Schizophr Bull 24(3):469–477

Prince M, Patel V, Saxena S, Maj M, Maselko J, Phillips MR, Rahman A (2007) No health without mental health. Lancet 370(9590):859–877

Rinaldi M, Perkins R (2007) Comparing employment outcomes for two vocational services: individual placement and support and non-integrated pre-vocational services in the UK. J Vocat Rehabil 27(1):21–27

Saraceno B (2014) Discorso globale, sofferenze locali. Analisi critica del Movimento di salute mental globale. il Saggiatore, Milano

Saraceno B, van Ommeren M, Batniji R, Cohen A, Gureje O, Mahoney J, Underhill C (2007) Barriers to improvement of mental health services in low-income and middle-income countries. Lancet 370(9593):164–1174

Saxena S, Maulik P (2003) Mental health services in low and middle income countries: an overview. Curr Opin Psychiatry 16:437–442

Saxena S, Thornicroft G, Knapp M, Whiteford H (2007) Resources for mental health: scarcity, inequity, and inefficiency. Lancet 370(9590):878–889

Sederer L (2010) Inpatient psychiatry: why do we need it? Epidemiol Psichiatr Soc 19:291–295

Skapinakis P, Bellos S, Koupidis S, Grammatikopoulos I, Theodorakis PN, Mavreas V (2013) Prevalence and sociodemographic associations of common mental disorders in a nationally representative sample of the general population of Greece. BMC Psychiatry 13(1):163

Sledge WH, Tebes J, Rakfeldt J, Davidson L, Lyons L, Druss B (1996a) Day hospital/crisis respite care versus inpatient care: I. Clinical outcomes. Am J Psychiatry 153:1065–1073

Sledge WH, Tebes J, Wolff N, Helminiak TW (1996b) Day hospital/crisis respite care versus inpatient care, part II: service utilization and costs. Am J Psychiatry 153(8):1074–1083

Solar O, Irwin A (2007) A conceptual framework for action on the social determinants of health. Available at http://whqlibdoc.who.int/publications/2010/9789241500852_eng.pdf. Accessed 29 July 2014

Stewart KA, Keusch GT, Kleinman A (2010) Values and moral experience in global health: bridging the local and the global. Glob Public Health 5(2):115–121

Stylianidis S, Peppou L, Drakonakis N (2014) Ethical and deontological issues relating to forced psychiatric hospitalisation. In: Douzenis A, Lykoura L (eds) Ethics and deontology in mental health. VITA Medical Press, Athens, in Greek

Susser E, Schwarz S, Morabia A, Bromet EJ, Begg MD, Gorman JM, King MCC (2006) Psychiatric epidemiology: searching for the causes of mental disorders. Oxford University Press, Oxford

Teague GB, Bond GR, Drake RE (1998) Program fidelity in assertive community treatment: development and use of a measure. Am J Orthopsychiatry 68:216–232

The Hellenic Ombudsman (2007) Ex Officio investigation by the independent authority, the Hellenic Ombudsman into involuntary hospitalisation of mental patients. Special Publication. Available at http://www.synigoros.gr/reports/Eidiki_Ekthesi_Akousia_Nosileia_17.5.07.pdf. Accessed on 28 July 2014 (in Greek)

Thornicroft G, Tansella M (2013) The balanced care model for global mental health. Psychol Med 43(04):849–863

Totman J, Mann F, Johnson S (2010) Is locating acute wards in the general hospital an essential element in psychiatric reform? The UK experience. Epidemiol Psichiatr Soc 19:282–286

World Bank (2010) World bank list of economies (http://data.worldbank.org/about/country-classifications). World Bank, Washington, DC

World Health Organization (WHO) (2001) The world health report: 2001: mental health: new understanding, new hope. WHO Press, Geneva

World Health Organization (WHO) (2003) Investing in mental health. WHO Press, Geneva

World Health Organization (WHO) (2005) Mental health atlas. WHO Press, Geneva, Revised Edition

World Health Organization (WHO) (2008a) The global burden of disease: 2004 update. WHO Press, Geneva

World Health Organization (WHO) (2008b) mhGAP. Mental Health Gap Action Programme: scaling up care for mental, neurological, and substance use disorders. WHO Press, Geneva

World Health Organization (WHO) (2010) Mental Health Gap Action Programme. mhGAP intervention guide for mental, neurological and substance use disorders in non-specialized health settings. WHO Press, Geneva

World Health Organization (WHO) (2011) Impact of financial crises on mental health. Available at http://www.euro.who.int/__data/assets/pdf_file/0008/134999/e94837.pdf. Accessed 29 July 2014

World Health Organization (WHO) (2013) Comprehensive mental health action plan 2013–2020. Available at http://apps.who.int/gb/ebwha/pdf_files/WHA66/A66_R8-en.pdf?ua=1. Accessed 28 July 2014

World Health Organization (WHO) (2014) Social determinants of mental health. Available at http://apps.who.int/iris/bitstream/10665/112828/1/9789241506809_eng.pdf. Accessed 29 July 2014

Psychiatric Reform in Greece

Panagiotis Chondros and Stelios Stylianidis

Abstract

This chapter presents the attempts to reform psychiatric services in Greece by making extensive reference to the historical-statutory framework, current conditions and the ethical basis of the change being attempted. It presents the achievements made and analyses the problems being faced. It includes information about the legislation and the rate at which structures have been developed. In the context of social psychiatry principles, reform is viewed from the following perspective: reform must seek to achieve a new form of psychiatric care which promotes tolerance of diversity and social integration by developing mental health networks and other forms of social networks. The discussion outlines factors which will assist in improving psychiatric care and raises questions that must concern stakeholders in the reform.

5.1 Introduction

The reform of psychiatric services in Greece is considered to be one of the most wide-ranging attempts at reform in Greece compared to reforms in other sectors, such as the education system or primary healthcare. Despite conflicting views, we cannot overlook the sheer duration of legislative, institutional and organisational changes which have occurred, the abolition of old organisations and the creation of new structures and workplaces.

P. Chondros (✉)
Association for Regional Development and Mental Health EPAPSY, Athens, Greece
e-mail: pan_ch@otenet.gr

S. Stylianidis
Department of Psychology, Panteion University, Athens, Greece
e-mail: stylianidis.st@gmail.com

© Springer International Publishing Switzerland 2016
S. Stylianidis (ed.), *Social and Community Psychiatry: Towards a Critical, Patient-Oriented Approach*, DOI 10.1007/978-3-319-28616-7_5

There has been extensive discussion about the reform philosophy, the degree to which targets have been achieved, as well as the completion of individual phases of the reform process. The problems (like the achievements) have been recorded to a satisfactory degree (Sakellis 2009, 2012; Ministry of Health and Social Security 2010, 2012; Deliverables for the project 'Evaluation of ongoing implementation of the National Action Plan' PSYCHARGOS; Stylianidis and Chondros 2011, 2012). The discourse which has emerged among direct stakeholders takes four very specific forms:

(a) The discourse which downplays reform efforts, transforming them from a complex scientific, social and organisational issues into a administrative issue.
(b) The discourse which expresses a strict, inflexible biomedical model, reflective of a conservative ideology, with emphases on strict evidence-based treatment and the issue of safety.
(c) The dogmatic left-wing discourse about liberation from mainstream psychiatric ideology that lacks any real scientific arguments, which results in a form of nihilism along the lines of "all or nothing", "all NGOs are forces for privatisation", "the EU doesn't help with reforms but only with driving home neoliberal policies" and so on.
(d) An alternative reform-based discourse derived from left-wing, social-democratic ideology which has become associated with the entire incomplete reform effort in Greece.

In the context of social psychiatry principles, reform is viewed from the following perspective: reform must seek to achieve a new form of psychiatric care which bolsters tolerance of diversity and social integration by developing mental health networks and other forms of social networks (Stylianidis and Chondros 2008). It must be psychiatric care of the subject, for the subject, involving the subject. As a break from both asylum-based culture and the biomedical model which classifies symptoms, it proposes biological treatments, downplaying emotional and mental communication, while promoting the attribution of meaning to suffering and the ability of new mental health professionals to feel empathy. Patel et al. (2006: 1315) succinctly put it as follows: "We believe that our ultimate professional goal as mental health professionals in a globalized world is to secure a reasonable opportunity for people with mental disorders to achieve better health outcomes. We already have the evidence we need to make the case for international mental health". The change in psychopathology, self-stigmatism among patients and mental function goes beyond the individual level and is directly associated with the reproduction of policies to counter social inequalities and market cynicism, by transforming social pain, fear, withdrawal and passivisation of the population into new networks and forms of solidarity, creativity and questioning of our role as "technicians" of psychiatric care (Basaglia 1982).

5.2 Historical: Institutional Framework

In the Greek healthcare system, the National Health System (NHS) (introduced in 1983) coexists with mandatory social security and a voluntary and the private health insurance system. It provides universal coverage of the population since it is based

Table 5.1 Selected data about resources in the health sector in Greece

National health spending	9,0 as a % of GDP (2006)
% of public health spending out of total spending	62.8 % (2005)
% of national budget set aside for mental health	None (2005)
Persons practising medicine	5 per 1,000 people (2005)
Hospital clinics	4,7 per 1,000 people (2005)

(From: Tountas (2008))

on the principles of equality, equal access to services for all and social cohesion. Private psychiatric clinics are regulated by two different laws, depending on the year in which they were founded (Law 235/2000, which has been suspended, and Law 517/1991), which lay down different operating requirements, thereby creating a serious institutional problem.

The health system has undergone continuous reform in terms of primary healthcare, regional administration, decentralisation, organisation and financing of hospital care (Table 5.1).

The process of psychiatric reform was given operational form when the PSYCHARGOS programme was established (Constantopoulos and Yiannoulatos 2004; Madianos 1994). It is important to stress that except from a few cases (such as the Direct Support Programme for the Dromokaitio Psychiatric Hospital in 2000), the development and operation of units specified in Regulation (EEC) No 815/1984 and thereafter and in the PSYCHARGOS programme were funded in part by the European Union (up to 75 % for a kick start, i.e. infrastructure and equipment and running costs for 1 or 1.5 years). One result of this, inter alia, was an emphasis on commitments to implement projects by applying agreed protocols specifically outlined in various operational programmes (combating exclusion from the labour market, health-welfare Programmes) rather than an emphasis on ensuring the maturity of stakeholders in psychiatric care to allow them to adopt and promote reform. The results of this special situation are numerous (and need to be documented). Among other things, one could include the quality of the units which were founded (under pressure of compliance with time frames) and the reactions and prejudices that led to certain of them not being allowed to open and operate.

A key turning point in how services are organised was Law 2716/1999 *on the development of mental health services and other provisions*, while another is the segregation of Greece into sectors (sectorisation) and the establishment of sectoral mental health committees which had to operate in accordance with the provisions of the law. The country has been divided into mental health sectors, with each prefecture forming a sector, except several prefectures with low populations which are placed in a sector along with another adjacent, more populous prefecture. Other exceptions were the prefectures of Attica and Thessaloniki, which are divided into several sectors, with additional specialist sectors for children and adolescents. Sectoral mental health committees have been set up nationwide, and all sectoral children and adolescent mental health committees have also been set up.

What is worth noting is that both the enactment of Law 2716/1999 (which is the first time a separate piece of legislation on mental health was enacted) and sectorisation were obligations Greece had made to the EU, rather than the result of major internal processes. Numerous articles of Law 2071/1992 relate to defending the rights of mental patients and the harmonisation of Greece's legal framework on psychiatric practice with modern scientific achievements. For those very reasons, it is a major turning point. Law 4074/2014 will also play a key role in the development of the legal and institutional framework. It was via this legislation that Greece ratified the Convention on the Rights of Persons with Disability (CRPD) and the Optional Protocol. That law, which has superior effect since it ratifies an international convention, addresses issues such as the ability to deprive someone of their freedom and therefore the involuntary hospitalisation of persons with disability, the involvement of persons with disability in decision-making and monitoring and the option to report violations of the rights of individuals with mental or other forms of disability. Table 5.2 sets out the texts which shape the legal framework for mental health services and mental healthcare in Greece.

Table 5.2 Legal framework for mental health and care services in Greece

Text	Description
Law 1397/1983	*National Health System, Government Gazette 143/A/7.10.1983*
	Introduced the right to health to the Greek legal system for the first time
Law 2071/1992	*Modernisation and organisation of the health system, Government Gazette 123/A/15.7.1992*
	Introduced mental health units and reformed the rules on involuntary hospitalisation
Law 2519/1997	*Development and modernisation of the NHS, organisation of health services, reforms pertaining of medicines and other provisions, Government Gazette 165/A/21.8.1997*
Law 2716/1999	*Development and modernisation of mental health services and other provisions, Government Gazette 96/A/17.5.1999*
Law 2447/1996	The concept of "judicial assistance" was introduced
Ministerial Decision No. A3α/οικ876/16-5-2000	Method for organising and running psychosocial rehabilitation units (boarding houses, hostels) and sheltered accommodation schemes pursuant to Article 9 of law 2716/1999, Government Gazette 661/B/23.5.2000
Ministerial Decision No. Υ5β/Γ.Π. οικ. 156618/ 25.11.2009	Method for organising and running daycare centres pursuant to Article 8 of Law 2716/1999, Government Gazette 2444/B/2009
Ministerial Decision No. Υ5β/οικ1662/21.5.2001	Method for running and staffing mobile mental health units pursuant to Article 7 of Law 2716/1999, Government Gazette 691/B/2001
Law 3418/2005	*Code of Medical Ethics (2005) Article 28*
	The framework for mental healthcare which the doctor is obliged to provide to his patient, Government Gazette 287/A/28.11.2005
Law 4072/2012	Ratification of the Convention on the Rights of Persons with Disability and the Optional Protocol to the Convention on the Rights of Persons with Disability, Government Gazette 88/A/11.4.2012

Other milestones in the reform process were the agreements between the European Commission and the Ministry of Health reached in 2009 and 2013. The first agreement has become known as the Spidla Agreement (from the name of the competent Social Affairs Commissioner who signed it) and was the result of institutional, administrative and economic problems which accumulated during implementation of the goals of the PSYCHARGOS programme and the consequent pressure exerted by various bodies on the Ministry of Health and above all by the Hellenic Ombudsman for Health and Social Protection. That pact specified the need for continuation of psychiatric reform and identified specific measures: the creation of a team of international independent experts, certification and licensing of all mental health structures operated by bodies governed by private law, the conclusion of agreements between the Ministry of Health and all stakeholders, secure financing, support for the social cooperatives and others. The relevant agreements must include the following as a minimum: quality standards for the services offered, costing data for the services depending on the type of services, as well as monitoring, evaluation and financial auditing criteria and procedures. The second was an update of the first and included a time frame for implementing the pact.

The key principles in the action plan for implementing the MoU are:

(a) The new system to be in place from January 1, 2016 must be sustainable and provide quality services which reflect the real needs of beneficiaries.
(b) Common operating standards must be adopted for all mental health units, irrespective of their legal format.
(c) Targets must be realistic, placing emphasis on financing interventions based on measureable results.
(d) Interventions must be comprehensive and cohesive, to ensure multiplier effects.
(e) The Ministry of Health must finance the specialised/individual needs of beneficiaries on the basis of cost per beneficiary and the type of mental health unit.
(f) The new system must be the product of consultation with stakeholders.

The first major developments in the field of social-community psychiatry in Greece date from the 1970s. In terms of service provision, the Mental Health Centre opened in Athens in 1956, and in 1972 the first daycare centre opened in Thessaloniki, in 1978 the first daycare hospital opened at the Aeginitio Hospital, in 1979 the Vyronas-Kessariani Community Mental Health Centre opened and in 1981 the Prefecture of Fokida began offering mobile mental health services. Negative developments in Greece were the establishment of the Leros Psychopaths Colony in 1958 and the Paedopsychiatric Hospital in 1959 (Public Paedopsychiatric-Neuropsychiatric Hospital with a 350-bed capacity, which was renamed the Attica Paedopsychiatric Hospital in 1986). From the mid-1970s, criticism about traditional psychiatry began to emerge in Greece, and groups to support psychiatric patients locked up in asylums were formed. At the same time, small organised groups/movements relating to the rights of mental patients appeared, but had no major ideological influence on the development of psychiatry, compared to similar movements in Western Europe. One move in this context was the Hellenic-French Social Psychiatry

Symposium (Lebovici and Sakellaropoulos 1984) held in 1981, at which criticism of traditional psychiatry and the asylum culture which was radical for its time was heard, and a working group was set up to take measures against the asylum on Leros and other asylums in Greece. In general terms, up to 1981 there was a significant lag in how psychiatry developed in Greece compared to other European countries (Madianos et al. 1999; Stylianidis et al. 2007; Ploumpidis 2009).

5.3 Regulation (EEC) No 815/84

When emergency financial aid from the former EEC was introduced (Regulation (EEC) No 815/84), Greece was the only case of direct financing to a member state: the process of deinstitutionalisation began, improvements to hospital care were made, preparations for shifting patients to protected or relatively autonomous homes in the community were made and new, socially focused mental health services were developed (Tsiantis 2004; Madianos 2005; Karastergiou et al. 2005).

As far as structures and services were concerned, the goal was to "develop a complete network of community services to ensure at a healthcare region level (mental health sector) operational capacity in terms of the needs of the local population, a goal which is clearly wider than treating illness" (Ministry of Health and Welfare 2001). At the level of service units, particular emphasis was placed on developing psychiatric departments at general hospitals and mental health centres, while on the other hand the burden fell on developing outpatient psychosocial rehabilitation units (hostels, boarding houses, sheltered accommodation) capable of housing a large number of chronic patients who had been locked up in psychiatric hospitals.

The new units also needed a wide range of mental health professionals in various areas of specialisation and a person-centre approach by those professionals towards the mental patient. For that reason, the necessity of major changes "in the training and life-long education of mental health professionals, and the know-how transfer procedures" was officially recognised (op. cit.). From the moment the system had to have a social focus, it was recognised too that "support for local communities and authorities, overcoming fear about mental illness which has shaped prejudice and stereotypes [is a condition] for gradually eliminating the social stigma associated with mental patients and their families, and comprehensive social support and solidarity towards mental patients must be a national priority" (op. cit.).

In short, the goals laid down for achieving psychiatric reform were:

To develop infrastructure and structures based on the principles of sectorisation and social psychiatry and to ensure the continuity of psychiatric care
Deinstitutionalisation, psychosocial rehabilitation and social reintegration for chronic patients in psychiatric hospitals
Ensuring full adequacy in terms of primary healthcare, outpatient care and hospital care at general hospitals

Developing mental health services to prevent, diagnose, treat and care for patients and to ensure psychosocial rehabilitation and social inclusion of persons with autism spectrum disorders and learning problems

To develop preventative and direct crisis intervention actions for users of addictive substances

5.4 Current Data

In Greece, the lack of epidemiological data remains a key problem. Until recently, in fact until the Panhellenic Adult Psychopathology Study was conducted by the University Psychiatric Clinic of the University of Ioannina (2009–2010) for the Ministry of Health (Skapinakis et al. 2013), there were few studies on the prevalence of mental disorders in the general population and those that existed primarily related to urban environments and limited geographic areas.

Older surveys have shown that 16 % of the general population in Greece suffers from some form of mental disorder (Mavreas et al. 1986), while women, widows and individuals in lower socioeconomic brackets have higher rates of psychiatric morbidity. In one epidemiological survey in the general population carried out in Evia, it was found that 29 % suffered from at least one mental disorder (Stylianidis and Stylianoudi 2008; Stylianidis et al. 2014), while a similar survey carried out in the general population on Paros-Antiparos in 2008 on a sample of 506 individuals showed that 22 % of the sample had clinically significant morbidity (Stylianidis et al. 2010). Women had significantly higher morbidity than men (30 % compared to 13 %). The prevalence of depression in women was 7.88 % compared to just 1.14 % in men. Harmful alcohol use was found to be 13.06 % and 23.86 % in men and 3 % in women. Another epidemiological survey in Greece carried out on the general population in rural communities in the northern Aegean, on a sample of 428 people, showed that 14 % of the population had some psychiatric symptoms, while women had almost twice the likelihood of men of presenting some psychiatric symptom (Skapinakis et al. 2007).

According to more recent epidemiological data (Skapinakis et al. 2013), 1 in 6 Greeks aged 18–70 have developed clinically significant psychopathology and 1 in 12 (600,000) have serious psychopathology. International data showing that in Greece 75 % of the population with some form of psychopathology do not receive any treatment for their problem have been confirmed. In addition, the suicide rate has risen from 2.8 per 100,000 in 2008 to 5.2 in 2010 (Giotakos et al. 2011; Economou et al. 2013). As far as adolescents are concerned, research data confirm that mental disorders, dominated by depression, affect 3–8 % of the population and are directly related with negative health behaviours such as smoking, use of psychotropic substances and alcohol abuse and with reduced performance at school, poor social relations, bullying, high-risk sexual behaviour and even suicidal tendencies (Giannakopoulos et al. 2009). A study conducted on Greek adolescents found that the rate of attempted suicide in 2007 was 13.4 % of the population (Kokkevi et al. 2010). According to a survey conducted by the National School of Public Health

(Zavras et al. 2012), between 2006 and 2011 an increase was noted in the use of both antipsychotics (+18/59 %) and antidepressants (+34.80 %). Hospital treatments have also increased significantly (24 %), while there has also been a constant drop in the use of private health services (Kentikelenis et al. 2011). See the relevant chapter for a detailed presentation of the epidemiological data.

The next key indicators of the rate of reform are the rate of change in psychiatric beds in use and the way in which they are allocated between hospitals and social care structures. In 2001, 49 % of psychiatric beds were in psychiatric hospitals, compared to 99 % in 1982. More specifically, 3 % were at general hospitals, 50 % remained in psychiatric hospitals and 47 % were in social structures (psychosocial rehabilitation centres) (Amaddeo et al. 2007: p. 237). In terms of the total number of psychiatric beds (irrespective of where they are located) per 100,000 people, Greece is close to the European average (10.2) at 8.7. There were 8,486 psychiatric beds in public psychiatric hospitals between 1981 and 1982, 5,007 in 1996 and 3,500 in 2000 (Stylianidis et al. 2009).

As far as all structures are concerned, in 2008 there were 410 accommodation facilities in operation (irrespective of the programme during which they were developed) designed to promote deinstitutionalisation, along with more than 180 community mental health structures and 14 social cooperatives (Stylianidis et al. 2009). The number of chronic patients in public hospitals in the 2-year period 1981–1983 was 5,677 but by the year 2000 that figure had dropped to 2,922 (Madianos 2005; Tountas 2008). Between 2001 and 2009 as part of phase II of the PSYCHARGOS programme, four of the nine psychiatric hospitals were shut down. As a result of the deinstitutionalisation programme, the number of mental patients living in 452 psychosocial rehabilitation centres stood at 2,689 in 2009 (1,289 patients in 2002 in 146 psychosocial rehabilitation centres), while the number of long-term patients being treated in psychiatric hospitals was below 2,000. In 2013 that figure had dropped further; however, there is a lack of updated data. Compared to the targets set in the National Plan for Psychiatric Reform (PSYCHARGOS), by 2008 78 % of the necessary accommodation structures had been completed, but only 28 % social mental health structures were in place (138 were missing) (these included psychiatric departments at general hospitals for adults and children, mental health centres, daycare centres, mobile units, short-stay hostels), and only 20 % of the 55 specialist structures for alcohol, substance dependence, autism and Alzheimer's disease were in existence (Stylianidis et al. 2009; Stylianidis and Chondros 2010).

A key fact that needs to be mentioned is the major increase in committals on orders from Public Prosecutors. The psychiatric reform committee of the Hellenic Psychiatric Association (2008) conducted research for 2 years and concluded in its report that in Greece there was a high rate of committals on orders from Public Prosecutors. In 2007 the Attica Psychiatric Hospital accepted 2,900 admissions, 52 % of which were involuntary, the Attica Dromokaitio Psychiatric Hospital had 1,554 admissions (50.2 % were involuntary) and the Thessaloniki Psychiatric Hospital had 3,770 admissions (28.9 % were involuntary). As the Committee pointed out, those high rates are fictitious to a large degree since recourse to use of Public Prosecutor orders is often abused to ensure a bed, which is otherwise hard to find in the public psychiatric system. However, it is a strong indication that both the mental health system and the welfare network in Greece are malfunctioning (Stylianidis et al. 2009). (See the relevant chapter on the issue of involuntary hospitalisation.)

In short, over the least three decades, some steps have been taken to improve and develop mental health services (Stylianidis et al. 2009):

Law 2716/1999 was enacted, which is a quite comprehensive framework law, which placed the development of community services on the Greek policy agenda.
The percentage of beds in psychiatric hospitals (out of all psychiatric beds) was reduced by almost half.
A large number of young professionals acquired initial training and practical experience in community settings, which is the start of a change in the model used to provide psychiatric care.
Examples of good practice at community level emerged, thanks to efforts to implement the principles of social psychiatric and provide comprehensive coverage for the local population.

However we cannot in any sense talk about a successful reform process since the problems at structural level and at the level of day-to-day functionality remain numerous and critical.

5.5 Problems with Reforming the Mental Health System

Stakeholders in the field (professionals, administrators, caregivers and above all patients) face shortages and policy contradictions in the entire psychiatric system despite the need for the adoption of rational rules and procedures to ensure a positive outcome for the reform process.

More specifically, one key mistake is the fragmentation of the system and the unequal allocation of services. Mental health services are provided by the NHS (psychiatric hospitals, general hospitals and various bodies governed by private law), the private sector, social security organisations such as the IKA social security fund, local government agencies, military agencies, the Ministry of Education and the Church. It is only logical that the lack of central co-ordination and the inability to attribute responsibility create an ineffective, non-accessible and costly system (Thornicroft and Tansella 2010).

The condition of political support for reform in effect came from "outside", from the officials and control mechanisms of the European Commission following international stigmatism of Greece when the international community "uncovered" the scandal on Leros (1988). To the extent that the demand for reform did not come as a social mandate backed by a wide-scale movement, but as a change imposed by others, the entire venture was only supported by a small minority of mental health professionals, who frequently face indifference, ambivalence or even outright hostility from trade unions in the sector. Experts with various different professional and institutional roles in the psychiatric sector have reached this conclusion about the key reasons for failure of reform, namely, lack of any social movement to support the philosophy underpinning the reform process (Madianos 2009; Stylianidis 2009; Megaloeconomou 2005; Sakellis 2009; Chondros 2009).

The basic requirements to support a movement for mental health are missing. There have been no collective demands for specific goals to be achieved. Only in the last 5 years have different activities been organised to support the reform process, such as demonstrations, meetings, official communication with the authorities and relevant documentation. The key elements of a movement are also missing (Tilly 2007), such as unity, involvement of a satisfactory number of individuals and long-term, systematic commitment from participants in the movement.

Another key mistake in how the reform was planned, which is frequently encountered in other similar experiences (Maj 2010), is that the provision of care and the way in which services are organised have been closely tied into ideological and political frameworks. The logic of party politics and vested interests and the prevailing culture of informal networks of corruption and intertwined interest for the two main political parties from the time of Greece's return to democracy after the dictatorship to the present day have resulted in the irrational use of resources without any targeting or any evaluation – monitoring of the actions taken. That led to a series of negative effects: it actually negated the expertise and continuous training of the human resources so vital for reform, there was resistance to adequate national resources being used (apart from financing from the EU), there was resistance to epidemiological studies in the general population and studies about how services operated and could be adjusted to the changing mental health needs of the population, guidelines for how services could operate properly were not adopted, and consequently there was no systematic monitoring and evaluation of services, and there was opposition to promote a culture of synergy, networking and complementary activities by the bodies involved at social level (Stylianidis 2009; Stylianidis and Chondros 2010).

The ethical and deontological basis of the changes attempted remained loose for a long time, to the extent that any official annual reports of the independent authorities responsible for protecting the rights of mental patients were not acted upon, neglected by the Ministry of Health. Another barrier to real change was the failure to implement existing legislation on mental health (Laws 2071/1992 and 2716/1999) [perhaps the most progressive legislative intervention in the post-dictatorship period that the lack of policy plan and the weakness of the reform movement turned it to yet another piece of legislation that remained inactive]. Another barrier was the failure to implement the sectorisation principle which only seemed to concern the Greek state when it had to manage complaints from international organisations about human rights violations. Note also that advocacy and empowerment of families and users of mental health services is perhaps considered a marginal activity for almost all the scientific community and is used more as a "democratic alibi" more than as a necessary form of ethical and scientific documentation of psychiatric practice. The increase in psychiatric treatments on the basis of Public Prosecutor orders, which is over 53 % of all admissions to psychiatric departments or hospitals, is scandalous. All this data paints a rather grim picture of a period of 20 years of precarious reform (1989–2010).

5.6 Discussion

Firstly, one needs to be careful about the expectation of purely technocratic resolution of particularly complex problems faced by the endeavour to change psychiatric care in Greece, given that we need to have a serious reflection on the conditions required for wide-ranging restructuring of the system which is needed in order to ensure that any reform effort is viable.

Key questions which arise are as follows: How can a modern state respond within the context of the globalisation of markets, to immense needs and new demands for health, mental health and social care which come from new emerging, socially excluded social groups, when its policy is dictated by a hostile neoliberal framework that promotes aggressive, lawless entrepreneurialism? How can the continuation and support for collapsing psychiatric reform and a holistic approach to the needs of individuals with severe mental disorders be propped up? How can this be done especially when innovative experiences of social entrepreneurship and pilot best practices with a positive cost-benefit result in terms of the social reintegration of vulnerable population groups are not being supported in political and financial terms? How can a new, valuable social and cultural movement emerge in Greece against the background of the growing capitalistic void, the rise of profit, unrestrained competition, egoism, individualism, illegality and the alienations of people's conscience, to retain a fluid, unsecure job, faced with the paralysing fear of threatened long-term unemployment?

A prerequisite for any new plans for changes in the mental health sector continues to be real interest by players in the sector in meeting the actual patient. Meetings must take place under the best possible actual, institutional and organisational conditions for services and be focused on understanding the psychopathology of the *Other*, on attempting to build together a new narrative about the mental disorder between the parties involved, in other words the patient and his family and the mental health professional, and the multidisciplinary treatment group he belongs to. Moreover, the logic around which new mental health services are organised cannot only be governed by administrative and quantitative criteria; instead mental health groups must be able to pose themselves continuous questions and adjust the treatment and care responses to the complex dialectic of needs, available resources and complex answers (Rotelli 1988).

The steps required have been examined and evaluated in practical terms in various health systems with different degrees of resource availability and varying social conditions. Thornicroft and Tansella (2010) provide us with an overview of how we can improve mental healthcare at local, regional and national level. Taking into account the special historical, social and political conditions, as well as the major objections to psychiatric reform taking place, we propose the following guidelines and plans of action for better mental health in Greece (Stylianidis and Chondros 2010):

- A public health perspective must be adopted along with a strategy for the entire population, a strategy which will tie treatment, holistic care and psychosocial rehabilitation together and will integrate all psychotherapeutic techniques and models into an individualised care plan for each patient.
- The gradual transfer of resources (financial and human resources) from institutional care to the community requires that institutional structures be completely replaced by an alternative network of community mental health structures. Preserving the present-day parallel system of institutional and community care for a period of two decades has not only been financially disastrous for the national budget, but has created confusing, conflicting messages about the entire reform effort. Funding for new services and support for existing ones must be tied into the achievement of objectives by each service based on evaluations. Planning effective services in the context of the economical crisis which requires constant cuts is feasible, provided it is accompanied by radical, innovative practices (McDaid and Knapp 2010). The attempt to abolish asylums cannot, of course, be taken to the other extreme of unplanned and hasty closure of structures (based on other political or fiscal interests) in a manner which could be characterised as *violent* on a political, social and organisational level.
- An updated national strategic plan for mental health needs to be drafted and prepared. Greece's emphasis must be on the concept of updating the plan (i.e. regularly reviewing the plan) via procedures that do not allow doubt regarding the work of all persons involved in drafting the plan.
- Statutorily mandated, real involvement by associations, families and users of mental health services in the planning, running and evaluation of mental health services is needed. Support for organised actions to empower those associations is needed.
- Regular epidemiological studies must be carried out on the general population and services to investigate the population's changing mental health needs and how services operate and their effectiveness. These studies must not merely be published in scientific journals but must be tools for changing and improving the day-to-day care offered by services.
- A system for monitoring and externally evaluating services must be put in place. The objective must be to operate a system of co-ordinated services.
- A new type of training for staff in services must be introduced, involving universities and other educational institutions (medical schools, psychology departments, social work schools, nursing schools, technological educational institutes, etc.) focused on modern aspects of social psychiatry and public health.
- Targeted actions are needed to educate the public about mental health and promote mental health issues (to combat the stigma of mental disease, prejudice, social exclusion) with a start, middle, end and a predefined evaluation method.

A policy of networking mental health services with primary healthcare and welfare in the context of the sectorisation.

Evidence-based best practices (psychosocial rehabilitation, social entrepreneurship, crisis interventions, cooperation with primary healthcare) are needed to ensure the transfer and multiplier effect of innovation throughout the entire system of services.

Existing legislation needs to be implemented in relation to hospitalisation procedures on the orders of the Public Prosecutor, and sectorisation needs to be fully implemented for the entire range of the population.

The independent authority responsible for protecting the rights of mental patients needs to be supported, with more extensive powers, in close cooperation between the Ministry of Health, the Ministry of Justice and the Ombudsman.

Achieving all these objectives goes well beyond the current state of know-how in the sector. It requires real involvement, not merely as a matter of choice, but as a stance which as J. P Sartre stressed is a material part of the human state. It also requires a responsible stance to defend not only universal values but the fate of specific mentally vulnerable individuals and fellow citizens, whom we should be genuinely concerned about.

References

Amaddeo F, Becker T, Fioritti A, Burti L, Tansella M (2007) Reforms in community care: the balance between hospital and community-based mental health care. In: Knapp K, McDaid D, Mossialos E, Thornicroft G (eds) Mental health policy and practice across Europe. The future direction of mental health care. Open University Press, Berkshire, pp 235–249

Basaglia F (1982) Crimini di pace. In: Scritti II 1968–1980. Einaudi, Torino, pp 237–338

Chondros D (2009) Lasting problems of psychiatric reform and actions planned under the National Structural Reform Plan 2007–2013. In: Sakellis G (ed) Psychiatric reform in Greece: needs – proposals – solutions. Sakkoulas Press, Athens, pp 157–167 (in Greek)

Constantopoulos A, Yannoulatos P (2004) Greek psychiatric reform. In: Kyriopoulos J (ed) Health systems in the world. From evidence to policy. Papazisis Publishers, Athens, pp 525–549

Economou M, Madianos M, Peppou LE, Theleritis C, Patelakis A, Stefanis C (2013) Suicidal ideation and reported suicide attempts in Greece during the economic crisis. World Psychiatry 12(1):53–59

Giannakopoulos G, Dimitrakaki C, Pedeli X, Kolaitis G, Rotsika V, Ravens-Sieberer U, Tountas Y (2009) Adolescents' wellbeing and functioning: relationships with parents' subjective general physical and mental health. Health Qual Life Outcomes 7:100

Giotakos O, Karabelas D, Kafkas A (2011) Financial crisis and mental health in Greece. Psychiatriki 22:109–119

Karastergiou A, Mastrogianni A, Georgiadou E, Kotrotsios S, Mauratziotou K (2005) The reform of the Greek mental health services. J Ment Health 14(2):197–203

Kentikelenis A, Karanikolos M, Papanicolas I, Basu S, McKee M, Stuckler D (2011) Health effects of financial crisis: omens of a Greek tragedy. Lancet 378(9801):1457–1458

Kokkevi A, Rotsika V, Arapaki A, Richardson C (2010) Changes in associations between psychosocial factors and suicide attempts by adolescents in Greece from 1984 to 2007. Eur J Public Health 21:694–698

Lebovici S, Sakellaropoulos P (1984) Hellenic-Greece social psychiatry symposium. Kastaniotis Press, Athens

Madianos M (1994) Psychiatric reform and its development. From theory to action. Ellinika Grammata Press, Athens (in Greek)
Madianos M (2005) Psychiatry and rehabilitation. Kastaniotis Press, Athens (in Greek)
Madianos M (2009) Adventures in incomplete reform: from the case of Leros to 'PSYCHARGOS'. In: Sakellis G (ed) Psychiatric reform in Greece: needs – proposals – solutions. Sakkoulas Press, Athens, pp 11–24 (in Greek)
Madianos MG, Zacharakis C, Tsitsa C, Stefanis C (1999) The mental health care delivery system in Greece: regional variation and socioeconomic correlates. J Ment Health Policy Econ 2(4):169–176
Maj M (2010) Mistakes to avoid in the implementation of community mental health care. World Psychiatry 9(2):65–66
Mavreas VG, Beis A, Mouyias A, Rigoni F, Lyketsos GC (1986) Prevalence of psychiatric disorders in Athens. Soc Psychiatry 21(4):172–181
McDaid D, Knapp M (2010) Black-skies planning? Prioritising mental health services in times of austerity. Br J Psychiatry 196(6):423–424
Megaloeconomou T (2005) Deinstitutionalisation as a treatment. The problem of power, social control and emancipation in the psychiatric reform process. In the Athens Psychiatric Hospital Scientific Association (ed) Psychiatry notes: 20 years of struggle in the field of psychiatry and society. Special edition of Psychiatry Notes (in Greek). pp 69–78
Ministry of Health & Social Solidarity (2010) Report evaluating the interventions to implement psychiatric reform for the period 2000–2009: http://www.psychargos.gov.gr/Documents2/Ypostirixi%20Forewn/Ypostirixi%20EPISTHMONIKH/Ex%20Post%20%CE%A0%CE%91%CE%A1%CE%91%CE%94%CE%9F%CE%A4%CE%95%CE%9F%202%20Teliko.pdf. Accessed on 20 Jul 2014
Ministry of Health & Social Solidarity (2012) Report of the working group to revise the PSYCHARGOS Programme – PSYCHARGOS III National Action Plan (2011–2020). Ministry of Health and Social Security, Athens, Available at: http://www.psychargos.gov.gr/Documents2/%CE%9D%CE%95%CE%91/%CE%A8%CE%A5%CE%A7%CE%91%CE%A1%CE%93%CE%A9%CE%A3%20%CE%93'%20(2011–2020).pdf. Accessed on 31 July 2014
Ministry of Health & Welfare (2001) Psychargos 2001–2010, programme to develop mental health sector structures and infrastructure. Ministry of Health and Social Security, Athens
Patel V, Saraceno B, Kleinman A (2006) Beyond evidence: the moral case for international mental health. Am J Psychiatry 163(8):1312–1315
Ploumpidis D (2009) Evaluation of psychiatric reform in Greece. Synapsis J 15(5):22–28 (in Greek)
Psychiatric Reform Committee of the Hellenic psychiatric Association (2008) 2006–2008 report, Athens (in Greek)
Rotelli F (1988) L'istituzione inventata. Per la salute mentale/for mental health, Rivista Centro Regionale Studi e Ricerche sulla Salute Mentale, (1)
Sakellis G (2009) Psychiatric reform in Greece: needs – proposals – solutions. Workshop conclusions. In: Sakellis G (ed) Psychiatric reform in Greece: needs – proposals – solutions. Sakkoulas Press, Athens, pp 119–128 (in Greek)
Sakellis G (2012 March). The welfare state in crisis. In Stylianidis S, Ploumpidis D (eds) Proceedings of the Panhellenic conference on psychosocial rehabilitation. Main recommendation of the Panhellenic conference on psychosocial rehabilitation: what changes for what new needs. Association for Regional Development and Mental Health (in Greek), Athens, pp 30–39
Skapinakis P, Zisi A, Savvidou M, Tseloni M, Chiou M (2007) Prevalence and socio-demographic correlations of psychiatric morbidity in rural communities in the Northern Aegean Region. Greek Med Arch 24(1):30–36 (in Greek)
Skapinakis P, Bellos S, Koupidis S, Grammatikopoulos I, Theodorakis PN, Mavreas V (2013) Prevalence and sociodemographic associations of common mental disorders in a nationally representative sample of the general population of Greece. BMC Psychiatry 13(1):163
Stylianidis S (2009) Stigmatising psychiatric reform. In: Sakellis G (ed) Psychiatric reform in Greece: needs – proposals – solutions. Sakkoulas Press, Athens, pp 43–58 (in Greek)

Stylianidis S, Chondros P (2008) An alternative psychiatric approach to the concept of community and mental health networks. In: Stylianidis S, Lily Stylianoudi MG (eds) Community and psychiatric reform: the experience of Evia, 1998–2008. Topos Press, Athens, pp 215–230 (in Greek)

Stylianidis S, Chondros P (2010) Mental health care in Greece today: current situation and critical aspects of health policy and social policy. Mod Issues 111:102–108 (in Greek)

Stylianidis S, Chondros P (2011) Crise économique, crise de la réforme psychiatrique en Grèce: indice de déficit démocratique en Europe? Inf Psychiatr 87(8):625–627

Stylianidis S, Chondros P (2012) La réforme psychiatrique en Grèce: quelques remarques à propos de la précarité Actuelle causée par la crise. VST-Vie Soc Traitements 1:128–134

Stylianidis S, Lily Stylianoudi MG (eds) (2008) Community and psychiatric reform: the experience of Evia, 1998–2008. Topos Press, Athens (in Greek)

Stylianidis S, Theocharakis N, Chondros P (2007) The suspended step of psychiatric reform in Greece: a timeless approach featuring topical questions. Archaeol Arts 105:45–54 (in Greek)

Stylianidis S, Gionakis N, Chondros P (2009) Greek psychiatric reform viewed from the perspective of Italian reform experience. Synapsis J 15(5):28–44 (in Greek)

Stylianidis S, Skapianakis P, Pantelidou S, Chondros P, Avgoustakis A, Ziakoulis M (2010) Prevalence of common mental disorders in an island area: needs assessment and planning of mental health actions. Greek Med Arch 27(4):675–683 (in Greek)

Stylianidis S, Pantelidou S, Chondros P, Roelandt J, Barbato A (2014) Prevalence of mental disorders in a Greek island. Psychiatrike = Psychiatriki 25(1):19–26

Thornicroft G, Tansella M (2010) In: Stylianidis S (ed) For better mental health care. Topos Press, Athens (originally published in 2009)

Tilly C (2007) Social movements 1768–2004. Savalla Press, Athens

Tountas G (2008) Healthcare services. Odysseas – New Health, Athens (in Greek)

Tsiantis I (2004) The first years of psychiatric reform in Greece. In: Essays in honour of Prof. K. Stefanis – scientific and social career. Arsenidis Press (in Greek), Athens, pp 135–140

Zavras D, Tsiantou V, Pavi E, Mylona K, Kyriopoulos J (2012) Impact of economic crisis and other demographic and socio-economic factors on self-rated health in Greece. Eur J Publ Health cks143

Further Reading

Examples of best practice from Greece:

Angelidis G, Giaglis C (2011) Petras olympos psychiatric hospital: closure of long-term psychiatric treatment departments and the transformation of the hospital into a network of social psychiatric services. Dodoni Press, Thessaloniki (in Greek)

Sakellaropoulos P (ed) (2010) The emotional bond between the therapist and patient as the foundations of psychiatry. Papazisis Press, Athens (in Greek)

Stylianidis S, Ploumbidis D (ed) (2014) Psychosocial rehabilitation under conditions of economic crisis. What changes for what new needs. Proceedings of the conference from 30–31 March 2014, Athens (http://www.me-psyxi.gr/images/proceedings_of_wapr%201.pdf) (in Greek)

Tsiantis I (ed) (1995) Children at the Leros psychopaths colony. Kastaniotis Press, Athens (in Greek)

The Contribution of Psychoanalytical Thinking and Practice to Social Community Psychiatry

6

Michael A. Petrou

Abstract

This chapter examines the concept of "subject" and "subjectivity" in relation to mental pain in the context of the development of psychiatry and psychoanalysis. The issue of the "subject" of mental pain is of tremendous interest both for the clinician and the human sciences, because the history of subjectivity is intimately tied into the adventures of psychiatric approaches to mental illness from the end of the nineteenth century to the present day.

We then go on to present the stance of psychoanalytical thinking and practice within hospital structures, and outside of them, in other words in the community, using illustrative examples, and the major, important role psychoanalysis played in the move for psychiatric reform in the last decades of the twentieth century.

An attempt is then made to (a) highlight the ways in which psychoanalysis is present in psychiatric care structures and (b) determine the conditions for establishing a mental health structure governed by the principles of psychoanalytical thinking. One part of this chapter is dedicated to depicting the aspects of how such a structure could work.

Before the general discussion, we propose a series of conditions about how individual and social pain are connected, which was an issue of concern to Freud from as early as 1880s, and which today in a period of generalised crisis is particularly acute and challenging for clinical thinking and practice.

M.A. Petrou
Clin. Psychologist, Soc. Anthropologist and Psychoanalyst (IPA)3,
Alcimachou Street, 11634 Athens, Greece
e-mail: petrou.mic@gmail.com

© Springer International Publishing Switzerland 2016
S. Stylianidis (ed.), *Social and Community Psychiatry: Towards a Critical, Patient-Oriented Approach*, DOI 10.1007/978-3-319-28616-7_6

6.1 Introduction

In the pages which follow, we examine how psychoanalysis, as a way of thinking and practice, contributed to the movement for psychiatric reform which commenced after WWII, which culminated in America and Europe in the 1960s and 1970s and which finally saw the light of day in Greece in 1985.

Although the founding fathers of psychiatry, who focused on objective nosography, did not lose sight of the patient as the subject of their interest, they needed many decades before innovative psychiatrists more inspired by psychoanalysis would manage to release mental patients from the alienating shackles of the asylum and attempt to reintegrate them back into society where they belonged.

This chapter starts by examining the concept of "subject" and "subjectivity" in relation to mental pain, and using illustrative examples presents the position of psychoanalysis within hospital structures, and outside of them, which is to say in the community. It then goes on to present psychoanalysis' contribution to the transformation of psychiatric asylums into primary and secondary care facilities for mental patients and ends with a set of conditions for connecting individual and social pain together.

6.2 Subject, Subjectivity and Mental Pain: The Subject of Mental Pain

Every culture, every society and every professional group have their own myths. As far as psychiatry is concerned, tradition has it that the doctor Philippe Pinel sets inmates at the Salpêtrière Asylum in the revolutionary Paris of 1795 free of their chains. The scene with Tony Robert-Fleury captured for all time in his famous painting shows one of the founding myths of social-community psychiatry.

During the early years of the modern period, madness had been transformed into a mental illness and had become firmly locked into the world of clinical medicine, as the classic works of Michel Foucault (1963, 1964) have shown: centuries-old madness became medicalised and the mad were locked up in medical institutions, hidden away for many decades in asylums. This final link resulted in perceptions and practices relevant to mental illness following the dominant medical standard in each case; today, for example, mental illness is suffocating within the narrow straits of pure biological and behavioural medicine within the biomedical model, an approach where the patient and his experience of pain are in effect absent.

On the contrary, the Age of Enlightenment placed man, thirsty for boundless knowledge and constant progress, at the centre of its interest: the being endowed with abilities, the producer of thoughts and deed who speaks in his own name, who wants self-determination, the being called the "subject".

The so-called human sciences, including psychoanalysis, derive from Enlightenment concerns, and their development has been marked by the refutation of the claims it made as modern history has unfolded.

Pinel's legendary gesture, so-called traitement moral which he developed, inspired by the practices of the hospital superintendant, and the no restraint idea of Englishman William Tuke were archetypal standards for dealing with the mentally ill, as mental patients were then called, in human and social terms. Even mental patients were entitled to participate in the revolutionary ideal of liberty, equality and fraternity.

Exactly one century later, the nosographical works of the founders of modern psychiatry Emil Kraepelin and Eugen Bleuler, and then of Karl Jaspers and Eugene Minkowski, took a phenomenological approach and are marked by a laborious effort to describe and classify psychoses and emotional disorders based on objective clinical criteria. Even through this insistence on objectivity, the subject is present in clinical practice. Mental patients are not just the object of the social practice charged with managing them, which was named psychiatry. They are, like every individual, subject to desires, knowledge, feelings and forms of behaviour, part of society as a whole and carriers of civilisation, just like their doctors, who together developed a special "social relationship" (Pouillon 1970, p. 77) which has been restrictively named "treatment".

At that same time, for Sigmund Freud, subjectivity became the central clinical issue and the involvement of the subconscious, a defining factor in how mental function was organised. For the father of psychoanalysis, mental pain did not lack meaning, no matter the extent to which the patient was unaware of it. It had meaning and content, and the patient was involved in the process of acquiring or attributing meaning to it and consequently was involved in his own treatment.

Two excerpts from his early work demonstrate the importance Freud attributed to the diagnostic and therapeutic value of the narration of mental pain.

Firstly, for the describing clinician (1893, p. 159–160):

> The case histories I write should read like short stories and that, as one might say, they lack the serious stamp of science. I must console myself with the reflection that the nature of the subject is evidently responsible for this, rather than any preference of my own … a detailed description of mental processes such as we are accustomed to find in the works of imaginative writers enables me, with the use of a few psychological formulas, to obtain at least some kind of insight into the course of that affection (he means the hysteria).

And clearly for the narrating patient (1893, p. 48, 62):

> "Keep still! Don't say anything! Don't touch me!" …. Then she said in a definitely grumbling tone that I was not to keep on asking her where this and that came from, but to let me tell her what she had to say. I fell in with this, and she went on without preface.

Thus, thanks to the exhortations of the patient Emmy von N., free association on the patient's part became the main instrument of treatment.

However, depending on its quality and severity, psychopathology affects, even disorganises, the processes and contents of thought, emotion and deed. Subjectivity, identity and relations with others are all called into doubt. For psychoanalysis, the meeting between the patient and clinician allows for the painful subjectivity of the former to be unfurled against the subjectivity of the latter, against the backdrop of immense risks for both.

The long European psychiatric tradition seeks to understand the patient's subjectivity through a thorough clinical approach and in terms of classification is governed by an internal cohesive reasoning, organised around the concepts of psychosis and neurosis.

On the contrary, current psychiatry, which has trapped itself within the so-called atheoretical classification system (DSM-V, ICD 10, etc.), has abandoned logical coherence in the organisation of diseases and has necessarily limited itself to the need to understand the multifarious mental pain of each individual subject. In effect, it is a system which is exclusively biomedical and behavioural, which psychiatrifies human experience in its entirety through empirical classification, which ignores the range of limits and the continuity between normalcy and morbidity (Canguilhem 1972) and the relations between diseases with similar sets of symptoms (Corcos 2013). How can one not raise the difference here with psychoanalytic thinking when McDougal (1978) wrote the *Plea for a Measure of Abnormality*?

Psychoanalysis is not just a treatment for mental pain. It is a process of exploration, a method for a therapeutic process and a theory (Freud 1923, p. 234) which rests on a central hypothesis, applicable to each individual, according to which the unconscious organises mental life, establishing conflict between diametrically opposed demands, which are seeking out equally different solutions.

As S. Stylianidis showed in two recent articles (2011, 2012), the quality of the clinical session is forged by a system which does not give the appropriate importance to the patient's thoughts, feelings and deeds because in the dominant perception of psychiatry, they lack objectivity! Recalling the work of Ricœur (1996), he notes the importance for the patient of establishing his role as narrator, through the potential to express his subjective pain given to him by the clinical process (2012, p. 17). In the author's view, subject-based clinical practice ought to be developed along four lines: patient experience, psychocognitive function, the conscious and unconscious meaning of the symptoms and the patient's position within the family and social milieu.

The recently published DSM-V has abandoned the decades old multiaxial system. In particular, the removal of the second axis, which described the patient's personality underlying the overt symptomatology, is another concession by scientific thinking to the pressure of circles outside of medicine (Hochmann 2010, p. 233). In contrast to the so-called atheoretical DSM, what is of immense importance is to highlight through clinical practice the latent structure of the patient's personality. That is because mental economy and dynamics are, according to Freud, determined by the latent structure of personality, which is shared both during the pre-morbidity period of the subject's life and upon onset of the illness, and after any possible recovery.

In lecture XXXI of the New Introductory Lectures, Freud describes the famous crystal metaphor (1933, p. 58):

> If we throw a crystal to the floor, it breaks; but not into haphazard pieces. It comes apart along its lines of cleavage into fragments whose boundaries, though they were invisible, were predetermined by the crystal's structure. Mental patients are split and broken structures of this same kind.

Instead of making a standard DSM-based diagnosis, highlighting the latent mental structure of the patient's personality (Bergeret 1974) and the individual dynamic lines which are present or potentially present (Roussillon 2007) and mobilising them can prevent, ameliorate and/or reverse the pathological course of the illness, in conjunction with the resilience to the illness the patient may demonstrate (Cyrulnik 2011). All these are vital clinical tools for a proper diagnosis, evaluation and prognosis, for understanding the patient and for developing a tailor-made care plan for him.

Consequently, the following dimensions are vital for a subject-based psychiatry (Stylianidis, op. cit., p. 20; 2012, p. 20):

> Psychodynamics like defence mechanisms, object relations, the intrapsychic conflicts approach, interaction methods, object investment and separation models, cognition and learning methods and procedures, the subject's position in the family and the socio-cultural context to which he belongs, different phenomenological aspects especially subjective pain and its connection to social pain, adaptation methods, personality types, available mental, family and social resources for preparing an tailor-made treatment and care plan for the subject.

Referring to Racamier (1993) we can define care as an organic, cohesive set of methods for a group governed by psychoanalytical thinking aimed at preserving and bolstering the mental health dynamic of patients and their families, as well as the inclusion of various psychotherapies and other treatment approaches.

6.3 Psychoanalytical Thinking and Practice in Hospital Services and in the Community

Psychoanalytical Institutes in the Community

When the first psychoanalytical institutes were set up to train new psychoanalysts and promote psychoanalytical thinking within the psychiatric and wider scientific community, the first institutes to care for patients based on the psychoanalytical approach were also set up. In this twofold way, psychoanalysis from the outset acquired a position in both society and the community.

Between 1886 and 1896, pre-psychoanalytical Freud was responsible for the Max-Kassowitz Institute's "neurotic patients" clinic. It was the first public centre set up in 1788 to provide care to indigent children in the Austro-Hungarian capital (de Mijolla 2002).

After Freud himself established the International Psychoanalytical Association (IPA) in Nuremburg in 1910 to safeguard the theoretical, clinical and educational unity of psychoanalysis, the expansion of the psychoanalytical movement allowed M. Eitingon, E. Simmel and K. Abraham to set up the Berliner Psychoanalytische Poliklinik in Berlin in the early 1920s, which was immediately renamed the Berliner Psychoanalytische Institut. It was the first institution which brought together educational activities (lectures, didactic analyses and supervised analyses) and wider mental care as part of a clinic. Just 2 years later came the Vienna Institute. Both closed their doors when Nazism took hold and were silent during the course of the war.

The Tavistock Clinic was founded in London in the same year as the Berlin Institute and since then has been providing diverse, top quality training and has been engaged in important research and treatment activities, while after WWI came the turn of Paris with the Société psychanalytique de Paris et Institut psychanalytique de Paris (1954), though the psychoanalytical movement had been active in the French capital from as early as 1926. This was followed by Frankfurt with the Sigmund-Freud-Institut, involved in training, providing services and doing research focused on psychosomatic issues and society.

Psychiatric Reform and Psychoanalysis

When WWII ended, against the backdrop of optimism and freedom which swept the post-war Western world, two things relevant to psychiatry changed rapidly: the first effective neuroleptic medicines were introduced (Chlorpromazine), and the antipsychiatry movement began to spread inspired by Laing, Cooper and Esterson in England, Szasz in America and Basaglia in Italy, while institutional psychotherapy began to be developed by Daumézon, Koechlin, Tosquelles and Oury in France. Many other psychiatrists, including psychoanalysts, although reserved about the activism and radical ideas of those named above, systematically expressed concerns which soon resulted in questions about the psychiatric status quo and in the asylum-centred structure of psychiatry being overturned. The time for psychiatric reform had come.

Deinstitutionalisation does not only mean abolishing or restricting the number of asylums or reducing the number of beds at psychiatric hospitals. Above all, it means developing psychiatric services within general hospitals and health centres as well as networks of outpatient structures that focus on prevention, treatment and psychosocial rehabilitation, working in cooperation with the relevant community structures and social institutions in each case. It means sectorising health services so that users can turn to services based in the area where they live.

Users of such services are not cut off from the fabric of society since they continue to maintain interpersonal ties to the extent possible and become named objects of new, real investments made by the staff of the structures, compared to the anonymity and mass nature of older-style psychiatric services. Moreover, since the number and importance of therapists increase by setting up a multidisciplinary treatment team, patients are released from the need to repeatedly see the single, traditional attendant doctor.

As far as the psychoanalytical movement is concerned, one illustrative example of this endeavour was the establishment of the renowned outpatient care centres in Paris' 13th arrondissement (in addition to the aforementioned institutes and clinics in the rest of the post-war Western world). The *L' Association de Santé Mentale du 13e arrondissement de Paris* was founded in 1958 by Professors P. Paumelle, S. Lebovici and R. Diatkine and was in effect the first attempt to "sectorise" care for each age group and pathology for individuals living in that area of Paris. These centres, working in partnership with public hospitals, also combined numerous educational activities in line with psychoanalytical tradition.

In Athens, D. Kouretas (at the Athens Psychiatric School), A. Potamianou (at the Centre for Mental Health and Research) and P. Sakellaropoulos (at the Theotokos Foundation) worked under adverse conditions to promote the psychoanalytical approach in Greece. Inspired by the French example, and with the active support of S. Lebovici, A. Potamianou set up the "Centre" which she has run since 1956, an innovative venue for psychiatric reform with psychoanalytical training provided within the unfavourable environment of post-civil war Greece which had been marked by exiles and psychiatric confinement.

> According to Anagnostopoulos et al. (2009, p. 348), greek psychoanalysts, indicating the intention to proceed to some theoretical and clinical adjustments, have since 1980s played a more active role in the development of public health services and, by extension, in psychiatric reform taking place in Greece. The most extensive psychoanalytical interventions relate to the supervision of clinical work, primarily at units where psychiatry is practiced in the community, and short-term psychotherapy, which is frequently provided in cooperation with treatment facilities.

Generally speaking, in the overall move for psychiatric reform and in modern attempts to sectorise psychiatric services, psychoanalysis has been present from the outset in all attempts to promote deinstitutionalisation in the Western world after WWII:

In hospitals: outpatient clinics, the placement of beds in general hospitals and liaison-based psychiatry between hospital clinics.
Outpatient facilities: mental health centres, adult and child treatment centres, crisis centres, psychosocial rehabilitation structures, mobile units in regions lacking any fixed psychiatric services, home intervention and treatment teams, assertive community treatment, outreach treatment, etc.
In the community: partnerships with local government authorities (welfare services) and with the Church.
In education: schools (to prevent bullying) and universities (such as counselling services for students).
In large-scale disasters and acts of violence: "the analysts are in the trenches" as B. Skarlew et al. (2004) so eloquently put in the title of their book.

Two Illustrative Examples

Daycare Centres for Autistic Children

The development of psychoanalytical clinical practice relating to child psychosis and autism based on the work of psychoanalysts Klein, Winnicott, Mahler, Meltzer, Tustin, Bettelheim and others has declined dramatically over recent decades, thanks to the global dominance of behavioural and cognitive methods such as ABA and TEACCH.

The fact that the older approach is receding has led us, as psychoanalysts, to reassess and update our assumptions about the pathogenesis and approach to treating child psychosis and autism. Today, daycare centres need to combine prevention, treatment and educational activities for children, support their families and build close partnerships with schools and the community. For Hochmann (2006, 2008), treatment, education and school integration are the three prongs of care for autistic children.

At daycare centres, in addition to the individual programme, method or technique used, it is the very organisation of the centre that allows treatment and educational activities to be developed. Different approaches, venues and people the child can interact with function (a) as acceptors of the different sides of each child and (b) create something like a "differential dynamic" that allows them to pass through one form of process to another. It is the lack of similarities, the breaks in continuity which create facts and the fact – when put together- which create opportunities for narration, for telling stories. In this way, the daily extracts from the story of each child become the object of a diverse process by different interlocutors, who work in partnership, until they reach the end recipient, the child, in their final form as a unit of meaning which can in time be appropriated.

Including children with autism in small groups of others of their own age, which operate on the basis of a well-structured daily schedule, allows each child to distinguish how to participate in different activities and to experience them as separate activities. These different experiences are, however, combined together through systematic communication with the child's various interlocutors, allowing the development of creativity and the production of meaning, which are equally essential, with the overriding goal being to create one's own personal story (Petrou and Doxiadi 2009).

What we know as art therapy is an internationally accepted way of working with children with emotional and mental difficulties. Cultural media (such as painting, music, etc.) are preferred educational means for each child and for offering the treatment to those who need it. They are mediation objects between the participants in an activity, in other words the child and the experts. They are a *pliable medium* to use Milner's (1993) apt expression: flexible and easily adjustable media, just as the instructor, the therapist, the partner and not only the child must be flexible.

When working with a child with pervasive developmental disorder, cultural media can (under certain frameworks and cooperation conditions) help the child give form and shape to aspects of himself and the world around him. The senses and movement are stimulated by the physical properties of the object, leading through the special relationship developed between the child and expert, to preverbal channels of communication and symbolisation, which can then be verbalised (Petrou 2010).

Halfway Houses

This term primarily means residential units and sheltered accommodation intended to accommodate patients after they leave psychiatric clinics, before they are fully integrated back into society, as well as any other structure which prevents patients from staying long term in psychiatric hospitals or a transitional space between the hospital and the community.

Serious psychiatric disorders require a relatively long-term stay in a clinic, frequently resulting in the patient being institutionalised (whether out of passivity, due to lack of initiative, etc.). If hospitalisation is coupled with the lack of any family support framework and/or job, the patient will need a halfway house to help him and to accompany him on the difficult path towards social reintegration.

During their stay in halfway houses, residents form a therapeutic community. They have a structured daily schedule to learn individual and social skills. They participate in individual and group meetings with staff, to take initiatives and analyse day-to-day difficulties they encounter with themselves, with others, with society, with the halfway house itself and with their process of social reintegration.

However, halfway houses which attempt to replace asylums and their problems frequently end up developing at least some of the same features of a total institution, to use the phrase from Goffman (1961) which describes asylums, namely, that many residential units have medical, nursing, occupational therapy, social work and administrative services, even though they are supposed to be "homes"! Residential units, even though they are halfway houses, frequently operate as a self-contained "whole" which disavows any sense of "elsewhere": an "elsewhere" where the management could be located, an "elsewhere" where the patient could meet his doctor or therapist, an "elsewhere" where the staff could gather, an "elsewhere" where one could report to, an "elsewhere" that the structure could be associated with and so on. As in the case with daycare centres for autistic children, diversity and connection – and not homogeneity – are the factors used to give meaning and to ensure mental integration and social reintegration (Petrou 2005).

The position of psychoanalysis in institutions

> Now let us assume that by some kind of organisation we were able to increase our numbers to an extent sufficient for treating large masses of people. Then, on the other hand, one may reasonably expect that at some time or other the conscience of the community will awake and admonish it that the poor man has just as much right to help for his mind as he now has to the surgeon's means of saving his life: and that the neuroses menace the health of a people no less than tuberculosis, ... Then clinics and consultation departments will be built, to which analytically trained physicians will be appointed ... This treatment will be free. It may be a long time before the State regards this as an urgent duty. Present conditions may delay its arrival even longer. Probably these institutions will first be started by private beneficence; some time or other, however, it must come.... It is very probable, too, that the large scale application of our therapy will compel us to alloy the pure gold of analysis with the copper of direct suggestion.

Those are Freud's own words from his introduction at a psychoanalytical conference in post-war Budapest in 1918 (Freud 1919, p. 166–7). This historical talk provoked a series of conflicts within the psychoanalytic community relating to the sort of mix Freud was talking about and about the position of psychoanalysis within institutions.

In any event, the link between psychoanalysis and public psychiatric care was already a well-established fact during WWII. The development of psychoanalysis is tied into the modern history of psychiatry, its practices and theoretical ideas and the very education and training of psychiatrists.

In 1917 Freud wrote (1917, p. 253–4):

> You will grant that there is nothing in the nature of psychiatric work which could be opposed to psychoanalytic research. What is opposed to psychoanalysis is not psychiatry but psychiatrists. Psychoanalysis is related to psychiatry approximately as histology is to anatomy: the one studies the external forms of the organs, the other studies their construction out of tissues and cells. It is not easy to imagine a contradiction between these two species of study, of which one is a continuation of the other.

To make this clearer from a pedagogical viewpoint, let's assume that psychoanalysis is present in three ways within psychiatric care structures, where it became one of the theoretical and clinical means for deinstitutionalisation:

1. As part of the treatment of psychiatric patients. It is the psychoanalytical psychotherapy of psychoses, where changes in the framework and technique are necessary in order to work with psychotic patients (Searles 1965a, b; Rosenfeld 1965; Bleger 1981; Racamier 1990; Mentzos 1991, 2008; Benedetti 1992; Schermer and Pines 1999; Tzavaras and Stylianidis 2002; Tzavaras, Vartzopoulos and Stylianidis (eds) 2008).
2. In the hands of enlightened psychiatrists-psychoanalysts, who were responsible for hospitals, clinics and so on, psychoanalysis becomes a working method within institutions and relates to all aspects of work within the institution. It is a *psychoanalyst without a couch*, to quote the eloquent title of the classic work by Racamier (1973). The psychiatric hospital has transformed from an asylum and place of restraint and confinement to the medium for therapeutic processes, and its spaces and the relationships which develop within it became institutional. What provides treatment is not the institution but the setting, to use Oury's classic phrase (2004), in other words the process of creation and deconstruction once the risk of fossilisation or hegemony of one or the other institution appears. It is the famous institutional psychotherapy, whose pioneers were G. Daumézon, P. Koechlin, F. Tosquelles, F. Oury and others.
3. As a way of thinking about the work done within institutions and of intervening in those cases where the work is blocked by conflicts, dichotomies, projections, projective identifications, denials and other widespread archaic defence mechanisms. It is all about supervision and more recently about institutional analysis and intervention (Hinshelwood 2001; Kaës 1987, 2005; Nicolle and Kaës 2008; Pinel et al. 2007; Boutin and Van der Stegen 2012 and others).

However, what are the aspects of the "model" and the conditions for introducing and running a mental health institution along the lines set out in psychoanalytical theory? For pedagogical reasons again, we can summarise them as follows:

The first, key condition is to allow the patient to have (perhaps for the first time) the experience of a framework where, in relation to others and the institution himself, desires, restrictions, frustrations, differences and conflicts are the object of a process and not something to be avoided, confronted or repressed.

The institution is not the structure, the therapeutic organisation. It is a total social fact, in the sense given to that term by the anthropologist M. Mauss, i.e. a fact which "mobilises all component parts" and which are at once legal, economic, religious, aesthetic, morphological and so on (1950, p. 274). It is a psychocognitive institution, as Hochmann (2008) demonstrated: "When we decide to abandon the comfort of an institution which is surrounded by walls and we open up, without any particular protection … we find ourselves in a particularly vulnerable position, in which we risk losing ourselves. In that case, we need to refer to a theoretical model, which gives meaning to what we are doing and who we are. A model that introduces a new institution against the ill, and against the rest of society, as employees who perform a standard task. The theory, what I call a psycho-cognitive institution (institution mentale) is in our eyes and in the eyes of others who define it, through its own special nature, the type of relations we develop during our practice" (1971 [2003], p. 462–3).

For Hochmann, there can be no therapeutic approach to psychotic patients outside of institutions. The subject himself is the *institution mentale* to the extent that he creates and organises his thoughts. A psychotic patient faced with the difficulty of organising them in a non-delirious manner is the subject "in search of an author". That author or narrator is none other than the institutional process: along the lines of motherly care, he gradually settles into the framework of a "narrative envelope" (Stern 1992), a reality where therapist and patient share meaningful relationships amid fragmented experiences and with each other. That is mental care for Hochmann: *consolation*, whose main instrument is narration, as he showed in his work of the same title (1994).

By multiplying their views (which Bion (1965, p. 90) called a vertex), the members of a treatment team can build from the pile of episodic remnants of everyday life and the biography of the patients, a history within which different events assume a place and acquire meaning. This is a playful procedure, in the same sense that Winnicott used when talking about therapy as a game (1971), giving particular pleasure because it activates a mental autoeroticism (Hochmann 2008). As something different from the satisfaction of release, it relates to a pleasant mental function. It is tried out initially as team work among therapists and is gradually shared with the patient, who discovers a way to overcome the agony of separation, fragmentation anxiety, persecution, etc., receiving pleasure from the processes of representation and symbolism which are the foundations of thought.

The main aim of the psychoanalyst within the institution is not to interpret and to highlight the unconscious meaning. It is to offer a panorama of images and tales as materials to create the patient's story, a creative process from which the patient can draw pleasure and relief. It is psychoanalysis as "meta-narration" to use Schafer's (1997) phrase, and the psychoanalyst is the person who embodies that story-creating function.

As Boutin and Van der Stegen (2012) have shown, the purpose is not to "play the psychoanalyst" of the staff, institution, relatives, patients, etc. The psychoanalyst in the institution is "the witness of what psychoanalysis has to say about being human"; in other words the human aspect must remain central, which allows everyone (therapist, patient or relative) to open up to life and each other.

The various mediation media (painting groups, music, drama, dance therapies etc.) which the institution provides are not activities in the service of sub-maniacal defences and therapist-patient activism. They create transitional spaces which allow the patient's mental reality to be externalised, to connect it to that of others and to the institution and to develop processes of shaping and connection, as we explained above are so central to daycare centres for children with autism.

The development of transference and counter-transference between patients, therapists and the framework is the means for recognising recurring patterns within which the patient is trapped and the lever for shifting out of them. If the institution's response is different from that of the archaic environment, rather than providing an interpretation (which is frequently ineffective), it is better for the patient to develop relations with himself and with others within the team, rather than within a misleading, overprotective, rejective or contradictory duality (Cahn 1991; Searles 1965).

Such laborious work, the Ego, especially that of someone with schizophrenia, cannot be completed unless supported by institutional processes that allow a connection between the inner mental world, the intra-family setting and the intra-institutional world and consequently integration of the fragmented parts of his psyche.

It is clear that an institution of this type must be able to distinguish between conflicts and dichotomies of the patient and those of the institution itself. The treatment group in such a context is called upon to be quite robust, to endure the large number of projections which it must separate from its own issues and call it into constant question. Supervision, institutional analysis and intervention focus precisely on those processes and the barriers that are encountered in working with psychotic patients.

6.4 Individual and Community Pain: Human Pain in Society

Freud's interest in understanding social and cultural phenomena from the viewpoint of psychoanalysis runs throughout all his work: from 1908 and the article entitled *"Civilised" sexual morality and modern nervous illness* (1908), and the books *Totem and Taboo* (1913), *Group Psychology and analysis of the Ego* (1921), *The Future of an Illusion* (1927), *Civilisation and its Discontents* (1930), to his final work *Moses and Monotheism* (1939).

Freud comes from the intellectual tradition of the Enlightenment and grew and developed like his contemporaries, within the context of the claims and teachings of that period. However, the neurotic individual of the previous century soon began to realise that instead of experiencing the promised happiness and endless progress, he was experiencing a sense of generalised discontent, doubt about meaning and a sense of threat, particularly in light of two destructive world wars and the subsequent Cold War: a discontent within civilisation, whose origin and effects were analysed by Freud in his work. He wrote that civilised man has swapped part of his potential happiness for some security (1930, p. 114). Consequently, on the Freudian hypothesis, civilisation was built on man giving up direct, complete satisfaction of his instinctual desires: erotic, destructive and narcissistic desires.

Giving up erotic desires frequently leads to neurotic inhibitions and symptoms. At the other extreme, any prevalence of destructive urges over the urge to live leads to the dissolution of primordial violence, sometimes at personal level (psychosis, destructive thinking), sometimes at interpersonal level (breaking of bonds, as in the case of the threat of social dissolution) and sometimes at state level (conflicts and wars). He emphatically stated that the battle between the urge to live and the urge to destroy is what life is really about generally speaking, and for that reason the development of civilisation ought bluntly to be described as the vital battle of the human species (1930, p. 138).

The concept of instinct indicates the constant and unavoidable pressure from instinctual drives that are at the basis of human sexuality, narcissism and destructiveness. The violence of instincts is more powerful than rational interests. Where the overvalued strength of rational discourse failed, Freud counter-proposed the mental process of unconscious forces. This task falls on the shoulders of culture, as he quite unexpectedly concludes at the end of New Introductory Lecture XXXI: "The therapeutic efforts of psychoanalysis, he writes, would consist in strengthening the ego, to become more independent over the Superego, widen the field of perception and transform its organization in order to appropriate more sections of the Other. Where the Other was, the Ego must reach. That is the cultural work, cultural activity, work of civilisation" (Es ist Kulturarbeit) (1933, p. 79).

What is civilisation? Is it not the regulation of desires a product of the mediation of the Ego between conflicting instinctual demands of the Other and prohibitions emanating from the Superego? What relationship can civilisation have with the Other, the Ego, Superego and the Id?

Kulturarbeit is a phrase which Freud did not explore in as much theoretical detail as he did with dream work and grief work, nor did it receive the appropriate attention from his followers. Despite that, it retains an important position in Freudian thinking. We consider that it is similar to and on a par with the mental work of the individual subject, but at a social level. Mental work cannot exist or be understood without *Kulturarbeit*, or vice versa (Petrou 2012).

If the Ego is present, he wrote in *An Outline of Psycho-Analysis* (1938), the Other and the Superego are the past. The Other is the hereditary disposition, the Superego is to be bequeathed. In New Introductory Lectures he once again said, the Superego is not formed in the image of the parents' prohibitions but by the content of the parents' Superego. It regulates social conduct, which represents tradition, the ideals of the past, and may withstand for some time the challenges of a new economic situation (p. 177). Humanity does not live only in the present; the past, tradition and civilisation survive via the Superego.

When he explores the ideology and influence of the leader in the book *Group Psychology and Analysis of the Ego*, he writes that each member of the group assigns part of his Id to the leader. That assignment gives rises to two identifications: one with the leader, who expresses the now common ideal, and the other, the inter-egoic one, between members, which is the foundation of group ties.

Kulturarbeit and mental work develop along two lines relevant to each subject: one outside of time which entails cross-generational ties and carries tradition and super-egoic identifications and one which is of this time, entailing ties with those existing at this time, inter-egoic identifications and narcissistic contracts.

The last decades of the postmodern world (Aubert 2004, 2010) led R. Kaës, thanks to his clinical-theoretical approach to groups (2007), to reassess Freudian views about the social origin of mental discontent which Freud had been talking about since as early as 1908. In his books about the discontent modern subject face, Kaës (2012) describes how psychoanalysis invents and works with those clinical-theoretical standards of understanding changes and transforming in time, space, ties, civilisations and mentalities. Those standards are clearly temporary and inadequate to allow us to think again about our relationship with the unknown.

The postmodern world violently and rapidly overturned the narcissistic basis of our subjective and social identity, our perceptions and the myths on which our sense of belonging and relations between members of society, civilisation and nature rest. In a community of individuals, where processes lack subjects, ties (whether intergenerational or intersubjective) are in deep crisis. Consequently, subjectification, socialisation and symbolisation (the only things which can process the dispersion, heterogeneity and gap between experience of the inner world and that of the external environment) are gaping, leaving the crevice from whence violence and destructiveness emerge, quite unprotected.

The author identifies four features of our postmodern civilisation as responsible for inadequate symbolisation:

A culture of control which pursues compulsory homogenisation and integration of everyone can only result in controlled violence applicable within its very structure and uncontrolled social violence which rejects all laws foreign to it (lawlessness, racism, terrorism).

A culture without limits which promises to promote exaggeration, omnipotence, "hubris" in a word: the idea that "everything is possible". The result: unthinking exposure to risk, ending in destructive injury.

A culture of urgency and immediacy, due to the shortening of our temporal horizons due to hubris: "we have to manage to get everything done". As a result, a specific tie is retained in the present, but it is not recorded in history. The inability to make medium-term plans further contributes to the disorganisation of thought, of the ability to choose and of grief.

Lastly, a culture of melancholy, in other words endless, unprocessed loss and grief, both personal and collective, at social level: the death of God, of man, of humanism, of ideologies, a culture of genocides, of destructive population shifts, etc.

Faced with this melancholic disenchantment with our culture, postmodernism also cultivates maniacal promises, dreams of hedonistic dominance and uncontrolled destruction. The massive changes relate primarily to large structures which frame and normalise social formations and processes: myths and ideologies, faith and religions and power and hierarchy. They are meta-social guarantors of the key structures of symbolisation, which is "culture" in its various manifestations and forms, in short *Kulturarbeit*.

The crisis of meta-social guarantors also drags meta-mental guarantors (which are the background of the psyche, the processes and environmental formations on which the psyche of each subject is based, the fundamental prohibitions, intersubjective conventions and pacts, etc.) into crisis.

As far as the mental pathologies we have been seeing for decades and the generalised discontent in both Western civilisation and in the entire Third World afflicted by famines, diseases, violence and fanaticism are concerned, social scientists have given us very useful methodological tools and well-documented analyses to help us understand these phenomena.

Limiting ourselves to the more classic authors, in *Suicide* (1897), Durkheim analyses the concept of social ties in relation to the forms of social solidarity and the termination thereof in the case of lawlessness. In the *Sociology of Mental Disorder* (1965) Bastide argued that the deconstruction of a social group and/or society is accompanied by mental deconstruction for its members. Castel (1978, 2005, 2009; Castel et al. 1979), working on the forms and processes of social exclusion, developed critical views about care institutions for mental patients and the relationship of mental illness with modern social circumstances.

The "Third Difference" and the Ethnopsychiatric Approach

Let us now turn our attention to refugees and migrants who are seeking out a better future in countries in the Western world. Whether these people are obviously patients or not, they carry within them immense mental pain: personal pain, family pain and cultural pain. The burden of those individuals raises serious questions about our own capacity for tolerance towards difference and our own personal and cultural pain compared to otherness in general and the ties and bonds within our own Western societies which are suffering too.

Understanding these individuals and dealing with them at an institutional, social and clinical levels are urgent and difficult, almost impossible one might say. If we limit ourselves to the clinical work needed, the difficulties are already immense (Kleinman 1980, 2008). Simplifying already difficult moral, epistemological and theoretical-clinical issues, we either need to treat them as if they are patients whose mental economy and dynamic we know or must work to understand the "third difference", after that of gender and generation, referred to by Kaës et al. (2012): cultural difference which gives rise of identification pain.

Thanks to the work of the ethnologist, psychoanalyst and Hellenist Georges Devereux (1970, 1972 etc.), since the 1960s and 1970s, we have had the necessary methodological tools to understand these people. It is called Psychoanalytic Ethnopsychiatry: a twofold, nonsimultaneous approach characterised by absolute respect for the autonomy of the conceptual and methodological framework of both anthropology and psychoanalysis, which demonstrates the complementary nature of these two systems of understanding. Devereux writes (1972, p. 10):

> The principle of dualist and non-simultaneous discourse categorically rejects all 'interdisciplinary' attempts to add, merge, combine or view things in parallel, in short to view each discipline 'as combined with' another… It makes every 'deduction' from ethnology and psychoanalysis or vice versa, utterly fraudulent.

This was supplemented by the anthropologist F. Laplantine, who stressed that the ethnopsychoanalytic methodology seeks to "avoid the double barrier of (a) fully relativising psychiatry and (b) psychiatrifing culture" (Laplantine 2007, p. 24).

Some of Devereaux's students, Nathan (1986, 1988, 2007), Moro (2002, 2004), Zajde (2005, 2011) and others set up a centre in Paris bearing their teacher's name, working with refugees, immigrants and second- and third-generation migrants, in order to continue his research. Another psychoanalyst and anthropologist, Douville (2000, 2007, 2014; Douville et al. 2012), has taken a different scientific path, studying violence in history and introducing the concept of "the melancholisation of social ties", working on social exclusion among European and African adolescents.

6.5 Discussion

What is the future of social-community psychiatry against the background of the endless, drastic cut in social spending, the drive for cost-effectiveness and the suffocating framework wherein a form of psychiatry aimed at psychiatrifying the human experience and suppressing it with medicines is coming to dominate?

It is beyond the bounds of a chapter like this to answer a question like that. However, we cannot ignore the fact that as long as these two constraints continue to play a decisive role in the future of the sector, we cannot overlook at least two internal limitations: our present identity and the very nature of psychosis.

In relation to the first, in one of his articles, Stylianidis (2012) raised the question of the extent to which it is not just society but also the dominant model of psychiatry that is afraid of psychoanalysis, and vice versa. "The presence of a psychiatric team which makes reference to psychoanalysis … faces numerous uncertainties". Referring to the work of Ehrenberg (2007) and Castel (2005, 2009) about the drop in the quality of day-to-day life and the rise in social pain and the sense of insecurity, he points out the unheard-of type of meeting between society and the psychoanalyst which entails strong moral, scientific and humanitarian (practical) dilemmas: "Issues of managing and understanding the needs of collective and individual pain are raised, which is not a well-known psychopathological subject area" (see 18).

As far as the second constraint is concerned, it has to do with psychosis per se. Depending on the country involved, asylums have either been completely done away with or have reduced in numbers. That was a major scientific and humanitarian necessity. However, one of the founding fathers of the movement to abolish asylums, Hochmann (1994), wrote of his disappointment and the risks entailed by the new structures that replaced asylums:

> All attempts encountered over the last quarter of a century in the entire Western World under different names: treatment communities, institutional psychotherapies, even antipsychiatry, end up with the same disenchantment. The asylum cannot change. It now tends to be quickly rebuilt even within the most cutting-edge or innovative institutions.

Hochmann bases this unfortunate finding on his immense clinical experience and active participation in the attempt to promote deinstitutionalisation: it is psychosis itself which "secretes the asylum which requires the conditions of the asylum". The projections that emanate from schizophrenics are recorded within the very matrix and form of the institution, which if left its own devices will work in favour of the psychosis. Counter to the violent acting out and extreme passivity of the schizophrenic (as a form of protection against fragmentation or annihilation anxiety), the institution has to choose between adopting an equally passive stance (which is often rejective) or an activist one (which often idealises the potential of psychosis and treatment communities) or giving the chance to develop painful thought processes and questioning of the framework and everything that happens in that context.

Mental health structures with a psychoanalytical focus cannot be the product of administrative decisions or so-called scientific discoveries. They must be institutions which do not institutionalise once and for all, where theories and practices are not infallible truths, where their truth is partial and revisable. In other words, they ought to be the product of innovative, radical, subversive thinking and above all open to the potential of being overturned by newer thinking, by newer standards which adopt new mentalities, new institutions and so on (Petrou 2005).

In recent years we have acquired the tools to advance, to move from theoretical speculation to testing them in clinical terms, to move beyond ideological delusions that came from previous decades and to think about our foundation myths, about *subjection* as Castoriadis (1975) has called it and about the function for which the institution is run by the institutional status quo.

One such tool is progress in understanding manifestations of the subconscious within institutions noted in recent decades by group psychoanalysis. According to Kaës this is a new methodological paradigm (2005, p. 8) within psychoanalytical theory and clinical practice, which demonstrates the processes of connecting the individual, as the subject of the unconscious and the group, with intersubjective wholes. Kaës' central hypothesis is that what is not symbolised by the mental pain of the subjects in an institution "comes back within the institution in a setting where mental reality is associated in a mixed up and confused manner with the realities of other classes ... It negates thinking and goal achievement, which are the main task and social function of the institution" (Kaës, op. cit., p. 47).

The balance achieved from time to time by an institution is ephemeral, because the mental ties (personal, interpersonal and institutional) are exceptionally prone to disconnect and to become rigidly locked into institutional processes. Institutional intervention seeks to analyse these fixating repetitions and to restart institutional processes, which Pinel has called *processuality* (Pinel and Morel 2001; Pinel 2005): the ability of the institutional group to preserve active processes for investing in the work done with patients, associates and the institution itself, the thinking process and the process of questioning practice.

In his book Darcourt (2006) asks "Are Psychoanalysis and Psychiatry Still Useful?" Psychiatry always gained from using different theoretical-clinical approaches, because on its own, none suffices to fully understand mental pain.

In short, psychoanalysis can contribute to releasing and freeing the dominant form of psychiatry from the suffocating bind in which it finds itself through:

Recognising the importance of mental pain and its processes, because the diagnosis cannot relate to a supposedly objectified body. Being empathic towards others is the means for diagnosis which makes the process become intersubjective understanding.

The therapeutic relief felt by the patient through the assignation of meaning to his experience and through developing a tailor-made care plan. Pain is placed within a narrative which tells the subject's own story, because narration is a treatment tool in the context of total care.

The satisfaction the therapist gets from working with mental patients and which is transmitted over to the patient, in terms of mental function.

Showcasing the connections between individual aspects of pain and the social factors which define, augment and ameliorate it.

The trials and tribulations which we are constantly obliged to subject our theories and clinical practice to and of course the constant development of networks of prevention, treatment and psychosocial rehabilitation along the lines outlined in this chapter.

References

Anagnostopoulos D, Christodoulou N, Ploumpidis D (2009) Psychoanalysis and the public health sector: the Greek experience. Psychiatriki 20(4):342–350
Aubert N (2004) L'individu hypermoderne. Édition Erès, Paris
Aubert N (2010) La société hypermoderne: ruptures et contradictions (No. 15). L'Harmattan, Paris
Bastide R (1965) Sociologie des maladies mentales. Flammarion, Paris
Benedetti G (1992) New paths in psychotherapy. Psychol Top 5(2):95–140
Bergeret J (1974) La personnalité normale et pathologique. Dunod, Paris
Bion WR (1965) Transformations: change from learning to growth. Heinemann, London
Bleger J (1981) Symbiose et ambiguïté (1967). PUF, Paris
Boutin M, Van der Stegen E (2012) Max ou la psychanalyse comme ouverture à une anthropologie. Coq Héron 209:26–35
Cahn R (1991) Adolescence et folie. PUF, Paris
Canguilhem G (1972) Le normal et le pathologique. PUF, Paris
Castel R (1978) L'ordre psychiatrique: l'âge d'or de l'aliénisme. Minuit, Paris
Castel R (2005) Risque, insécurité sociale et psychiatrie. Entretien Joubert M. et Louzoun C. (sous la direction de): Répondre à la souffrance sociale. Erès, Paris
Castel R (2009) La montée des incertitudes. Travail, protections, statut del' individu. Le Seuil, Paris

Castel F, Lovell A, Castel R (1979) La société psychiatrique avancée: le modèle américain. Bernard Grasset, Paris

Castoriadis C (1975) L'institution imaginaire de la société. Seuil, Paris

coll Roussillon R (2007) Manuel de psychologie et de psychopathologie clinique générale. Masson, Paris

Corcos M (2013) L'homme selon le DSM. Le nouvel ordre psychiatrique. Albin Michel, Paris

Cyrulnik B (2011) Resilience: how your inner strength can set you free from the past. Penguin, New York

Darcourt G (2006) La Psychanalyse peut-elle encore être utile à la psychiatrie? Odile Jacob, Paris

de Mijolla A (2002) Dictionnaire international de la psychanalyse. Hachette, Paris

Devereux G (1970) Essais d'Ethnopsychiatrie générale. Gallimard, Paris

Devereux G (1972) Ethnopsychanalyse complémentariste. Flammarion, Paris

Douville O (2000) Pour introduire l'idée d'une mélancolisation du lien social. Clin Méditerr 63:239–261

Douville O (2007) De l'adolescence errante: Variations sur les non-lieux de nos modernités. Pleins feux, Paris

Douville O (2014) Les figures de l'Autre: Pour une anthropologie clinique. Dunod, Paris

Douville O, Benhaim M, Boukobza C, Cousein M et al (2012) Clinique psychanalytique de l'exclusion. Dunod, Paris

Durkheim E (1897 [1976]) Le Suicide: étude de sociologie. PUF, Paris

Erhenberg A (2007) Épistémologie, Sociologie, sante publique. Tentative de clarification. Neuropsychiatr Enfance Adolesc 55:450–455

Foucault M (1963) Naissance de la clinique. Une archéologie du regard médical. PUF, Paris

Foucault M (1964 [1972]) Histoire de la folie à l'âge classique. Folie et déraison. Gallimard, Paris

Freud S (1893) Studies on hysteria. S E 2:1–305

Freud S (1908) "Civilized" sexual morality and modern nervous illness. S E 9: 177–204

Freud S (1913) Totem and taboo. S E 8:vii–162

Freud S (1917) Introductory lectures on psycho-analysis. S E 16:241–463

Freud S (1919) Lines of advance in psycho-analytic therapy. S E 17:157–168

Freud S (1921) Group psychology and the analysis of the ego. S E 18:65–144

Freud S (1923) Two encyclopaedia articles: (a) psycho-analysis. SE 23:233–260

Freud S (1927) The future of an illusion. S E 21:1–56

Freud S (1930) Civilization and its discontents. S E 21:57–146

Freud S (1933) New introductory lectures on psycho-analysis. S E 22:1–182

Freud S (1938) An outline of psycho-analysis. S E 23:139–208

Freud S (1939) Moses and monotheism. S E 23:1–138

Goffman E (1961) Asylums: essays on the social situation of mental patients and other inmates. Doubleday, New York

Hinshelwood RD (2001) Thinking about institutions. Jessica Kingsley Publishers, London

Hochmann J (1971 [2003]) L'institution mentale. In: La psychiatrie communautaire. Le Seuil, Paris

Hochmann J (1994) La consolation. Essai sur le soin psychique. Odile Jacob, Paris

Hochmann J (2006) Soigner, éduquer, instituer, raconter. Histoire et Actualité des traitements institutionnels des enfants psychiquement troublés. Rev Fr Psychanal 70(4):1043–1063

Hochmann J (2008) Soin institutionnel aux enfants et aux adolescents souffrant de troubles graves et précoces du développement (autismes et psychoses de l'enfance). Encyclopédie Médico-Chirurgicale, Psychiatrie/Pédopsychiatrie, 37-210-A-10

Hochmann J (2010) Histoire et Actualité du concept de psychose de l'enfant. L' inf Psychiatrique 86:227–235

Kaës R (ed) (1987) L'Institution et les institutions: études psychanalytiques. Dunod, Paris

Kaës R (ed) (2005) Différence culturelle et souffrances de l'identité. Dunod, Paris

Kaës R (2007) Un singulier pluriel. Dunod, Paris

Kaës R (2012) Le malêtre. Dunod, Paris

Kaës R, Pinel JP, Kernberg OF (2012) Souffrance et psychopathologie des liens institutionnels. Dunod, Paris

Kleinman A (1980) Patients and healers in the context of culture: an exploration of the borderland between anthropology, medicine, and psychiatry, vol 3. University of California Press, California

Kleinman A (2008) Rethinking psychiatry. Simon and Schuster, New York

Laplantine F (2007) Ethnopsychiatrie psychanalytique. Beauchesne, Paris

Mauss M (1950) Essai sur le don. In Sociologie et Anthropologie. PUF, Paris

McDougall J (1978 [2013]). Plea for a Measure of Abnormality. Routledge, London

Mentzos S (1991) Psychodynamische Modelle in der Psychiatrie. Vandenhoeck & Ruprecht, Göttingen

Mentzos S (2008) New trends in psychoanalytical psychotherapy for schizophrenia. In: Tzavaras N, Vartzopoulos I, Stylianidis S (eds) Psychoanalytical psychotherapy for schizophrenia. Kastaniotis Press, Athens, pp 51–84, (in Greek)

Milner M (1993) The role of illusion in symbol formation. In: Rudnytsky P. (ed)., Transitional objects and potential spaces: Literary uses of DW Winnicott, Columbia University Press, pp 13–39

Moro MR (2002) Enfants d' ici venus d'ailleurs: naître et grandir en France. La découverte

Moro MR (2004) Psychothérapie transculturelle de l'enfant et de l'adolescent. Dunod, Paris

Nathan T (1986) La folie des autres. Traite d'Ethnopsychiatrie clinique. Dunod, Paris

Nathan T (1988) Psychanalyse païenne. Essais ethnopsychanalytiques. Dunod, Paris

Nathan T (2007) Nous ne sommes pas seuls au monde: les enjeux de l'ethnopsychiatrie. Le Seuil, Paris

Nicolle O, Kaës R (2008) L'institution en héritage. Mythes de fondation, transmissions, transformations: mythes de fondation, transmissions, transformations. Dunod, Paris

Oury F (2004) Institutions: de quoi parlons-nous? Institutions 34, retrieved: http://ressources-cemea-pdll.org/IMG/pdf/institutions_de_quoi_parlons_nous.pdf. Accessed 15 July 2014

Petrou M (2005) New structures, yet. But are they new institutions? Psychiatry Notes 9:19–29 (in Greek)

Petrou M (2010) Intermodality and intersubjectivity. Paper at the 1st international psychoanalysis and the group conference. Athens 12 Nov 2010 (in Greek)

Petrou M (2012) Abuse: stimulation and collapse of the symbolic class. (Keynote speech) Manifestations of abuse workshop. Processes and changes through psychoanalytical psychotherapy. Cyprus Association for Psychoanalytical Psychotherapy Studies Nicosia, 21 Jan 2012 (in Greek)

Petrou M, Doxiadi A (2009) Perivolaki III. Psychiatry Notes 107:123–124 (in Greek)

Pinel J-P (2005) La déliaisons pathologique des liens institutionnels dans les institutions de soins et de rééducation. In: Kaës R, Pinel J-P, Kernberg OF (eds) Souffrance et psychopathologie des liens institutionnels. Dunod, Paris

Pinel J-P (2007) La supervision d'équipes institutionnelles. In: Lipianski M, Delourme A et al (eds) La supervision. Dunod, Paris

Pinel J-P, Morel S (2001) Psychose et institution: défenses paradoxales, anti-processualité et originaire évidé. Rev Psychothér Psychanal Group 1(36):133–145

Pouillon J (1970) Malade et médecin: le même et/ou l'autre? (remarques ethnologiques). Nouv Rev Pychanalyse 1:77–98

Racamier PC (1973) Le Psychanalyste sans divan. La psychanalyse et les institutions de soins psychiatriques. Payot, Paris

Racamier PC (1990) En psychanalyste et sans séances. Rev Fr Psychanal 54(5):1165–1183

Racamier PC (1993) L'art de soigner. Gruppo, 9. Apsygée, Paris

Ricœur P (1960) Soi-même comme un autre. Le Seuil, Paris

Ricœur P (1996) Les paradoxes de l'identité. L' Inf Psychiatrique 72(3):207–210

Rosenfeld HA (1965) Psychotic states: a psycho-analytical approach. International University Press, New York

Schafer R (1997) Tradition and change in psychoanalysis. International University Press, New York
Schermer VL, Pines ME (1999) Group psychotherapy of the psychoses: concepts, interventions and contexts. Jessica Kingsley Publishers, London
Searles H (1965 [1985]) The contribution of familial treatment to the psychotherapy of schizophrenia. In: Boszormenyi-Nagy I, Framo J (eds) Intensive family therapy: theoretical and practical aspects. Harper & Row (Second edition, New York, NY: Brunner/Mazel), New York
Searles H (1965 [1986]) Collected papers on schizophrenia and related subjects. International University Press, New York
Sklarew BE, Twemlow SW, Wilkinson SM (2004) Analysts in the trenches: streets, schools, war zones. Analytic Press, California
Stern D (1992) The 'pre-narrative envelope': an alternative view of 'unconscious fantasy' in infancy. Bull Anna Freud Cent 15(4):291–318
Stylianidis S (2011) The clinical practice of the ephemeral. Views on individual and social pain. Clinical and social questions from a psychoanalytical viewpoint. Oedipus 5:229–249 (in Greek)
Stylianidis S (2012) Subjective pain compared to the simplified reductionism of modern classificatory psychiatry: towards a psychiatry of the person. Synapsis J 24(8):16–21 (in Greek)
Tzavaras N, Stylianidis S (2002) Psychotherapy and transference in psychotic illnesses: references to text by Freud and this followers. In: Tzavaras N, Ploumpidis DN, Stylianidis S (eds) Schizophrenia: a phenomenological and psychoanalytical approach. Kastaniotis Press, Athens, pp 65–86 (in Greek)
Tzavaras N, Vartzopoulos I, Stylianidis S (eds) (2008) Psychoanalytical psychotherapy for schizophrenia. Kastaniotis Press, Athens (in Greek)
Winnicott D (1971) Playing and reality. Tavistock, London
Zajde N (2005) Enfants de survivants. La transmission du traumatisme chez les enfants des Juifs survivants de l'extermination nazie
Zajde N (2011) Psychotherapy with immigrant patients in France: an ethnopsychiatric perspective. Transcult Psychiatry 48(3):187–204

Part II
Applications of Social Psychiatry

Promoting Mental Health: From Theory To Best Practice

Stelios Stylianidis, Pepi Belekou, Lily Evangelia Peppou, and Athina Vakalopoulou

Abstract

Health is not just a biological matter (in the sense of the absence of illness) but also a social phenomenon, since it incorporates the quality of relations individuals have with each other and with their environment. The importance of mental health, its interdependence on physical health and the burden that mental disorders cause on a personal, family and social level have gained increasing recognition both by the relevant policymakers and by the general public.

Mental health is defined as the state of emotional well-being which prompts individuals to recognise their skills, to effectively deal with stressful life situations, to work to produce results and to contribute to the society in which they live. In our times, man appears to be particularly vulnerable in terms of mental health, and the frequency with which mental disorders are appearing is constantly on the rise. Both promoting health and preventing illness seek to ensure the common goal of maintaining and improving health.

Late diagnosis of mental problems in the young can very likely lead to serious mental illnesses in adult life with long-term effects. The World Health Organisation (WHO) has highlighted the importance of promoting mental health and prevention in children and adolescents and urges governments worldwide to include mental health as a key part of their primary healthcare. However, there is nonetheless an immense gap between needs and resource availability. However, in all European Union countries, there is some activity in terms of mental health

---

S. Stylianidis (✉)
Department of Psychology, Panteion University, Athens, Greece
e-mail: stylianidis.st@gmail.com

P. Belekou • L.E. Peppou • A. Vakalopoulou
Association for Regional Development and Mental Health (EPAPSY), Athens, Greece
e-mail: p.belecou@hotmail.com; lilly.peppou@gmail.com; athenaki83@hotmail.com

© Springer International Publishing Switzerland 2016
S. Stylianidis (ed.), *Social and Community Psychiatry: Towards a Critical, Patient-Oriented Approach*, DOI 10.1007/978-3-319-28616-7_7

prevention and promotion. The availability of the practices, resources and infrastructure which has been developed varies from country to country reflecting different situations in healthcare systems, political history and traditions and their understanding of both mental and public health.

A literature review highlights examples of best practices and evaluation of the effectiveness of measures to promote mental health among individuals of school age, since it recognises that education contributes to the prevention of the onset of mental illnesses.

The *programme to promote mental health in children and adolescents in selected areas of Greece* ran for the period 2011–2013. It was financed by the Stavros Niarchos Foundation and implemented by the Association for Regional Development and Mental Health on the islands of the NE and Western Cyclades. The measure sought to ensure primary protection of the mental health of children and adolescents. It included awareness-raising and counselling groups for parents of children in each age group, awareness-raising and counselling groups for adolescents about mental health issues and awareness-raising and support groups for teachers in preschool, primary and secondary education.

The awareness-raising groups performed an educational support role. The principles of assertive-experiential learning were chosen for the methodological approach. The results were particularly encouraging in all sectors of intervention. The chapter highlights the epistemological and social need for holistic interventions on interactive local systems, to ensure the best outcome of programmes to promote mental health.

7.1 Introduction

Health is a wide-ranging concept which can include positive, negative, functional and experiential definitions. The historic definition of health as the absence of illness is clearly an example of a negative definition. On the contrary, an example of a positive definition is the one from the WHO (1948) which states that health is a complete state of physical, mental and social well-being. A functional definition would refer to the ability to participate in normal social roles while an experiential definition would take into account one's sense of self (Kelman 1975).

Consequently, health is not just a biological but also a social phenomenon, since it incorporates the quality of relations individuals have with each other and with their environment (Tountas 2001). It can be depicted as a complex model which reflects the physical, mental and social dimension of well-being and illness.

The importance of mental health, its interdependence on physical health and the burden that mental disorders cause on a personal, family and social level have gained increasing recognition both by the relevant policymakers and by the general public. According to the Mental Health Declaration for Europe, "mental health -representing a state wellbeing in which the individual realises his own abilities, can cope with the normal stresses of life, can work productively and fruitfully, and is able to contribute to his community- has been recognised as fundamental to quality of life, enhances social cohesion, enhances peace and stability in the environment and contributes to the economic development of societies" (Jané-Llopis and Anderson 2006).

7.2 Concepts and Definitions: Historical Background

According to the World Health Organisation (WHO 2003a), mental health is defined as the state of emotional well-being which prompts individuals to recognise their skills, to effectively deal with stressful life situations, to work to produce results and to contribute to the society in which they live.

In our times, man appears to be particularly vulnerable in terms of mental health, and the frequency with which mental disorders are appearing is constantly on the rise. According to a recent health report, in the USA one in five Americans suffers every year from a diagnosable mental disorder, while 50 % of the American population will present such a disorder during their life time (Sultz and Young 2010). It also mentions that one in ten people will become ill with depression at some time in their life. It is estimated that around 6 % of the general population suffers from depression, in other words around 350 million people on the planet, 550,000 of whom are in Greece (Skevington and O' Connell 2004). One should not ignore the fact that mental disorder, which reflects a social pathology and is the result of the interactions of the psychobiological substrate with the natural environment, increases in periods of economic recession and social crisis, like the one we are currently experiencing.

According to research carried out in all EU countries (Wittchen et al. 2011), 38 % of the population (including those in childhood) are estimated as presenting some mental disorder every year. As far as adolescents are concerned, around one in five has been diagnosed with some form of mental disorder. It is no coincidence that mental disorders appear for the first time in adolescence or in early adult life (WHO 2009) since they may be an early sign of the appearance of mental disorders in adult life. According to the results of one study, 75 % of individuals with a diagnosed mental disorder at the age of 26 had been diagnosed for the first time during adolescence (WHO 2005). Around the world, almost 20 % of children and adolescents suffer from some mental illness, which degrades their quality of life, while also raising social and economic barriers for them. WHO surveys argue that mental illnesses and their symptoms are accompanied by mental, social and economic burdens of a scale of € 240 billion in the EU. In Europe 20 % of children and adolescents face developmental, mood-affective and behavioural disorders, while 4 % of children aged 12–17 years old suffer from depression (SOU Report 2006).

According to more recent epidemiological data (Mavreas et al. 2010), one in six Greeks aged 18–70 have developed clinically significant psychopathology and 1 in 12 (600,000) have serious psychopathology. International data showing that in Greece 75 % of the population with some form of psychopathology do not receive any treatment for their problem have been confirmed. In addition, the suicide rate has risen from 2.8 per 100,000 in 2008 to 5.2 in 2010 (Giotakos et al. 2011). As far as adolescents are concerned, research data confirm that mental disorders, dominated by depression, affect 3–8 % of the population and are directly related with negative health behaviours such as smoking, use of psychotropic substances and alcohol abuse and with reduce performance at school, poor social relations, bullying, high-risk sexual behaviour and even suicidal tendencies (Giannakopoulos et al. 2009). A study conducted on Greek adolescents found that the rate of attempted suicide in 2007 was 13.4 % of the population (Kokkevi et al. 2010).

7.3 Promoting Health and Preventing Illness

During the 1980s, and on November 21, 1986, in particular, the first international conference to promote health was held in Ottawa, Canada, under the aegis of the WHO, where the charter to develop actions to achieve health for all from 2000 onwards was presented. At that conference, a wide-ranging definition of health promotion was presented and then adopted:

> Health promotion is the process of enabling people to increase control over, and to improve, their health. A necessary tool in health promotion is health education, which is can be defined as a process which helps individuals take decisions, adopt behaviours and act in accordance with the need to safeguard and promote their own health. (Tountas 1994)

Health promotion includes all aspects which affect the individuals' choices about his behaviour such as values, beliefs, attitudes and incentives which prompt them towards a special form of health behaviour. In addition, it recognises that individuals do not make choices on their own but based on interactions with their environment (family, friends, social and community milieu, economic and political environment). Consequently, health promotion requires an exploration of the methods used by social policy such as laws and regulations about how the state operates, and social structures can change or support the positive dimension of health. Health promotion activities seek to support individuals and their social environments, to organise and set priorities and take action on health issues in line with social needs (Whitehead 2004).

On the other hand, illness is defined as an interruption or irregularity in bodily functions which causes pain or weakness. Anything that negatively affects the physical functionality of the body can be considered to be an illness. Although most people do not try to get ill, they do adopt day-to-day habits which are harmful to health, such as smoking or not exercising.

Illness prevention relates to any attempt to stop the onset of a specific illness or condition, such as heart conditions, diabetes or cancer, for example (Breslow 1999). In addition, prevention can include identifying illnesses during their early-onset phase. Such types of prevention are considered to be more effective than any other health promotion or behavioural strategy.

Both promoting health and preventing illness seek to ensure the common goal of maintaining and improving health. The difference lies in the fact that health promotion activities can be more general and seek to improve the individual's overall wellbeing. Illness prevention, on the other hand, focuses on preventing a specific disease. Moreover, health promotion arises from the needs and priorities of each distinct community, while illness prevention will most likely be based more on general data which show the importance of a health problem in the community such as depression levels in the elderly, for example.

7.4 The Importance of Promoting Mental Health

Late diagnosis of mental problems in the young can very likely lead to serious mental illnesses in adult life with long-term effects. Moreover, disorders that have not been identified and treated can seriously reduce the abilities of adolescents in becoming productive members of society and can lead to high levels of crime, major family conflicts, destructive substance abuse, low self-esteem and alcoholism (ASTHO 2002; WHO 2003b). The current socioeconomic crisis, the high demands of modern life, the incomplete parenting, changes in the family structure, dysfunctional interpersonal relations and new demands on adolescents have made it essential to identify mental health problems among adolescents in good time and provide them with support (Patel et al. 2007). However, for that to happen, one must first fully understand and approximate the environment of adolescents in terms of family and school, since mental health problems which prevent functionality are reflected in their reactions to social/environmental stressors (Appleton and Hammond-Roley 2000).

The World Health Organisation (WHO) has highlighted the importance of promoting mental health and prevention in children and adolescents and urges governments worldwide to include mental health as a key part of their primary healthcare (WHO 2004, 2011). However, there is nonetheless an immense gap between needs and resource availability (Keiling et al. 2011). However, in all European Union countries, there is some activity in terms of mental health prevention and promotion. The availability of the practices, resources and infrastructure which has been developed varies from country to country reflecting different situations in healthcare systems, political history and traditions and their understanding of both mental and public health.

7.5 Best Practices for Promoting Mental Health: International Standards

A literature review highlights examples of best practices and evaluation of the effectiveness of measures to promote mental health among individuals of school age, since it recognises that education contributes to the prevention of the onset of mental illnesses. In fact, programmes that are implemented in schools that focused on promoting general psychological skills (coping skills) for adolescents appear to be more effective than those which focus on specific problematic forms of behaviour (Mentality 2003). This approach includes interactive and participative methodologies, which have been confirmed as being more effective (Tobler et al. 2000).

After running the Responding in Peaceful and Positive Ways (RIPP) programme on 600 adolescents to develop socio-cognitive skills to promote non-violent conflict resolution and positive communication among them and teachers and parents, it appears that the participants acquired important knowledge about how to effectively communicate, manage anger, be empathic and control urges (Farrell et al. 2001).

The interpersonal cognitive problem-solving programme (ICPS) appeared to be equally important. It was run by teachers in the classroom to train adolescents about effective thinking, listening and interpersonal skills for solving problems using techniques such as dialogue, role playing, team spirit and relaxation (Shure and Spivack 1988). The participants appeared to significantly improve their cognitive conflict resolution skills and inhibitions, and spontaneity was significantly reduced. The intervention had a major effect on the role of teachers and also contributed to a reduction in psychological distress.

The Promoting Alternative Thinking Strategies (PATHS) programme was aimed at educating adolescents within structured groups to recognise, understand and self-regulate their emotions (Greenberg and Kusche 1998). For more positive results, printed materials were provided to teachers and parents about how to manage adolescents. The results of the programme confirm improve self-efficacy and positive mental health among the adolescents.

Hains and Ellmann (1994) designed an intervention programme for adolescents to reduce negative emotional arousal and other psychological consequences of stress. The adolescents participated in 13 groups overall which were briefed about stress and its harmful effects of health and were trained in stress management and problem-solving techniques. After the end of the intervention, stress levels reduced but not to such an important degree as the improvement in their attitude towards seeking health from mental health specialists. The awareness-raising and information campaign applied to 472 adolescents in England contributed significantly to the reduction in stigma about mental illness (Pinfold et al. 2003).

The WHO has shown the importance of integrating health services into the context of the school environment, which to a large extent is based on training the trainers (WHO 2010). Job satisfaction has been shown by many studies to positively affect teachers' ability to manage stress (Bindhu and Sudheeshkumar 2006) while fostering self-efficacy and positive health among teachers who protect both their own professional commitment and the mental balance of adolescents (Brouwers and Tomic 2000).

In one programme to promote mental health in the school environment run for adolescents, parents and teachers (Webster-Stratton and Hammond 2001), the results were positive for all three target populations: after counselling groups, parents appear to have lower levels of negative parenting and higher levels of positive parenting. Moreover, the ties between school and family and the partnership between teachers and parents improved, behavioural problems of children at home and school declined and the role of teachers and how they managed classes were improved.

In another interventionist programme to bolster the educational role and well-being of teachers (Wyn et al. 2000), the latter participated in a total of ten group sessions lasting 30 h which included experiential exercises such as exchanging professional experiences with colleagues, recognising specific stressors and potential coping strategies, using alternative ways of thinking and analysing specific methods for dealing with unruly students in the classroom. After the end of the programme, teachers noted a drop in psychological distress, improved social relations with each other and a drop in levels of burnout.

Another programme for parents and teachers of primary school pupils used teach learning methods to prevent early aggression in children and prepare them for higher school classes (Hawkins et al. 1991). At the end of the programme, teachers acquired stronger skills for teaching social skills to children and more effective knowledge dissemination methods. For their part, parents improved communication skills with their children, learned how to implement home discipline techniques and increased their knowledge about adolescent issues.

In 2008 the WHO in partnership with the International Association for Child and Adolescent Psychiatry organised an interventionist programme for adolescents, parents and teachers and government bodies to provide information and raise awareness about mental health issues faced by children and adolescents (Hoven et al. 2008) in nine countries. Positive changes were recorded in terms of the knowledge acquired by all participants, while the stigma attached to mental illness dropped and mental health issues were integrated into public debates and media coverage.

7.6 Best Practices in Greece

Programme to Promote Mental Health in Children and Adolescents

The programme to promote mental health in children and adolescents in selected areas of Greece ran for the period 2011–2013. It was financed by the Stavros Niarchos Foundation and implemented by the Association for Regional Development and Mental Health on the islands of the NE and Western Cyclades, where two mobile mental health units have been in operation for the last 10 years. These island areas are remote, meaning that social services either operate below capacity or do not exist at all, and the problems frequently encountered by health services make it difficult if not impossible to prevent and deal with mental health problems.

The intervention was aimed at primary protection of the mental health of children and adolescents and consisted of three levels, to support adolescents and children within frameworks which are important for their development: (a) interventions for the adolescents themselves, (b) interventions at school by working with teachers and (c) interventions in the family. The programme was designed as follows:

(a) Awareness-raising and counselling groups for parents of children in each age group (parents of children of preadolescent and of adolescent age). The main goal of the parents' intervention group was to improve positive mental health and reduce mental distress (by focusing on promotion and prevention, respectively). In addition, specific goals of the intervention were to reduce parental stress, to cultivate coping skills, to expand social networks and to improve attitudes towards mental health professionals and the idea of seeking out help for psychological difficulties.
(b) Awareness-raising and counselling groups for adolescents about mental health issues and theatrical play meetings, where the central goal was to improve positive mental health and reduce mental disorders. Secondary goals included improving the degree of self-efficacy, cultivating coping skills and improving attitudes towards mental health professionals and the idea of seeking out help for psychological difficulties.
(c) Awareness-raising and support groups for teachers in preschool, primary and secondary education. The main goal of this intervention was to improve the ability of teachers to identify mental stress in children and adolescents and to improve their professional self-efficacy. Secondary goals included learning coping skills and expanding social networks.

Planning the Intervention

The plan was that teacher and parent groups would attend nine 2-h long meetings and adolescents would attend 18 meetings with two facilitators in each group (expert mental health trainers specialised in group work). The groups were to meet every 15 days. Each of the meetings per group sought to address specific issues and cover a particular topic. A manual was drawn up for each group meeting which consisted of two parts: (a) a seminar-like presentation on the topic presented using interactive media and (b) an experiential part to ensure deeper assimilation of the topic through experience.

Preparing the manuals was the tool and joint basis for the interventions. The content and subject matter was determined by an informal exploration of needs done by a focus group of school advisors and educational bodies during the preparatory phase. Members of the teams across the entire programme were also asked at the first meeting as part of a brainstorming exercise. The final subject matter was approved by the editorial committee, having taken into account the information generated by the focus groups. The manuals were written by committees of group facilitators appointed depending on the area of specialisation each one had. The editorial team then edited the texts. Each manual was different and aimed at a specific target group. Depending on the subject examined, the epistemological focus of the manual differed (psychoanalytical, systemic, cognitive-behavioural).

The content of the manuals was revised during the programme in line with the intervention's quality control process. The diaries designed as part of the programme's internal evaluation process to be filled out by the group therapists with information about the process indicators for each meeting (a) ensured the uniformity of the intervention at different stages of the programme and (b) allowed one to identify weaknesses in the meetings and correct them later (such as subject matter might have needed to be explored in more detail or required more time or fewer experiential exercises may have been needed).

Methodology: Awareness-Raising and Counselling Groups: Assertive, Experiential Learning

The awareness-raising groups performed an educational support role. Their primary target was to create a framework to activate the individual as a "whole" (Senge et al. 2008). Implementing the project utilised key principles of group dynamics, such as interaction, building a team spirit, developing social networking, creating familiarity, developing communication and cooperation skills, expressing emotions and connecting to personal meaning (Navridis 2005). Consequently, the educational process also aided the personal growth of those who participated.

The principles of experiential learning were chosen for the methodological approach. As stated above, the structured group interventions followed a manual which included presentations and experiential techniques, such as how to present the topic of small groups, role play games, case studies, simulations (goldfish bowls), communication exercises and use of the group as a forum for social learning about the target group. The approach was experiential and integrated the concept of assertive learning and was aimed at the ability of participants to learn through experience.

Yalom (1995) states that the group process on its own has an experiential character. In addition, experiential learning places emphasis on the important role played by experience in the learning process and provides intellectual and emotional stimulation seeking to integrate intellectual and emotional processes (Evans 1994). At the same time, it is based on initiative and assertive involvement of the individual, which gives the chance to act and take responsibility for the process (Mulligan 1993) and covers a longer time period since it mobilises the individual as a "whole". Learning is in depth and can help the individual grow, affecting his attitudes and personality.

Results

A multifaceted approach was used to evaluate the programme in an attempt to remain in keeping with the complexity of the programme itself and each such mental health prevention and promotion programme. In particular, indicators relating to structure, procedure and outcomes of the programme were included, and information was collected in various ways relating to the outcome indicators: number of referrals to mobile units, use of self-reporting scales, questions to subjects benefiting from the programme, focus groups and open-ended questions about satisfaction with the programme. A brief presentation of the results is set out below.

Overall 1,259 received services as part of the programme over 2 years, and 66 individuals (teachers in the second round) participated in the programme in both years. One thousand and twenty-three people received programme services in the Cyclades, 140 in Evia and 96 in the northern suburbs of Athens. In each target group, the figures for those who received services were 585 teachers, 513 parents and 161 adolescents. The lower number of adolescents compared to other groups can be explained by the difficulty in approaching and retaining the specific population group in long-term, stable prevention measures, especially when the programme is run outside of school hours.

As far as referrals to mobile units are concerned, there was a significant increase which reflects the positive impact of the specific programme on the local communities in the Cyclades where it was run. In the first year, 23 % of referrals to paedo-psychiatric services offered by the mobile unit came from the programme while the corresponding figure for adult services was 16 %. In the second year, 29 % of referrals to paedo-psychiatric services came from the programme and 17 % of referrals for adult services.

As far as adolescents are concerned, the interventions generated the following statistically significant differences compared to the scales before and after the intervention:

Improved self-efficacy (theatrical games and counselling groups)
Reduced symptoms of stress (theatrical games)
Reduced social dysfunction (counselling groups)
Increased use of emotional and practical support as coping strategies (counselling groups)
Reduced mental stress in general (theatrical games)

Adolescents considered that the interventions helped them improve self-confidence, learn more about themselves, become able to express their thoughts and emotions without problems, make new friends and seek out help if they needed it. The interventions do not appear to have improved their positive mental health (mental well-being) but that change may require time to take place.

As far as parents were concerned, the intervention succeeded in large part in its individual goals as is clear from the statistically significant changes noted between the two points in time when the evaluation tools were used (before and after the intervention). The following findings were recorded:

A reduction in psychological distress (psychopathologies of a neurotic type using the GHQ scale)
Improved positive mental health
Reduced parental stress
Expanded social networks
More frequent use of coping skills

As far as teachers are concerned, the internal evaluation and quality control processes resulted in the targets for the specific intervention being redefined as well as in a change in methodology from year 1 to year 2. The lack of a statistically significant impact of the intervention in year 1, the focus groups with group facilitators and a supervisor and the focus groups with the teachers themselves held at the end of year 1 led to a change in focus. During year 1 the intervention primarily related to emotional difficulties faced by teachers themselves and to raising of awareness about mental health issues. In year 2, however, the intervention focused on issues such as identifying mental disorders, managing difficulties in the classroom and fostering the role of the teacher so that he/she could provide effective, real support to students.

The evaluation of that year, which also included teachers who had taken part in year 1 and some who had taken part in year 2 (deeper examination of issues and focus of specific school-based issues), showed that during year 1, teachers had learned about mental health issues and awareness of them had increased, while in year 2 they were given the opportunity to use that knowledge, to better organise and manage their own issues in terms of their tendency towards emotional over-involvement and their position in relation to the student, parent, colleagues and headmaster.

The intervention led to better identification and recognition of mental health issues among students, greater professional self-efficacy, better social networking and cultivation of better coping skills.

The programme's successes include the involvement and high response rate among local communities which were helped in actively participating in all stages of programme implementation. All procedures were made easier, since facilities were provided for the interventions, thereby raising awareness and informing the population and using the local process to spread news about the programme. For the purposes of the programme, psychometric tools were translated and localised for the Greek population, which can now be used to conduct other research into related topics, and the scientific process used to document the manuals means they can now be used for other mental health working groups, agencies and organisations.

Consequently, the programme's contribution and effectiveness was evaluated on many levels, since the programme itself appears to have benefited the attendees, local communities, mental health services in the local area, mental health professionals and the scientific community in general.

7.7 Discussion

The literature and history of psychiatric reform in Greece shows that the reform process was not accompanied by programmes of this sort which would have improved primary prevention in the population against mental illnesses. Even agencies which could have presented examples of good social psychiatry did not adopt a structured programme to promote mental health.

The programme we implemented had positive effects on local communities, as we mentioned, but also had specific constraints and limits. In many cases we have seen islands of psychiatric reform collapse in the past because of lack of resources and because of the medical focus of the culture within agencies/services, professionals and the wider healthcare system. (See the chapters on psychiatric reform in Europe and Greece.) Reality has taught us that certain synergies are needed at institutional level to run programmes of this kind and that networks of services (networking) are needed to (a) ensure that reform is not put at more risk and (b) ensure that it does not remain suspended in mid-air. Moreover, one disadvantage of the situation in Greece is that mental health promotion and health education are not taught in educational institutes, except in some isolated postgraduate courses. Professionals therefore lack the ability to acquire the necessary tools and skills for the relevant practices.

Talking about local communities, it is essential to stress the multifaceted aspect of interventions of this kind, as well as the complex interactions between the individual, family, wider community (local authorities, services, agencies) and the wider framework to which the community belongs. Fritjof Capra, an important systems theorist, highlighted the idea of the web of life. For major social issues such as health, he refers to direct connections and interactions with living systems: individuals, social systems and ecosystems (Capra 1997, 2004). The concept of the web of life in the humanities demonstrates the use of network networks at all system levels. It is a dynamic process with numerous individual levels, which are both affected and affect the system. We can identify the benefits of an intervention on all the levels referred to but contrariwise the fact that the same benefits may also be needed to affect the culture of the scientific sector, to shape policy, and the content of interventions. Living systems respond to the effects they are subject to from their environment by making structural changes (Bateson 1979; Maturana and Varela 1987).

At the same time, the concept of interdependence of all phenomena allows us to understand the multiplier effect of positive results on the members of a community, and outside of it, by connecting the local with the global. Modern theories of networks talk about the "human superorganism" where local contributions to the human social network can have global consequences (Christakis and Fowler 2010). Consequently, interventions to promote mental health need to take these fundamental changes in the theory of humanities and the connections between phenomena which were until now treated as "separate" into account and must approach the individual from a holistic scientific perspective.

References

Appleton P, Hammond-Roley S (2000) Addressing the population burden of child and adolescent mental health problems: a primary care model. Child Psychol Psychiatry Rev 5:9–16

Association of State and Territorial Health Officials (ASTHO) (2002) Mental health resource guide. Child and Adolescent Mental Health, Washington, DC

Bateson G (1979) Mind and nature: a necessary unity. Dutton, New York

Bindhu C, Sudheeshkumar P (2006) Job satisfaction and stress coping skills of primary school teachers. Education Resources Information Centre, available at: www.eric.ed.gov

Breslow L (1999) From disease prevention to health promotion. JAMA 281(11):1030–1033

Brouwers A, Tomic W (2000) A longitudinal study of teacher burnout and perceived self-efficacy in classroom management. Teach Teach Educ 16(2):239–253

Capra F (1997) The web of life: a new scientific understanding of living systems. Anchor Books, New York

Capra F (2004) The hidden connections: a science for sustainable living. Anchor Books, New York

Christakis NA, Fowler JH (2010) Connected: the amazing power of social networks and how they shape our lives. HarperPress, London

Evans N (1994) Experiential learning for all. Cassell, London

Farrell AD, Meyer AL, White KS (2001) Evaluation of Responding in Peaceful and Positive Ways (RIPP): a school-based prevention program for reducing violence among urban adolescents. J Clin Child Psychol 30(4):451–463

Giannakopoulos G, Dimitrakaki C, Pedeli X, Kolaitis G, Rotsika V, Ravens-Sieberer U, Tountas Y (2009) Adolescents' wellbeing and functioning: relationships with parents' subjective general physical and mental health. Health Qual Life Outcomes 7:100. doi:10.1186/1477-7525-7-100

Giotakos O, Karabelas D, Kafkas A (2011) Financial crisis and mental health in Greece. Psychiatriki 22:109–119

Greenberg MT, Kusche CA (1998) Promoting social competence and preventing casebook for practitioners. American Psychological Association, Washington, DC, pp 69–82

Hains AA, Ellmann SW (1994) Stress inoculation training as a preventative aggression: results of a primary prevention program. J Am Acad 3:43–50

Hawkins JD, Von Cleve E, Catalano RF (1991) Reducing early childhood maladjustment in school-aged children: the effects of the PATHS curriculum, Manuscript Mentalities Briefing Paper 1. Mentality, London

Hoven CW, Doan T, Musa GJ, Jaliashvili T, Duarte CS, Ovuga E, … Task Force WA (2008) Worldwide child and adolescent mental health begins with awareness: a preliminary assessment in nine countries. Int Rev Psychiatry 20(3):261–270

Jané-Llopis E, Anderson P (eds) (2006) Mental health promotion and mental disorder prevention across European Member States: a collection of country stories. European Communities, Luxembourg

Kelman S (1975) The social nature of the definition problem in health. Int J Health Serv 5(4): 625–642

Kieling C, Baker-Henningham H, Belfer M, Conti G, Ertem I, Omigbodun O, … Rahman A (2011) Child and adolescent mental health worldwide: evidence for Action. Lancet 378(9801): 1515–1525

Kokkevi A, Rotsika V, Arapaki A, Richardson C (2010) Changes in associations between psychosocial factors and suicide attempts by adolescents in Greece from 1984 to 2007. Eur J Public Health. doi:10.1093/eurpub/ckq160, 1–5, advance Access published Nov 26, 2010

Maturana H, Varela F (1987) The tree of knowledge. Shambhala, Boston

Mavreas et al (2010) Epidemiological research in Greece. (Unpublished data)

Mentality (2003) Making it effective: a guide to evidence-based mental health promotion. Radic Child Adolesc Psychiatry 30:208–217

Mulligan J (1993) Activating internal processes in experiential learning. In: Boud D, Cohen R, Walker D (eds) Using experience for learning. The Society for Research into Higher Education and The Open University Press, Milton Keynes

Navridis K (2005) Group psychology. Ellinika Grammata Press, Athens (in Greek)

Patel V, Flisher A, Hetrick S, McGorry P (2007) Mental health of young people: a global public-health challenge. Lancet 369(9569):1302–1313

Pinfold V, Toulmin H, Thornicroft G, Huxley P, Farmer P, Graham T (2003) Reducing psychiatric stigma and discrimination: evaluation of educational interventions in UK secondary schools. Br J Psychiatry 182:342–346

Report SOU (2006) Youth, stress and mental problems – analyses and health promotion issues

Senge P, Scharmer O, Jaworski J, Flowers B (2008) Presence. Exploring profound change in people, organisations and society. Nicolas Brealey, London

Shure MB, Spivack G (1988) Interpersonal cognitive problem solving. In: Price RH, Cowen EL, Lorion RP, Ramos-McKay J (eds) Fourteen ounces of prevention: a casebook for practitioners. Aldine, Hawthorne, pp 69–82

Skevington SM, O'Connell KA (2004) Can we identify the poorest quality of life? Assessing the importance of quality of life using the WHOQOL-100. Qual Life Res 13(1):22–34

Sultz H, Young K (2010) Health care, USA: understanding its organisation and delivery, 7th edn. Jones & Bartlett Learning, Sudbury

Tobler NS, Roona MR, Ochshorn P, Marshall DG, Streke AV, Stackpole KM (2000) School-based adolescent drug prevention programs: meta-analysis. J Prim Prev 20:275–336

Tountas G (1994) Health education. In: Kaklamanis E, Frangouli-Koumantaki Y (eds) Preventative medicine and health education. P. C. Paschalidis Medical Press, Athens (in Greek)

Tountas G (2001) Society and health, 2nd edn, Social Factors. New Health, Athens, p 140, in Greek

Webster-Stratton C, Hammond M (2001) Preventing conduct problems, promoting social competence: a parent and teacher training partnership in head start. J Clin Child Psychol 30: 283–302

Whitehead D (2004) Health promotion and health education: advancing the concepts. J Adv Nurs 47(3):311–320

Wittchen HU, Jacobi F, Rehm J, Gustavsson A, Svensson M, Jönsson B, … Steinhausen HC (2011) The size and burden of mental disorders and other disorders of the brain in Europe 2010. Eur Neuropsychopharmacol 21(9):655–679

World Health Organisation (WHO) (1948). Preamble to the Constitution of the World Health Organisation as adopted by the International Health Conference, New York, 19–22 June, 1946; signed on 22 July 1946 by the representatives of 61 States (Official Records of the World Health Organisation, no. 2, p. 100) and entered into force on 7 April 1948

World Health Organisation (WHO) (2003a) The solid facts. WHO Regional Office for Europe, Denmark

World Health Organisation (WHO) (2003b) Caring for children and adolescents. Conclusions from Pre-conference Luxembourg, Denmark

World Health Organisation (WHO) (2004) Prevention of mental disorders: effective interventions and policy options: summary report. World Health Organisation, Geneva

World Health Organisation (WHO) (2005) Health Evidence Network (HEN) What are the main factors that influence the implementation of disease prevention and health promotion programmes in children and adolescents? WHO Regional Office for Europe, Copenhagen

World Health Organisation (WHO) (2009) WHO calls for action on world autism awareness day, News release 2 Apr 2009, Geneva, World Health Organisation

World Health Organisation (WHO) (2010) Youth-friendly health policies and services in the European Region. WHO Press, Geneva

World Health Organisation (WHO) (2011) Young people: health risks and solutions. World Health Organisation (WHO), Geneva

Wyn J, Cahill, Holdsworth R, Rowling L, Carson S (2000) Mind matters, a whole-school approach promoting mental health and wellbeing. Aust N Z J Psychiatry 34:594–601

Yalom ID (1995) The theory and practice of group psychotherapy. Basic Books, New York

Social Suffering and Mental Health in Metropolitan Athens: A Qualitative Approach

8

Stelios Stylianidis, Athina Vakalopoulou, and Lily Evangelia Peppou

Abstract

Modern metropolises have now transformed into anonymous zones without history, similar to anywhere else in the world, overcrowded with various people who do not know each other and who have never come into contact. Social inequalities in such environments and the consequent social exclusion have a negative effect on health, mental health and the well-being of the population. The aim of this study is to explore social exclusion in metropolitan Athens and in particular to record its socio-demographic profile, its self-image, experiences of social racism and health problems for the homeless in the centre of the Greek capital. The homeless characterise themselves as unfortunate and unlucky, and some have experienced others as being indifferent towards them or have suffered social racism, while others have described a completely positive response from others. At the same time, they have quite a few health problems, and almost one in two has a clear sense of sadness and stress. A major percentage also report substance and alcohol abuse, while quite a few appear to use alcohol as a form of self-treatment. In conclusion, the city generates alienation, fear, insecurity and unhappiness. Every community ought to use any resources it has to implement organised policies and create social networks to address the complex needs that arise.

S. Stylianidis (✉)
Department of Psychology, Panteion University, Athens, Greece
e-mail: stylianidis.st@gmail.com

A. Vakalopoulou • L.E. Peppou
Association for Regional Development and Mental Health (EPAPSY), Athens, Greece
e-mail: athenaki83@hotmail.com; lilly.peppou@gmail.com

8.1 Introduction

It is widely known that the migration movement mushroomed after the end of the Cold War. It emerged as part of globalisation processes and lead to a deep restructuring of the social geography of metropolitan areas. "The world became a city", said the historian Lewis Mumford in a characteristic phrase in 1961. Indeed his forecast has become a reality, in the sense that the entire world was transformed into an immense array of large urban areas, which have seen a shift from South to North: social inequalities and exclusion, the stigmatism of poverty and the increasing complexity of social suffering (Castells 1989). The city offers the ability to adapt for survival, concealment and communication. However, it does not have the suitable institutions and does not have any potential for gradual integration into the urban space (Saraceno 2010). Marc Augé (1992), one of France's best-known anthropologists, used the term "non-place" (non-lieu) to refer to anonymous places without history, similar to anywhere else in the world, overcrowded with various people who do not know each other and who have never come into contact. That definition clearly reflects the social reality of metropolitan areas in Europe and more widely.

This trend began to dominate in the first decade of the new millennium, and for metropolises with global influence, the specific movement was named "super-diversity" (Vertovec 2007). The phenomenon of social fragmentation and marginalisation has spread not just to the metropolises of the South but to large Northern European cities as well, despite the fact that they developed under completely different conditions compared to those of South America and the European metropolises. "Rounded" approaches to dealing with this complex problems by formulating proposals and guidelines for changes in social and sanitary policy have failed to provide persuasive answers at local level, such as the problems of social suffering and social exclusion in the world's metropolitan centres (Thomas et al. 2005; Saraceno 2014; Stewart et al. 2010).

The gap between generalised declarations and announcements by the planning authorities to relieve the vulnerable populations who live in a constantly ephemeral reality and understanding of the specific impact at local level are now immense (Appadurai 2002). In the harsh and chaotic reality of modern metropolises, social suffering is bound up with mental pain and psychiatric disorders and abandonment with the lack of rudimentary care for individuals with problems of public health work, identity and survival. The violence which exists in this context is not just suppression, ghettoisation, social exclusion and lack of access to health, welfare and mental health services and breach of all fundamental rights for a decent life: It is also symbolic, mental, emotional, cultural violence and a lack of any investment in the future (Bourdieu 1991). Pain in a metropolitan setting, in no man's land, is a new "paradigm" within which situations of pain are interdependent (Stylianidis et al. 2011). The responses are fragmented and noncontinuous, and respect for rights is an "insignificant" problem compared to the "health bomb" waiting to go off that these people represent, as a threat to public health. As B. Saraceno (2010) writes, the North (no matter where it is located geographically) has its very own South.

The social inequalities of these metropolises have a negative impact on health, mental health and well-being to a greater degree. Quite a few studies confirm the fact that they are accompanied by mental disorders, with most common ones being stress and depression, followed by addiction and dependence problems and by cardiovascular conditions (Stuckler et al. 2009). The most powerful risk factors are unemployment, low levels of education, low income and degraded living conditions (Fryers et al. 2003). The loss of work and long-term poverty impact even more on individuals from minorities, such as migrants (Doorslaer et al. 1997; Wilkinson 2002), with depressive symptoms appearing often, especially in men (Stansfeld et al. 2003). In addition, those individuals are twice as much as risk of early mortality and have increased morbidity (Bartley et al. 1997; Blane et al. 1997).

Greece, well known for its migrant flows, has today become a "host country" for migrants with an inadequate migration policy (The World Bank 2011). The majority of migrants in Greece are Albanian (Ventura 2006). This chapter will attempt to show based on recent research data that there is a need for holistic, multifaceted and integrated responses to such complex problems, in contrast to the fragmented responses from services that are limited in a piecemeal fashion to looking at the individual level only.

8.2 Observations About the Description of Metropolitan Athens

Athens has a diverse distribution of different classes and ethnic minorities. The city centre (Omonoia Square) is literally "abandoned" to the hands of various ethnic groups including quite a few Greeks in an exceptionally perilous state.

Agios Panteleimonas Square is an extreme case study (Arapoglou 2006) which allows us to understand in depth the complexity of conflicts within the endogenous population. According to the mayor of Athens, Kaminis (2011), "both legitimate migrants and migrants without anywhere lawful to stay enter the country, while 300 of them gather in the city centre every day". He also states the constant stream of migrants without a lawful right to stay leads to an increase in the number of victims of the general social crisis. As a result, a new category of homeless people has emerged, the new homeless: educated people, possibly with families, who suddenly found themselves faced without a job or home. It is worth noting that in 2011 the competent authorities recorded 25,000 homeless people who took shelter in abandoned buildings, squares and pavements in Attica alone (Giannarou 2012).

The link between fluidity and pain and crime rates is undisputed. It is illustrative that in a recent evaluation by Mercer in 2011 (Global 2011), Athens "fell" eight places in the rankings for safety and quality of life and is now in bottom place in terms of European capitals. The increasing levels of migrants and the homeless population in general have also led to a corresponding rise in crime levels. Recent research by Kapa Research showed that 79.3 % of those questioned felt at risk because of cases of violence happening daily involving migrants without any papers (Tryfonas 2012). Migrants are pushed towards illegal acts because their fundamental rights have been infringed and because of their position in the social pyramid. They are perpetrators of crimes against property, such as theft, and crimes involving the trafficking and use of drugs and prostitution, primarily involving women (Bui and

Thongniramol 2005). Official data from the Hellenic Police shows that of the 12,250 people detained in Greece's prisons, 7,700 are foreigners (Souliotis 2012).

The sense of failure, deriving from the inability to meet basic needs, and the sense of isolation and being cut-off from the social fabric lead the homeless to low self-esteem, despair and a total lack of incentives to survive. Poverty has a direct psychological impact on the sense of shame, low self-worth and stigmatism (Patel and Kleinman 2003). On the other hand, social stigma lies not only in the lack of work and poverty but also in the personal characteristics of the homeless person, such as use of drugs, alcoholism and mental illness, trapping them in a single "identity", that of social suffering (Major and O'Brien 2005). Because of the nature and heterogeneity of the homeless situation, their only name is "the others". Studies on the homeless (Harter et al. 2005) have shown that self-stigmatism is intimately bound up with low self-esteem, loneliness, the sense of being trapped, suicidal ideation and the sense of guilt and low self-worth because the situation they are in appeared to affect mental illness variables such as stress and depression. The majority of the mass media and key figures who shape public opinion transform this phenomenon into images and dialogues about extremely stigmatised ghettos, which in turn form the cultural concept of homeless people for us.

8.3 Research Design

Against this background, the Regional Development and Mental Health Association, working in partnership with the Panteion University, carried out a study to explore social exclusion in Metropolitan Athens. The specific aims of the study were:

(a) To identify and capture the socio-demographic characteristics of homeless people in the centre of Athens
(b) To explore the image they have of themselves and the image others have of them
(c) To record and capture key health and mental health problems they report

To achieve those objectives, a qualitative approach was adopted for three main reasons. The study's primary aim was to explore views, feelings and experiences of the homeless in depth, spontaneously and freely, without the restrictions a quantitative approach imposes. At the same time, the limited literature on the topic in Greece meant that the study was more exploratory and less an attempt to verify or reject some research hypothesis. Lastly, the absence of a weighted clinical tool for migrants would limit the validity of the results.

Method

Sample
Feasibility sampling was used in this study to record a wide range of views, experiences and emotions. Participants were recruited from various places where the homeless congregate in Athens: in Koumoundourou, Amerikis, Koliatsou, Viktorias, Vathi, Liossion, Acharnon, Exarchia, Omonia, Stournai, Polytechnio, Metaxourgio

Table 8.1 Interview topic guide

Questions:
1. How would you characterise yourself?
2. How do people treat you?
3. How is your health?
4. How is your mental health? (how are you psychologically?)

and Agios Panteleimonas Squares. We approached both Greek and migrant homeless people. The only criterion for inclusion in the study was their willingness to participate, and the sole exclusion criterion was the lack of an ability to communicate with the investigators in either Greek or English. The participants received coffee and cigarettes for taking part.

Interview Tool

The interviews were semi-structured and included open-ended questions that primarily focused on the socio-demographic profile of the homeless, their self-image, experiences of social exclusion they may have had and their state of health, including their mental health.

The interview tool (a topic guide) was developed by the investigating team and is summarised in Table 8.1.

The face-to-face interviews were conducted by 11 final year students of psychology at the Panteion University after a 3-day training course about the research methodology and interview techniques using cultural competence tools (Gionakis 2010). The students were supervised once a month.

Due to participants being suspicious about the use of recording devices, the students noted the responses down on paper. Participants were approached by pairs of students: one to conduct the interview and the other to keep notes.

Data Analysis

Thematic analysis was used to interpret the data in line with and Interpretative Phenomenological Approach (IPA) to the narratives (Smith et al. 2009). Initially, the two investigators read the narratives independently numerous times, noting down the thematic titles in the margins which could be used to summarise them. Then the themes in each narrative were tied together and classed, and in the final stage, the investigators tried to identify recurring and new themes, taking into account overlapping data from the narratives in the sample. The two investigators found similar themes (reliability), and if they disagreed, the theme was determined after a discussion held with the entire research team.

8.4 Results

Socio-demographic Profile of the Population

Table 8.2 shows the socio-demographic characteristics of the participants.

In total, 329 people participated in the study. 14.28 % of the people in the study were aged 18–22, and a similar figure applied to the 28–32 age bracket. This was

Table 8.2 Socio-demographic characteristics of the people in the study

Distribution	N=329	%
Age		
18–22	47	14.28
23–27	41	12.47
28–32	47	14.28
33–37	39	11.85
38–42	34	10.33
43–47	24	7.3
48–52	25	7.6
53–57	15	4.56
58+	42	12.46
No response	1	0.3
Gender		
Male	251	76.2
Female	78	23.7
Nationality		
Greece	137	41.6
Lebanon	5	1.5
Afghanistan	27	8.2
Pakistan	29	8.8
Iran (Persia)	6	1.8
Iraq	6	1.8
Morocco – Tunisia	9	2.7
Africa	23	7
Bangladesh	16	4.8
Romania	5	1.5
Albania	15	4.5
Bulgaria	13	3.9
Nigeria	1	0.3
Pontus – Caucasus	1	0.3
Algeria	3	0.9
Syria	10	30.4
Latvia	1	0.3
India	5	1.5
Georgia	2	0.6
Palestine	4	1.2
Ukraine	1	0.3
China	2	0.6
Undisclosed	5	1.5

followed by 12.46 % for the over 58 age bracket. Moreover, 76 % of the sample consisted of men and around half the participants were Greek (42 %), which confirms the state of crisis and utter uncertainty in modern Greek society.

Axis 1: Self-Image

The thematic analysis of the narratives showed that 36.7 % of the sample focused on unhappiness, poverty and misfortune. Quite a few said they felt "hurt, afraid, unfortunate and without hope" (N18, N69). Family relations were quite illustrative of their overall condition: "My parents never wanted me, my father used to beat the living daylights out of me whenever he drank" (N60). On the contrary, 14.5 % of the population characterised themselves as "good people" struggling to get by and hoping for something better: "I'm optimistic, I've got dreams for the future" (N51), "I'm a good person, why do I have to endure all this?" (*N117*) and "I'm good, spontaneous, hard-working" (*N93*). They have experienced pain and instability as well as separation, situations which have activated feelings of guilt and low self-esteem: "I've messed up. My parents don't even want to see me" (*N56*), "I feel like a great big nothing" (*N92*), "I feel like an idiot. I didn't grab opportunities" (*N107*) or "I'm ruined and I have myself to blame for that" (*N87*). Lastly, a small part of the sample (9.5 %) considered themselves to be happy, lucky and proud: "I'm not some random guy, I know who I am" (N97) and "I'm a proud person. I don't beg. If someone wants he will give me money" (N13).

Axis 2: Treatment by Others

It is noteworthy that around 24 % of the sample gave conflicting responses. Seventy seven of the 329 participants reported that people "help, give you coffee, cigarettes and food" (N7) and "give you clothes and food" (*N114*), while on the other hand, 79 participants described extremely stigmatising behaviour from other people: "They don't see as any different from dogs" (N33), "there's racism. They say I stink because I'm black" (N70) and "They look down on us because we are on the margins" (N62). 10.9 % of the population responded that sometimes people treat them well other times with racism, while 8 % said that people were indifferent: "No one pays attention. And rightly so, why should they care?" (N76) and "People don't care about me. It's like I'm invisible to them" (N69).

Axis 3: Physical Illnesses

Of the 329 participants, 121 replied that they have physical illnesses (36.7 %), the most common being muscular-skeletal problems (13.6 %) because of their terrible living conditions. That was followed by cardiovascular conditions (6.3 %) and dental issues (3.3 %). 32 % of the sample denied any physical illnesses, while 8.5 % did not respond.

Axis 4: Mental Illnesses

Of the 329 people in the sample, only 16 (4.9 %) replied that they did not have any problem or felt happy/hadn't given up hope when asked how they felt psychologically. On the contrary, almost one in two (188 people, 54.7 %) described a palpable sense of sadness/worry/melancholy: "I feel really sad and worried. I want to cry all the time. I wish I'd just die in my sleep so that I wouldn't understand a thing" (N13), "I think I've probably got depression. It's like I feel unhappy all the time and can't escape from it. Sometimes I'm so upset I want to throw up" (N99), "I usually feel melancholic at night. I cry almost every night because of how unhappy I feel. Sometimes I dream about getting away from all this, but the next evening it's the same thing over again, … trapped in the same situation, without being able to escape" (N183) and "Sadness like a shadow over me every day. That follows me wherever I go, whatever I do. I feel empty" (N305).

In parallel, a large percentage (154, 46.8 %) described intense and palpable stress/anxiety: "All day I feel that I'm wound up, my nerves are on edge, I feel I can't calm down at all, that nothing can relieve me" (N113), "I'm stressed, very stressed and anxious, about what to do, how I can escape from all this" (N278) and "I'm in a bad way psychologically, I'm stressed out all the time. I can feel my heart racing from the stress and panic, like I have a weight on my chest, a knot, I feel like I'm boiling inside… I walk so I won't have to think, but I can't calm down… the worst thing is when I can't manage to sleep at night with my thoughts and the anxiety" (N311). In addition to palpable sadness and stress which dominates the stories from participants, a large portion of the sample (119 people, 36.2 %) had pessimistic thoughts about the future and/or ideas of unworthiness: "I feel that everything is a mountain … I don't know if and how I will manage to overcome all these difficulties that have arisen … I'm overcome with despair" (N98), "I've lost all trust in myself and all self-esteem. Basically, I hate myself. I'm a piece of rubbish" (N106), "I feel helpless, I'm not worth anything, I'm nothing" (N250) or "I'm very disappointed by myself, I feel a failure, that I've come to this point, that I cannot overcome my problems, that I can't do anything" (N288). Lastly, a small percentage (around 17 %, 56 people) reported physical symptoms such as sweating, rapid heartbeats and breathing difficulties and/or disturbed sleep. It is worth noting that 12 participants had been hospitalised at some point in a psychiatric department of a general hospital or in a psychiatric hospital and received medication for their mental health problems (primarily: psychosis, anorexia nervosa, personality disorders and depression).

Axis 5: Substance Dependence

As far as substance dependence is concerned, 121 people said that they never used substances or alcohol. However, 51 participants (15.5 %) reported using substances, heroin, hashish, cocaine and LSD primarily, and 45 (13.6 %) frequently used alcohol: "I love alcohol" (N34) or "Alcohol is my only prop" (N67). A small percentage (around 9.4 %, 31 people) reported occasional use of alcohol mainly for self-medication to deal with stress, the cold or insomnia: "Alcohol is the only medicine" (N7), "I drink alcohol occasionally, it helps with the void and mood" (N80), "I drink win to forget" (N110) or "sometimes I drink beer to get rid of the stress" (N218).

8.5 Discussion: Conclusions

Reformulating the experiences and comments from this study, it is clear what the key aspects of social suffering in the urban environment are. As far as the socio-demographic profile of this population is concerned, the study has confirmed that there is a mosaic of socially vulnerable groups in the centre of Athens. Migrants from countries such as Albania, Afghanistan, Pakistan, Bangladesh, Iraq, Iran, Turkish Kurdistan, Palestine, Sudan and Somalia form the vast majority of those living in Metropolitan Athens without valid paperwork. The idea of a homeland differs and is complicated in the minds of those people because they are "on the move". On a symbolic, psychoanalytical level, this process has been described as abandonment of an all-containing idea (Stylianidis 2011, 2012), such as the homeland, community, family, mother and the social roles assumed. They come via dangerous, often fatal, routes.

The fragility of their personality and adjustment difficulties are balanced by "proud isolation" from the wider society of the country they establish themselves in, which is a condition for psychological self-protection (Stylianidis 2012).

As far as the mental health problems they face are concerned, almost one in two homeless people found it difficult to function satisfactorily, mainly due to the palpable sense of depression and/or stress. The extent to which that depression or stress meets specific diagnostic criteria was not examined in this study, which aimed primarily at recording the subjective views of the participants in the study. The palpable social suffering identified in the sample in this study cannot be medicalised – psychiatrified and codified in terms of symptoms, to bring it into line with the findings of modern epistemology (DSM) (Stylianidis 2012). Subjective mental pain is tied into a wider framework of social suffering, which is being explored by modern classificatory psychiatry (Stylianidis 2011). It has, in fact, been found that interculturalism is tightly bound up with stress-related disorders and depression and that the length of time migrants stay in Greece, without a family, without a legal right of residence or right to work, significantly affects their depressive symptoms (Madianos et al. 2008).

The fragmentation of government bodies and services which was noted confirms the gap which exists. Primary healthcare and welfare services look down on and stigmatise marginalised individuals, which has further repercussions on the continuity of their health, psychiatric and social care. At the same time, fear from residents and the sense of being trapped inside their own homes create the phenomenon of polarised social exclusion.

Government policies on the various forms of social exclusion appear pointless in the sense that they only provide piecemeal, ineffectual solutions. One could say that the state appears unable to take action to effectively address the special, different needs of this population and to create specialised services like mobile mental health units for cities.

Cities undoubtedly generate fear, discrimination and a sense of insecurity. Despite that, in every society (even in times of crisis) there is a wealth of sources, technologies and social ties that could be used to implement organised policies and to establish networks to address these complicated needs. Developing new networks would be possible if the political authorities, citizens and those directly involved focused on the key problems of those excluded from society, irrespective of the environment where one lives and works, thereby creating a new democratic and participative local culture.

This study had specific methodological constraints. Because of the qualitative approach adopted, the findings are not considered representative of the population overall and cannot therefore be generalised for Athens' entire homeless population (sampling was not done in a randomised fashion) or the homeless of other large cities in Greece. At the same time, the findings describe or attempt to systematically present some in-depth observations rather than quantify the scale of the problem and/or the phenomenon. As already mentioned, because of the explanatory nature of the study and the fact that there was a large number of migrants in the sample, a clinical tool for identifying mental disorders tailored to other population groups (like migrants) was not included. A supplementary epidemiological study could be carried out later, which would focus on all the issues thrown up by this study: a valid distinction between social suffering and mental disorders, differences between Greek and migrant homeless people, the profile of homeless people who have to face social racism and the tie between social racism and mental illnesses.

References

Appadurai A (2002) Deep democracy: urban governmentality and the horizon of politics. Public Cult 14(1):21–47

Arapoglou VP (2006) Immigration, segregation and urban development in Athens: the relevance of the LA debate for Southern European metropolises. Greek Rev Soc Res 121:11–38

Augé M (1992) Non-lieux: introduction à une anthropologie de la surmodernité. Seuil, Paris

Bartley M, Blane D, Montgomery S (1997) Health and the life course: why safety nets matter. Br Med J 314:1194–1196

Blane D, Bartley M, Smith GD (1997) Disease aetiology and materialist explanations of socioeconomic mortality differentials. Eur J Public Health 7(4):385–391

Bourdieu P (1991) Language and symbolic power. Harvard University Press, Cambridge, MA

Bui HN, Thongniramol O (2005) Immigration and self-reported delinquency: the interplay of immigration generations, gender, race, and ethnicity. J Crime Justice 28(2):71–99

Castells M (1989) The informational city: information technology, economic restructuring, and the urban-regional process. Blackwell, Oxford

Fryers T, Melzer D, Jenkins R (2003) Social inequalities and the common mental disorders. Soc Psychiatry Psychiatr Epidemiol 38(5):229–237

Giannarou L. (2012, Apr 1) Alarm over illegal immigrants. Kathimerini Newspaper (in Greek), Athens

Gionakis N (2010) Cultural heterogeneity awareness guide (in Greek). Vavel Day-care Centres run by Syneirmos-AMKE Social Solidarity, Athens

Harter LM, Berquist C, Scott Titsworth B, Novak D, Brokaw T (2005) The structuring of invisibility among the hidden homeless: the politics of space, stigma, and identity construction. J Appl Commun Res 33(4):305–327

Kaminis G (2011) Aiming for good governance – the future: which political models to follow? In 1st International Scientific Forum Souq (SOUQ: Centro Studi Sofferenza Urbana). Milano

Kidd SA (2007) Youth homelessness and social stigma. J Youth Adolesc 36(3):291–299

Madianos GM, Gonidakis F, Ploumpidis D, Papadopoulou E, Rogakou E (2008) Measuring acculturation and symptoms of depression of foreign immigrants in the Athens area. Int J Soc Psychiatry 54(4):338–349

Major B, O'Brien LT (2005) The social psychology of stigma. Annu Rev Psychol 56:393–421

Mercer's Quality of Living ranking highlights – Global (Cited 11 June 2011). Available at: www.mercer.com/qualityofliving (retrieved 05.06.2012)

Mumford L (1961) The city in history: its origins, its transformation, and its prospects. Harcourt Brace, New York

Patel V, Kleinman A (2003) Poverty and common mental disorders in developing countries. Bull World Health Organ 81(8):609–615

Saraceno B (2010) The paradigm of urban suffering. Centro Studi Sofferenza Urbana (SOUQ), 2. http://www.souqonline.it/public/html-asp(287130).pdf

Saraceno B (2014) Discorso globale, sofferenze locali. Analisi critica del Movimiento di salute mentale globale. Il Saggiatore, Milano

Smith JA, Flowers P, Larkin M (2009) Interpretative phenomenological analysis: theory, method and research. Sage, London

Souliotis G (2012, Apr 22) Detention centres … in prisons. Kathimerini Newspaper (in Greek), Athens

Stansfeld SA, Head J, Fuhrer R, Wardle J, Cattell V (2003) Social inequalities in depressive symptoms and physical functioning in the Whitehall II study: exploring a common cause explanation. J Epidemiol Community Health 57(5):361–367

Stewart KA, Keusch GT, Kleinman A (2010) Values and moral experience in global health: bridging the local and the global. Global Pub Health 5(2):115–121

Stuckler D, Basu S, Suhrcke M, Coutts A, McKee M (2009) The public health effect of economic crises and alternative policy responses in Europe: an empirical analysis. Lancet 374(9686):315–323

Stylianidis S (2011) The clinical practice of the ephemeral. Views on individual and social pain. Clinical and social questions from a psychoanalytical viewpoint. Oedipus 5:229–249 (in Greek)

Stylianidis S (2012) Subjective pain compared to the simplified reductionism of modern classificatory psychiatry: towards a psychiatry of the person. Synapsis J 24:16–21 (in Greek)

Stylianidis S, Koutsosimou M, Vakalopoulou A (2011) The "no man's land" of the metropolitan area of Athens: research data and future challenges. Centro Studi Sofferenza Urbana (SOUQ), 4. http://www.souqonline.it/home2_2_eng.asp?idtesto=829

The World Bank (2011) Migration and remittances factbook 2011. The World Bank publications, Washington, DC

Thomas P, Bracken P, Cutler P, Hayward R, May R, Yasmeen S (2005) Challenging the globalisation of biomedical psychiatry. J Public Ment Health 4(3):23–32

Tryfonas G (2012, Apr 8) Throw them all out of the country. Vima tis Kyriakis newspaper (in Greek), Athens

Van Doorslaer E, Wagstaff A, Bleichrodt H, Calonge S, Gerdtham UG, Gerfin M et al (1997) Income-related inequalities in health: some international comparisons. J Health Econ 16(1):93–112

Ventura L (2006) Diaspora, globalisation and collectivities. Mod Issues 92:31–39 (in Greek)

Vertovec S (2007) New complexities of cohesion in Britain: super-diversity, Transnationalism and civil-integration. Report written for the Commission on Integration and Cohesion (CIC)

Wilkinson RG (2002) Unhealthy societies: the afflictions of inequality. Routledge, London

The Recovery Model and Modern Psychiatric Care: Conceptual Perspective, Critical Approach and Practical Application

Stelios Stylianidis, Michail Lavdas, Kalomira Markou, and Pepi Belekou

Abstract

The recovery model is a model that allows an individual to take back control of his life. It was primarily developed for serious mental disorders for which the biomedical model precluded any possibility of "real recovery" and control over life by individuals with mental disability. From a biopsychosocial viewpoint, the recovery model shifts the treatment objective from reducing symptoms to real integration and assignment of meaning of the life of individuals and their participation on equal terms in society. In other words, the perception is that recovery-as-healing goes beyond the concept of "therapeutic accompaniment" and "care", as formulated by Racamier (Le psychanalyste sans divan. La psychanalyse et les institutions de soins psychiatriques. Payot, Paris, 1970, Les schizophrènes. Payot, Paris, 1980, Le génie des origines: psychanalyse et psychoses. Payot, Paris, 1992), and is transferred into modern psychotherapeutic concerns about psychoses. In any event, that requires a change in culture and how psychiatry is practised. In other words, it requires the individual to function as a user of mental health services, as an "expert user" when it comes to his own illness and not as a passive user who complies with treatment guidelines. This change must be accompanied by a simultaneous change in the way services are structured and operate, and in the more general attitude of the community, so as to accept difference and to make individuals adjust to the "norm" of a condition for integration.

S. Stylianidis (✉)
Department of Psychology, Panteion University, Athens, Greece
e-mail: stylianidis.st@gmail.com

M. Lavdas • K. Markou • P. Belekou
Association for Regional Development and Mental Health, Athens, Greece
e-mail: p.belecou@hotmail.com

© Springer International Publishing Switzerland 2016
S. Stylianidis (ed.), *Social and Community Psychiatry: Towards a Critical, Patient-Oriented Approach*, DOI 10.1007/978-3-319-28616-7_9

This chapter explores the history and conceptual meaning of the recovery model and ends with critical remarks about how it has been applied at both Greek and international level. This path is accompanied by presentation of a clinical case to show how the recovery model can be used in practice.

9.1 Introduction

The concept and practice of *recovery* appears to have been gaining ground over the last decade, particularly in the best practices of Anglo-Saxon countries and the experiences of deinstitutionalisation and critical psychiatry in Europe.

The plethora of references in the literature to the concept of recovery and the different perspectives of those involved in psychiatric care and psychosocial rehabilitation (mental health professionals, families, users of services, volunteers, managers of mental health services) have frequently caused confusion and a sense of fluidity about the real meaning of recovery and how it can be applied in practice.

This chapter attempts to clarify the conceptual confusion which exists about recovery and how it has been perceived in Greece. Moreover, a systematic literature review enables us to comment on objections to its adoption in practice by looking at clinical examples, in the context of psychosocial rehabilitation at the Regional Development and Mental Health Association.

9.2 Conceptual Framework and Definitions of Recovery

Laird (2002) proposes four different definitions for recovery: (a) returning to a normal state; (b) an act, instant, process or period of recovering; (c) something gained or restored in the process of recovering; and (d) an act of acquiring useful substances from untreated sources, such as scrap.

These four definitions (Davidson et al. 2005) can be used to clearly and accurately identify four different categories in the context of holistic healthcare such as (a) acute physical conditions, (b) injury and its consequences, (c) disorders caused by substance usage and (d) serious mental disorder.

Babiniotis (2002) defines the Greek word for "recovery" (*anarrosis*) as "the gradual rehabilitation of health after an illness" which is similar to the definition [a] in the Webster dictionary which relates to physical health, even if chronic such as asthma, diabetes, cancer etc. Likewise, Babiniotis (2002, p. 767) tells us that the Greek word *iasis* (healing) makes a "rehabilitation of health".

We can see that the concept of rehabilitation appears in both the definitions of the Greek words for *recovery* and *healing*, but this cannot fully capture the fourth definition of recovery contained in the Webster dictionary. However, given the wider heterogeneity of serious mental illnesses both in terms of diagnosis and treatment, recovery is seen as having different meanings for people who have experienced or are experiencing different developments and outcomes for their illness.

Despite the lack of uniformity, most definitions of recovery include the elements of acceptance of the illness, hope for the future and the search for renewable self-meaning and a different identity. Three of the most frequently citied definitions of recovery in the literature are provided below:

1. Recovery presupposes the development of new meaning and life purpose for an individual, as he grows beyond the destructive results of psychiatric disability (Anthony 1993).
2. Recovery relates to the actual life experience of individuals who accept and move beyond the challenge their disability poses (Deegan 1988).
3. Recovery is a process via which individuals with psychiatric disabilities can rebuild and develop important personal, environmental, social and spiritual ties and come to terms with the destructive effects of discrimination by integrating them (Spaniol and Koehler 1994).

Definitions of this type, which clearly converge and complement each other, differ from the definition used in clinical research. In that perspective, recovery is defined as the disappearance of the symptoms which caused the individual disability or, in the case of physical health, a return to the previous state (Young and Ensing 1999). Consequently, *recovery* in clinical research is the absence of some unwanted points or situations, such as illness or symptoms, or the disappearance of some problem that was not part of the individual's life before the illness, by using medication or hospitalisation (White 2000; Whitwell 2001).

Although this model can include positive improvement indicators, such as work and home, the focus nonetheless remains on overcoming barriers and on a return to the previous state of health (Davidson and Strauss 1995).

From the viewpoint of users of mental health services and professionals involved in psychosocial rehabilitation, recovery cannot be viewed as a "static situation or result" (Deegan 1996a, b) nor is it the same as treatment; instead it is a life process which involves an increasing number of steps towards different life levels (Jacobson and Curtis 2000). The outcome of all this is that recovery, in Greece, has begun to be experienced by the movement of users of mental health services and their families more as an attitude, a way of life, a feeling, a vision or experience (Deegan 1988, 1996a, b), rather than as a type of clinical outcome per se.

Restoring the state prior to illness is a one-dimensional view of one's overall self-meaning, which is capable of forming an identity and of attempting to achieve goals which have meaning for oneself, rather than merely the persistent, frequently tortuous existence of the results and side effects of mental illness (Davidson 2003; Davidson and Strauss 1992).

Combining the bibliographical references together, we suggest that *recovery*, for the purposes of Greece, be seen as a continuous process of getting better that leads to healing or in short "recovery-as-healing".

9.3 Concerns About Recovery-as-Healing and the Biomedical Model

The focus of the process of recovering from an illness includes, among other things, the idea of the individual reacquiring habits and a life plan, which can be used to define his personal identity day by day.

The aim of recovery, which does not include "healing here and now" as a goal of the doctor-patient therapeutic relationship, presupposes a shift in attention from the illness and its development factors to what is really in question: reinvestment in an active life, improving to the maximum degree possible for the individual his day-to-day conditions and social life. That presupposes that we rely on those "unused resources" that allow us to overcome the consequences of illness, to highlight our personal goals, and the role of faith or hope that a recovery/healing is possible.

This approach presupposes conscious "disconnection" of the history of the illness and the factors that affect it from the individual's past, which also includes a series of other definitive factors (Bowie et al. 2010). The perception is that recovery-as-healing goes beyond the concept of "therapeutic accompaniment" and "care", as formulated by Racamier (1980), in contradistinction to the one-sided view of treatment which has been transferred into the modern concerns of the psychotherapy of psychoses (Mentzos 2008; Benedetti 1992; Hochman 1986; Rosenfeld 1965; Searles 1965; Vartzopoulos and Stylianidis 2008).

Personal initiative and the individual assigning meaning in the recovery-as-healing process, developing or redefining a life plan (Sartre 1985), which was brutally interrupted by the onset of a serious psychiatric disorder, is a modern development and transformation of the substance of deinstitutionalisation, as formulated by F. Basaglia and the Italian Psichiatria Democratica (Basaglia 2005) movement. This disconnection of illness from the individual's life plan also includes other factors. Psychopathological factors are not adequate to interpret the phenomenon of day-to-day life being temporalised, increased barriers to full psychosocial rehabilitation and more so the future and personal life of the individual (Gerard 2011; Pachoud 2012; Warner 2004).

Even the disconnection of the clinical approach and holistic outcome for the individual is not widely recognised in the international scientific community and literature, but it is "familiar" to many clinicians. Take, for example, the many patients with serious psychiatric disorders who present no symptoms after effective treatment using psychotropic drugs but face immense difficulties in finding an active social and personal life again. In any event, the so-called negative symptoms of schizophrenia are a critical enigma and challenge in clinical psychopharmacology. On the other hand, we have those patients who despite the chronic presence of productive psychotic symptoms, such as delusions (audio, visual, sensory etc.), manage to achieve a stable life and relative autonomy, with social ties and a job, and participate in a process of persons improvement of their cognitive and social skills (Liberman et al. 2002, 2008).

Recognising and accepting this "mismatch" between the biomedical model and the process of recovery/integration/healing necessarily leads us to adopt two discrete strategies which must operate as a complement to each other, to promote the holistic approach to patients' needs: in addition to the traditional medical strategy which aims to address the symptoms of the disease and maximise the potential for a positive outcome, it is also necessary to implement a strategy of equal importance that supplements one's clinical practice and which methodically aims at maximising the individuals' potential for recovery/healing/social integration. A key role in the recovery strategy is held by life experience, testimony and narratives, which in terms of qualitative research have the same important scientific value as epidemiological studies about the prevalence and outcome of schizophrenia.

The study and practical implementation of projects in this direction, such as the very important synthesis done by Amering and Schmolke (2009), highlight important aspects of the recovery process, such as empowerment and the ability to choose, or the role of self-determination, hope and in particular narrative ability and reformulation of the subject's identity (Giddens 2004). Narration and the creation of a framework for highlighting and listening are for certain writers the preferred way of describing human experience and changing the individual's perspective and stance towards the prospect for re-establishing his identity and life plan, while minimising the consequences of mental disability (Davidson 2003).

This interpretation of the stories of users of services and the perception of mental health professionals about recovery and psychosocial rehabilitation can give us the opportunity to improve the qualitative methodology and document the implementation of recovery plans in a mental health service (Greacen and Jouet 2012).

9.4 Modern Developments in Recovery

Recovery from a mental illness, as narrated by Pat Deegan through her description of her psychotic experience, is a process of personal development and growth, a way of life (Deegan 1988, Deegan 1996a, b) and not a return to the situation prior to the illness. Such testimony from other individuals who have experienced a serious mental illness and long-term studies over the last three decades opened the way for further research and applications in the field of recovery, demonstrating that individuals who suffer from schizophrenia can recover and enjoy positive results in a life full of meaning (Anthony et al. 2003).

The findings of research show good long-term results for the majority of people with serious psychiatric disorders. The best known research is by Harding et al. (1987) which monitored a group of 269 individuals who on average had 10 years of absolute disability and 6 years of continuous hospitalisation. Those individuals participated in a dynamic psychosocial rehabilitation programme, completed it and then received community mental health services. The results from the 10-year follow-up showed that although 2/3 of the group lived in the community, they were utterly dependent on services and were socially isolated, which was not particularly encouraging. However, the second follow-up at 20–25 years showed that around 55 % of the individuals had regained functionality to a significant degree, did not have problems or had very few problems and had recovered. At the same time, a study carried out globally by the WHO into schizophrenia (Harrison et al. 2001) followed up individuals diagnosed with schizophrenia in numerous countries after a 15- and 25-year gap. The results show that 56–60 % of those individuals had recovered.

After these developments, interest began to grow in the recovery model as a re-exploration of psychiatric care and its practices (Roberts and Wolfson 2004). Major attempts to implement the recovery model have been made around the world in the mental health sector, showing a clear trend of moving away from traditional, biomedical models. Some US states, New Zealand, Australia and more recently European countries, like England, have begun to plan and develop mental health services focused on the recovery model. In the USA, for example, the recovery model was adopted as the central policy on mental health in 2003, as part of the reform of the mental health system. We also have the example of states like Massachusetts, Florida and Ohio which designed and developed recovery model-based services. Likewise, in 2001 New Zealand and England integrated the concept of recovery as central to the planning of mental health services.

Even though some of those services at first sight have not familiarised themselves with these concepts, and may appear to be services provided in a traditional setting by many mental health systems, there is no such thing as a recovery-oriented service whose central idea is not that recovery is possible and whose goals are to foster hope, healing, empowerment and connection.

Since the experience of recovery from a mental illness is essentially personal and individualised, and is something much wider than the remission of symptoms, we see a constant need on the part of researchers to develop research tools to respond to the sheer breadth of definitions of recovery. Despite that, the methodology of traditional documented research cannot respond and evaluate new practices – methods for developing mental health services, like recovery (Anthony 2000). Most researchers stress that qualitative methods will play an important role, making it clear what the recovery process includes in order to achieve the transformation of mental health services in that direction.

Personal narratives are particularly valuable here. Individuals narrate their stories explaining their personal journey over the course of their recovery and talk about what has helped them. Those narratives, and the internal dynamic they have, open the path to demystifying mental illness, demonstrating a dynamic path towards achieving goals (MHC 2005).

The perceptions of mental health professionals and the culture of organisations that provide services are very important factors since one needs to create such environments or systems that favour the recovery process. The literature identifies recovery-oriented services as those within which individuals are supported as they grow and implement their personal recovery plans, which can encourage their personal preferences and allow the user of services to assume risks and move forward (Weaver 1998).

In the systems providing mental health services referred to, employees are trained in the principles of the recovery model to achieve two objectives: to explore the concept of recovery and at the same time to explore the role of the mental health professional in this case. In addition, these systems integrate services provided by mental health professionals, services provided by service users and services provided by a combination of the two.

9.5   Case Study: Implementation of the Recovery Method

Case
A.G. is 50 years old and suffers from organic psychotic disorder. The problem presented at the age of 35 following excessive alcohol consumption. He presented symptoms of aggression, mainly verbal aggression, persecution complex, suspiciousness and lack of trust in all around him. He has finished junior high school and completed his military service, has worked and has been married. When the problem started he separated, was left homeless and was treated at Dafni Psychiatric Hospital where he received medication. He did not follow medical guidelines and his situation deteriorated. After his last period of treatment at Dafni, he was transferred to the Paleo Penteli Residential Unit at the age of 47.

Problems the resident faced:

- Alcohol addiction
- No insurance coverage (for health insurance)
- No financial support (no job and no benefits)
- No family support
- No social contact with friends
- No love life

Treatment plan for the recovery process and to improve the quality of life

- Take medication and stop alcohol consumption
- Obtain a health insurance booklet and welfare benefits
- Pscyhoeducation
- Re-connect with family
- Social skills training
- Work
- Sheltered accommodation

A.G. is 50 years old, comes from Athens and suffers from organic psychotic disorder. According to his own testimony, the problem presented at the age of 35, at a time when he was consuming excessive quantities of alcohol to escape difficult situations in his day-to-day life. When he drank, he would have symptoms of aggression, mainly verbal aggression towards parents, friends or unknown people, whom he would shout at and pester. Often his outbursts of "anger" (as he called it) would be accompanied by ideas of suspicion, persecution or lack of trust. He had finished junior high school and done his military service and when he came back after the army went to an iron and aluminium design school. His training helped him work as an ironsmith sometimes in private companies and sometimes in his family's business, alongside his brother. At the age of 33, he married a foreign woman from Sri Lanka and stayed with her for 6 years. However, when A.G. began to cause problems due to his drinking, his wife was forced to leave because she could not stand a life like that. However, they continued in law to be married since they had not divorced, because his former wife needed him to renew her visa and residence permit in the country.

After they separated, he returned to his family home where he lived with his brother and mother. His father had died a year earlier, when A.G. was 37. Cohabitation was not an easy affair at all. He continued to drink and stopped working, and his brother was forced to seek a Public Prosecutor's order to have him admitted to the Dromokaitio Psychiatric Hospital. He stayed there a few days, was given medication and returned home. When leaving the hospital, he asked his family for money to go and live on his own, since he would cause problems if he continued to live with them. He did in fact rent an apartment, but did not keep up with his obligations (he didn't pay the rent or bills), and the owner evicted him. Since he had no other choice, he returned to his family home again. However, because of the incidents he caused, this time the neighbours obtained a Public Prosecutor's order and he was taken to the Athens Psychiatric Hospital at Dafni. Once again the doctors administered medication but he did not take it.

When he was discharged, he did not return home. He remained homeless and made a small shelter under the stairs of a church so he could sleep. He stayed there for around 2 years and was cared for and supported by women from the neighbourhood, who gave him food and money which enabled him to buy cigarettes and drink. He enjoyed that period because he felt free to do what he wanted and did not have to give account to anyone, especially not his family. After much discussion and exhortation from others, he decided to voluntarily admit himself to hospital so be able to be transferred to some psychosocial rehabilitation unit. In April 2009, he was transferred to the Palia Penteli residential unit; the scientific treatment team there came into contact with the hospital, his family and residents of the area where he lived to collect information, and this played a vital role in designing his individual treatment plan and implementing the recovery model.

When collecting all the information about his story, the team initially recorded his problems, invited him to tell them why he had been transferred to the residential unit and attempted to understand from the discussion whether he accepted that he was suffering from a serious mental illness and needed help. A.G. accepted that he had had a bad time and that all the negative things in his life had started from the time he started drinking. He wanted to lay a new foundation and start over afresh, which would allow him to acquire a normal, decent life. His "acceptance" of the problem was the springboard for starting the treatment process.

Relying on the basic principles of the recovery-as-healing model (the recovery model) which preach a renewal of hope and decisiveness, regaining of social position, managing symptoms, overcoming stigma and redefining oneself, the team explained to A.G. that the path to recovery is a constant struggle which goes through various stages before the goal is reached. In those stages of recovery, mental health professionals are there to help and guide. They offer hope and the belief that recovery can happen; they train, support, inform and design the individual treatment plan and focused on a structured programme that helps the individual improve his quality of life in the community.

Taking into account the user of services' problems, the team set a series of priorities and started from the easiest and most achievable, which would bolster self-confidence and provide satisfaction and the hope that the objective could be achieved. For example, A.G.:

Was addicted to alcohol and was not taking medication
Did not have social security (to cover medical treatment)
Did not have financial support (or a job or benefits)
Did not have family support
Did not have social contacts

The team's primary, main goal was to administer medication and get A.G. off alcohol, and it proposed that he attend a detox programme and enrol with Alcoholics Anonymous. He did not agree, insisting that he could manage on his own and that he should stay at the residential unit. The initial period was not at all easy. He found it difficult to sleep, had headaches, asked for painkillers to calm down and did not participate in outings to avoid contact with places selling food and drinks since he feared he would only be incited to drink. Every week he met with his psychiatrist, and every day the scientific team talked with him and supported him as he continued his efforts. It took about 6 months for him to come off alcohol, and during that entire period, he received medication which he now continues.

He had no insurance coverage as mentioned. He did not appear to be registered with any social security provider and that created problems because he had no Medicare. Since he did not have access to public services, while he was receiving training, the scientific team told him about his rights, and with the help of a social worker, he collected together all the paperwork needed and submitted it to the welfare department to get a welfare book and a welfare allowance. The allowance was a small amount of financial aid, since at that time he did not have any financial resources, other than the small amount of help he continued to receive from the Church.

Seeing that he could resolve important practical issues, he began to trust himself, to have hope and have an incentive to continue his attempts to regain a normal life. Once he was able to recognise reality and set realistic goals, he started psychoeducation. The purpose was to use face-to-face sessions with his psychologist to be able to understand the situation he was in before the treatment; to place emphasis on the continuity of care by continuing his medication, which was vital; and also to evaluate his needs, interests and wishes, so that he could continue to improve his quality of life.

The next step was to reconnect with his family, who had pulled away and did not want any contact with him because it could not manage the problems his behaviour created. When he entered the residential unit, his brother was quite distrustful and appeared disappointed and considered that nothing would change, since this was a tried and tested pattern of behaviour. The scientific team advised him to give A.G. time, to visit him with their mother more frequently at the residential unit and to have a positive outlook on the efforts A.G. was making, because this time he was inside a structured framework now. A.G. received indirect support from the family visits, tried harder and believed that he could regain their acceptance. In fact, their relations today are back to normal and A.G. visits his family at regular intervals, wants to help his brother and takes care of his mother. His circle still cannot believe the change: it's as if they are seeing another person.

A.G. lacked much in terms of social contacts and social skills. As an individual, during his early days at the residential unit, we noticed that he was quite shut off and solitary and found it difficult to speak, and there were days he only wanted to sleep and the expression on his face was melancholic, as if something was missing. By giving him time to adjust and by talking to him and ensuring he attended a social skills training course, he managed to acquire friends, to go out, to attend social events, to be more communicative and to be expressive. Having been able to work in his past life (and having given that up because of drinking), we discussed with him how interested he would be in working again. He thought that would be impossible because of his medication, but it was something he wanted a lot. It was explained what the role of social partnerships is, and he became a member and for a year now has been working in a cleaning team at the Ministry of Labour.

Having taken quite a few steps, only the last, most difficult one remained: the preparations for him to be able to become autonomous and live in the community, either with a foster family or in sheltered accommodation. One year before this happened, with the help of staff, he began his training for living on his own and became involved in all the relevant aspects of such a life (e.g. personal hygiene, maintaining and cleaning his own space and communal areas, preparing meals, using public transport and social services to deal with issues that arose etc.). Since last June, A.G. has been living in sheltered accommodation with two roommates.

His own active involvement in planning his treatment, based on teamwork and cooperation, and his incentive to change and rehabilitate himself, brought about the desired result and one can talk of recovery here. According to Anthony (1993), "recovery can be described as a deep personal process unique to the individual, during which perceptions, values, emotions, goals, abilities and/or roles change. It is a way of living a satisfactory, hope-filled, contribution-packed life even given the constraints the illness imposes. Recovery includes developing new meaning and life purpose, as the individual grows beyond the destructive consequences of the mental disorder".

Having said that, the positive outcome for this user of mental health services entails several difficulties in implementing the recovery model. In addition to his disappointment and withdrawal when did not manage to reach a target, which is something the scientific team could deal with, there were serious issues faced by staff. Since they did not have the necessary knowledge and training, they were distrustful about whether he could recover and considered that he would not achieve anything and clearly expressed this sense of pessimism.

In this case the head of the unit and scientific team had a dual role to play. On the one hand, he had to encourage A.G. when he lost faith, and on the other, he had to provide on-the-job training about the principles of the recovery model and our role as mental health professionals. Of course it was only to be expected that this would happen, and the employees were not directly responsible. The root of the problem lies in the public mental health system which does not ensure that people are recruited to these services based on specific criteria, nor does it ensure they receive continuing training, meaning that they have erroneous perceptions, they have no hope and their stigma about mental patients remains undiminished.

One should remember that individuals with mental problems may have special characteristics and resistances to change, which are frequently viewed by the biomedical model as irreversible and which in quite a few cases are not even taken into consideration. The fact is that such individuals continue to have abilities and skills to relearn things and to adjust to the circumstances of their life plan. It is not the diagnosis which defines the needs of the individual but the description of his needs, functionality and the constraints the illness imposes.

9.6 The Recovery Model and Its Relationship to Public Mental Health in Greece: Final Remarks

Implementing the recovery model as described above is a goal officially set out in the report of the working group on revision of the PSYCHARGOS programme (Ministry of Health and Social Solidarity 2012). The section referring to the structure of mental health care units and the functions of the overall mental health system, in terms of service provision, highlights the importance of promoting the recovery of patients and restoring them to their social roles and of social (re-)integration (p. 94). It is also included as one of the three main planks of education and training. In conjunction with key issues in social psychiatry and quality of care in mental health services and best practices for mental health promotion and education in the community, the aim of education must be to "firmly establish reform in the mental health sector, by disseminating cutting-edge examples of best practices in vital sectors relating to the organisation of services and their adoption by employees in the mental health sector" (p. 223). This is the PSYCHARGOS III Report and was approved by Ministerial Decision No. Υ5β/Γ.Π./οικ 46769 as the National Action Plan and sets out a series of actions over a 10-year horizon which seek to gradually address all needs in the mental health sector at the national level. The Ministerial Decision states it is "the operational arm of the Greek State's policy on psychiatric reform, deinstitutionalisation and modernisation of the system for providing mental health services".

Key aspects of deinstitutionalisation and real psychiatric reform are changes in culture about how psychiatric care is provided. Four different approaches are needed here (a) in the culture of care which must provide assistance and protection, but frequently limits the autonomy of the patient; (b) the culture of care which places trust in experts and requires "compliance" (not negotiation) by patients in the context of the biomedical model; (c) in the culture of education which uses training methods to achieve goals in a friendly, structured manner; and (d) in the culture of empowerment which favours the transfer of power from experts to users of mental health services, creating a balanced relationship which seeks to safeguard resources and the environment, which are vital elements for the autonomous growth and development of users of services. The recovery model demands this shift in power and the commitment from the user of services to treatment via a process of negotiation and joint decision-making. This process is the opposite of compliance, which is defined as one-sided obeisance of medical orders and is a doubtful treatment goal since it does not appear to take into account concepts such as empathy and building up the importance of treatment (Molodynski et al. 2010). The special features of each user of services and the fact that his personality is taken into account are equally important factors as the skills and experience of doctors. Unfortunately, in Greece there have been shortfalls in and objections to adopting a culture which promotes real recovery, since the system has a lack of coordination, services are unequally deployed, there are insufficient links between services and services cannot network, all of which have negative repercussions on the continuity of care and all of which are coupled with the lack of any increase in financing which would ensure the viability of the system (Ministry of Health and Social Solidarity 2010). The structural problems which external evaluation identified in the period 2000–2009 also compound the difficulties in implementing the recovery model. More specifically, the involvement of users of services and advocacy was found to be underdeveloped, and there were major inadequacies in the destigmatisation of mental illness.

The inflexibility of the public system and its inability to support the culture of empowerment and recovery became particularly clear during the ongoing evaluation for the 2010–2015 period (Ministry of Health and Social Solidarity 2013) during which the scientific team from the Institute of Psychiatry found major problems in how the mental health system is organised and noted that the organisational structure has not improved in real terms compared to the findings of the ex-post evaluation (2010) which were presented above. It stated that "the system remains highly fragmented and without coordination, without linkages between the agencies and organisations involved. Users of services do not receive services in the context of the Mental Health Region in which they live, meaning valuable human and economic resources are not used rationally or efficiently". The picture of the public system in decline under current socioeconomic conditions (Kentikelenis et al. 2011; Stylianidis and Chondros 2011) is supplemented by the lack of participation by users of services since "users continue not to be involved in decision-making, in the control of units and on sectoral mental health committees". In addition, the high number of involuntary admissions to hospitals noted by the external evaluation and confirmed by Drakonaki et al. (2012) shows a major shortfall both in relation to the rights of persons with mental problems and the real implementation of the culture of empowerment and recovery.

9 The Recovery Model and Modern Psychiatric Care

In conclusion, using the recovery model, one does not just recover from mental health problems but also manages the fact that one has lived in a psychiatric institution and endured the consequences of the stigma of mental illness and isolation from society and work. However, the chronicity does not only lie in cases of long-term hospitalisation in an institution but also in cases of "institutionalised day-to-day life", with its painful repetitiveness. A key principle of the recovery model is that the chronicity of illness does not also mean that the situation has to be incurable, which is a prejudice a significant portion of mental health experts have, not just experts but all those directly or indirectly involved in or called upon to shape the "common language" which will create the conditions for implementing the recovery model, free of personal expectations which prevent recovery. We have identified a jigsaw of opposing views and expectations which is presented in diagram form below.

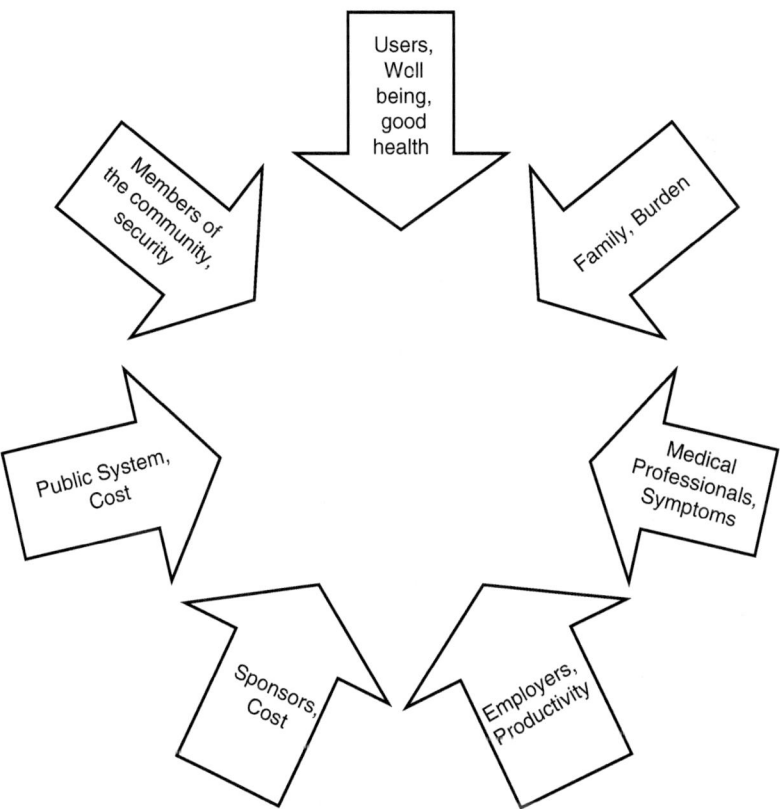

Consequently, the development of a common language between users of mental health services and mental health professionals is vital so that everyone can realise that mental health concerns us all, as the WHO recommends, and for each partner to shift his view of treatment from discouraging pessimism towards reasonable optimism of creative risk and change.

9.7 Uses and Abuses of the Term *Recovery* (Slade et al. 2014)

Abuse 1. Recovery Is the Most Cutting-Edge Model Around

Constant dissemination of the recovery model and recovery-oriented services means the risk of fragmentary changes in the structure and function of an organisation without that entailing a change in the culture, which is essential, is common. For example, 13 of the US states have committed to hiring users of mental health services via a national security system. Placing individuals with mental health problems in paid jobs is in line with the principles of the recovery model but does not mean on its own that it is sufficient. They may be hired but they are subsequently marginalised by colleagues, and the duties they are assigned to do not match their skills or are the minimum ones possible. In this way, empowerment through work operates independently of recovery objectives and does not promote equal participation, more hope and self-determination while also transforming culture.

Abuse 2. Recovery Isn't Applicable to "My Patients"

The ideology of recovery and the practice of achieving it have primarily developed through clinical work with psychosis. However, a major portion of mental health professionals declare that the model isn't suited to their own patients who they considered to be "too ill" to respond or unfit for recovery due to a diagnosis that doesn't match psychosis.

However, the recovery model has shown that it can be directly applicable even for individuals in crisis, while the literature also shows that the model can be applied to individuals who are not suffering from mental problems in the psychosis category, such as personality disorders and eating disorders, and to individual of different ages and nationalities.

Abuse 3. Services Can Help Individuals Recover Through Effective Treatment

Mental health professionals are more used to the clinical interpretation of recovery which relates to recovery from the symptoms of an illness and to the "clinical treatment" of an individual. However, the main meaning of recovery is to regain control of one's life – which anyone can do – and to give meaning to the roles one performs.

These two approaches (the clinical and the more personalised) may be complementary but one may experience one independently of the other. Traditionally, mental health services either supported the clinical aspect of recovery or (in the worst case scenario) adopted the belief that recovery of any form is not possible for individuals with mental health problems.

To fully support the real sense of recovery, services and the mental health system need to break away from the dominant biomedical model, which entails medication and "compliance", even if administered without the patient's volition. Mental health services must constantly invest in hope in individuals, helping them define themselves, secure access to the entire range of social services (accommodation, education, work, self-help, crisis support and support in day-to-day life, psychological treatments and advocacy), improve their social integration and protect their human rights. Consequently, the treatment method can improve the personal growth of the person in recovery but impede attempts to achieve self-determination if tied into forced compliance practices.

Abuse 4. Forced Detention and Treatment Promote Recovery

Forced treatment is proposed as an effective way of dealing with an individual who cannot take care of himself. The idea of a Community Treatment Order was introduced in England in 2008, to reduce the number of involuntary admissions to the psychiatric department, but it has not had the expected results and in fact the number of committals has increased from 2007/2008 to 2011/2012 (44,094 in 2007/2008 to 48,631 in 2011/2012). The issue of a Community Treatment Order entailing forced treatment or committal was proposed as a less restrictive alternative solution that forced psychiatric treatment in an institution or psychiatric department of a general hospital. Despite the ethical, moral and legal problems of limiting the individual's freedom in the community, the idea has come to prevail in Anglo-Saxon countries that the key advantages of this solution, such as secured living for chronic patients in the community, a reduction in the "revolving door" phenomenon and the multiplication of patient's skills through social integration, could offset the disadvantages (Lawton-Smith et al. 2008; Monahan 2011). However, Stylianidis et al. (2013) have raised questions about the measure, criticising it for the following reasons: (a) lack of persuasive documentation, (b) a risk of increased use of coercive measures during the practice of psychiatry, (c) unresolved ethical and moral aspects of the entire procedure for the time being and (d) the potential to limit other alternative social care solutions.

A systematic review of the literature on Community Treatment Orders (Kisely et al. 2005) shows that there is little support for its effectiveness in terms of the use of health services, social functionality, the state of mental health, quality of life and satisfaction with care. Researchers have also shown that 85 Community Treatment Orders have prevented one readmission, 27 have prevented one individual from remaining homeless due to mental illness and 238 have prevented one arrest.

Community Treatment Orders appear to be becoming more common even though recent studies show that it is ineffective in preventing readmission (Burns et al. 2013). In addition, Community Treatment Orders work counter to the process of regaining a life with meaning, a process which requires self-determination and respect for the individuality of the person as a citizen in society.

Abuse 5. Focusing on Recovery Means That Services Need to Close

Focusing on the recovery model is certainly not an adequate excuse for making cutbacks. It's not reasonable for one to assume that a meaningful life for an individual is not one lived within the narrow confines of a mental health service, and the view is frequently expressed towards users of mental health services that their contact with services unrelated to mental health and with informal forms of care is more important. The gradual reduction in contact with official mental health services and the transfer of support to informal support-in-the-community networks (friendships, self-help groups, community groups, work etc.) could possibly bolster the recovery process.

However, that process is not linear and services must be available for whenever they are needed again. The continuity of care means that someone may move from an informal type of care to a more specialised one and vice versa. The doors of communication must remain open to ensure continuous support for the individual, who depending on his state of health and life circumstances may choose a different form of support.

Clearly, ineffective services must be replaced or must adapt to the needs of users of services via a continuous process of evaluation and monitoring, in which beneficiaries themselves must be involved. A reduction in services is not justified under any circumstances by a focus on recovery, which requires constant support for individuals in the process of regaining control of their life using different services depending on their needs.

Abuse 6. Recovery Means Making People Independent and "Normal"

The clinical aspect of mental health services that offer services to integrate people into society primarily identifies problems those individuals have. Consequently, clinical interventions seek to bring about changes through treatment so that they can "fit in" and function "as normal" and "independent" individuals in the community. However, recovery does not simply mean "getting better" or no longer needing support. It means "regaining control of one's life" and the right to participate in all cultural and economic activities as a subject of law and equal citizen. It requires a system for providing services to be organised that is based on the principles of human rights and the social model for addressing exclusion. Integration and citizenship do not mean "becoming normal like others" but creating societies and communities that accept the integration of those who are different, where everyone has a place.

Abuse 7. One Only Contributes to Society Having Fully Completed the Recovery Process

Work (whether paid, voluntary or in the home) is the main way of contributing to the community. Work supports recovery. Most people who use mental health services are able to work, but the rate of unemployment among this specific group is over 70–80 %, which is much higher than in any other disability category.

Self-stigmatisation, expected discrimination and prejudice from services and the community are key factors in the higher unemployment rates, while the benefits offered are a factor promoting exclusion rather than mobilising such individuals to find work. However, one needs to stress that society as a whole benefits from accepting and recognising the equal right to work and equal opportunities for work for persons with mental disabilities.

9.8   Annex 1. Key elements of the recovery model

Key elements of the recovery model		
Element	Description	Sources
Renewed hope and commitment	The feeling of hope and trust in the probability of a renewed sense of self and purpose, which is accompanied by a desire and incentive to do things, is vital for recovery. This sense of hope can come from within oneself or from others who believe in the potential of the individual, even if he does not believe in himself	Davidson et al. (1997, 2001), Deegan (1996a, b), Fisher (1994), Jacobson and Curtis (2000), Jacobson and Greenlay (2001), Mead and Copeland (2000), Smith (2000), and Young and Ensing (1999)
Redefining oneself	The most essential aspect of recovery is perhaps the one relating to redefining oneself and re-evaluating mental illness as a part of a diverse identity that each of us has and not as the dominant social role of the "mental patient"	Davidson and Strauss (1992), Deegan (1996a, b), Fisher and Ahern (2000), Hatfield (1994), Pettie and Triolo (1999), Ridgeway (1999), Spaniol and Koehler (1994), and Young and Ensing (1999)
Reintegrating the illness	The first step towards recovery is frequently described as recognition and acceptance of the limitations the illness imposes and discovering talents, gifts and abilities that allow the individual to pursue and achieve life goals despite the existence of the disability	Deegan (1988, 1993), Hatfield (1994), Munetz and Frese (2001), Ridgeway (1999), Sayce and Perkins (2000), Smith (2000), Sullivan (1994), and Young and Ensing (1999)
Involvement in activities and roles that provide meaning	By expanding into and occupying normal, functional social roles (such as spouse, employee, student, taxpayer, friend) and contributing creatively to the community which the individual himself chooses, the patient lays the foundations for his own recovery	Anthony (1993), Davidson et al. (2001), Jacobson and Greenley (2001), Lunt (2000), Ridgeway (1999), and Young and Ensing (1999)

Key elements of the recovery model

Element	Description	Sources
Addressing stigma	Individuals must recover from the social consequences and social stigma and from the effects of the illness itself. Recovery includes developing resilience to stigma and/or actively fighting against it	Deegan (1996a, b), Houghton (2004), Perlick (2001), and Ridgeway (1999)
Regaining control	Individuals must take primary responsibility for transforming themselves from people with disability into people in recovery. Regaining control over one's own life contributes to the treatment through a redefined sense of self as an agent and effective subject. Opportunities must be available to people who make choices and people who need to have choices, from which they can choose. People must also be given opportunities to succeed and fail	Anthony (1993), Bassman (1997), Baxter and Diehl (1998), Deegan (1988, 1996b), Fisher (1994, n.d.-a), Frese et al. (2001), Hatfield (1994), Jacobson and Curtis (2000), Jacobson and Greenley (2001), Leete (1994), Lehman (2000), Lovejoy (1982), Lunt (2000), Mead and Copeland (2000), Munetz and Frese (2001), Ridgeway (1999), Smith (2000), Walsh (1996), and Young and Ensing (1999)
Empowerment and exercising rights of citizenship	As the sense of empowerment and control over one's own life emerges, people in recovery begin to demand their rights (such as the right to decide where they will live, who they will love, how they will spend their lives) and assume responsibility for themselves (by paying taxes, voting, volunteering) like any other citizen does	Fisher (1994, n.d.-b), Jacobson and Greenley (2001), Munetz and Frese (2001), Ridgeway (1999), Walsh (1996), and Young and Ensing (1999)
Managing symptoms	Although full remission of the symptoms is not necessary, the ability to manage one's symptoms in some way is a vital condition for recovery. Recovery includes good and difficult times, setbacks and successes and moments when the symptoms may be more or less under control. The change lies in the individual's active involvement in the treatment and his choice to manage his own symptoms, so that they are under his control instead of him passively accepting the services he receives	Deegan (1996b), Fisher (1994), and Ridgeway (1999)
Support from others	Recovery does not happen in isolation. Showing independence in the community where someone has chosen to live and the support he may received from others and from the models one chooses for oneself, be they family members, friends, professionals, members of the community or peers, encourages the individual to overcome difficult moments and reinforces good ones	Baxter Diehl (1998), Fisher (1994), Jacobson and Greenley (2001), Mead and Copeland (2000), Ridgeway (1999), Smith (2000), Sullivan (1994), and Young and Ensing (1999)

This table has been adapted from Davidson et al. (2005)

References

Amering M, Schmolke M (2009) Recovery in mental health: reshaping scientific and clinical responsibilities, West Sussex: Wiley-Blackwell

Anthony WA (1993) Recovery from mental illness: the guiding vision of the mental health service system in the 1990s. Psychosoc Rehabil J 16(4):11–23

Anthony WA (2000) A recovery-oriented service system: setting some system standards. Psychiatr Rehabil J 24(2):159–168

Anthony W, Rogers ES, Farkas M (2003) Research on evidence-based practices: future directions in an era of recovery. Community Ment Health J 39(2):101–114

Babiniotis G (2002) Dictionary of the modern Greek language with comments on how to use words correctly: interpretative, etymological, orthographic dictionary featuring synonyms, opposites, proper nouns, scientific terms and abbreviations. Athens: Lexicology Centre [in Greek]

Basaglia F (2005) L'utopia della realtà, vol 296. Torino: Giulio Einaudi

Bassman R (1997) The mental health system: experience from both sides of the locked doors. Prof Psychol Res Pract 28(3):238–242

Baxter EA, Diehl S (1998) Emotional stages: consumers and family members recovering from the trauma of mental illness. Psychiatr Rehabil J 21(4):349–355

Benedetti G (1992) New paths in psychotherapy. Psychol Top 5(2):95–140

Bowie CR et al (2010) Prediction of real-world functional disability in chronic mental disorders: a comparison of schizophrenia and bipolar disorder. Am J Psychiatr 167(9):1116–1124

Burns T, Rugkåsa J, Molodynski A, Dawson J, Yeeles K, Vazquez-Montes M, Voysey M, Sinclair J, Priebe S (2013) Community treatment orders for patients with psychosis (OCTET): a randomised controlled trial. Lancet 381(9878):1627–1633

Davidson L (2003) Living outside mental illness: qualitative studies of recovery in schizophrenia. NYU Press, New York

Davidson L, Strauss JS (1992) Sense of self in recovery from severe mental illness. Br J Med Psychol 65(2):131–145

Davidson L, Strauss JS (1995) Beyond the biopsychosocial model: integrating disorder, health, and recovery. Psychiatry Interpersonal Biol Processes 58(1):44–55

Davidson L, Chinman M, Kools B, Lambert S, Stayner DA, Tebes JK (1997) Mental illness as a psychiatric disability: shifting the paradigm toward mutual support. Community Psychol 30:19–21

Davidson L, O'Connell MJ, Tondora J, Lawless M, Evans AC (2005) Recovery in serious mental illness: a new wine or just a new bottle? Prof Psychol Res Pract 36(5):480

Davidson L, Stayner DA, Nickou C, Styron TH, Rowe M, Chinman ML (2001) Simply to be let in: inclusion as a basis for recovery. Psychiatric rehabilitation journal, 24(4):375

Deegan PE (1988) Recovery: the lived experience of rehabilitation. Psychosoc Rehabil J 11:11–19

Deegan PE (1993) Recovering our sense of value after being labelled. J Psychosoc Nurs 31(4):7–11

Deegan PE (1996a) Recovery and the conspiracy of hope. Pat Deegan, PhD & Associates, LLC

Deegan PE (1996b) Recovery as a journey of the heart. Psychiatr Rehabil J 19:91–97

Drakonakis N, Spourdalaki E, Tsaousaki K, Peppou L, Stylianidis S (2012) The legislative framework for involuntary psychiatric hospitalisation in Greece: the gap between the law and how it is implemented and the system's "grey areas". Synapsis J 8(27):32–37 (in Greek)

Fisher D (1994) Health care reform based on an empowerment model of recovery by people with psychiatric disabilities. Hosp Community Psychiatry 45(9):913–915

Fisher DB, Ahern L (2000) Personal assistance in community existence (PACE): An alternative to PACT. Ethical Human Sciences and Services, 2(2):87–92

Frese FJ, Stanley J, Kress K, Vogel-Scibilia S (2001) Integrating evidence-based practices and the recovery model. Psychiatr Serv 52(11):1462–1468

Gerard V (2011) L' experience morale hors de soi. PUF, Paris

Giddens A (2004) La Transformation de l'intimité. Sexualité, amour et érotisme dans les sociétés modernes

Greacen T, Jouet E (Dir.) (2012) Pour des usagers de la psychiatrie Acteurs de leur proper vie. Rétablissement, inclusion sociale, empowerment. Érès, Toulouse

Harding CM, Brooks G, Ashikaga T, Strauss J, Breier A (1987) The vermont longitudinal study of persons with severe mental illness, 1: methodology, study sample and overall status 32 years later. Am J Psychiatr 144(6):718–726

Harrison G, Hopper K, Craig T, Laska E et al (2001) Recovery from schizophrenia, a 15 and 25 year international follow up study. Br J Psychiatry 178:506–517

Hatfield AB (1994) Recovery from mental illness. J Calif Alliance Mentally Ill 5(3):6–7

Hochman J (1986) Realité partagée et traitement des psychotiques, Revue française de Psychanalyse, 1643–1665

Houghton F (2004) Flying solo: single/unmarried mothers and stigma in Ireland. Ir J Psychol Med 21(1):36–37

Jacobson N, Curtis L (2000) Recovery as policy in mental health services: strategies emerging from the states. Psychiatr Rehabil J 23(4):333–341

Jacobson N, Greenley D (2001) What is recovery? A conceptual model and explication. Psychiatr Serv 52(4):482–485

Kentikelenis A et al (2011) Health effects of financial crisis: omens of a Greek tragedy. Lancet 378(9801):1457–1458

Kisely S, Campbell LA, Preston N (2005) Compulsory community and involuntary outpatient treatment for people with severe mental disorders. Cochrane Database Syst Rev 20;(3):CD004408

Laird C (2002) Webster's new world dictionary and thesaurus. New World Dictionaries, New York

Lawton-Smith S, Dawson J, Burns T (2008) Community treatment orders are not a good thing. Br J Psychiatry 193:96–100

Leete E (1994) Stressor, symptom, or sequelae? Remission, recovery, or cure. J Calif Alliance Mentally Ill 5(3):16–17

Lehman AF (2000) Putting recovery into practice: a commentary on "What Recovery means to us." Community Mental Health Journal, 6(3):329–331

Liberman RP, Kopelowicz A (2002) Recovery from schizophrenia: a challenge for the 21st century. Int Rev Psychiatry 14:245–255, http://www.tandf.co.uk/journals/titles/09540261.html

Liberman RP, Kopelowicz A, Ventura J, Gutkind D (2002) Operational criteria and factors related to recovery from schizophrenia. Int Rev Psychiatry 14(4):256–272

Lieberman J, Drake R, Sederer L, Belger A, Keefe R, Perkins D, Stroup S (2008) Science and recovery in schizophrenia. Psychiatr Serv 59(5):487–496

Lovejoy M (1982) Expectations and the recovery process. Schizophr Bull 8(4):605

Lunt A (2000) Recovery: moving from concept toward a theory. Psychiatr Rehabil J 23(4):401

Mead S, Copeland ME (2000) What recovery means to us: consumers' perspectives. Community Ment Health J 36(3):315–328

Mental Health Commission (MHC) (2005) Quality in mental health – your views. Mental Health Commission, Dublin

Mentzos S (2008) New trends in psychoanalytical psychotherapy for schizophrenia. In: Tzavaras N, Vartzopoulos I, Stylianidis S (eds) Psychoanalytical psychotherapy for schizophrenia. Kastaniotis Press, Athens, pp 51–84 (in Greek)

Ministerial Decision No. Υ5β/Γ.Π./οικ 46769. 10-year programme to develop mental health units and action (PSYCHARGOS III) (2011–2020). Ministry of Health & Social Solidarity

Ministry of Health & Social Solidarity (2010) Report evaluating the interventions to implement psychiatric reform for the period 2000–2009. Ministry of Health and Social Security, Athens

Ministry of Health & Social Solidarity (2012) Working Group report on revision of the PSYCHARGOS Programme. Ministry of Health and Social Security, Athens

Ministry of Health & Social Solidarity (2013) Report evaluating the interventions to implement psychiatric reform for 2012. Ministry of Health and Social Security, Athens

Molodynski A, Rugkåsa J, Burns T (2010) Coercion and compulsion in community mental health care. Br Med Bull 95(1):105–119

Monahan J (2011) Mandated psychiatric treatment in the community – forms, prevalence, outcomes and controversies. In: Kallert TW, Mezzich JE, Monahan J (eds) Coercive treatment in psychiatry: clinical, legal and ethical aspects. Wiley, Chichester

Munetz MR, Frese FJ III (2001) Getting ready for recovery: reconciling mandatory treatment with the recovery vision. Psychiatr Rehabil J 25(1):35

Ohio Department of Mental Health (2003) Ohio mental health recovery and consumer outcomes initiative, http://www.mh.state.oh.us/initiatives/outcomes/outcomes.html

Pachoud B (2012) Se rétablir de troubles psychiatriques: un changement de regard sur le devenir des personnes. Inf Psychiatr 88(4):257–266

Perlick DA (2001) Special section on stigma as a barrier to recovery: introduction. Psychiatr Serv 52(12):1613–1614

Pettie D, Triolo AM (1999) Illness as evolution: the search for identity and meaning in the recovery process. Psychiatr Rehabil J 22(3).255–262

Presidents New Freedom Commission on Mental Health (2003) Achieving the promise: transforming mental health care in America, http://www.mentalhealthcommission.gov/reports/Finalreport/Fullreport.htm

Racamier PC (1970) Le psychanalyste sans divan. La psychanalyse et les institutions de soins psychiatriques. Payot, Paris

Racamier PC (1980) Les schizophrènes. Payot, Paris

Ridgeway PA (1999) Re-storying psychiatric disability: learning from first person narrative accounts of recovery. University of Kansas School of Social Welfare, Lawrence

Roberts G, Wolfson P (2004) The rediscovery of recovery: open to all. Adv Psychiatr Treat 10:37–49

Rosenfeld HA (1965) Psychotic states: a psycho-analytical approach. Intern. Univ. Press, New York

Sartre JP (1985) Existentialism and human emotions. New York: Citadel

Sayce L, Perkins R (2000) Recovery: beyond mere survival. Psychiatr Bull 24(2):74–74

Searles HF (1965) Collected papers on schizophrenia and related subjects. Karnac, London (reprinted 1986)

Slade M, Amering M, Farkas M, Hamilton B, O'Hagan M, Panther G, Perkins R, Shepherd G, Tse S, Whitley R (2014) Uses and abuses of recovery: implementing recovery-oriented practices in mental health systems. World Psychiatry 13(1):12–20

Smith MK (2000) Recovery from a severe psychiatric disability: findings of a qualitative study. Psychiatr Rehabil J 24(2):149–158

Spaniol L, Koehler M (eds) (1994) The experience of recovery. Centre for Psychiatric Rehabilitation, Boston

Stylianidis S, Chondros P (2011) Crise économique, crise de la réforme psychiatrique en Grèce: indice de déficit démocratique en Europe? Inf Psychiatr 87(8):625–627

Stylianidis S, Zoumpourli L, Mazaraki N (2013) Community treatment orders. ATH 6:17–22 (in Greek)

Sullivan WP (1994) A long and winding road. Process Recover Sev Ment Illn Innov Res Clin Serv Community and Rehabil 3:19–27

Vartzopoulis I, Stylianidis S (2008) Psychoanalytical psychotherapy for schizophrenia. Kastaniotis Press, Athens (in Greek)

Walsh D (1996) A journey toward recovery: from the inside out. Psychiatr Rehabil J 20(2):85–89

Warner R (2004) Recovery from schizophrenia: psychiatry and political economy. New York: Brunner-Routledge

Weaver P (1998) Recovery: Plain and simple. In Keynote Address, State Case Management Conference, Tulsa, Oklahoma, Oklahoma Department of Mental Health

White W (2000) Toward a new recovery movement: historical reflections on recovery, treatment and advocacy. Recovery Community Support Program (RCSP) Conference, April 3-5. Retrieved from www.facesandvoicesofrecovery.org

Whitwell D (2001) Recovery as a medical myth. Psychiatr Bull 25(2):75–75

Young SL, Ensing DS (1999) Exploring recovery from the perspective of people with psychiatric disabilities. Psychiatr Rehabil J 22(3):219–231

Mobile Mental Health Units on the Islands: The Experience of Cyclades

10

Stelios Stylianidis, Stella Pantelidou, Antonios Poulios, Michail Lavdas, and Nikos Lamnidis

Abstract

Mobile mental health units were first introduced in Greece in 1981 and they were later extended to geographically remote areas where there were inadequate mental health services, as part of the process of psychiatric reform. The key aims of such mobile units are to record needs; to provide timely diagnosis and intervention; to offer psychosocial support, counselling and psychotherapy to adults and children, as well as home interventions; to train volunteers; to liaise with local bodies; and to develop actions to promote mental health. Against that background, we present the experience from 10 years of running mental health units in the Northeastern and Western Cyclades. Emphasis is placed on the special features of this intervention in the local community on the islands, and the factors defining needs, as well as the requests which emerged. Clinical work is also presented and the special features of the psychosocial and psychotherapeutic interventions which were used are pointed out. Measures to promote mental health which were implemented are also described, and future targets for these sectors based on new socioeconomic circumstances are sketched.

S. Stylianidis (✉)
Department of Psychology, Panteion University, Athens, Greece
e-mail: stylianidis.st@gmail.com

S. Pantelidou • M. Lavdas • N. Lamnidis
Association for Regional Development and Mental Health (EPAPSY), Athens, Greece

A. Poulios
Clinical Psychologist, National and Kapodestrian University of Athens, Athens, Greece

10.1 Historical Background

1981 was a turning point, when mobile mental health units were introduced to Greece's public mental health system. The Social Psychiatry and Mental Health Association founded by Panagiotis Sakellaropoulos began operating in the Prefecture of Fokida, where a system for in-time intervention for acute cases was set up, i.e. for individuals who suddenly or gradually went into crisis.

The chronicles of that Association (Sakellaropoulos 2011) state that "mobile units work at the home of the patient in an acute phase and work with the family. An attempt is also made at the same time to ensure that relatives and neighbours become allies in the whole endeavour right from the outset. This means that from phase one the patient calms down and is able to take part in his own treatment. It means that the family trusts the treatment team and relies on it. It also means that the social milieu is assisted in demystifying the risk from madness and can change its attitude towards it". The home intervention model was known as "psychiatric care at the patient's home" and was organised by the Association in rural areas based on the model used in Athens, with the aim of preventing patient's having to be forcibly hospitalised.

The key issues which emerged from pilot use of mobile units in the Prefectures of Fokida, Evia and Thessaloniki (Ierodiakonou 1982, 1983; Ierodiakonou et al. 1983; Sakellaropoulos et al. 1983, 1987; Sakellaropoulos 1984; Dambassina et al. 1987) were (a) there was a need for psychiatric assistance in remote rural areas and (b) the treatment responses had to be culturally compatible with the socio-cultural environment and local community networks (Stylianidis 1989).

The model of mobile mental health units was developed with certain modifications and adjustments, depending on the theoretical approach of the body involved and the special features of each area based on geographical, social and cultural criteria. These units were a key element in how mental health services were organised in the Greek regions as part of psychiatric reform. The result of long-term operation of mobile mental health units was that they were incorporated into the legal framework in Law 2716/1999 as autonomous mental health units as part of the psychiatric reform process. Compared to other mental health units, these mobile mental health units have certain special features, since they operate in the manner outlined below (as is clear from Ministerial Decision No. Υ5β/οικ.1662 (Government Gazette 691/B/5.6.2001) laying down the modus operandi and staffing requirements for mobile mental health units specified in Article 7 of Law 2716/1999 and all other modalities required to give effect to that Article):

(a) In mental health sectors whose geographical area and layout, residential diversity and social, economic and cultural conditions coupled with the nature of mental disorders make it difficult for residents of those areas to access mental health services
(b) In neighbouring mental health sectors when there are no adequate mental health services

Consequently, the key aim in setting up mobile units was to meet mental health needs in geographically remote areas, where there were either no mental health services or existing ones were not adequate, by using the minimum own infrastructure and maximising use of infrastructure belonging to other healthcare services.

The precise work done by mobile mental health units was identified in Law 2716/1999 and in subsequent texts such as the ex ante evaluations (Ministry of Health & Social Solidarity 2010). Their task is:

In-time diagnosis – intervention to prevent the onset of disease or a remission
Home intervention to deal with and manage crises
Home treatment and monitoring of medication, follow-up of the course of the illness at regular intervals, and to ensure the continuity of psychiatric care for the patient
Help and support for the patient in meeting his practical needs with emphasis on teaching him skills and preparing him for the end goal, which is an independent life
Counselling – support for the family of the patient to ensure better communication and reduce stress for both the family and the patient
Training volunteers
Combating social stigma through community training programmes

The mobile units operated under a scientific officer. A multidisciplinary intervention team was also appointed by the management team of the body to which the mobile mental health units belonged, following a recommendation from the scientific officer. The staff comprising that multidisciplinary intervention team could include a psychiatrist, psychologist, social worker, nurse, industrial therapist and health visitor, as well as administrative and auxiliary staff who were suitably trained, an expert pedagogue, speech therapist or other healthcare professional. However, the key function of these mobile units is determined by local needs and the resources available to run them. In Greece, there are a total of 27 mobile mental health units being operated by not-for-profit private bodies as hospital units.

10.2 Key Principles and the Running of Mobile Mental Health Units

The key principles relating to the design and running of community mental health services like mobile units, broken down into sections, are presented below (WHO 2001; Mechanic 2001; Thornicroft and Tansella 1999):

A. Deinstitutionalisation
   A shift in core psychiatric care from the psychiatric hospital to the community
   Synergy with local social policies
   Respect for human rights
B. Effectiveness
   Treatment method that includes the patient's families
   Development of programmes to promote mental health
   Evaluation of services provided

Equality of access and provision of care
   Development of self-help resources for patients
   Ensuring the continuity of care
C. Liaising
   Interdisciplinary approach to the provision of services
   Working in networks
   Interconnection between mental health services and primary healthcare
D. Demedicalisation
   A shift in the interest of mental health professionals from illness to the person himself and his social disadvantage.
   An individualised care plan based on the special needs of each patient (Stylianidis and Pantelidou 2006a).

Based on these principles, mobile units primarily focused on:

(a) Providing diagnoses and treatment for mental health problems and the psychosocial problems of children, adolescents and adults at individual and family level
(b) Assessing and recording mental health needs within their area of remit, to plan interventions focused on specific needs (Slade et al. 1999)
(c) Developing mental health education and promotion programmes in the community
(d) Liaising with primary healthcare and social and educational bodies in the community
(e) Mobilising local authorities and integrating the activities of units into the social policy of each municipality (Stylianidis and Pantelidou 2006b; Stylianidis et al. 2007)
(f) Training volunteer local support groups
(g) Developing evaluation activities for the services provided
(h) In-time diagnosis and prevention of relapses and hospitalisation for serious psychiatric cases

10.3 The Liaison Model for Mobile Mental Health Units and Primary Healthcare

Primary healthcare is the first line of contact for patients and consequently for mental disorders which are in an early stage or an advanced – yet undiagnosed – stage. Primary healthcare means "the general system of providing outpatient healthcare services, which ensures equal access for the entire population at individual and family level of primary healthcare services. The system seeks to prevent, maintain, promote, restore and bolster health, by providing certified medical services, tests and medicines, and by adopting common primary healthcare rules".

Cooperation with primary healthcare bodies is a top priority, since patients with ordinary mental disorders such as depression with chronic physical illness in co-morbidity or with the presence of psychosomatic symptoms come to this level of care to receive suitable assistance. Primary healthcare coordinates the individual's healthcare, has direct access to the patient and his family and ensures the continuity of case is the entry point for more specialised care (Barbato 2008). Consequently, the timely identification and handling of a psychiatric problem is a priority in attempts to integrate mental health into primary healthcare. Mental health in primary healthcare is defined by the WHO as "providing basic preventive and curative mental healthcare at the first point of entry in the health system". The "best" outcome in terms of health and mental health is ensured by identifying and dealing with mental disorders and cases of co-morbidity in good time, with the aim of really reducing the treatment gap in mental health (see the Chapter 4). The diagram below allows us to comprehend the importance of integrating mental health into primary healthcare for achieving a "smooth outcome" for disorders (adapted from WHO, WONCA 2008):

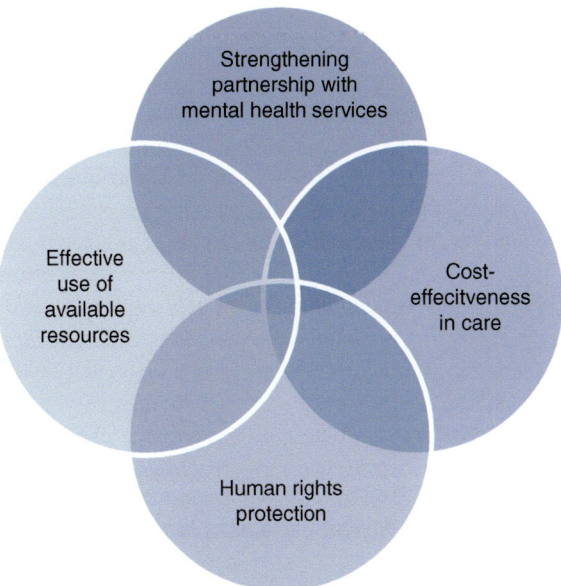

Different interfaces with primary healthcare have been proposed depending on the responsibility and competence of healthcare professionals working in primary healthcare in relation to psychiatric illness and the accompanying symptoms.

The main cooperation and interface models are listed below:

(a) The training model which stresses the improvement in knowledge and skills of primary healthcare professionals in recognising and managing mental disorders (WHO 2001; Thompson et al. 2000; Bower and Gilbody 2005).
(b) The consultation-liaison model based on mental health professionals acquiring a training relationship with the primary healthcare team and providing

counselling and supervision in the management of difficult cases (Gask et al. 1997; Bower et al. 2004).
(c) The collaborative model which combines elements of the two previous models in changing the role of primary healthcare professionals and mental health professionals in general healthcare (Bower and Gask 2002; Simon et al. 2001).
(d) The replacement/referral model which focuses on the psychiatric problem being managed by mental health professionals while having primary healthcare professionals has general clinical responsibility (Bower 2002). In Greece, psychiatric disorders are primarily managed by mental health professionals, but frequently the role of GPs is undervalued, with the recognition level for psychiatric disorders in primary healthcare being quite low (Mavreas et al. 1986). Nonetheless, in remote rural or island areas with few to now specialised mental health services, the role of primary healthcare remains central, since it is the first line for dealing with and for contact with patients.

Although great emphasis was initially given to a model of interface between mobile mental health units and primary healthcare, quite a few difficulties arose in practice from implementing this model, mainly due to problems associated with primary healthcare. The inadequate development of primary healthcare structures in Greece and the lack of networking between services and inadequate training for primary healthcare professionals about mental health issues, coupled with the lack of psychiatric departments at general hospitals in the regions and understaffed primary healthcare structures, contribute to the role of primary healthcare as a gatekeeper being weakened and had downplayed the role of the GP as someone in the first line for psychiatric disorders. Such a role would have included initial diagnosis, basic treatment, and referral to a specialised service or mental health professional (when that was considered necessary) to ensure the continuity of care and provide suitable specialised treatment in keeping with subsequent levels of care.

10.4 Examples of How Mobile Mental Health Units Operate in Europe

Lausanne's pilot experience of mobile units, which has been in operation since 2002, uses Assertive Community Treatment (ACT) as its theoretical basis. The multidisciplinary team which intervenes in rural areas of the Canton of Vaud ensures psychiatric follow-up for the community of patients suffering from serious psychiatric disorders with a high drop-out rate from routine psychiatric follow-up (Bonsack 2008). After that experience, the investigators identified three target populations: (a) patients considered to be "frequent consumers of care" who visited the emergency psychiatric care department quite frequently or who were hospitalised without being put into any real care plan, (b) patients who refused all care despite the intervention of the primary healthcare network or secondary healthcare in the area and (c) patients who presented symptoms of the onset of psychosis and did not seek help of their own initiative nor on the initiative of their family. The mobile mental health units in the Vaud Canton covered patients in all age groups.

In Belgium (Jacob 2014), mobile mental health units have also been deployed in the context of psychiatric reform. There are two types of mobile units:

(a) Mobile mental health units for intensive follow-up purposes used to deal with crises and acute cases
(b) Mobile mental health units for continuous follow-up of individuals with chronic and complex problems

Mobile units were introduced as part of the process of deinstitutionalisation and a reduction in the number of psychiatric beds in hospitals. In doing so, the economic and human resources saved were transferred to the innovative concept of mobile mental health units.

The role of these units in Belgium complements the psychiatric system of care which is focused on reform with the aim of providing mental health services in the community, recovery, empowerment of local networks and liaising with primary healthcare. The country currently has 40 mobile mental health units and the process of evaluation is underway to determine the size of the network needed to cover the entire territory of Belgium. Early results indicate that the units have contributed to a reduction in hospitalisations and to keeping individuals in the community.

The WHO pyramid (2009) helps us better visualise the position of mobile mental health units and the linkage to lower and more specialised levels of healthcare, in conjunction with the cost required to run them and the needs of the population covered.

10.5 Experiences and Best Practices

The Regional Development and Mental Health Association (a NGO) is responsible in scientific and administrative terms for two mobile mental health units in the Cyclades (whose permanent recorded population within the area of remit is 78,267). The NE Cyclades mobile mental health unit commenced operations in June 2003 and the one in the Western Cyclades in January 2004. Financing to run the mobile units comes from national resources (MHSS), European funding, local government authority resources, donations and other specialised European programmes and multidisciplinary partnerships. The NE Cyclades mobile unit is based on Paros and is responsible for the islands of Syros, Andros, Mykonos, Tinos, Paros and Antiparos. Likewise, the Western Cyclades mobile unit is based on Milos and is responsible for the islands of Milos, Kimolos, Sifnos, Serifos, Kea and Kythnos. In terms of how the two mobile units work, every 15 days, a team comprised of a psychiatrist, child psychiatrist, psychologist and social worker visit the islands referred to (the specialisations are determined based on needs and available financial resources). Sessions are held at the unit's headquarters in premises provided by health centres of local government authorities. Experts also make home visits. In addition to their clinical work, a variety of mental health education and promotion activities take place on each island, based on the operating targets of the mobile units, and there is also a central secretariat in operation on Paros which organises treatment and community work.

It should be stressed that these two mobile units are special in that they cover island areas that are difficult to access, especially during winter months. The 12 islands within the remit of the units do not have any other mental health services to deal with psychiatric and child psychiatric cases. There is only one child psychiatrist at the Syros General Hospital. In addition, social services are limited and health centres and regional medical surgeries are now understaffed. Before the mobile units commenced operations, one key feature of local communities was a lack of any cultural or well-designed activities relating to public mental health and social exclusion. In addition, difficulties in access to and lack of an adequately organised communication network reinforced the insecurity of residents and fostered an inward-looking outlook, apparent self-sufficiency and in some cases discrimination and social exclusion (Stylianidis and Pantelidou 2006a).

The special features of each local community determined the mode of intervention at clinical and community level when the mobile units became operational:

Interventions were tailored to the special needs of each island.
Using an ethnopsychiatric approach, the socio-humanitarian features of each community were identified: specific cultural codes, attitudes towards differentness, prejudice about mental health issues and all factors which play an important role in shaping psychiatric requests and how symptoms manifest.

The activities of the mobile units in the NE and Western Cyclades are presented by looking at the following areas: (1) needs, (2) clinical work, (3) interface with primary healthcare, (4) mental health promotion and networking with local bodies and (5) evaluation.

Needs

A key condition in designing and developing special actions (treatment, social, etc.) for a mental health services is to assess the needs in the area of remit (Thornicroft and Tansella 1999). In the case of the mobile mental health units for the NE and Western Cyclades, needs were initially assessed at empirical level when the units became operational and an epidemiological study was carried out into the prevalence of mental disorders in the general population on Paros and Antiparos.

The needs assessment began by collecting data from primary healthcare and social services on the islands. Working groups were also set up with key persons in the community: local government representatives, doctors, teachers, priests and policemen. This process allowed important information to be recorded on each island relating to:

- Chronic psychiatric cases in the community
- Cases of families with severe psychosocial problems
- The frequency of Public Prosecutor orders for involuntary hospitalisation

- The frequency of requests for intervention in cases of child abuse – negligence
- Needs and requests relating to children and families which come through schools
- Problems faced by vulnerable groups, such as migrants, and people with chronic physical conditions
- The need for mental health promotion activities

In addition, in 2007, an epidemiological study was carried out to examine the prevalence of common mental disorders on Paros and Antiparos (Stylianidis et al. 2010). The study was carried out in partnership with the University of Ioannina (Psychiatric Department, Medical School) and the Panteion University.

The primary synchronic study was conducted on a sample of 506 people from the general population chosen by ordinary random sampling (from 776 people chosen, 506 agreed to participate, which is a 65 % participation rate). Psychiatric morbidity was assessed using a fully structured interview, namely, the Clinical Interview Schedule Revised (CIS-R, Lewis and Pelosi 1990; Singleton et al. 2003). The average age of the sample was 44 (age range 18–74). Clinically significant psychiatric morbidity was found in 22 % of the sample. Women had significantly higher morbidity than men (30 % compared to 13 %). In addition, the prevalence of major depression of at least average severity was 0.6 % in men and 3.6 % in women, while mild depression was 1.1 % in men and 7.8 % in women. In contrast with the often more frequency prevalence of depression in women compared to men (1:7), the harmful use of alcohol assessed by AUDIT (Babor et al. 1992) showed a figure higher than the general population (13 %) which the vast prevalence being in men (23.8 %) in the sample compared to woman (3 %). Anxiety disorders and clinically significant stress had a prevalence of 6.8 % in men, 12.73 % in women and 10 % overall. As far as correlations with socio-demographic variables were concerned, it was found that women, single people and the unemployed had a higher rate of morbidity, while individuals with higher and university level education and individuals with a high reported family income had lower morbidity.

A similar study on the prevalence of common mental disorders was also carried out on a sample of 323 high school pupils on Paros (Stylianidis et al. 2010) and the results are presented in the next chapter.

Moreover, a descriptive study of the prevalence of mental disorders in migrants being followed up by the Paros-Antiparos team was also carried out in the period 2004–2006 (Pantelidou et al. 2008). In total, 43 adult migrants (81 % of Albanian descent) received services from the mobile unit on Paros and Antiparos between 2004 and 2006, accounting for 8 % of all users of the service at that time. Of that figure, 48 % were men and 62 % women, aged 20–40. The most frequent requests from migrants related to psychiatric symptoms, mainly mood (affective) disorders (30 %), psychotic syndrome (14 %) and problematic family relations (18 %). As the results clearly show, high percentages of migrants contacted the service about severe mental disorders and relationship problems (including domestic violence problems) compared to the percentages for the total patient population who received services over that period. The study showed the need to develop actions focused on the special features of minorities in island areas, taking into account the serious social problems they face in certain cases (Pantelidou et al. 2010).

Table 10.1 Absolute frequencies of the number of persons receiving services during the first decade the NE and Western Cyclades mobile units were in operation

Users of services	NE Cyclades	Western Cyclades	Total
Adults	4.636	1.547	6.183
Children/adolescents	1.339	567	1.906
Total	5.975	2.114	8.089

Since the main aim of the mobile unit was to prevent recurrences and avoid hospitalisation for severe psychiatric cases, in 2005, a study was launched to record problems associated with the process of involuntary hospitalisation and to record the number of hospitalisations from the Cyclades (Stouraitou et al. 2009). During the first years of the study, an increase in hospitalisations was noted, which may have been associated both with highlighting severe psychiatric cases that had remained untreated in previous years (since there were no mental health providers before 2003) and with the general trend towards higher involuntary hospitalisations in Greece at that time. The study is under way still in order to capture the trend in subsequent years. From the information collected, we also noticed difficulties associated with the detention and transfer of patients, for whom the Public Prosecutor had issued a hospitalisation order. Due to the geographical isolation of some islands and the lack of a psychiatric department at the Syros General Hospital, patients were transferred from the islands to Syros in order for a first expert opinion to be provided by the hospital's psychiatrist and were then sent on to Athens. That resulted in long waits (due to the absence of frequent sailings to and from Syros) for patients in detention cells, especially on islands that did not have health centres, coupled with long journeys on ships. Following an intervention from the mobile unit which worked with the Syros Public Prosecutor's Office, a request was made for patients to be sent directly to Athens, and not via Syros. Moreover, when psychiatrists from the mobile unit are on the islands, they play the role of expert report-writer in the case of Public Prosecutor orders for hospitalisation, which has also significantly improved the procedure.

Clinical Work

The mobile units' clinical work includes diagnostic assessments, individual counselling and psychotherapy sessions, group psychotherapy, family and couples counselling sessions, setting up a social club for individuals with severe psychosocial problems, carrying out social studies into cases of child abuse, psychosocial support for families facing numerous problems (psychiatric symptoms, socioeconomic problems), as well as home interventions.

From the time when mobile units commenced operations up to 2013, a total of 6,109 adults and 1,891 children and adolescents had received services. As far as the NE Cyclades are concerned, 4,580 adults and 1,327 children and adolescents received services. In the Western Cyclades, 1,529 adults and 564 children and adolescents received services (see Table 10.1). As far as demographic data for the

Table 10.2 Demographic data pertaining to adult users of services from the NE and Western Cyclades mobile units while in operation ($N = 6.183$)

Variable	F	%
Gender		
Male	1988	32.2
Female	4186	67.8
Origin		
Greek	5581	92.5
Other	455	7.5
Marital status		
Single	1218	21.1
Married	3246	56.4
Divorced	556	9.7
Widowed	654	11.4
Cohabiting/living together	80	1.4
Employment		
Employee	3849	77.7
Unemployed	414	8.4
Working occasionally	690	13.9
Visited mental health professional in the past		
Yes	2189	40.5
No	3213	59.5

service users was concerned, for adults the average age was 49.7 years ($SD = 18.8$ $min = 18$ $max = 104$) and for children and adolescents it was 9.2 years ($SD = 4.1$ $min = 1$ $max = 18$). Table 10.2 summarises the other data about adults (the next chapter presents more data about children and adolescents). It is worth noting that around 10 % of the permanent population on the areas these mobile units covered have benefited from the services they offer.

Table 10.2 shows an increase in the influx of new cases in the first 2 years, which reflects the fact that communities were learning that the mobile units were in operation, which was achieved through mobilisation at community level, contacts with local professional bodies operating in the communities and through specific mental health promotion activities. The consequent drop, with the lowest absolute frequency point after the commencement of operations being achieved in 2009, can be explained by the increased financing difficulties at that time, which made it difficult for mental health bodies to operate and made their operations more precarious, undermining plans and making it difficult to keep adequate staff levels up, having adequate budget to pay accommodation of staff, make more trips to distant islands (etc).

From 2010 onwards, an increased influx of new cases was noted. This was the time when the socioeconomic crisis began and consequently, as is well-known, psychosocial difficulties increased as is clear from the demand for such services. Note that in 2012, another serious difficulty in financing brought another drop in new cases, but figures recovered the following year. The flow of cases was partially determined by the continuity of funding and the continued assurance of the problem-free operation of teams on each island.

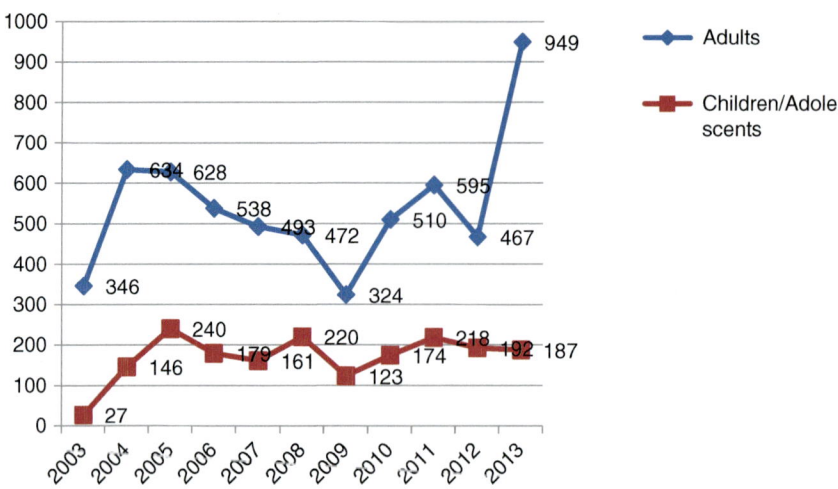

Fig. 10.1 Absolute frequencies of new cases for adults and children/adolescents while the Northeastern and Western Cyclades mobile units were in operation (N=6,182 and 1,906 for adults and children/adolescents, respectively)

Table 10.3 Relative frequencies of diagnostic categories for adults (ICD10) who received services at the Northeastern and Western Cyclades mobile units during their first decade in operation (N=4,636 and 1,547 respectively)

Diagnostic category	NE Cyclades	Western Cyclades
Organic mental disorders (F00-F09)	7.8 %	12 %
Disorders due to substance use (F10-F19)	2.4 %	1.2 %
Schizophrenic, delusional disorders (F20-F29)	6.9 %	3.4 %
Mood (affective) disorders (F30-F39)	28.2 %	27.9 %
Neurotic, stress-related disorders (F40-F48)	18.5 %	23.4 %
Eating disorders, non-organic sleep disorders (F50-F59)	0.7 %	0.7 %
Disorders of personality and behaviour (F60-F69)	2.4 %	4.7 %
Mental retardation (F70-F79)	1.1 %	1.9 %
Disorders of psychological development (F80-F89)	0.2 %	0.4 %
Unspecified mental disorder (F99)	0.1 %	0.1 %
Counselling (Z71)	6.6 %	4 %
Relations problems – social issues (Z60-F63)	18.1 %	13.8 %
No psychopathology – certificates – other	7.1 %	6.5 %

Although there were also fluctuations noted in relation to children and adolescents as well, the fluctuations were not so intense. That could be explained by the fact that (a) the population is more limited and (b) by the fact that the caregivers for children are usually mobilised to seek out help if problems arise, irrespective of socioeconomic conditions (Fig. 10.1).

Looking at diagnoses for adults who have received services so far (see Table 10.3), the most frequent diagnoses relate to mood (affective) disorders and nervous disorders and disorders associated with stress, as one might have expected based on

Table 10.4 Relative frequencies of diagnostic categories for children and adolescents (ICD10) who received services at the Northeastern and Western Cyclades mobile units during their first decade in operation ($N=1,339$ and 567 respectively)

Diagnostic category	NE Cyclades	Western Cyclades
Organic mental disorders (F00-F09)	0.3 %	0.2 %
Disorders due to substance use (F10-F19)	0.1 %	
Schizophrenic, delusional disorders (F20-F29)	0.3 %	0.9 %
Mood (affective) disorders (F30-F39)	4.1 %	5.7 %
Neurotic, stress-related disorders (F40-F48)	11.4 %	13.4 %
Eating disorders, non-organic sleep disorders (F50-F59)	1.8 %	1.4 %
Disorders of personality and behaviour (F60-F69)	1.7 %	1.1 %
Mental retardation (F70-F79)	2.4 %	3.9 %
Disorders of psychological development (F80-F89)	25.2 %	19.6 %
Behavioural and emotional disorders with onset usually occurring in childhood and adolescence (F90-F98)	22.2 %	21.6 %
Unspecified mental disorder (F99)	0.1 %	
Relations problems – social issues (Z60-F63)	25.9 %	26 %
No psychopathology – certificates – other	4.7 %	6.2 %

Table 10.5 Relative frequencies of sources of referrals to the Northeastern and Western Cyclades mobile units during their first decade in operation

Source of referrals	NE Cyclades	Western Cyclades	Total
Self-referral	48.9 %	30.6 %	44.4 %
Primary healthcare	23.3 %	26.6 %	24.1 %
Private doctor	5 %	2.9 %	4.5 %
Community body	6.8 %	5.1 %	6.4 %
Public authorities	1.5 %	3.8 %	2.1 %
Church	0.3 %	0.3 %	0.3 %
Educational body	6.1 %	22.3 %	6.6 %
Other	8.1 %	8.4 %	11.6 %

previous epidemiological studies (Skapinakis et al. 2013). That was followed by requests relating to relationship and social problems, which emphasises the necessity of adopting a biopsychosocial approach to providing mental health services in the community. Although there is no epidemiological data for the Cyclades as a whole, the numbers do appear to reflect the relevant frequencies of organic and psychotic disorders which could possibly apply to a population overall which under other conditions would need to travel to the capital or even endure involuntary hospitalisation while in crisis.

Likewise, Table 10.4 relating to the diagnoses of children and adolescents shows that the most frequent diagnoses had to do with psychological development and behavioural and emotional issues which onset during childhood and adolescence, along with relationship problems and other social issues.

As is clear from Table 10.5, most referrals came to mobile units of their own initiative. One could argue that this was based on social mobilisation of the staff of public services and the dissemination of information about how mobile units operate by persons who received services, i.e. word of mouth. The next source of referrals was primary healthcare providers. Although the second highest figure, this percentage does not reflect what was initially expected. In reality it appears that a multidisciplinary structure, like the mobile units, partially mobilised the referrals from primary healthcare due to the dysfunction arising from the crisis in the public health system. It appears that (a) primary healthcare is not operating properly in Greece's regions, in contrast to the massive enlargement of secondary and tertiary care in the capital, and (b) there is a potential lack of training among doctors in the interface between primary healthcare services and mental health and chronic welfare cases.

Of course, having said that, one cannot assume that within a decade of mobile units being in operation, a system of liaisons with primary healthcare providers operating within the territorial remit of the mobile units has not been built up. The lowest frequency for sources of referrals was for the Church. Here we can see a lack of information as well as the systematic preparation work that needs to be done in order for a different culture (relating to prejudice, different conceptual approaches to these matters and mutual resistance) not to be a barrier for many priests referring individuals with psychosocial problems to mental health services. However, given the close contact between priests and the community, especially in areas outside of urban centres, an attempt has been made in terms of community activities in cooperation with the local dioceses, to offer training seminars for priests run by experts from the mobile units. The "Other" source of referrals relates primarily to referrals in the context of community activities such as workshops, mental health promotion teams and local mental health teams.

Looking more deeply at the issue of sources of referrals, it is clear that over time they differ in a statistically significant manner (*chi-square statistical verification* $(18) = 295.69, p < 0.001$). As Table 10.5 shows, the assumption about self-referrals and referrals from primary healthcare has been confirmed. In addition, there was an initial stability in the frequency of self-referrals in the first 6 years; the mobile units were in operation, which was then followed by a major rise, which corresponds to a drop in referrals from primary healthcare providers.

Certain other conclusions could be drawn by exploring the longitudinal changes in adult diagnoses, which were statistically significant (*chi-square statistical verification* $(24) = 477.51, p < 0.001$) (Fig. 10.3). In all cases, relatively lower frequencies were noted in the distribution of each diagnostic category in the period 2007–2009. In some cases, such as psychoses and organic psychotic disorders, this could be explained by the fact that the majority of these cases were identified when the mobile units commenced operations, to the extent that one of the aims of this intervention in relation to such psychopathologies was to reduce hospitalisations and relapses. Moreover, during that 3-year period, the first serious difficulties in terms of organising and funding mental health structures were dealt with, which had made it difficult for the structures to operate and consequently to accept new cases.

As is the case with any community intervention where there are no other mental health services, the frequency of psychotic disorders dealt with by the service will

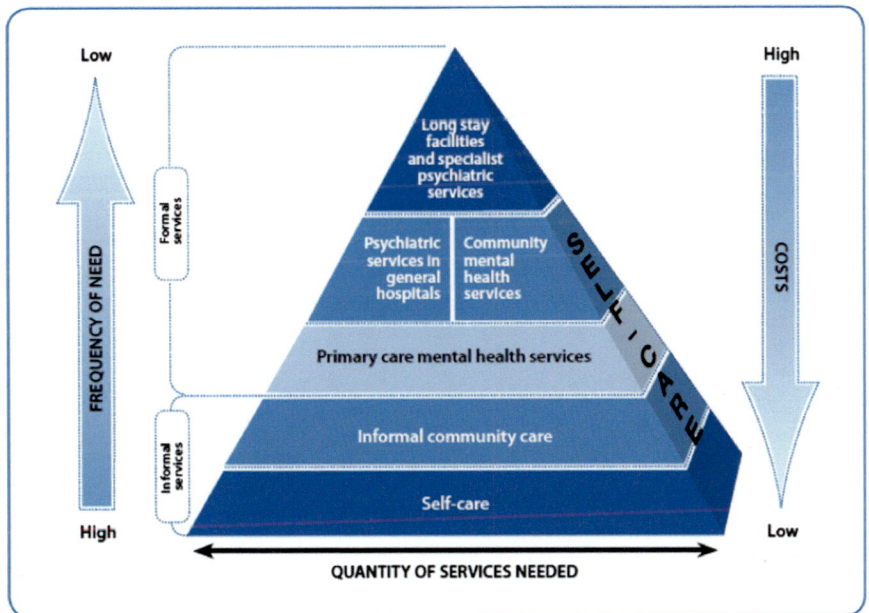

Fig. 10.2 WHO Service Organization pyramid for an optimal mix of services for mental health (WHO 2009) (Reprint from http://www.who.int/mental_health/policy/services/mhsystems/en/. Accessed on 14th January 2015)

initially be higher and will then gradually decrease. According to Peritogiannis and Mavreas (2014), individuals suffering from psychotic disorders have greater needs and also greater difficulties in receiving mental healthcare. At the same time, serious psychiatric disorders in areas which do not have specialised psychiatric care at primary healthcare level are frequently not diagnosed and are undertreated (Tylee and Walters 2006), and systematic attempts are then required to effectively deal with this through early intervention. The special feature of the clinical and statutory framework within which the mobile mental health units operates is that there is no direct possibility of referral to a specialised psychiatric unit or psychiatric department in a general hospital, meaning that it is vital to utilise mobile support networks in the community and for the multidisciplinary team to be "clinically inventive" in order to reduce relapses and to manage them as best as possible in the community context. Current socioeconomic conditions which are associated with the onset or increase in factors burdening mental health, such as financial debt, lack of resources to access private mental health services, lack of resources for medication, unemployment, etc., make individuals more vulnerable to the development of mental disorders. Recent studies show an increase in psychiatric problems in relation to these factors (Economou et al. 2011, 2012; Giotakos 2011; Skapinakis et al. 2013).

The data for the populations within the mobile units' territorial remit show that the increase relates to mood (affective) disorders, neurotic, and stress-related and

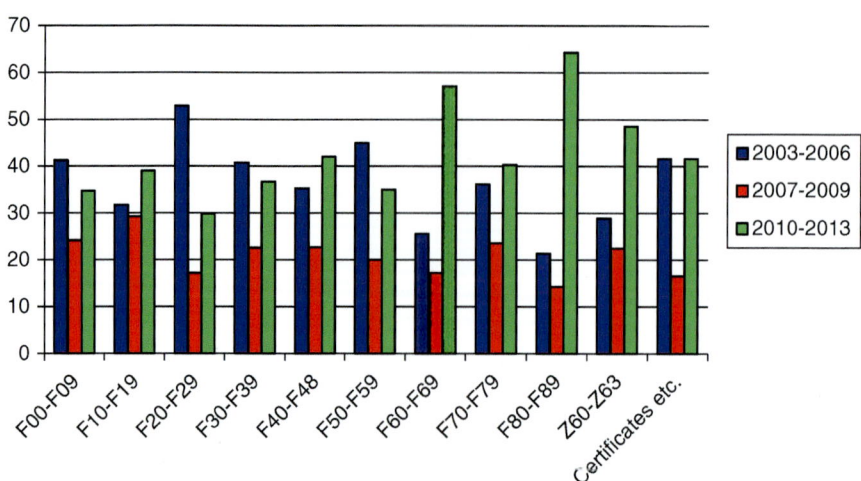

Fig. 10.3 Relative frequencies of diagnoses while mobile units were in operation in the Northeastern and Western Cyclades for adults who received services ($N=6,183$, the relative frequencies have been calculated for each diagnostic category)

somatoform disorders, to behavioural and physiological-related disorders and syndromes associated with physical factors, and to problems associated with the primary support framework, which includes family circumstances. As far as the latter category is concerned, one may also need to add that the increase for such requests may be attributable to raise awareness due to the mental health promotion programme for groups of parents, teachers and adolescents, funded by the Stavros Niarchos Foundation.

Clinical observations about psychosocial-psychotherapeutic interventions and the current status of the mobile units. Examination of the clinical treatment work done by the mobile units revealed a series of interesting indications about the forms that psychopathology can take and about the course of treatment and the final outcome on the islands where the units are engaged in clinical activities. We will refer to just some of these and set out a series of hypotheses to be explored, relating to their emergence, and the beneficial consequences of psychotherapeutic management.

Borderline personality disorders. Despite morphological differences, given that a borderline individual on Milos will not be as openly suicidal as a borderline individual in New York (Clarkin et al. 2004), the fundamental hallmark signs of the disorder remain unchanged. Traumatic stress in light of (real or threatened) loss of an object (vital for mental "survival") remains the core of the disorder. What the most common "threatened loss curves" are is a complex matter which includes modern Greek customs and habits (Kapsomenos 2008) and systematic social traumas (Hopper 1996) which have reached a climax now with the current economic and social crisis. Closeness to school age for each child, and especially the last child in the birth order, makes a vulnerable mother, in terms of capacity for mentalisation and reflectivity, a suitable candidate to fall ill (Fonagy et al. 2002). Even if such vulnerability has been associated with genetic predisposition (Lieb et al. 2004), the onset of the illness will almost always be the direct consequence of psychotraumatic burdens. This point is exceptionally important for psychotherapeutic interventions and for more the systematic psychotherapies which take place in the context of mobile units. Moderation and realism in treatment goals and a balanced ratio between empirical clinical approaches (such as treatment as usual, TAU), psychoanalytic theorising – which is sometimes backed up by cognitive or systemic theorising or even ordinary behavioural approaches Kernberg et al. 2008) – and evidence-based approaches help contribute to optimum formulation of these clinical cases. The countertransference risks (Rosenfeld 1987) from the therapist being merged into and absorbed in the treatment situation are reduced in this way, and it becomes easier to implement a sort of phased step psychotherapy which is a key part of what Thomä and Kächele had to say about psychoanalysis (1987): a continuing series of variable duration short-term psychotherapies which can be renewed or terminated at critical points. Thus, psychotherapy can last a few months (given that the frequency at which therapists visit each island is every 2 weeks, the maximum number of sessions could be 2 on the weekend of the visit, or 4 a month, or a total of 20–25 sessions overall) up to 4–5 years (i.e. almost 200 sessions). It is important to note that the total cost of relatively "long-term" psychotherapy provided by mobile units continues to be much less than the amount required to pay for even a small part of any long-term hospitalisation. As is well known, it is highly likely that some of those patients will also require additional treatment for various other cases such as anxiety crises, intense stomach pains (which may even require investigative laparoscopy), psychiatric hospitalisation or depression and attempted suicide even (Kienast et al. 2014). Consequently, further research is needed with a long-term follow-up period to show that such psychotherapy cannot only improve the patient's quality of life but also to a large extent reduce co-morbidity (Leuzinger-Bohleber et al. 2003) and the cost corresponding to it.

Depression. This was the most common disorder which came in a number of "disguises" associated with physical complaints, paranoid ideation or behavioural disorders, requiring detailed clinical investigation in order to establish the diagnosis. Middle-aged women who need to deal with the gradual loss of their reproductive capacity are a group vulnerable to the onset of depressive disorders, in addition to other burden factors. In some cases, responsiveness to antidepressants may affect the diagnosis, thereby requiring frequent collaboration between the therapist and psychiatrist.

Suicidality is once again relatively limited and complex nosological-anthropological studies need to be carried out to show what share of the affected population is at a higher risk of suicide.

Of the various types of psychotherapy that exist, it appears that the relational approach (Diamanti 2014) has a very good response rate for certain categories of depression (Blatt and Luyten 2009), on a par with that of the CBT approach (Tzanoulinos 2014).

Narcissistic disorders of personality and psychopathy. A frequent initial finding in this category of disorders is the charm and allure exerted on the supervising team when such patients are presented by their therapist. They are men and women with a reported "rich" sex life, who frequently defraud their milieu and who have been involved in crime and with reported cases of marginal or threatened violence and systematic (projective) attribution of responsibilities to members of the family environment; with a background of involvement with the police or judicial authorities; and with complex psychosocial-cultural difficulties which are interwoven with social services provided by local government authorities (which are very poorly organised in any event).

It is not at all uncommon for a careful study of the background of such cases to show complex traumatic burdens that could even relate to previous generations, a background that may only be obtained after quite a few sessions and quite a few months of meetings and may often be hidden or more often involve dichotomies, denials and refusals (Hatziandreou 2012). In this case, the search for help is associated with a recent psychotraumatic event which sits atop the unconscious traumatic substrate.

In cases like these, it is possible for the patient to seek help because of depressive complications, which spring from unconscious wounds from pathological narcissism which can create exceptionally dangerous situations of threatened suicide.

Usually all this is attributed to significant others. There is relatively low compliance with treatment, frequent dropouts and a restoration of the treatment relationship when new difficulties arise. It is not at all rare hallmark of such cases for the police, Public Prosecutor, therapist, local doctor and parents to be involved. Potentially, at least one part of the population in subsequent criminal or illegal activity may consist of individuals with such disorders.

A very large part of the treatment in cases like these is recognition and awareness of the innate psychological factors and personal contribution/responsibility of the patient for what is happening to him (since this primarily affects males) or her (which is a much rarer case).

Developmental disorders. These disorders are common in such populations given the low level of psychiatric services, especially primary, prevention-oriented care. Children and adolescents with psychopathology are not diagnosed and are not dealt with, meaning we have clinical pictures of chronic regression, neglect and sometimes mental decline.

Even if such patients are lagging behind in terms of family and social relations, they can remain functional and achieve a degree of adjustment which in some cases is far from negligible. Here traditional societies may be "better" (from a wider anthropological viewpoint) than "hyper-diagnostic" modern Western societies (Kessing 2005).

Psychoses. It is critical for them to have adequate follow-up so that schizophrenic and bipolar disorders can be distinguished from psychotic episodes (Kessing, op. cit.) which need a different psychotherapeutic approach. A real diagnostic and treatment question is when is the right time to start antipsychotic treatment and provide short-term hospitalisation, if it is considered necessary.

The Interface with Primary Healthcare

Taking into account the problems relating to how primary healthcare operates in Greece and the difficulty in developing and evaluating a model of cooperation between the mobile units and primary healthcare, quite a few measures were taken to lay the foundations for a more effective interface in the future.

Major emphasis was placed on training primary healthcare professionals in how to prevent, recognise and manage mental disorders. Training included regular seminars held locally on each island or conferences arranged in cooperation with the Hellenic Society for Genetic/Family Medicine, aimed at all doctors and nurses involved in primary healthcare in the Cyclades. In addition to seminars held at health centres at regular intervals, a total of four training workshops were held centrally on Paros and Syros over the course of 2 days for primary healthcare doctors in the Cyclades, in cooperation with the Hellenic Society for Genetic/Family Medicine and the participation of Greek and foreign experts (e.g. from the WHO).

In a qualitative study which employed semi-structured interviews carried out by the Regional Development and Mental Health Association in cooperation with the University of the Aegean to evaluate the first training seminar held on Syros, views about mental disorders and the educational needs of 17 staff in primary healthcare were recorded (Stylianidis and Zisi 2005). All those questioned agreed that users of services frequently contacted primary healthcare services to deal with their mental health problems. The responses showed that in the case of adults, depression and anxiety disorders were the most frequent, while in children, behaviour and speech problems were the most common. The treatments proposed by those questions included counselling and referral to a mental health professional, especially to deal with schizophrenia and when the treatments of GPs failed or when the symptoms were persistent, with a poor response to medication. However, most doctors agreed that the treatments at primary healthcare level were not sufficient and emphasised the need to organise training on mental health issues. When asked about their views on depression and schizophrenia, there appeared to be a relative inability to scientifically formulate the nature of these disorders. The seminar which was held was viewed in a positive light by primary healthcare staff (Stylianidis and Zisi 2005).

In addition, over the last 3 years, the WHO's MhGap guide (WHO 2010) has been translated into Greek and is being used in training. This guide has been used to successfully carry out training seminars for primary healthcare doctors on Syros, Tinos and Paros. It is essential to remind readers that during the first years that the units were in operation, a system of referrals to and from the primary healthcare using special forms had been put in place. Over time, referrals and cooperation on cases being followed up were primarily done via regular meetings with doctors at health centres.

Promoting Mental Health and Networking with Local Bodies

Networking with local bodies on the islands and developing activities to promote mental health are an integral part of the mobile units' activities, which are primarily community-focused services operating in the context of the public mental health system (Stylianidis and Pantelidou 2006b; Pantelidou et al. 2010; Pantelidou et al. 2012). In general terms, these actions included:

Workshops and other special events (such as a mental health festival and activities of a cultural and sporting nature) aimed at the residents of each island, to provide information about the mental health of children, adolescents and adults. The aim of these measures was to reduce stigma about mental illness and to provide information and allow for the timely search for help from mental health experts. One or two such activities take place on each island every year.

Special events with a less theoretical and more experiential character relating to specific population groups: the elderly, the disabled, people with physical illnesses, parents, children, etc. For example, over the last 3 years, parent support groups, support groups for relatives of patients with dementia and empowerment groups for women who have suffered domestic violence have been held.

Programmes aimed at providing information and training for specific professionals in the community: training groups to provide information about key psychopathology issues in children and adolescents and issues of how to deal with behavioural problems, training seminars for GPs, training for police officers about how to handle Public Prosecutor orders for involuntary hospitalisation and cases of domestic violence and training for priests about key aspects of mental health.

Planning and development of voluntary support groups comprised of patients, relatives and other individuals from the local community. Once such group was recently launched on Paros, after a seminar held in cooperation with the National Disabled Confederation (May, 2014) to provide information about the rights of individuals with mental disability and how to organise self-advocacy measures.

A network of local bodies was developed which entails regular meetings of local groups of representatives from health services, social services, educational bodies, local government authorities and public authorities whose aims are (a) to improve networking between local services, (b) to continuously record needs, (c) to cooperate in managing serious psychiatric cases in the community, (d) to cooperate in the planning and implementation of mental health prevention and promotion measures and (e) to develop broad institutional synergies on wider local development issues along with local government authorities and other bodies (whether formal or not) in each community, taking into account special cultural and social features.

Assessment

A key aspect of how mobile mental health units operate is evaluation of the services they provide in order to use those results to improve how the service functions (Pantelidou et al. 2010).

During the second year that the mobile units were in operation, a pilot study was conducted (in cooperation with the Universities of Ioannina and the Aegean) to assess levels of satisfaction among patients and their relatives with the services provided by mobile units. A Patient/Relative Mental Health Services Satisfaction Scale (based on the Verona Service Satisfaction Scale-VSSS, Ruggeri and Dall'Agnola 1993) was used which was filled out by a sample of 126 individuals, users of services from the start of operations until the time of the study (ordinary random sample). Eighty-one percent of the sample was women and 19 % men, and

67 % were still using the service, while the others had received services in the past. The majority of those questioned (78 %) said they were quite satisfied or very satisfied with the effectiveness of the service in handling their requests and with the ability and behaviour of staff (94 %). A large percentage of those questioned (63 %) said they disliked sessions being cancelled because of problems therapists had in travelling to the islands (difficulties in accessibility of the islands because of weather conditions in winter months).

The services provided continue to be evaluated even today and in 2012 a process of assessing the clinical interviews on a systematic basis was launched. In this context, each new recipient of services is evaluated when he starts using services and then 6 months later, and when he finishes using them. The following scales have been used in this context: World Health Organisation Quality of Life-Bref (WHOQOL-bref) (WHOQOLGroup 1998; Ginieri-Coccossis et al. 2009), the revised version of the Symptom Checklist-90 (SCL-90-R) (Derogatis and Savitz 2000; Donias et al. 1991) and the Strength and Difficulties Questionnaire (SDQ) (Goodman and Goodman 2009; Giannakopoulos et al. 2009) for children and adolescents.

Conclusions

It is important to examine whether the mobile mental health units model could be spread in order to firmly establish psychiatric reform in the difficult socioeconomic period of crisis by taking a different perspective: (a) the mental health needs of the population in remote areas and in the rest of the country are rapidly increasing, and consequently the line-up of the multidisciplinary team would in turn have to be bolstered in order to be rudimentarily adequate to address the needs which arise; (b) the current crisis in the public health system overall and in primary healthcare in particular (the National Healthcare Service Provider, known by its Greek abbreviation EOPYY, and the National Primary Healthcare Network, known by its Greek abbreviation PEDY) coupled with the dramatic reduction in staff, the decline in working conditions and the increased needs because of the crisis have made it significantly more difficult to organise a strategy to integrate mental health into primary healthcare; and (c) the innovative aspect of best practices need to be showcased and documented in cooperation with Greek and European networks.

Taking into account the new conditions which have shaped socioeconomic circumstances over recent years, the challenges and future goals for how mobile units can operate include:

Developing specialised measures for vulnerable population groups affected by the economic crisis, such as families with members suffering from serious physical or psychiatric conditions and who also face socioeconomic problems, unemployed support groups, etc.
Measures relating to the prevention and handling of mental health problems and the social problems of immigrants
Developing actions to evaluate special treatment interventions for special psychopathologies

Carrying out economic studies, cost-benefit analyses and efficiency analyses into the long-term operation of mobile units

Organising self-help groups for individuals suffering from depression and other mental disorders

Empowering patients and relatives to take steps to defend their rights and promote self-advocacy

Developing programmes aimed to assisted work for individuals with mental health problems

Liaising with European mental health service networks which offer mobile units in remote areas to provide theoretical and scientific documentation of best practices

Bibliography

Babor TF, De la Fuente JR, Saunders J, Grant M (1992) The alcohol use disorders identification test: guidelines for use in primary health care (WHO publication No. 92.4). World Health Organisation, Geneva

Barbato A (2008) Mental health care in primary care, Presentation at the Educational Workshop for Primary Health Care and Mental Health professionals. Paros, Greece

Blatt S, Luyten P (2009) Depression as an evolutionarily conserved mechanism to terminate separation distress: only part of the biopsychosocial story? Neuropsychoanalysis 11:52–61

Bonsack C (2008) Equipes de psychiatrie mobiles pour les trois âges de la vie: l'expérience lausannoise. Psychiatrie 171(33):1960–1969

Bower P (2002) Primary care mental health workers: models of working and evidence of effectiveness. Br J Gen Pract 52(484):926–933

Bower P, Gask L (2002) The changing nature of consultation-liaison in primary care: bridging the gap between research and practice. Gen Hosp Psychiatry 24(2):63–70

Bower P, Gilbody S (2005) Managing common mental health disorders in primary care: conceptual models and evidence base. BMJ Br Med J 330(7495):839

Bower P, Jerrim S, Gask L (2004) Primary care mental health workers: role expectations, conflict and ambiguity. Health Soc Care Community 12(4):336–345

Clarkin JF, Levy KN, Lenzenweger MF, Kernberg OF (2004) The personality disorders institute/borderline personality disorder research foundation randomised control trial for borderline personality disorder: rationale, methods, and patient characteristics. J Pers Disord 18(1): 52–72

Dambassina L, Stylianidis S, Sakellaropoulos P (1987) Réflexions sur l'expérience d'une Unité Mobile dans une région rurale en Grèce. In: Chanoit PF, De Verbizier J (eds) Recherches en Psychiatrie Sociale. Érès, Paris, pp 107–114

Derogatis LR, Savitz KL (2000) The SCL–90–R and Brief Symptom Inventory (BSI) in primary care. In: Maruish ME (ed) Handbook of psychological assessment in primary care settings. Lawrence Erlbaum Associates Publishers, Mahwah, pp 297–334

Diamanti A (2014) The progress of treating ... Clinical presentation at the mobile units training seminar. April 2014 (in Greek)

Donias S, Karastergiou A, Manos N (1991) Standardisation of the symptom checklist-90-R rating scale in a Greek population. Psychiatriki 2(1):42–48

Economou M, Madianos M, Theleritis C, Peppou L, Stefanis C (2011) Increased suicidality amid economic crisis in Greece. The Lancet 378:1459

Economou M, Madianos M, Peppou LE, Theleritis C, Stefanis CN (2012) Suicidality and the economic crisis in Greece. Lancet 380(9839):337

Fonagy P, Gergely G, Jurist EL, Target M (2002) Affect regulation, mentalisation and the development of the self. Other Press, New York

Gask L, Sibbald B, Creed F (1997) Evaluating models of working at the interface between mental health services and primary care. Br J Psychiatry 170(1):6–11

Giannakopoulos G, Tzavara C, Dimitrakaki C, Kolaitis G, Rotsika V, Tountas Y (2009) The factor structure of the Strengths and Difficulties Questionnaire (SDQ) in Greek adolescents. Ann Gen Psychiatry 8:20

Ginieri-Coccossis M, Triantafillou E, Tomaras V, Liappas IA, Christodoulou GN, Papadimitriou GN (2009) Quality of life in mentally ill, physically ill and healthy individuals: the validation of the Greek version of the World Health Organisation Quality of Life (WHOQOL-100) questionnaire. Ann Gen Psychiatry 8:23. doi:10.1186/1744-859X-8-23

Giotakos O, Karabelas D, Kafkas A (2011) Financial crisis and mental health in Greece. Psychiatriki 22:109–119

Goodman A, Goodman R (2009) Strengths and difficulties questionnaire as a dimensional measure of child mental health. J Am Acad Child Adolesc Psychiatry 48(4):400–403

Hatziandreou M (2012) Intergenerational trauma and ideology. Oedipus 8:371–380 (in Greek)

Hopper E (1996) The social unconscious in clinical work. Group 20(1):7–42

Ierodiakonou C (1982) The current turn towards social psychiatry. Greek Med 48:80–83 (in Greek)

Ierodiakonou C (1983) Mobile units in the context of the community mental health centre in rural areas. Medicine 44:225–232 (in Greek)

Ierodiakonou C, Iakovidis A, Bikos K (1983) Mobile mental health units associated with general hospitals in the countryside. Mater Med Greca 11:518–522

Jacob B (2014) La Réforme des soins en santé mentale en Belgique. Available at: http://www.psy107.be. Accessed 30 July 2014

Kapsomenos G (2008) Pierre Bourdieu's theory of practice. http://praxeologysocial.wordpress.com/2008/02/23/bourdieu-theory-of-practice/ (in Greek)

Kernberg OF, Yeomans FE, Clarkin JF, Levy KN (2008) Transference focused psychotherapy: overview and update. Int J Psychoanal 89:601–620

Kessing LV (2005) Diagnostic stability in bipolar disorder in clinical practice as according to ICD-10. J Affect Disord 85(3):293–299

Kienast T, Stoffers J, Bermpohl F, Lieb K (2014) Borderline personality disorder and comorbid addiction: epidemiology and treatment. Dtsch Arztebl Int 111(16):280

Leuzinger-Bohleber M, Stuhrast U, Rüger B, Beutel M (2003) How to study the 'Quality of Psychoanalytic Treatments' and their long-term effects on patients' well-being. Int J Psychoanal 84:263–290

Lewis G, Pelosi AJ (1990) Manual of the revised clinical interview schedule (CIS-R). Institute of Psychiatry, London

Lieb K, Zanarini MC, Schmal C, Linehan MM, Bohus M (2004) Borderline personality disorder. Lancet 364:453–461

Mavreas VG, Beis A, Mouyias A, Rigoni F, Lyketsos GC (1986) Prevalence of psychiatric disorders in Athens. Soc Psychiatry 21(4):172–181

Mechanic D (2001) The scientific foundations of community psychiatry. In: Thornicroft G, Szmukler G (eds) Textbook of community psychiatry. Oxford University Press, New York, pp 41–52

Ministry of Health & Social Solidarity (2010) Report evaluating the interventions to implement psychiatric reform for the period 2000–2009. Ministry of Health and Social Security, Athens, Available at: http://www.psychargos.gov.gr/Documents2/Ypostirixi%20Forewn/Ypostirixi%20 EPISTHMONIKH/Ex%20Post%20%CE%A0%CE%91%CE%A1%CE%91%CE%94%CE%9 F%CE%A4%CE%95%CE%9F%202%20Teliko.pdf. Accessed on 30 July 2014

Pantelidou S, Stylianidis S (2009) Best practice models in the field of mental health promotion: the experience of mobile mental health units in the NE and Western Cyclades run by the Regional Development & mental health Association. Nea Hygeia 68:2 (in Greek)

Pantelidou S, Tsiolka E, Stylianidis S (2008) Prevalence of mental disorders in migrant users of the services of mobile mental health units in the NE Cyclades, on Paros and Antiparos. Poster, 20th Panhellenic psychiatry conference, Hellenic Psychiatry Association. Hania, Crete (in Greek)

Pantelidou S et al (2010) Innovative actions, challenges and prospects for mobile mental health units in the NE Cyclades run by the Regional Development & Mental Health Association:

the example of Paros and Antiparos. In: Koulierakis G (ed) Clinical psychology and health psychology. Papazisis Press, Athens, pp 309–323 (in Greek)

Pantelidou S, Vakalopoulou A, Stylianidis S (2012) Development of special prevention programmes and how domestic violence cases were dealt with by mobile mental health units in the NE Cyclades run by the Regional Development and Mental Health Association. Proceedings of the 4th Panhellenic mobile mental health units conference. University of Ioannina, Ioannina (in Greek), pp 45–49

Peritogiannis V, Mavreas V (2014) Community mental health groups in Greece. The example of mobile mental health units. Greek Med Arch 31(1):71–76 (in Greek)

Rosenfeld H (1987) Impasse and interpretation. Tavistock, London

Ruggeri M, Dall'Agnola R (1993) The development and use of the Verona Expectations for Care Scale (VECS) and the Verona Service Satisfaction Scale (VSSS) for measuring expectations and satisfaction with community-based psychiatric services in patients, relatives and professionals. Psychol Med 23(02):511–523

Sakellaropoulos P (1984) Rural mobile psychiatric care unit in the prefecture of Fokida. Tetramina 27(1):1729–1856 (in Greek)

Sakellaropoulos P (2011) Social Psychiatry and Mental Health Association, Chronicles. Retrieved August 6, 2014, from http://www.ckpsegr/history.html (in Greek)

Sakellaropoulos P, Zikos N, Frangouli A, Papanikolaou P (1983) Organising mental health services in a rural area. Proceedings of the 10th Panhellenic neurological Psychiatry Conference, Thessaloniki, 1 (pp 399–405) (in Greek)

Sakellaropoulos P, Frangouli A, Dragona T, Zikos N (1987) Les experiences l'une unité psychiatrique mobile dans une region rurale. In: Chanoit PF, De Verbizier J (eds) Recherches en Psychiatrie Sociale. Érès, Paris, pp 179–194

Simon GE, Katon, WJ, VonKorff M, Unützer J, Lin EH, Walker EA, …, Ludman E (2001) Cost-effectiveness of a collaborative care program for primary care patients with persistent depression. Am J Psychiatry 158(10):1638–1644

Singleton N, Bumpstead R, O'Brien M, Lee A, Meltzer H (2003) Psychiatric morbidity among adults living in private households, 2000. Int Rev Psychiatry 15(1–2):65–73

Skapinakis P, Bellos S, Koupidis S, Grammatikopoulos I, Theodorakis PN, Mavreas V (2013) Prevalence and sociodemographic associations of common mental disorders in a nationally representative sample of the general population of Greece. BMC Psychiatry 13:163

Slade M, Thornicroft G, Glover G (1999) The feasibility of routine outcome measures in mental health. Soc Psychiatry Psychiatr Epidemiol 34(5):243–249

Stouraitou S, Stylianidis S, Pantelidou S, Stavroyannopoulos P, Chondros P, Drakonakis N, Dromboni F, Papasaika E (2009) Involuntary psychiatric hospitalisations in the Prefecture of the Cyclades: the situation and comments. Psychiatry Notes 107:66–79 (in Greek)

Stylianidis S (1989) Culture of models and techniques, intervention methods and experience of the community psychiatry in rural areas in Greece. Lectures Reports, Simposio Regional W.P.A., ASAM, Granada, pp 109–113

Stylianidis S, Pantelidou S (2006a). Implementing case management in psychosocial rehabilitation and social psychiatry. Psychiatriki 17(2):113–121 (in Greek)

Stylianidis S, Pantelidou S (2006b) Mobile mental health units in the Cyclades (Regional Development and Mental Health Association) as multipliers of public mental health actions. Psychiatry Notes 96:18–24 (in Greek)

Stylianidis S, Zisi A (2005) The importance of continuing training in psychiatry for primary healthcare professionals: the example of mobile mental health units in the NE and Western Cyclades. Protovathmia Frontida Hygeias 17(4):165–174 (in Greek)

Stylianidis S, Pantelidou S, Chondros P (2007) Des unités mobiles de santé mentale dans les Cyclades: le cas de Paros. Inf Psychiatr 83(8):682–688

Stylianidis S, Skapianakis P, Pantelidou S, Chondros P, Avgoustakis A, Ziakoulis M (2010) Prevalence of common mental disorders in an island area: needs assessment and action plan. Greek Med Arch 27(4):675–683 (in Greek)

Thomä H, Kächele H (1987) Psychoanalytic practice. Springer, Berlin

Thompson C, Kinmonth AL, Stevens L, Pevele RC, Stevens A, Ostler KJ, ..., Campbell MJ (2000) Effects of a clinical-practice guideline and practice-based education on detection and outcome of depression in primary care: Hampshire Depression Project randomised controlled trial. Lancet 355(9199):185–191

Thornicroft G, Tansella M (1999) Translating ethical principles into outcome measures for mental health service research. Psychol Med 29(04):761–767

Tylee A, Walters P (2006) Underrecognition of anxiety and mood disorders in primary care: why does the problem exist and what can be done? J Clin Psychiatry 68:27–30

Tzanoulinos G (2014) The progress of treating ... Clinical presentation at the mobile units training seminar. Apr 2014 (in Greek)

WHOQOL Group (1998) The World Health Organisation quality of life assessment (WHOQOL): development and general psychometric properties. Soc Sci Med 46(12):1569–1585

World Health Organisation (WHO) (2001). Mental health: new understanding, new hope. Geneva: WHO Press. Available at: http://www.who.int/entity/whr/2001/en/whr01_en.pdf?ua=1. Accessed 30 July 2014

World Health Organisation (WHO) (2009) Organisation of services. Mental health policy and service guidance package. WHO Press, Geneva

World Health Organisation (WHO) (2010). mhGAP intervention guide for mental, neurological and substance use disorders in non-specialised health settings: mental health Gap Action Programme (mhGAP). Available at: http://whqlibdoc.who.int/publications/2010/9789241548069_eng.pdf. Accessed 6 Aug 2014

World Health Organisation (WHO). World Organisation of Family Doctors (Wonca) (2008) Integrating mental health into primary care: a global perspective. WHO, Geneva

Community Child Psychiatry: The Example of Mobile Mental Health Units in the NE and Western Cyclades

11

Stella Pantelidou, Vicky Antonopoulou, Antonios Poulios, Jenny Soumaki, and Stelios Stylianidis

Abstract

This chapter outlines innovative measures in the field of community child psychiatry in Greece and abroad, with emphasis on the special features of interventions in geographically remote areas. It presents the work done by mobile mental health units in the NE and Western Cyclades in the child psychiatry sector. Reference is made to the clinical work and the differences noted in terms of new cases, initial requests, referrals and diagnoses over the 10 years the units have been in operation. In addition it presents measures taken to record needs, promote mental health among children and adolescents, and in terms of the prevention and management of abuse. The data and the measures taken are directly tied into the new conditions which have emerged in Greece as a result of the socio-economic crisis.

11.1 Introduction

Good mental health is essential to the development processes of children and adolescents. It ensures optimum psychological and social functionality (WHO 2005a) and plays an important role in the development of identity and healthy interpersonal

---

S. Pantelidou • V. Antonopoulou • JennySoumaki
Association for Regional Development and Mental Health (EPAPSY), Athens, Greece
e-mail: stpantelidou@hotmail.com; v_antonop@yahoo.gr; soumakijenny@gmail.com

A. Poulios
Clinical Psychologist, National and Kapodestrian University of Athens, Athens, Greece
e-mail: antpls@yahoo.gr

S. Stylianidis (✉)
Department of Psychology, Panteion University, Athens, Greece
e-mail: stylianidis.st@gmail.com

© Springer International Publishing Switzerland 2016
S. Stylianidis (ed.), *Social and Community Psychiatry: Towards a Critical, Patient-Oriented Approach*, DOI 10.1007/978-3-319-28616-7_11

relationships, bolsters learning ability and the ability to manage developmental or other challenges on the path towards adulthood.

Using international literature (WHO 2005b) we can document the reasons why it is necessary to develop and implement effective interventions for children and adolescents:

A large percentage of the psychopathology which manifests in an individual's adult life starts in the early development stages, during which it is feasible to prevent future psychopathology.

The value of early intervention in mental disorders is particularly important and reduces the likelihood of chronic mental disability.

Effective interventions to promote the mental health of children and adolescents reduce the burden of psychiatric disorders in the individual and his/her family, thereby reducing the cost of long-term care for the health system.

Available research data supports the view that the prevalence of mental disorders in children and adolescents is high internationally, at around 10–20 % (Kieling et al. 2011). Studies point out that in geographically isolated areas, in particular, the occurrence rates for mental disorders are clearly higher (Ellis and Philip 2010), mainly where there are other risk factors as well, such as low socioeconomic levels, parental psychopathology and the effect of stressors.

It is also a fact that only 10–22 % of all those suffering from child and adolescent mental disorders can be identified by primary healthcare, which shows the inadequate levels of human resources and know-how in public mental health and the particularly significant treatment gap (WHO 2005a; Saxena et al. 2007). In addition, only the minority of high-risk children are monitored by mental health experts (Belfer 2008; NIMH 2001; Brugman et al. 2001). However, mood (affective) and behavioural problems of children appear to be stable over time, affect their quality of life and tend to develop into psychiatric disorders in adult life especially when there is no suitable intervention (Costello et al. 2003).

In a previous chapter, we reported on psychiatric reform in Greece and the essential change in the model from the provision of psychiatric care in asylums to community psychiatric care. However, as the national action plan PSYCHARGOS III (2011–2020) has recorded, "psychiatric reform has made deinstitutionalisation of chronic adult patients and the abolition of psychiatric hospitals a priority, with the result that few mental health structures have been created for children and adolescents" and concludes in relation to the modern Greek situation that "existing structures do not under any circumstances constitute an adequate network, while large geographical regions of the country have no child psychiatric services at all".

One can therefore understand that in order to abolish institutional care for children and adolescents, it would be necessary to operate an effective network of child and adolescent mental health services which would ensure that comprehensive child psychiatric care is provided at all levels of care, in the context laid down by international conventions and declarations on the protection of the rights of children (MHSS 2012).

As Kolaitis and Tsiantis (2013) have noted, "the lack of an adequate number of specialised community structures and services for child psychiatric care in Greece, which are suitably staffed by well-trained child psychiatry experts in adequate numbers, is a major barrier to the protection of the rights of children". The rights of children and adolescents may be neglected or violated in various ways, from the prenatal stage (such as great poverty in the family, socioeconomic inequalities), at the time of birth (such as inadequate health services in remote areas), during infancy (such as inadequate mental healthcare for young mothers) and during childhood and adolescence. In this regard Anagnostopoulos and Soumaki (2012) have pointed out that the methods of violating rights may be clear-cut as in the case of abuse or less obvious in the context of family conflicts and divorces. These situations can have physical and psychological effects and frequently lead to poor educational adjustment, low performance and early dropout from school with clear, long-term repercussions in terms of economic cost. It can also lead to increased levels of unemployment and reduced social integration and participation (Kolaitis and Tsiantis 2013).

The development of services to care for the mental health of children requires specific organisational plans as a starting point, with the aim of recording needs and developing and disseminating services to cover geographically remote areas as well, and to ensure that they are accessible to all citizens. If this is not done, there is a risk of services being created in a piecemeal manner, offering ineffective, expensive or hard-to-access care (WHO 2005a).

This chapter will place particular emphasis on community-focused child psychiatry services and the special features of interventions in geographically remote areas by looking at how mobile mental health units operate.

11.2 Definitions

Child psychiatry refers to services provided to children and adolescents and their parents that relate to:

Child psychiatry services in the community/at the child's place of residence based on the principles of sectorisation
Recording the mental health needs of children and adolescents, to develop services tailored to the special needs of each community
Child psychiatric evaluation and development of a customised treatment plan in cooperation with other bodies in the community such as schools, health services and social services
Actions for mental health education and promotion for children in the community
Prevention of relapses in cases of severe child psychiatric disorders

These points reflect the principles in the UN Convention on the Rights of the Child and aim to promote emotional well-being and the right to multifaceted development on an emotional, social and cognitive level to promote his/her abilities to the greatest extent possible while taking into consideration "his/her interest" (WHO 2005b).

The framework within which mobile mental health units operate (which is the prime example of community-focused services) is a basic example of how child psychiatry services can be provided in the community. As a form of organising psychiatric care and treatment, mobile mental health units' key features are that they provide comprehensive, quality mental health services while interfacing with primary healthcare and cooperating with existing health, educational and social services. Another feature is that they require minimal infrastructure of their own and maximise existing infrastructure which either belongs to other health services or local government authority services or agencies. Under Law 2716/1999 (Government Gazette 691/A), mobile mental health units provide services:

(a) In mental health sectors whose geographical area and layout, residential diversity and social, economic and cultural conditions coupled with the nature of mental disorders make it difficult for residents of those areas to access mental health services
(b) In neighbouring mental health sectors when there are no adequate mental health services there

Mobile mental health units are aimed at children and adolescents and adults suffering from mental disorders and/or psychosocial problems or who are in groups at high risk of manifesting mental disease. They are also aimed at the healthy population, through the mental health prevention, education and promotion programmes they run. Mobile mental health units operate in line with the principles and philosophy of social psychiatry (Mechanic 2001; Tansella and Thornicroft 2001).

11.3 Historical Background

Innovative steps towards psychiatric reform first began to be taken in Greece in the 1960s. During the 1970s and 1980s, community services were set up, cut off from traditional academic psychiatry, and the prime player in this field was Professor T. Sakellaropoulos. The Institute of Social Psychiatry was set up first in Pagrati followed by the Social Psychiatry Association, the first mobile unit in the Prefecture of Fokida (in 1981) and various structures in Evros (Livaditis 1995). At the same time, other social psychiatry services were set up such as:

The Paediatric Psychology Department at the Agia Sofia Children's Hospital in Athens
The Community Mental Health Centre in Thessaloniki
The University Clinic of the Ioannina Medical School
The University Mobile Unit for the Thessaloniki Region
The Vyronas – Kessariani Community Mental Health Centre

These structures provided satisfactory public care within their area (at that time the psychiatric sector as an area of remit was considered to be an innovation) to only 8 % of the country's population, due to the failure to complete sectorisation of services, the real lack of a central plan for deploying services in the regions, the absence of sufficient structures and the lack of coordination and cooperation (Sakellaropoulos 1995).

Today, the continued implementation of psychiatric reform is at risk both because of the economic crisis and its effects (Anagnostopoulos and Soumaki 2012, 2013b) and because of the attitude of public bodies to issues relating to how mental health services are deployed and organised (see the chapter on psychiatric reform in Greece and the chapter on the economic crisis and mental health: key issues).

The aim of modern child psychiatry is that all mental health problems are dealt with by keeping the children and adolescents in the community, providing them with the entire range of specialised psychosocial care and rehabilitation services they need (Anagnostopoulos and Lazaratou 2005).

Even though the system of mental health services for children and adolescents developed in a positive manner, it continued to be inadequate and limited in terms of development compared to the modern needs of children and adolescents and their families, while services are mainly focused in large urban centres, with the result that 30 prefectures in Greece do not have any child psychiatry services at all, and therefore a large proportion of the Greek population has no child psychiatry services at all (Asimopoulos 2007).

11.4 Current Situation

The current socioeconomic and cultural crisis (from 2009 onwards) highlighted a series of chronic dysfunctions which have hindered – but above all divided and fragmented – the psyche of individual subjects and of Greek society overall. These chronic defects in the structure and organisation of the very state and government have resulted in inadequate institutional functions and have also highlighted a plethora of contradictory forms of behaviour at social and individual level.

The combination of these factors, which are associated with the crisis, such as unemployment, insecurity, the abolition of institutions, continuous defeated expectations, lack of boundaries, serious conflicts and lack of a harmonious family life, has led to a major increase in new cases and therefore for demand for child psychiatry services and to a qualitative change in the psychopathology being encountered in day-to-day clinical practice.

Constant cuts in general spending on health and welfare have led to a shrinking in the already inadequate child psychiatry services offered by the Greek NHS and the abolition or reduction in real childcare policies for vulnerable groups of children and adolescents.

11.5 Literature Review

In one European study which covered 36 countries, it was found that the number of community child psychiatry units and the number of children and families treated were lower in general terms than the corresponding services for adults (Levav et al. 2004) even though the majority of mental disorders have the age of 14 as their starting point (Kessler et al. 2005). In addition, only 7 % of countries worldwide have enacted a comprehensive plan for their child and adolescent mental health policy (Shatkin and Belfer 2004). As far as access to existing community child psychiatry services is concerned, a key barrier – in addition to the stigma over mental disorders – is geographical inequality in the spread of such services, with non-urban areas being at a clear disadvantage (WHO 2005b).

Based on this data, increasing emphasis is being placed on developing community-focused child psychiatry services in geographically remote areas, which is a need the Greek mobile mental health units were called upon to meet in large part. The philosophy behind the mobile mental health units derives from the principles of assertive cooperation between mental health experts in all available agencies operating in a community.

The relevant literature relating to the provision of child psychiatry services by mobile mental health units abroad is relatively limited. Mobile mental health units have been deployed in Switzerland targeted specifically at adolescents who are either in high-risk groups for the development of serious psychopathology or who refuse to continue treatment after hospitalisation or who find it difficult to access child psychiatry structures. Bonsack et al. (2008) described an intervention model based on Assertive Community Treatment. The model is based on setting up and implementing a customised, holistic intervention plan which involves the reporting child psychiatrist, mental health experts operating the relevant community and the school and the parents of each adolescent. An essential factor in each intervention is to develop a robust treatment alliance and cultivate a climate of trust with families and to gradually empower the socialisation of, and development of activities by, each adolescent. To achieve these goals, the treatment plan also includes specialist carers (nurses) who make daily home visits and provide real help in implementing the treatment plan. In addition, clinical meetings are held weekly, to help assess each intervention and redefine treatment targets. The results of interventions are considered to be satisfactory, when there is a clear improvement in the adolescent's level of functionality.

In the USA, the charity the Children's Health Fund provides funding for mobile medical units that focus on the child population in areas where such services do not exist. Fifty mobile units operate in 16 states in the USA to provide services to poor families and minorities (Brito et al. 2010). To effectively run the mobile units, they have adopted a holistic programme and integrative approach. Paediatricians, nurses and mental health experts cooperate to develop intervention protocols whose primary aim is to identify mental health problems and increase referrals to specialised treatment. The main principles of the holistic model they follow are (a) ensuring accessibility, (b) ensuring the continuity of the intervention, (c) liaising with other services, (d) getting families and schools involved in the treatment plan, (e) making it easy to travel to and carry out medical tests and children's hospitals and (f) tailoring the intervention based on the special cultural features of each area covered.

Similar mobile units have also been deployed in the USA so that they are ready at any time to travel to areas affected by natural disasters (Madrid et al. 2008). In the field of child and adolescent mental health in particular, a model is used which posits the coexistence of mental health experts and paediatricians to deal with problems arising from a natural disaster from different angles. The initial focus takes into account the basic needs, while, as the programme continues, emphasis is placed on training professionals in the community and teachers to identify any mental health problems in children and adolescents in good time, as they emerge.

Although the existing literature is limited, it is clear that the key aspects of how mobile mental health units operate are that they must reflect the principles of primary, secondary and tertiary prevention, bearing in mind well-documented practices in the field of modern child psychiatry.

Interventions by community child psychiatry services such as those provided by mobile units must necessarily include programmes to deal with negative, stereotypical views in the community about the mental disorders of children and adolescents, in order to enable specialised help to be sought in good time (Naylor et al. 2009).

In addition, a key part of community interventions by mental health services for children and adolescents is to develop a stable partnership with schools and teachers (Bailey 1999; Eskin 1995). Schools are one of the most important community structures where mental health promotion programmes have a definitive impact (a) on combating stigma and (b) on improving the emotional and social functionality of students and (c) on identifying children with mental health problems (Rowling 2002; Zins et al. 2004; Payton et al. 2008). Early interventions to address emotional and behavioural problems and to train teachers to integrate techniques to promote student skills lead to long-term benefits in the field of child and adolescent mental health (Tennant et al. 2007; Wells et al. 2001).

Another feature of community-focused mental health services for children and adolescents, such as mobile units, according to the international literature is that the intervention team must have a multidisciplinary line-up which will enable it to target its work on the entire family. Some researchers have argued that in order for a child psychiatric diagnosis to be submitted, it is essential to know about and examine the interaction each child has with his family (Carr 2000; Cicchetti and Tucker 1994). A successful outcome from each treatment approach ought to include parental involvement, and when this is achieved, the results of treatment are clearly better (Dowell and Ogles 2010; Karver et al. 2006).

Another key area of intervention for child psychiatry services in the community is training primary healthcare doctors to identify children and adolescents with mental health problems early on (Hagan et al. 2008). This is vital since primary healthcare doctors tend to under-diagnose mental health problems in children and adolescents (Hickie et al. 2007) and consequently limit the number of referrals to mental health experts (Warfield and Gulley 2006).

Best practices: the example of mobile mental health units in the NE and Western Cyclades operated by the Regional Development and Mental Health Association.

A key priority of the mobile mental health units in the NE and Western Cyclades during their 10 years in operation has been to develop special prevention and promotion measures for the mental health of children and adolescents in the community within their territorial remit and to implement special treatment measures for children and adolescents and their families.

The child psychiatry department of the mobile units employs child psychiatrists, clinical psychologists specialised in children and social workers. The services are provided fortnightly, primarily at premises provided by health centres on the islands, at specially designed spaces in town halls and at the headquarters of the units. In addition, there is a special Family Clinic on Paros for children and adolescents with mental health problems. Systematic supervision of child psychiatry cases is also provided.

In short the operating targets for mobile units when providing services relating to children and adolescents can be summarised as follows (Pantelidou and Stylianidis 2010; Stylianidis and Pantelidou 2006; Stylianidis et al. 2007):

(a) To assess and record mental health needs for this age group
(b) To provide child psychiatry evaluation, diagnosis and treatment services for mental disorders and the psychosocial problems of children and adolescents
(c) To prevent, educate and promote mental health for children and adolescents by implementing special programmes and training groups of professionals working with children and adolescents and parents and to identify mental health problems in good time and refer them to a specialised service
(d) To liaise with primary healthcare, social and educational bodies in the community and to more effectively record needs and provide comprehensive interventions
(e) To develop specialised measures to prevent and deal with child abuse and victimisation

The section below provides a brief overview of the activities of mobile units in relation to those goals.

Clinical Treatments

During the 10 years the mobile mental health units have been in operation, they served a total of 1339 children and adolescents in the NE Cyclades and 567 in the Western Cyclades, whose average age was 9.2 years old ($SD=4.1$, $min=1$ $max=2$). The key demographic characteristics of children and adolescents who attended the units are presented in Table 11.1.

Monitoring the change in new cases over time, as shown in Fig. 11.1, during the first years in operation, there is a gradual increase in new cases. There was then a drop in new cases which probably reflects changes from funding cuts (reduced numbers of staff). There was another drop in new cases attending the units in 2009 for the same reasons. This was followed by a gradual rise in requests, which is probably associated with the impacts of the socioeconomic crisis and also with the activities the mobile units had engaged in relating to prevention and awareness raising about the psychosocial health of adolescents and their families (due to the increased number of requests from the community for actions of this sort). It is also worth noting that the influx of new cases in the Western Cyclades had fewer fluctuations over time compared to the

Table 11.1 Demographic characteristics of children and adolescents who received services from the mobile mental health units in the NE and Western Cyclades in the first 10 years they were in operation (N=1906)

Demographic variables	f	%
Gender		
Boy	1121	58.8
Girl	785	41.2
Country of origin		
Greece	1728	90.7
Abroad	178	9.3
Prior contact with a mental health expert		
Yes	391	24.5
No	1199	75.3

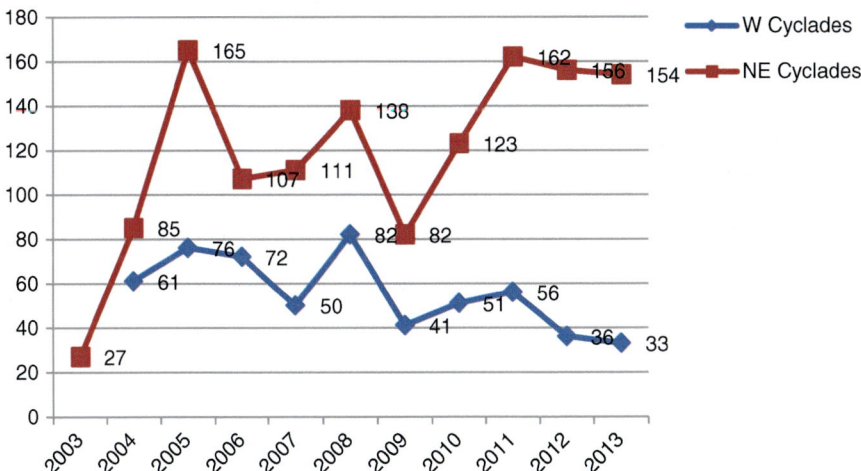

Fig. 11.1 Absolute frequencies of new cases of children/adolescents during the time the NE and Western Cyclades mobile units were in operation (N=1.339 and 567, respectively)

NE Cyclades, even though increases and reductions in new cases probably follow the same trend. This can be attributed to the fact that this area has a clearly smaller population and consequently the corresponding fluctuations are smaller.

As far as diagnoses are concerned, it appears that frequencies follow a similar trend for both mobile units. More specifically, as one might have expected, the most frequent diagnoses related to psychological development disorders, behavioural and emotional disorders normally diagnosed in childhood and adolescence and psychosocial problems, followed by mood (affective) disorders (see Fig. 11.2).

Monitoring the distribution of diagnoses over the time period the mobile units were in operation (chi-square statistical verification (24) = 132.7, $p<0.001$) (Fig. 11.3), one can see that in the last 4 years, the frequencies of psychopathologies of almost all types have increased. Exceptions are organic psychotic disorders, substance dependence and abuse and psychoses, possibly due to their low prevalence in the general child and adolescent population. As far as cases of developmental

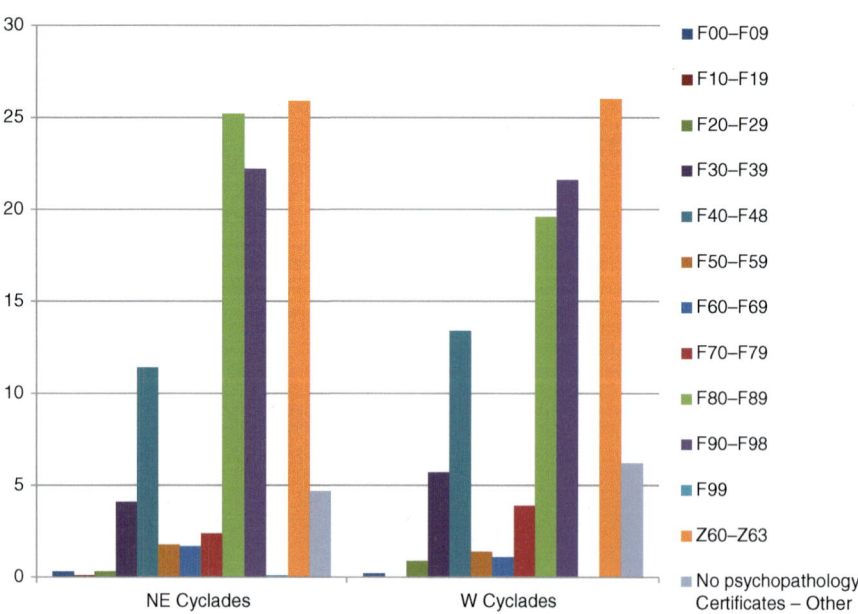

Fig. 11.2 Relative frequencies of diagnoses for children/adolescents who visited the NE and Western Cyclades mobile units during their first decade in operation ($N=1.339$ and 567, respectively)

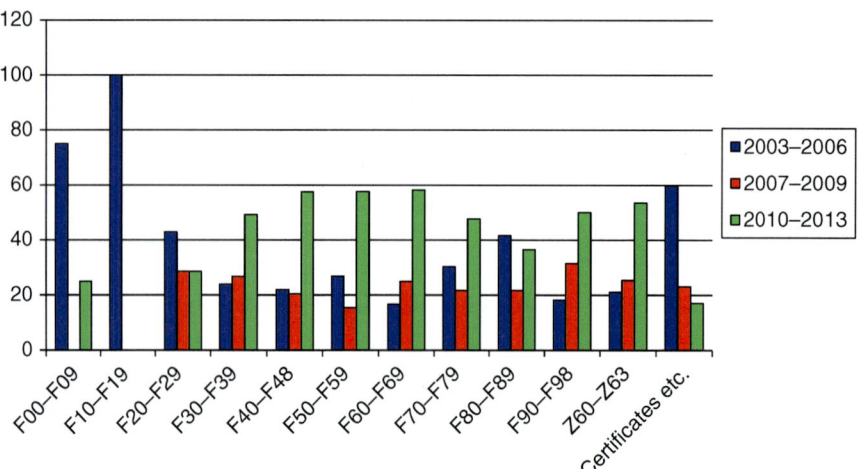

Fig. 11.3 Relative frequencies of diagnoses during the period the NE and Western Cyclades mobile units were in operation ($N=1906$)

disorders are concerned, one can see a drop in frequency and then a rise over the last 4 years, which could be attributed to the raised awareness of parents and teachers about such matters.

As Table 11.2 shows, the most frequent source of referrals was self-referral, which in the case of children and adolescents in effect means requests originating from their parents. The second most frequent source of referral was the school, which is the prime place outside the family where psychosocial difficulties become perceptible, which emphasises the need for close cooperation between community mental health structures and schools. The phenomenon of primary healthcare somehow being bypassed by mental health structures also appears in the case of children and adolescents since the frequency of referrals by this source (third in the rankings) could be characterised as rather lower than expected, which is perhaps indicative of the problems in the running of primary healthcare (reduced staff levels, lack of paediatricians on most islands within the area of remit, etc.).

By comparing the sources of referrals separately for the two mobile units, one can see that self-referrals were more frequent in the NE Cyclades than in the Western Cyclades, where the percentage of referrals from "other" sources is clearly higher, which may show another form of social networking in place in the Western Cyclades, in what are mostly more closed communities with a smaller population. The lower frequency of referrals from primary healthcare and private doctors in the Western Cyclades reflects the dearth of health professionals in those areas. The higher frequency of referrals from community bodies in the NE Cyclades may reflect the larger number of services on those islands.

Reviewing the sources of referral over time, which revealed a statistically significant change, $\chi^2 (14) = 83.7$, $p<0.001$ (see Fig. 11.4), shows that over time self-referrals increased and in fact that increase was higher over the last 4 years, i.e. since the socioeconomic crisis started. The crisis may have led a large portion of the population to seek out psychosocial help given the impacts it has had, and in the last 2 years in particular, the population has become more aware, thanks to mental health promotion programmes aimed at parents, adolescents and teachers. Those programmes also explain the increase in schools as a source of referrals. After 10 years of the mobile mental health units in operation, the number of self-referrals has increased significantly, which indicates an improvement in the level of basic trust between the multidisciplinary child psychiatry team and the population receiving services, the more pressing nature of requests due to the

Table 11.2 Relative frequencies of sources of referrals to mobile units in the NE and Western Cyclades in the first decade in operation ($N=1339$ and 567, respectively, 1906 in total)

Source of referrals	NE Cyclades (%)	Western Cyclades (%)	Total (%)
Self-referral	49.3	34.3	45.2
Primary healthcare	11.6	8.7	10.9
Private doctor	3.9	1.3	3.3
Community body	4.6	2.3	3.9
Public authorities	0.9	4.6	1.5
Church	0.2	0	0.1
Educational body	22.5	25	23.3
Other	6.9	23.7	11.8

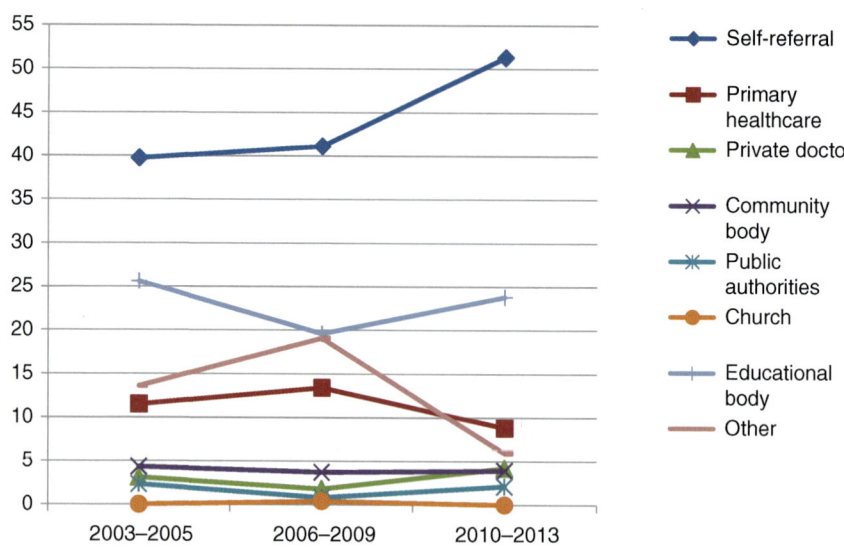

Fig. 11.4 Relative frequencies of sources of referral during the period the NE and Western Cyclades mobile units were in operation ($N=1906$)

Table 11.3 Relative frequencies of initial requests made to mobile units in the NE and Western Cyclades in the first decade in operation ($N=1339$ and 567, respectively, 1906 in total)

Initial request	NE Cyclades (%)	Western Cyclades (%)	Total (%)
Psychiatric symptoms	18.8	15	17.5
Learning problems	15.3	29.1	19.8
Behavioural problems	27.6	20.6	25.2
Substance dependence/abuse	0.2	0	0.1
Problems with family relations	16.4	14	15.6
Speech problems	5.8	6.2	5.9
Developmental disorders	1.9	1	1.6
Eating disorders	1.1	1.2	1.2
Mental retardation	0.4	0.8	0.5
Certificates, etc.	1	2.3	1.5
Social surveys	11.4	9.9	10.9
Medical report/certificate	0.1	0	0.1

socioeconomic crisis and the way the units operate in the networks within local communities.

As is clear from Table 11.3, initial requests made by individuals who contacted the mobile units most frequently related to psychiatric, learning and behavioural problems. That was followed by family problems and social studies, which is clear from the fact that over the last years mobile units undertook to carry out social studies on certain islands in cooperation with the public authorities on Syros. Comparing the two mobile units, one can see that a higher frequency of requests related to learning difficulties in the Western Cyclades, which is due to the fact that this mobile unit carried out interventions of this type in its first years in operation. However, over time those interventions were limited in number, thanks to a rise in other types of interventions, as is clear from a look at the types of requests over time. So it is clear that in the last 4 years, behavioural problems rose to a large degree as the type of requests made, as did psychiatric symptoms, since the initial requests differed in a statistically significant manner in the period under examination (chi-square statistical verification $(22) = 148.62$, $p<0.001$). These phenomena can clearly be associated with the impact on the socioeconomic crisis on the family.

Special Measures

A Family Clinic opened on a pilot basis on Paros in 2012, funded for the first year by the Stavros Niarchos Foundation. It offered family therapy from therapists specialised in the systemic approach. Families were referred here by the Child Psychiatry Department of the mobile unit and by other community bodies working with children and families.

The need to develop a specialist family therapy programme on islands like Paros and Antiparos emerged, thanks to increased needs for interventions on multiple levels for individuals and families, the constantly increasing number of requests related to the economic crisis and the well-known effectiveness of family therapy in dealing with child and adolescent mental disorders (Campbell et al. 2003; Carr 2000; Tomaras and Pomini 2007). At the same time, family therapy seeks to improve the quality of life of the family and support all its members (not just the child/adolescent who has presented some symptoms).

During the first year, 60 sessions were held with families and the intervention was evaluated. The intervention's specific goals were (a) to reduce the psychopathology of children, (b) to reduce parental stress, (c) to improve family functioning and (d) to improve the family's quality of life.

To evaluate the intervention, the following scales were presented to six families which took part on the pilot operation of the family clinic (the scales were administered at the start and end of the intervention):

(a) Parental Stress Questionnaire (Berry and Jones 1995) to assess parental stress
(b) Family Assessment Device (FAD) (Epstein et al. 1983) to assess family functionality
(c) WHOQOL Bref (WHOQOL Group 1998; Ginieri-Coccossis et al. 2009) to assess the quality of family life
(d) Strengths and Difficulties Questionnaires (Goodman and Goodman 2009; Giannakopoulos et al. 2009)

A total of 9–11 sessions were held with each family. The initial results show that there was an improvement in the level of family functionality, and the symptoms of emotional disorders and behavioural problems that children and adolescents initially presented declined, and their clinical picture overall improved. Parental stress decreased by the end of the intervention, but it appears that there was not a major change in the quality of the family's lives. The evaluation process is under way at present since the Family Clinic is still in pilot mode.

The Role of Supervision

A child psychiatry team working in the community needs to follow specific principles and practices, such as providing services with the maximum therapeutic benefit in the shortest time period and the least possible cost and ensuring the continuity of care, availability and the type of treatment approach which the individual or family is entitled to have.

Another important issue is to ensure accessibility since the layout of the service must allow for easy access both for users of the service and therapists.

However, the most difficult subject is the principle of dialectical interaction, which relates to ongoing interaction between the mental health expert and each community, since he needs to understand cultural values and habits, applied health policies and the economic and ideological viewpoints they serve, in order to be able to assess real needs and prepare the corresponding programmes (Madianos 1994).

The child psychiatry team meets the child and the institutions and is required to synthesise all the relevant types of thinking (medical and therapeutic, psychological, pedagogical and institutional) which do not all operate according to the same rules, and do not all have the same influence, even though they intersect and are interwoven.

The importance of supervision, i.e. of continuous analysis of the team's actions, is vital so that everyone is aware of the difficulties arising from working in the community, in order to reveal the conscious and unconscious barriers and the synthesis going on. It is a process which seeks to promote the mutual exchange of information and views and the sharing and collective processing of day-to-day treatment practice and experience.

In this special setting, the supervisor will need to bear in mind the real conditions of the *setting* and balance them out, as well as the needs of the therapists being supervised, group and community dynamics which give rise to mass projections and multiple transferences.

Frequently, in difficult situations where the case is severe or the bodies involved face specific difficulties, it is easy for the institution to be considered as the only, undisputed objective value and for members to adopt "easy" solutions such as the suggestion of hospitalisation without adequate interaction with the child/adolescent's support network, or a shift in treatment responsibility to another specialised service in an urban centre, or for there to be divided opinions between therapists about the type of treatment or competition between institutions.

It is clear from this how essential supervision is as a complex process of learning and education, which can provide greater awareness of the counter-transference emotions of the therapists, as a meeting, as a body of experience and as a "space" for analysing and bringing together the child's and family's narrative in the social setting they belong to.

Assessment and Recording of Needs

It is important for the plan to deploy mental health services to be based (a) on epidemiological data about the prevalence of mental health problems that children and adolescents face and (b) on the assumption that each problem must be explored by taking into account the cultural, geographical, social and family environment of the child (Grimes 2004).

The methodology employed over the 10-year period the mobile units have been in operation to assess and record needs includes the following:

Focus groups with teachers within schools. These groups discuss issues relating to child and adolescent behavioural problems as seen at school, cases of school violence and cases of possible neglect – abuse – and record teachers' requests to mobile units for support to manage such problems. After the groups are finished, needs and requests formulated by teachers are officially recorded.

Meetings with other professionals working with children in the community: paediatricians, speech therapists, occupational therapists and social workers (at health centres or social services) during which an empirical picture of needs in terms of mental health problems and the social problems faced by children and adolescents is obtained.

Systematic analysis of data relating to the reason why children and adolescents and parents have come to the units and the psychosocial profile of people receiving services from the mobile units.

Needs are recorded for this age group, especially via research activities which have been carried out over recent years in the context of how the mobile units operate. For example, on Paros a study was carried out to assess the prevalence of common mental disorders on 323 adolescents at the island's two high schools (among 16–18 year olds). The study was carried out in 2007 in cooperation with the Psychiatry Department of the University of Ioannina Medical School and is part of a wider epidemiological study on a sample of 5614 adolescents from schools in Epirus, Etolo-Akarnania and Attica (Skapinakis et al. 2011; Magklara et al. 2010, 2012). For Paros in particular, the key finding was that the prevalence of depression among adolescents who participated in the study was 12.7 % (the figure was almost twice as high in girls as in boys ($OR = 7.12$, $CI = 3.42$–14.82). The highest percentage was noted in students in the final year of high school and in students whose performance was average ($OR = 4.31$, 95 % $CI = 0.97$–19.13). A high positive correlation existed between reported victimisation in cases of school violence and the onset of depression ($OR = 3.47$, 95 % $CI = 1.04$–11.63). The use of cannabis also positively correlated with depression ($OR = 4.23$, 95 % $CI = 1.29$–13.89).

The general results of the nationwide study found that 32 % of adolescents have symptoms of psychological stress (42 % of girls and 20 of boys, $p < 0.01$) and there was a statistically significant correlation between mental health and the subjective assessment of the family's economic difficulties (Magklara et al. 2010). It was also found that the likelihood of the onset of suicidal ideation was higher for adolescents who reported that they were victims of school violence especially when it happened weekly and that finding is independent of the existence of any psychiatric symptoms (OR = 7.78, 95 % CI = 3.05–19.90).

Mental Health Prevention and Promotion Actions in Cooperation with Community Bodies

As part of their operations, the mobile units place particular emphasis on developing mental health prevention and promotion measures in the community (Pantelidou and Stylianidis 2009). Just some of these are listed below:

- In the period 2011–2013, a special 2-year programme was implemented to promote the mental health of children and adolescents funded by the Stavros Niarchos Foundation. During the programme groups were run for parents, teachers at all levels and adolescents on the Cyclades (within the remit of the mobile mental health units operated by the Regional Development and Mental Health Association). More than 900 people took part in the programme over the 2 years.
- The aim of the monthly parent groups was to brief them about child and adolescent mental health problems, improve communication and parent-child relations, support them in their parental role, identify child and adolescent mental disorders in good time and refer them to specialised services.
- Likewise, teacher groups were also held monthly, and they were able to learn about child and adolescent mental health issues so that they could recognise behavioural problems and emotional difficulties in good time. Particular emphasis was placed on communication between the school and family, on supporting them in organising actions to promote child and adolescent mental health at school and on prevention measures and measures to address school bullying. During the 2 years of the intervention, supervision groups for teachers were also in operation.
- Support groups for adolescents were also run twice a month as well as a theatrical play workshop to promote mental health.
- All special measures at schools included frequent meetings with teachers in order to ensure cooperation in supporting children with mental health problems and in dealing with cases of school bullying. In addition, special measures were taken to address the stigma of mental illness at school and workshops held to prevent school bullying for primary school pupils. Other special measures included organising workshops for teachers in cooperation with the Theseus Centre for the Prevention of Use of Addictive Substances in the Cyclades and the Prefecture of the Cyclades Health Prevention and Promotion Network based of Syros. The workshops held over the last 2 years were focused on prevention and dealing with problems of behaviour in the classroom and on prevention and managing cases of child abuse and victimisation.

In cooperation with health centres on the islands, training courses were held for paediatricians, GPs and rural doctors, to enable them to identify child psychiatric disorders in good time and refer them.

A total of ten workshops are held a year on the islands covered by the mobile units featuring theoretical presentations and experiential seminars to brief parents and teachers about child and adolescent mental health issues.

All these measures were implemented in cooperation with community bodies, especially schools, health providers and social services, with the support of local government and the Southern Aegean Region.

Preventing and Dealing with Child Abuse

Over recent years, because of the increase in requests for intervention in cases of child abuse and neglect, particular emphasis has been given to the development of measures to prevent and address those cases. In the 3-year period 2010–2013 in particular, experts at the mental health units dealt with 40 cases of child abuse. In cooperation with the Public Prosecutor and the competent community bodies in Syros and in Athens, social studies were carried out by social workers from the mobile units, and specialised intervention plans were drawn up to support the children and their families. Special educational seminars were organised to raise awareness among the police, so that they could suitably handle such cases, and special workshops have been held for teachers and doctors to brief them about how to identify such cases, how to suitably intervene and about the statutory framework. Cooperation with schools and community bodies was also important in developing the treatment plan. Working groups have also been set up with all local bodies on the islands (health services, social services, public authorities, educational bodies) in cooperation with the Ombudsman and Children's Ombudsman, to provide better liaisons with bodies so as to more effectively manage cases of child abuse and neglect.

11.6 Conclusions: Challenges and Prospects

In light of these points, it is essential to adapt how the community child psychiatry services provided by mobile mental health units are run in geographically remote areas to the new social and economic circumstances and the emerging needs in each community.

The challenge when faced with a lack of resources and the lack of consistency in institutional terms from the Greek state is to bolster the inventiveness of the multidisciplinary team in its dealings with local networks to implement innovative initiatives to deal with the complexity of requests for treatment and with societal demands.

In terms of secondary prevention, the importance of timely intervention in populations at high risk of developing mental disorders is well documented. Studies show that children with parents with severe mental disorders are vulnerable to the development of emotional, behavioural, social and learning difficulties due to the simultaneous impact of genetic, environmental and psychosocial factors (Royal College of Psychiatrists 2010). Consequently, it is important to develop interventions targeted at parents with such problems and their children.

To that end, emphasis needs to be placed on interventions aimed at vulnerable population groups which are more affected by the economic crisis, who also have difficulty in accessing services: families with severe economic problems and unemployed parents, families of migrants, children who have been abused, children of parents with severe health problems and single-parent families (Tsiantis and Asimopoulos 2009; Reiss 2013). Specialised programmes relating to these population groups are expected to be launched soon on Andros as part of the operations of the NE Cyclades mobile mental health units, funded by the Moraitis Foundation. These programmes will include prevention actions and interventions at family and individual level (by setting up a Family Clinic).

Over recent years, research has also focused on identifying the qualitative criteria that ought to govern how community-oriented child psychiatry services operate (Bickman 2008; Warren et al. 2010). One key issue in increasing the quality of care provided is to ensure the commitment of children and families to treatment, since studies stress that a percentage of around 40–60 % terminate treatment at community services early (high dropout) (Gopalan et al. 2010). To that end it is vital to train mental health professionals on evidence-based treatment choices and to integrate research methods to evaluate the services provided (Glisson et al. 2010).

Finally, it is necessary to extend mental health promotion measures for children and adolescents, via special programmes aimed at the general population and vulnerable groups, which could be implemented in cooperation with educational bodies and community health providers (Hoagwood et al. 2001; Hooven et al. 2011) and in cooperation with bodies from abroad which have implemented and evaluated similar actions already.

Bibliography

Anagnostopoulos D, Lazaratou E (eds) (2005) Introduction to social child psychiatry. Psychiatric Clinic, Medical School, National and Capodistrian University of Athens, Athens (in Greek)

Anagnostopoulos D, Soumaki E (2012) The impact of the socio-economic crisis on the mental health of children and adolescents. Psychiatriki 23(1):13–16 (in Greek)

Anagnostopoulos D, Soumaki E (2013a) The state of child and adolescent psychiatry in Greece during the international financial crisis: a brief report. Eur Child Adolesc Psychiatry 22(2):131–134

Anagnostopoulos D, Soumaki E (2013b) The mental health condition of children and adolescents in Greece in the time of crisis. Synapsis J 9(29):11–16 (in Greek)

Asimopoulos Ch (2007) Psychosocial rehabilitation of children and adolescents with mental health problems in Greece. Necessity, current situation, prospects. In: Issues in psychodynamic and psychosocial child psychiatry. Kastaniotis Press, Athens, pp 323–341, (in Greek)

Bailey S (1999) Young people, mental illness and stigmatisation. Psychiatr Bull 23:107–110

Belfer ML (2008) Child and adolescent mental disorders: the magnitude of the problem across the globe. J Child Psychol Psychiatry 49(3):226–236

Berry JO, Jones WH (1995) The parental stress scale: initial psychometric evidence. J Soc Pers Relatsh 12:463–472. doi:10.1177/0265407595123009

Bickman L (2008) A measurement feedback system (MFS) is necessary to improve mental health outcomes. J Am Acad Child Adolesc Psychiatry 47(10):1114–1119

Bonsack C, Holzer L, Stancu I, Baier V, Samitca M, Charbon Y, Kock N (2008) Equipes de psychiatrie mobiles pour les trois âges de la vie: l'expérience lausannoise. Rev Med Suisse 4:1960–1969

Brito A, Khaw AJ, Campa G, Cuadra A, Joseph S, Rigual-Lynch L, Olteanu A, Shapiro A, Grant R (2010) Bridging mental health and medical care in underserved paediatric populations: three integrative models. Adv Pediatr 57(1):295–313

Brugman E, Reijneveld SA, Verhulst FC, Verloove-Vanhorick SP (2001) Identification and management of psychosocial problems by preventive child health care. Arch Pediatr Adolesc Med 155:462–469

Campbell D, Bianco V, Dowling E, Goldberg H, McNab S, Pentecost D (2003) Family therapy for childhood depression: researching significant moments. J Fam Ther 25:417–435. doi:10.1111/1467-6427.00259

Carr A (2000) Evidence-based practice in family therapy and systemic consultation. J Fam Ther 22:29–60

Cicchetti D, Tucker D (1994) Development and self-regulatory structures of the mind. Dev Psychopathol 6:533–549

Costello EJ, Mustillo S, Erkanli A, Keeler G, Angold A (2003) Prevalence and development of psychiatric disorders in childhood and adolescence. Arch Gen Psychiatry 60:837–844

Dowell K, Ogles B (2010) The effects of parent participation on child psychotherapy outcome: a meta-analytic review. J Clin ChildAdolesc Psychol 39(2):151–162

Ellis IK, Philip T (2010) Improving the skills of rural and remote generalists to manage mental health emergencies. Rural Remote Health 10(3):503–1508

Epstein N, Baldwin L, Bishop D (1983) The McMaster family assessment device. J Marital Fam Ther 9:171–180

Eskin M (1995) Suicidal behaviour as related to social support and assertiveness among Swedish and Turkish high school students: a cross-cultural investigation. J Clin Psychol 51:158–172

Giannakopoulos G, Tzavara C, Dimitrakaki C, Kolaitis G, Rotsika V, Tountas Y (2009) The factor structure of the Strengths and Difficulties Questionnaire (SDQ) in Greek adolescents. Ann Gen Psychiatry 8:20

Ginieri-Coccossis M, Triantafillou E, Tomaras V, Liappas IA, Christodoulou GN, Papadimitriou GN (2009) Quality of life in mentally ill, physically ill and healthy individuals: the validation of the Greek version of the World Health Organisation Quality of Life (WHOQOL-100) questionnaire. Ann Gen Psychiatry 8:23

Glisson C, Schoenwald S, Hemmelgarn A, Green P, Dukes D, Armstrong KS et al (2010) Randomised trial of MST and ARC in a two-level evidence-based treatment implementation strategy. J Consult Clin Psychol 78:537–550

Goodman A, Goodman R (2009) Strengths and difficulties questionnaire as a dimensional measure of child mental health. J Am Acad Child Adolesc Psychiatry 48(4):400–403

Gopalan G, Goldstein L, Klingenstein K, Sicher C, Blake C, McKay M (2010) Engaging families into child mental health treatment: updates and special considerations. J Can Acad Child Adolesc Psychiatry 19:182–196

Grimes K (2004) Systems of care in North America. In: Remschmidt H, Belfer ML, Goodyer I (eds) Facilitating pathways: care, treatment and prevention in child and adolescent mental health. Springer, Berlin, pp 35–41

Hagan J, Shaw J, Duncan P (eds) (2008) Bright futures: guidelines for health supervision of infants, children, and adolescents. American Academy of Pediatrics, Elk Grove Village

Hickie IB, Fogarty AS, Davenport TA, Luscombe GM, Burns J (2007) Responding to experiences of young people with common mental health problems attending Australian general practice. Med J Aust 187(7):S47–S52

Hoagwood K, Burns BJ, Kiser L, Ringeisen H, Schoenwald SK (2001) Evidence-based practice in child and adolescent mental health services. Psychiatr Serv 52(9):1179–1189

Hooven C, Walsh E, Willgerodt M, Salazar A (2011) Increasing participation in prevention research: strategies for youth, parents and schools. J Child Adolesc Psychiatr Nurs 24(3): 137–149

Karver M, Handelsman J, Fields S, Bickman L (2006) Meta-analysis of therapeutic relationship variables in youth and family therapy: the evidence for different relationship variables in the child and adolescent treatment outcome literature. Clin Psychol Rev 26:50–65

Kessler RC, Berglund P, Demler O, Jin R, Merikangas KR, Walters EE (2005) Lifetime prevalence and age-of-onset distributions of DSM-IV disorders in the National Co-morbidity Survey Replication. Arch Gen Psychiatry 62(6):593–602

Kieling C, Baker-Henningham H, Belfer M, Conti G, Ertem I, Omigbodun O, Rohde LA, Srinath S, Ulkuer N, Rahman A (2011) Child and adolescent mental health worldwide: evidence for Action. Lancet 378:1515–1525

Kolaitis G, Tsiantis I (2013) Mental health of children and adolescents: issues of rights, ethics and deontology. Synapsis J 27(8):38–41 (in Greek)

Levav I, Jacobsson L, Tsiantis J, Kolaitis J, Ponizovsky A (2004) Psychiatric services for children and adolescents in Europe: results of a country survey. Eur Child Adolesc Psychiatry 13(6):395–401

Livaditis M (1995) Psychiatric service structures in Thrace and how they operate. In: Lemperière T, Féline A (eds) Adult psychiatry manual. Papazissis Press, Athens, pp 321–323, in Greek

Madianos M (1994) Psychiatric reform and its development. Ellinika Grammata Press, Athens (in Greek)

Madrid P, Sinclair H, Bankston A, Overholt S, Brito A, Domnitz R, Grant R (2008) Building integrated mental health and medical programs for vulnerable populations post-disaster: connecting children and families to a medical home. Prehosp Disaster Med 23(4):314–321

Magklara K, Skapinakis P, Niakas D, Bellos S, Zissi A, Stylianidis S, Mavreas V (2010) Socioeconomic inequalities in general and psychological health among adolescents: a cross-sectional study in senior high schools in Greece. Int J Equity Health 9:3

Magklara K, Skapinakis P, Gkatsa T, Bellos S, Araya R, Stylianidis S (2012) Bullying behaviour in schools, socioeconomic position and psychiatric morbidity: a cross-sectional study in late adolescents in Greece. Child Adolesc Psychiatry Ment Health 6:8

Mechanic D (2001) The scientific foundations of community psychiatry. In: Thornicroft G, Szmukler G (eds) Textbook of community psychiatry. Oxford University Press, New York, pp 41–52

Ministry of Health & Social Solidarity (2012) Report of the working group to revise the PSYCHARGOS Programme – PSYCHARGOS III National Action Plan (2011–2020). Ministry of Health and Social Security, Athens, Available at: http://www.psychargos.gov.gr/Documents2/%CE%9D%CE%95%CE%91/%CE%A8%CE%A5%CE%A7%CE%91%CE%A1%CE%93%CE%A9%CE%A3%20%CE%93'%20(2011-2020).pdf. Accessed on 31.7.2014

Naylor PB, Cowie HA, Walters SJ, Talamelli L, Dawkins J (2009) Impact of a mental health teaching programme on adolescents. Br J Psychiatry 194(4):365–370

NIMH (2001) The National Advisory Mental Health Council Workgroup on child and adolescent mental health intervention development and deployment, Blueprint for Change: Research in Child and Adolescent Mental Health. NIMH, Washington

Pantelidou S, Stylianidis S (2009) Best practice models in the field of mental health promotion: the experience of mobile mental health units in the NE and Western Cyclades run by the Regional Development and Mental Health Association. Nea Hygeia 68:2 (in Greek)

Pantelidou S, Stylianidis S (2010) Innovative actions, challenges and prospects for mobile mental health units in the NE Cyclades run by the Regional Development and Mental Health Association: the example of Paros and Antiparos. In: Koulierakis G et al (eds) Clinical psychology and health psychology. Papazisis Press, Athens, pp 309–323, in Greek

Payton J, Weissberg RP, Durlak JA, Dymnicki AB, Taylor RD, Schellinger KB, Pachan M (2008) The positive impact of social and emotional learning for kindergarten to eight-grade students: findings from three scientific reviews. Collaborative for Academic, Social, and Emotional Learning, Chicago

Reiss F (2013) Socioeconomic inequalities and mental health problems in children and adolescents: a systematic review. Soc Sci Med 90:24–31

Rowling L (2002) Mental health promotion. In: Rowling L (ed) Mental health promotion and young people: concepts and practice. McGraw-Hill, Australia, pp 10–23

Royal College of Psychiatrists (2010) CR164 parents as patients: supporting the needs of patients who are parents and their children. URL: www.rcpsych.ac.uk/publications/collegereports/cr/cr164.aspx

Sakellaropoulos P (ed) (1995) Adult psychiatry manual. Aspects of social psychiatry and their application to Greece. Papazisis Press, Athens (in Greek)

Saxena S, Thornicroft G, Knapp M, Whiteford H (2007) Resources for mental health: scarcity, inequity, and inefficiency. Lancet 370(9590):878–889

Shatkin J, Belfer M (2004) The global absence of child and adolescent mental health policy. Child Adolesc Mental Health 9(3):104–108

Skapinakis P, Bellos S, Gkatsa T, Magklara K, Lewis G, Araya R, Stylianidis S, Mavreas V (2011) The association between bullying and early stages of suicidal ideation in late adolescents in Greece. BMC Psychiatry 11:22

Stylianidis S, Pantelidou S (2006) Mobile mental health units in the Cyclades (Regional Development and Mental Health Association) as multipliers of public mental health actions. Psychiatry Notes 96:18–24 (in Greek)

Stylianidis S, Pantelidou S, Chondros P (2007) Des unités mobiles de santé mentale dans les Cyclades: le cas de Paros. L' Information psychiatrique 83:682–688

Tansella M, Thornicroft G (2001) Mental health outcome measures. Gaskell, London

Tennant R, Goens C, Barlow J, Day C, Stewart-Brown S (2007) A systematic review of reviews of interventions to promote mental health and prevent mental health problems in children and young people. J Publ Ment Health 6(1):25–32

Tomaras V, Pomini V (2007) Family therapy for the problems of adolescence. In: Issues in psychodynamic and psychosocial child psychiatry. Kastaniotis Press, Athens (in Greek), pp 623–635

Tsiantis I, Asimopoulos C (2009) Mental health of children and adolescents: the need for development and not backtracking (regression). In: Sakellis G (ed) Psychiatric reform in Greece: needs – proposals – solutions. Sakkoulas Press, Athens, pp 86–97 (in Greek)

Warfield M, Gulley S (2006) Unmet need and problems accessing specialty medical and related services among children with special health care needs. Matern Child Health J 10(2):201–216

Warren J, Nelson P, Mondragon S, Baldwin S, Burlingame G (2010) Youth psychotherapy change trajectories and outcomes in usual care: community mental health versus managed care settings. J Consult Clin Psychol 78:144–155

Wells J, Barlow J, Stewart-Brown S (2001) A systematic review of universal approaches to mental health promotion in schools. Health Service Research Unit, Oxford

WHOQOL Group (1998) The World Health Organisation quality of life assessment (WHOQOL): development and general psychometric properties. Soc Sci Med 46(12):1569–1585

World Health Organisation (WHO) (2005a) Child and adolescent mental health policies and plans. WHO Press, Geneva, Available at: http://www.who.int/mental_health/policy/services/9_child%20ado_WEB_07.pdf, accessed: 31.7.2014

World Health Organisation (WHO) (2005b) Atlas: child and adolescent mental health resources: global concerns, implications for the future. WHO, Geneva

Zins J, Weissberg R, Wang M, Walberg H (2004) Building academic success on social and emotional learning: what does the research say? Columbia University, Teachers College Press, New York

A Modern-Day Community Daycare Centre in Operation

12

Stelios Stylianidis and Dimitris Trivellas

> **Abstract**
> This chapter presents the complexity of definitions for and operations of a day hospital and a daycare centre, their historical development within social psychiatry and the main features of a well-designed framework for running and operating such structures. Those features include a multidisciplinary team and the use of mental institution, case management, psychotherapy interventions, psychosocial rehabilitation and recovery programmes as well as the essential networking of services offered. A detailed presentation of the Franco Basaglia Daycare Centre run by the Rural Development and Mental Health Association in the Northern Suburbs of Athens highlights the need for a change in the biomedical paradigm, as well as the clinical, institutional and theoretical prerequisites for avoiding the phenomena of chronicity and neo-institutionalisation in the community.

12.1 Introduction

For many years, the well-established thinking in the mental health sector was that serious mental illnesses unavoidably worsen and become chronic. The practice which was based on that perception was that professionals focused on only managing the psychopathology and the symptoms. Over time a wider perspective focused its interest on a new approach which singled out the effectiveness of outcomes and

---

D. Trivellas (✉)
Psychiatrist, Day Centre EPAPSY Scientific Assistant, 1st Department of Psychiatry, Eginition Hospital, University of Athens, Athens, Greece
e-mail: dtrivellas@gmail.com

S. Stylianidis
Department of Psychology, Panteion University, Athens, Greece
e-mail: stylianidis.st@gmail.com

patient care, in addition to the clinical side of things. Functionality in assuming social roles, in relationships, in work and in leisure, in quality of life and in family burden all became areas of major interest (Rössler 2006; Lieberman et al. 2008).

Empirical data and narratives direct from the mouths of patients now support the idea that recovery is possible (Farkas et al. 2007; Anthony 2000; Deegan 1988). The recovery model includes elements of acceptance of the illness, hope for the future and the search for renewable self-meaning and a different identity. Recovery cannot be understood as a static process or end result, nor is it the same as treatment; instead it is a life process which involves successive steps at different stages of life. Viewed from this perspective, it can be seen more as an attitude towards life or lifestyle, as a feeling, a vision or an experience. In recovery-oriented services, people are supported as they develop and implement their own personal recovery plans, are encouraged in their personal preferences and are allowed to move ahead while accepting uncertainty and potential risks (Stylianidis et al. 2013).

According to the WARP Declaration, psychosocial rehabilitation methods include ways of organising services to maximise the continuity of care, treatment and integrated interventions that foster the abilities of individuals and ameliorate the excessive pressure they are under, so that it is possible to avoid relapses and to promote optimum economic and social involvement. It is a joint effort between professionals and service users aimed at transforming the social roles of service users. Psychosocial recovery seeks to reduce stigmatism and disability, promotes equal opportunities and aims to help individuals fully enjoy their rights (WHO 1996).

Continuing day treatment (CDT) programmes focus on community stabilisation through comprehensive individualised rehabilitation and provide a unique level of care. CDT programs promote recovery through a variety of practical clinical therapeutic interventions. They are designed to "maintain or enhance current levels of functioning and skills, to maintain community living, and develop self awareness and self esteem through the exploration and development of strengths and interests" (Handa et al. 2009).

The aim of psychosocial rehabilitation at a daycare centre is to help individuals with persistent, serious mental disorders develop the emotional, social and cognitive skills they need to live, learn and work in the community with the least possible support from professionals. Without denying the existence and effect of the mental illness, psychosocial rehabilitation changes the way in which the illness is approached (Rössler 2006).

Although the majority of individuals in psychosocial rehabilitation programmes have been diagnosed with schizophrenic disorder, other groups of patients with psychotic and nonpsychotic disorders also make up the population rehabilitation is aimed at. According to a 2009 study in the USA, serious mental illness relates to 4.8 % of the adult population, while in the age group 18–25, it relates to 7.3 % of the population and rises to 9.1 % in adults living in poverty (Substance Abuse and Mental Health Services Administration 2012). All patients suffering from serious mental disorders need rehabilitation. The core group includes patients with persistent psychopathology, major instability, frequent relapses and difficulties in social integration (Rössler 2006).

12.2 Definitions

Psychosocial recovery programmes designed to offer daycare come under many different names. Partial care programmes, psychosocial programmes, daycare centres, social clubs, day hospitals or daycare units are just some of the terms frequently used. The situation is complicated further since structures with the same name differ considerably. In their endeavour to offer effective services, programmes develop and incorporate elements from different structures and innovative practices, which to a certain degree justify their diversity (Pratt et al. 2007).

Day hospitals or daycare units have been described as hospitals without treatment beds, as a structure which provides medical follow-up and a series of leisure and skills-cultivation activities (life, social and professional skills) to individuals who need intensive, short-term support, as an alternative to inpatient treatment or as a continuation of care after a period of hospitalisation has ended. They are aimed at the general population, which includes persons recently hospitalised, those in crisis who would otherwise need to be hospitalised and those suffering from chronic and serious mental disorders (Torrey and Fisher 1998). The term "day hospital" incorporates a heterogeneous set of mental health services, reflecting multiple functions and goals, even within the same organisation. That fact can be seen as an attempt to respond to multiple needs and as an inability to clarify its role in the spectrum of a modern social network for providing mental health services (Briscoe et al. 2004; Wilson 2008). The confusion in definitions has been confirmed in practice by researchers who have not identified differences in the symptoms of patients in hospitals and daycare centre examined and proposed two terms which could be used in the alternative (Holloway 1991; Briscoe et al. 2004). Research at a day hospital in Great Britain showed that a small percentage of available spaces were being used as an alternative solution to inpatient treatment. The majority of places were being used for "rehabilitation", but almost half of the patients with psychotic disorders only received general support. Those patient's needs could have been addressed by a daycare centre (Mbaya et al. 1998).

To more clearly define the content and role of complementary services necessary for a comprehensive care network, the literature has proposed, as distinction be drawn between day hospitals dealing with acute cases as an alternative to admission, transitional day hospitals to reduce the length of hospitalisation, daycare centres for rehabilitation and stabilisation and day treatment programmes to support outpatient treatment (Marshall et al. 2001).

It is important to distinguish day hospitals from daycare centres, whose primary aim is to provide social support to individuals with chronic and persistent mental disorders and to promote rehabilitation, social integration and recovery (Ives 1975). In the view of both those who receive services and those making referrals, day hospitals offer short-term, more intensive "treatment" in acute cases that need close follow-up of mental health. Daycare centres are perceived as a structure that offers more long-term psychosocial support to individuals with more resistant and longer-term problems, who are normally suffering from psychotic disorders (Catty et al. 2005).

Service users at daycare centres acting of their own accord as "volunteers" plan, choose and implement a series of activities and participate in and enjoy a social experience. As transitional structures, daycare centres promote liaisons with the family and social environment, so that they function and serve as a place aiding the return to normal living and working conditions.

Daycare centres can be divided up depending on the population they are aimed at:

Daycare centres for individuals with mental disorders or serious psychosocial needs which include:
   (a) Daycare centres for children and adolescents
   (b) Daycare centres for adults
Daycare centres for individuals with autism spectrum disorders
Daycare centres for sufferers of Alzheimer's disease and related disorders (Guide for organising and running daycare support and follow-up centres/PSYCHARGOS Phase II 2005)

Social clubs are a different model of psychosocial rehabilitation. They are organised by their members, offer a meeting place for socialising and function independently of the mental health system and may offer leisure, education, work opportunities, support on housing issues and other services the members decide on. The philosophy and development of the social club model is described in more detail in the following section (Novotny 2011).

12.3 Historical Development

Partial hospitalisation and social clubs are two different historical approaches that date back to the early movement that eventually led to modern-day all-day psychosocial rehabilitation programmes.

In the USSR in the 1930s, Dzhagarov, director of the Moscow Psychiatric Hospital, introduced the concept of partial hospitalisation. A number of patients at the hospital returned home in the evening. This innovation may have been prompted by increasing demands and limited resources, and Dzhagarov noted that the results of partial hospitalisation were similar to those of traditional hospitalisation. Industrial therapy was the basis of partial hospitalisation. In 1946 the first daycare centre in the Anglo-Saxon world opened in Montreal, Canada, to encourage social life. Attendance at the programme during the day and the return home in the evening was similar to being absent at work and did not cut the individual off from aspects of his day-to-day life (Cameron 1947). That was followed a short time later by the first day hospital in England aimed at patients who needed support after being discharged from hospital (Bierer 1948). One of Bierer's innovative ideas was to ameliorate the mass psychotic transference by setting up a multidisciplinary team (Chevallier-Fougas 2009). Similar structures were also in operation in the USA at that time at Yale University and the Menninger Clinic (Barnard et al. 1952). The first day hospital opened in Paris, France, in 1962 (Hôpital de jour de l'Élan). The director, Prof. Sivadon, influenced by the ideas of Bierer had initially set up a multidisciplinary team within his department which transformed into a treatment and social reintegration centre. Professional reintegration was the main aim of Sivadon's efforts (Bleandonu and Despinoy 1974). Early programmes took a psychiatric approach and placed emphasis on individual and group therapy and expressive therapies using art. They predated the deinstitutionalisation movement and were aimed at less burdened patients, compared to those for whom asylum-based treatments were reserved (Pratt et al. 2007; Mak 1994). In the 1960s the closure of large hospitals in the USA led to a boom in daycare programmes, with an emphasis on deinstitutionalisation.

In the 1940s former patients from the Rockland Psychiatric Center in New York set up a self-help group. In 1948 private resources were secured to house their endeavours in a building named Fountain House, which was a social meeting and support venue for its members, which operated outside the mental health system and became known as a social club. Participants were members, not patients, and remained for as long as they wanted, as is the case with any club. The initial aim was to improve the quality of life and satisfy basic needs, like housing, work, socialisation and leisure. As the club expanded, its members decided in 1955 to engage professionals without changing the atmosphere and philosophy of their endeavour. The basic principles governing the venture, which were later adopted by modern rehabilitationists, were an emphasis on the important role of individuals and their own responsibility for their own life in the rehabilitation process, recognising their abilities and right to live a normal life, and the value of voluntary participation. The way in which Fountain House operated met the basic human needs of belonging to a community and being productive. The emphasis on work was provided both in the club via teams responsible for caring for the space, cleaning and preparing meals and by placing members in jobs in the community with the support of the club's staff. Fountain House was the inspiration for the development of the social club model. In the 1970s there was a national training programme based on this approach, and 10 years later the model expanded abroad with similar structures being developed in many countries (Raeburn et al. 2013; Edward 1994; Warner 2006).

The first daycare centre opened in Greece in 1971 at the Thessaloniki branch of the Mental Health and Research Centre. It was followed by the first day hospital in 1978 (Mantonakis et al. 1994) and in 1984 came the psychosocial rehabilitation unit of the Vyronas-Kessariani Community Mental Health Centre (Madianos 2005), operating under the aegis of the University Clinic of the Eginition Hospital.

12.4 Theoretical Model

Work in a daycare centre requires the integration of different psychotherapy models to meet the individualised needs of the person and promote social integration in line with the principles of psychosocial rehabilitation and recovery. It requires a combination of strategies aimed at developing skills which allow interaction in a stressful environment and strategies to mobilise resources and change the environment, making it more facilitative and supportive for patients to gradually become autonomous.

Milieu therapy, CBT techniques, psychodynamic understanding and family and psychoeducational interventions enrich the theoretical armoury of the multidisciplinary team at the daycare centre. The modern outlook dictates that we develop an approach that integrates different psychotherapy schools and techniques bearing in mind the complexity of patient needs and the coherent use of case management in the context of how the multidisciplinary team works.

Milieu therapy relates to a supportive interpersonal environment which teaches, creates standards and bolsters healthy interaction between individuals. The term was introduced by A. Aichom in the early twentieth century (Shorter 2006). From the viewpoint of milieu therapy, any interaction between members and staff contains the therapeutic potential for self-awareness and the adoption of new, more functional ways of interacting and negotiating. It is inspired by the assumption that an individual's difficulties are born and expressed in their relations with other people. Each interaction ought to help create an environment of mutual trust, respect and support. Gunderson (1978) described five key elements of milieu therapy:

(a) Containment (the sense of support and control from the environment)
(b) Support
(c) Structure (an organised and predictable environment)
(d) Involvement (participation and integration into the environment)
(e) Reassurance (confirmation for the individual from his environment)

Washburn and Conrad (1979) proposed another element, negotiation, referring to the process of intermediation whereby members and staff set targets and devise a treatment plan (Pratt et al. 2007).

The therapeutic community is a small, cohesive community where members have a high degree of involvement in decision-making and the practical running of the unit. Based on the ideas of collectivity and empowerment, the ability for each one to enjoy his rights as a citizen, therapeutic communities are structured to encourage personal responsibility and to prevent dependence on professionals. Members/patients are viewed as sources of strength and creative energy for the treatment framework, and equality in relations within the team is considered to be the basis for a strong therapeutic relationship. Horizontal hierarchies and collective decision-making can wrongly be seen by some external observer as chaotic functioning of the group, but the staff of modern-day therapeutic communities are aware of the need for strong leadership and their responsibility for providing a safe framework for therapeutic work (Association of Therapeutic Communities 1999). The practice of therapeutic communities aims to be something more than a mere framework hosting patients with serious disorders who happen to be in therapy. In 1960 in his work *Community as Doctor* ..., Rapoport described four principles which define work in the therapeutic community (Dickey and Ware 2008):

Table 12.1 Therapeutic community principles

Theoretical principal	Origin in development	Culture in a community	Structures in a community	Rapoport's original community themes
Attachment	Primary bond, losses as growth	Belonging	Referral, joining, leaving	
Containment	Maternal and paternal holding	Safety	Support, rules, boundaries	Permissiveness
Communication	Play, speech, others as separate	Openness	Groups, ethos, visitors	Communalism
Involvement	Finding a place among others	Living-learning	Community meeting: agenda and structure	Reality confrontation
Agency	Establishing self as seat of action	Empowerment	Votes, decisions, seniority	Democratisation

From Haigh (1999: p. 257). Source: Haigh (1999, p. 257)

(a) The principle of democratisation
(b) The principle of permissiveness
(c) The principle of communalism
(d) The principle of reality confrontation

Later, Haigh (1999) attempted to define the substance of milieu therapy. He described five key qualities and presented them as a continuum, associating them with developmental stages, culture and structures of a community which adopts and serves them. The table above correlates these to Rapoport's principles cited above (Campling 2001) (Table 12.1).

The psychoanalytical perspective helps us attribute meaning to what we are doing in each moment both for the patient and in terms of organisation, administration and team work and the relationship between the institution and the community itself. What models could provide guidance and what metaphorical references could be used to provide care? Winnicott's holding, Bion's containment and the concepts of attachment have already been associated with the running of a therapeutic community (see the table above). The protective sheath that involvement at the level of therapy techniques with the patient's actual body offers must not be ignored especially in pathologies which are exceptionally regressive. Talking therapies provide us with resources for action and, according to P.C. Racamier, are acts which give meaning and which talk to the patient, his family, staff and the team more widely speaking.

The psychoanalytic literature on the theoretical understanding, technique and treatment of psychosis is very significant and useful. It includes not just the classic authors (S. Freud, P. Federn, O. Fenichel, M. Klein, K. Abraham, D. Winnicott,

S. Arieti, M. Balint), the British Kleinian and post-Kleinian school of object relations (W. Bion, H. Rosenfeld, H. Segal, B. Joseph, B. Hinshelwood, J. Steiner, N. Symington, J. Gottstein) and the contribution of French social psychiatry (psychiatry without a couch) which developed after WW II (J. Hochmann, P.C. Racamier, S. Lebovici, R. Diatkine, M. Bouvet) (Hatzistavrakis and Sakellaropoulos 2010). The contribution of psychoanalysis to applied social psychiatry is explored in more detail in the relevant chapter.

The need to refer to a theoretical model which gives meaning to the work and identity of the therapeutic team was stressed by J. Hochmann (2003a), a theory which he calls mental institution. It starts off from the risk of the asylum being reborn within the modus operandi of new community structures which were intended to abolish the asylum. The source of the rebirth of the asylum function lies in the "fear of madness" which is attributed to feelings of being invaded, of emptiness and of futility born from contact with psychosis. Those feelings are probably responsible for the tendency of the person to defend his mental space from the group of patients using artificial boundaries and distinctions, to avoid therapeutic activism, and for the prevalence of a type of anti-thinking which paralyses the structure and makes it appear to be an imitation, a parody of life, dominated by stereotypes and the bureaucratic handling of relationships (Hochmann 2003a).

J. Hochmann understands psychosis primarily as a defence rather than as a deficit or failing. The task of the preconscious, thanks to which we can think and also envisage what we are perceiving, is the transformation and representation of stimuli and unification of stimulus with the representation. Bion (1955) introduced beta elements to describe the clear sense that has not been reproduced by the sensory organs and alpha elements for those transformed in such a way that they are recognised by consciousness. Transformation takes place in the preconscious of the mother where the child projects unprocessed materials. Through reveries the mother associates and favours the projections, which are returned to the child in an acceptable form. Through those representations of an object, the preconscious of the child – his own alpha function – is formed. Following that approach, it is considered that in a psychotic function the preconscious is reversed in structure, causing fragmentation in relationships, attacking connections, projecting and fighting symbols, instead of connecting, introjecting and symbolising.

The psychoanalytical theoretical approach, described by J. Hochmann, leads him to a view of care where through daily interventions he attempts to modify the preconscious' defences and function. He considers care to be a mental activity whose object is to put the activity of thinking, the associative process, back into operation. That attempt may be made via numerous transactions, whether verbal or nonverbal, structured in the form of psychotherapy, or through day-to-day activities like play, hobbies or a shared meal. The therapeutic process begins when these transactions place priority on the symbolic aspect. The cognitive substrate, whether explicitly expressed or not, exists as a fantasy in the therapist's thoughts, pleases him, gives him meaning and satisfies him since it associates the events and builds a single story. Intellectual processing within the therapist presupposes the existence of a model he can refer to. For the therapist this interplay with the model is equivalent to the mother's reveries, when she transforms beta elements into alpha elements. It is an "alchemy" which occurs in the mind of the therapist and resembles the pleasure which he receives when he communicates a clinical case to colleagues or to his supervisors (Hochmann 2003b).

The cognitive model of psychotherapy on the other hand applies the initial ideas of Beck to understanding and treating psychosis (Beck et al. 2009). In this model, the way in which we interpret facts affects the way in which we feel and behave. These interpretations are frequently maintained by unhelpful thoughts, prejudices and behavioural reactions and are affected by core beliefs which are formed as a result of life experiences. Various cognitive models of psychosis and psychotic symptoms or experiences have been developed by writers such as Chadwick, Garety and Morrison who argue that the way people interpret psychotic phenomena rather than the psychotic experiences themselves cause a sense of malaise and disability (Morrison 2008). Cognitive-behavioural therapy (CBT) is proposed as an effective way of dealing with the symptoms of schizophrenia, particularly in patients with persistent symptoms, coupled of course with suitable medication. The extent of the effectiveness of this approach has been explored in later studies (Jones et al. 2012; Jauhar et al. 2014).

According to Beck, cognitive therapy cannot affect the basic neurophysiological predisposition or vulnerability involved in schizophrenia, but can modify the resulting dysfunctional beliefs and consequently provide better protection from stress. Psychotherapy and medication can ameliorate overactive cognitive schemata and free up resources for further control of reality (cognitive compensation) (Beck et al. 2009).

Negative beliefs about oneself, the world and others (such as "I am vulnerable", "other people are dangerous"), and beliefs which reinforce the adoption of paranoia as a strategy for managing interpersonal threats, are associated with psychosis. From the cognitive viewpoint, psychosis may be seen as a primary physiological experience with comprehensible consequences for the emotions and behaviour, consequences which are due to evaluation and handling of those experiences and not as an illness. Destructive or negative inferences drawn from experiences cause burden and a sense of malaise. It has been assumed that cognitive and behavioural responses, such as selective attention, repressing thoughts and safety behaviours, preserve psychotic experiences and the consequent burden (Jauhar et al. 2014).

The theory of social learning and the study of behaviour have significantly affected the development of psychosocial rehabilitation programmes. The functionality of patients with schizophrenia and their quality of life is significantly degraded because of difficulties that they have in social contact. The social deficits in patients with schizophrenia include difficulty in starting and keeping a conversation going and an inability to achieve goals or satisfy needs in situations which require social interaction. These difficulties significantly reduce their ability to respond in adult roles. Poor social functionality and stigmatising experiences in the past, coupled with stress in social contexts, contribute to social isolation and inadequate social support which in turn limit the individual's ability to develop and improve his social skills.

The social skills model offers a different perspective on how to approach social functionality. In this model, adequate social interaction is based on a set of three constitutive skills: (a) social perception or inference skills, (b) social cognition or processing skills and (c) behavioural response or expression skills (Liberman 2008; Vyskocilova and Prasko 2012).

The use of the term "skills" stresses the view that social interaction is based more on a set of learned abilities than on any fixed features, needs or internal processes. The relevant literature and research data argue that behaviours can be modified through experience and learning. So learning social skills is a structured educational process which can use teaching guidelines, imitation of models, breaking skills down into their component parts, role play and positive social support in order to teach social behaviour (Jauhar et al. 2014).

12.5 Features of How Daycare Centres Operate

The Space: The Infrastructure

The daycare centre must allow groups to be held and numerous day-to-day activities to be carried on in parallel. In addition, it must ensure privacy for one-to-one meetings. It is essential for the centre to have adequate space for all members and staff to meet, ancillary areas for preparing meals, etc. Adequate lighting, ventilation and heating, security and cleanliness are all conditions for a therapeutic space being suitable. It is also important for the centre to be sited within the fabric of the community and for it to be easily accessible by public transport (Pratt et al. 2007).

Staff

The daycare centre's scientific officer plays a critical role. He is responsible for annual planning, organising and ensuring the problem-free running of the centre. His duties include being responsible for organisation, continuing training, evaluation of staff and services provided and for drawing up the annual report on evaluation of the unit which is submitted to the management body to check if targets set have been met. Along with the multidisciplinary team, he prepares the overall schedule and the individual treatment plans for each attendee. He is also responsible for co-ordinating and implementing the work of the multidisciplinary team (Guide for organising and running daycare support and follow-up centres/PSYCHARGOS Phase II 2005).

The Multidisciplinary Team

The creation of multidisciplinary teams was proposed since different approaches to therapy by professionals from different areas of specialisation are required to meet the needs of mental patients. Psychiatrists, psychologists, psychiatric nurses, social workers and industrial therapists comprise the multidisciplinary team.

Multidisciplinary team working is described by Jefferies and Chan (2004) as:"the main mechanism to ensure truly holistic care for patients and a seamless service for patients throughout their disease trajectory and across the boundaries of primary, secondary and tertiary care".

Carrier and Kendall (1995) described a team as "a group of people with complementary skills who are committed to a common purpose, performance goals, and approach, for which they hold themselves mutually accountable".

The research evidence supports multidisciplinary team working as the most effective means of delivering a comprehensive mental health service to people with mental health problems, especially those with long-term mental health problems (Tyrer et al. 1998).

It is not just a matter of getting different mental health professionals together and magically multidisciplinary team working happens. Teams need to have shared goals and values, need to understand and respect the competencies of other team members, need to learn from other disciplines and need to respect their different views and perspectives.

Multidisciplinary teamwork and support from colleagues is often cited as an important source of reward to team members (Onyett and Ford 1996). While many multidisciplinary team members experience the work as demanding, job satisfaction and personal accomplishment tend to be high (Carson et al. 1991; Onyett et al. 1995).

The advantages to mental health professionals of multidisciplinary working include:

(a) Close-knit peer support for all health professionals and consideration for the complex and sometimes distressing clinical work to be done, i.e. involuntary admissions, violence, suicide, etc.
(b) Division of labour to ensure multidisciplinary service delivery, i.e. ensuring that all "biopsychosociocultural" components of intervention and care are delivered
(c) Ensuring that all members of the multidisciplinary team are used in a way that is maximally effective, i.e. service users who need a specific input/skill set can have access to that immediately, rather than having multiple assessments
(d) Cross-fertilisation of skills between professionals (Hoult 1986)
(e) Multidisciplinary peer review of all casework at team meetings
(f) Staff acquire new skills, participate in decision-making and take on more responsibility leading to increased job satisfaction (Onyett and Smith 1998)
(g) Delivering services that are planned and co-ordinated (Ovretveit 1993)
(h) Delivering services that are cost-effective (Knapp et al. 1994)
(i) Enhancing information sharing and streamlining work practices (Hornby 1993)

Working in teams also presents challenges to the mental health professionals involved and the mental health services, particularly around management, leadership, confidentiality and conflict management and resolution. Creative tension between disciplines can easily give rise to conflicts between them (Norman and Peck 1999). Team members typically place varying degrees of emphasis on the distinct elements of the biopsychosocial model of mental health and ill health (Hannigan 1999), so much so that there may be divisive debate about treatment approaches (Norman and Peck 1999). Hence, clear mechanisms for conflict resolution are required (Onyett et al. 1997; Byrne 2005), preferably through multi-professional consensus. Recognition of some authority structures to resolve disagreements may be required (Burns 2004). Having such clear mechanisms may in and of itself predispose to less conflict (Onyett et al. 1997).

The Services Provided

In close cooperation with other units in the sector, the daycare centre provides care and treatment on an individual, family, group and community level. According to the Guide for organising and running daycare support and follow-up centres/PSYCHARGOS Phase II, these services are primarily those listed below:

Needs assessment, preparation and implementation of individualised care and rehabilitation plans
Treatment interventions at individual and group level, with emphasis on training in social and individual skills
Developing and promoting professional skills to promote employment and integration into the labour market
Preparing meals and catering for beneficiaries
Leisure and cultural activities
Running a social club
Family support programmes and special treatment interventions (such as psychoeducation)
Training courses for staff and new professionals
Ongoing evaluation of activities and corresponding research activities
Community info programmes to address social stigma and prejudice associated with mental disorders

Services are planned by the scientific officer and multidisciplinary team and cover a 6-month period. Depending on the type of service, they are offered at individual and/or group level, at the daycare centre's facilities or elsewhere, with each member participating in selected activities for a specific time, based on the individualised care plan. Preparation, implementation and evaluation of the plan must take into account interventions relating to the individual himself which are being implemented at other mental health units (such as mental health centres, the psychiatric department of the general hospital, etc.). To that end, the multidisciplinary team cooperates closely with other mental health units to jointly prepare an individualised care plan which needs to be unique and uniform for the entire sector. In areas where there are no other mental health services, the daycare centre can meet the psychiatric follow-up needs to patients and implement treatments provided staff in the relevant areas of specialisation exist.

Case management plays an important role here, not just in co-ordinating and integrating mental health services but in mobilising community resources, in support for housing, work and other aspects of the individualised care plan, as described in detail in the section below.

12.6   Case Management

Case management is considered to be a relatively old methodological tool for organising community mental health services. In Greece this methodology is not widely used in a systematic way and has not been widely evaluated, despite similar concepts being described in the Greek literature: individualised care plan, individual treatment plan and co-ordination and integration of community mental health services. However, these have not been clearly formulated, other than in general principles of social psychiatry, both in relation to the theoretical model which dictates case management and the specific targets it sets, in order to be implemented and evaluated in the context of how the multidisciplinary-interdisciplinary mental health team which intervenes at various community units operates: daycare centres or day hospitals, ACT units or outreach teams or mobile units, as described in the relevant chapters of this book.

Theoretical Model and Principles

Parsons' (1977) model organises the information the team collects into the following levels: (1) values, (2) processes and (3) interactions. This model presupposes that each organisation is defined by a continuous feedback loop. The values create a frame of reference for actions. Procedures are the means for implementing actions. Interactions are the effects actions have on the environment. In a two-way manner, these interactions have an impact on the frame of reference and in turn modify the values.

For example, (1) the asylum model's basic principle was to promote the "good" of the ill person and to "protect" him, even though that meant sacrificing his autonomy. In "benign" cases of asylums, the institution had to do everything for the good of the "ill" who had psychiatric disorders, frequently against their will and by depriving them of their liberty. Those values required hierarchical functions (2), in the context of which preserving and safeguarding the status quo and security were of primary importance, even if it meant ignoring the fundamental rights of patients. The interaction with the environment (3) created the impression from the 1960s onwards of negative effects of asylums and institutionalisation, such as stigmatism and self-stigmatism, loss of autonomy and dominant social exclusion. As is well known, these findings lead to the logic of asylums and the culture which defined the operation of these "total institutions" being condemned (see Goffman, Basaglia); to the idea of moving beyond asylums; to the emergence of concepts such as autonomy, recovery and advocacy for the rights of the mentally ill; and to the structural changes in the entire system of psychiatric care. We need to change our practice, our thinking and our services and to raise certain fundamental questions. Who does what? With whom? For what purpose? To what end? Using what values? With what ability to learn from his experiences and above all from his mistakes? Have there been enough declarations about psychiatric reform and about showcasing of recovery as a new concept which in practical terms can promote empowerment and the life plans of patients? Taking these questions into account, we believe that case management can be a valuable methodological guide and a framework for thinking about change: change in our identity, development and transformation of our services and our psychiatric culture.

The values which define the use of case management as a tool for continuous monitoring and evaluation of psychiatric care in the community can be presented in very general form as follows:

(a) The transition from the concept of chronicity to psychosocial rehabilitation and a continuous recovery process
(b) Criticism in theoretical and methodological terms of clinical practice and the biomedical model
(c) The necessity for critical time intervention for an individual after hospitalisation (see the historic use of the ACT model)
(d) Dissemination of the recovery model to all parties involved in the social psychiatric care of the individual
(e) Changes to the life care plan of the individual based on this treatment plan
(f) The primary role the patient has in his own narrative despite institutional, cultural, therapeutic, social and contextual barriers and objections

Procedures are aimed at patients who are in the process of deinstitutionalisation or in follow-up after hospitalisation, such as individuals with severe psychopathology in the community. The targets are intended (a) to ensure the continuity of care and to establish a psychosocial support network, (b) to improve professional and social reintegration and (c) to prevent relapses, new periods of hospitalisation or a worsening in the individual's condition.

Six steps are normally followed by the mobile units of the University Psychiatric Clinic in Lausanne (Bonsack et al. 2013) to successfully prepare for case management:

1. *Application*: All patients who were hospitalised voluntarily or involuntarily at the psychiatric department or in the psychiatric hospital in that area are safely identified.
2. *First contact with patient*: The patient is briefed about the follow-up plan and accompaniment in the community, in cooperation with the hospital team at first.

3. *Evaluation*: The patient's clinical situation, family situation, support network and the resources needed for case management are evaluated.
4. *First counselling session during hospitalisation*: A necessary step to ensure that it is possible for the patient to return to the normal environment and that the support network is aware and on stand-by.
5. Adjustment of optimum case management in conjunction with individual needs and the needs of the actual support network.
6. Evaluation at 1 month and joint preparation of and consent to a new plan by the hospitalisation team and the case management team.

12.7   Objectives of Case Management Intervention

Intervention objectives – areas	Description and objectives	Example of various actions that can be taken
1. Co-ordination of the care system	Co-ordination of all health, mental health and social care services ensured by the case manager for the patient's benefit	Information provided about objectives, boundaries and responsibilities of each individual or body information Case manager appointed List of individuals who can be involved in the network prepared, and all of them are contacted
2. Commitment to the care plan	Commitment to each individual objective and reduction in the length of the recovery process Prevention of barriers and objections	Interventions with negative representations of traditional and asylum-based psychiatry Actions to promote destigmatisation, psychoeducation and connection of patient complaints to his pain, functional difficulties and symptom management
3. Commitment to and consent for medication	Long-term commitment to take medication	Briefing about and management of the day-to-day aspects of medication Monitoring of unwanted side effects, changes in treatment when needed, management of difficulties arising from side effects, cooperation with family members
4. Support from and involvement of the patient's environment	Support for and empowerment of relatives' skills Prevention of exhaustion and domestic violence	Information provided about smart ways to manage upsets in day-to-day life Showcasing "lost" skills and evaluating the need to support/rehabilitate members of the support network for a transitional period

Intervention objectives – areas	Description and objectives	Example of various actions that can be taken
5. Support for professional integration	Evaluation of skills to integrate into an appropriate work or professional activity or initially volunteer work which would open up the potential for employment (such as social cooperatives)	Raising the employer's awareness to prepare for the patient's return to his previous post Preventing failure short, medium and long term The patient may need a transitional period by joining an industrial therapy group
6. Day-to-day skills	Support, empowerment and development of day-to-day skills	Preparing and setting objectives in a daily schedule while respecting existing limitations in that phase and support from analogous resources Exploration of alternative solutions from the support network
7. Ties to the community	Improvement of existing ties, contribution to reactivating older ties, development of new ones to promote social reintegration	Accompanying the patient in the process of reactivating his contacts or creating new ties Training in communication skills, participation in service recipient groups or self-help groups, development of communication skills via role playing
8. Support and supervision of day-to-day care	Ensuring that the patient receives all the help and care he needs Finding auxiliary or complementary resources	Daily "at-home" evaluation, inclusion of volunteers into the case management process, support for the legal, social and insurance rights of service users, etc.
9. Prevention of relapses	Ensuring the continuity of the recovery process Preventing suicidality/suicide Preventing any possible return to substance and alcohol use	Evaluation of suicidality Use of appropriate tools, scales Limitation of dangerous equipment Development of a strategy to manage stress and adjustment difficulties Learning relaxation techniques, participation in sporting activities, daily exercise, etc. Psychoeducation about decision-making depending on the assessment of the patient's skills and abilities in each case Activation and co-ordination of services if readmitted to hospital

Intervention objectives – areas	Description and objectives	Example of various actions that can be taken
10. Conveying information – communication	Ensuring the continuity, flow and quality of information Supporting the integration and comprehension of information	Crisis plan: open discussion with the patient about the flow of information Organising the network and evaluating it Information exchange forms Joint assessment of the situation by all stakeholders, including the case manager, and agreement on supplementary, integrated action by all

Mapping out the network may be a useful tool in ensuring a successful outcome for case management. It is a graphic depiction – photograph of the network at the time of the first intervention:

A. The primary network consists of the individual's milieu and is not limited to his family, contrary to the belief commonly held by mental health professionals. It may consist of neighbours, colleagues, pets or even individuals who are no longer alive!
B. The secondary network may be formal or informal and includes health, mental health and social care professionals. While the formal network is mapped out in terms of services, the informal network is created on the initiative of members of the primary network, in order to find answers and solutions to their needs (such as associations for the family, service users, volunteers, etc.).
C. The tertiary network consists of services and organisations who exercise political, judicial, health or welfare powers. All these institutions are directly or indirectly involved in patients' rights. Consequently, it is self-evident that members of the case management team or case manager need to cooperate, intervene and/or exert pressure in the process of defending patients' rights.

The Example of How the Franco Basaglia Daycare Centre Operated by the Regional Development and Mental Health Association Works and Has Developed

The Melissia Daycare Centre was set up in 2004 as part of the PSYCHARGOS programme/Phase II. It offered services to 15 members aged 18–45 from the fifth Psychiatric Region, offering comprehensive psychosocial rehabilitation services. During the first 8 years, it was in operation, 42 patients received services.

In 2013 the Franco Basaglia Daycare Centre was upgraded when a centre providing community mental health services to residents in the fifth Psychiatric Region was developed in the context of the HR Development Operational Programme 2007–2013 in priority area 14 "Consolidating reform in the mental health sector".

Table 12.2 ICD 10 Diagnosis of attendees

Diagnosis	ICD 10 code	% of attendees at the Franco Basaglia Daycare Centre (2013–2014) (%)	% of attendees at mental health centres (1997); (Madianos 2010) (%)
Organic mental disorders	F00–09	2	3
Mental and behavioural disorders due to psychoactive substance use	F10–19	0	2.2
Schizophrenia, schizotypal and delusional disorders	F20–29	30	17.8
Mood [affective] disorders	F30–39	25	20
Neurotic, stress-related and somatoform disorders	F40–49	13	22
Behavioural syndromes associated with physiological disturbances and physical factors	F50–59	0	–
Disorders of adult personality and behaviour	F60–69	10	–
Mental retardation	F70–79	4	–
Disorders of psychological development	F80–89	0	–
Behavioural and emotional disorders with onset usually occurring in childhood and adolescence	F90–99	5	–
Others/not diagnosed		11	35

The centre is cofinanced by the Ministry of Health and the European Union. The aims of the 2-year pilot programme were to provide psychosocial interventions in the community, to reduce the number of hospitalisations and their duration to network services and to limit the treatment gap between needs and services provided in the region.

Diagnoses of attendees at the Franco Basaglia Daycare Centre, as shown in the diagram, appear to be dominated by schizophrenia spectrum disorders (F20–29) (30 %) followed by emotional disorders (F30–39) (25 %) and neurotic, somatomorph and stress disorders (F40–49) (13 %).

Table 12.2 attempts to compare the available data from 24 mental health centres in Greece for 1997. Differences exist because of the different classifications used and the significantly higher percentage of attendees at the Franco Basaglia Daycare Centre suffering from schizophrenia, schizotypal and delusional disorders (30 % compared to 17.8 %). That difference could be explained by the tradition in the previous operating period (2004–2012) where the daycare centre was aimed at individuals with psychotic disorders, but also perhaps by the emphasis given in the second phase of pilot operation (2013) to caring for individuals with serious and persistent mental disorders, by networking with inpatient psychiatric services and close cooperation with the psychosocial rehabilitation unit and the Assertive Community Treatment (ACT) team.

The extended services the Franco Basaglia Daycare Centre (run by the Regional Development and Mental Health Association) offers include:

The psychosocial rehabilitation unit for patients with serious and persistent mental disorders
Psychiatric and psychological assessment
One-to-one and group psychotherapy, art psychotherapy
Psychiatric follow-up – prescriptions
Assertive Community Treatment (ACT)
Social club
Networking, promoting mental health
Research, evaluation, documentation

12.8 Intervention Areas and Networking at the Franco Basaglia Daycare Centre

The Psychosocial Rehabilitation Unit

Getting a member to successfully commit to a treatment relationship is the first step towards rehabilitation. The clinician needs to build a constructive relationship with members and their families. Professionals and patients need to identify the other's agenda and seek out some common ground to develop a comprehensive care plan, an individualised recovery-focused plan (Sadock and Sadock 2008).

The process of rehabilitation and developing and implementing the individualised care plan includes the following stages:

(a) *Assessment/Diagnosis*: This helps the member identify or cultivate his readiness for rehabilitation, to set general goals and to identify skills, resources, and strengths and weaknesses relating to those goals.
(b) *Planning*: He works out in detail how to cultivate the skills and obtain the necessary support to achieve his goal, ties assessment into the intervention and develops a schedule for starting and ending the intervention.
(c) *Intervention*: This includes developing skills in an individual or group context and planning how to use them in vivo, co-ordinating and modifying the environment and available resources (Anthony and Farkas 2009).

In developing individualised care plans at the daycare centre in cooperation with the Istituto Mario Negri in Milano, the innovative methodology and technique called "Shared Care Pathways" (derived from the Italian method known as Percorsi di Cura Condivisi) is used, which empowers a change in the patient's position and involvement in the treatment process and follow-up which monitors the symptoms and functionality, as assessed and managed by all those involved and cooperating with him in this process (Biasi et al. 2006).

The innovation lies in the involvement of users and their families in jointly managing the treatment contract, in planning, in implementation and in the prevention of any possible future relapses. A third party, the guarantor, is involved in this model and takes part in the joint management plan.

To implement the plan a team needs to be set up which agrees joint practices set out in the plan and cooperates in making the plan a reality. The team members are the patient, the professional (the point of reference at the daycare centre), the relative or caregiver and the guarantor. The guarantor helps participants periodically verify the plan. The guarantor's role can be taken up by a mental health professional or not, provided he has no professional other relationship with the patient the plan relates to. His presence guarantees equality between team members and confirms the reliability of assessments. The presence of a third party in the customised psychosocial rehabilitation plan of the patient ensures the greatest possible democratic guarantee and defence of the patient's rights as a citizen with a mental disorder. The main objective is to place the patient in a more assertive and adult position, *assigning* him a significant part of the responsibility for self-assessment of his mental condition and his treatment choices. The concept of the reality of the therapeutic relationship is introduced in a clear, but controlled, nonthreatening way for the patient, thereby preventing reversion to psychotic defence mechanisms as much as possible. In addition, the patient is not alone in dealing with the burden of mental pain. The presence of third-party guarantors balances out the therapeutic process, ameliorating any paranoia towards the therapist and the patient's family environment, which frequently emerges during relapses. The presence of the family in the team is also very important since they actively participate but do not have an exclusive or primary role and do not receive all the violence of the psychotic process which they cannot handle and which is frequently returned to the patient in an unhealthy manner.

The "Shared Care Pathways" approach consists of three contracts (forms which are read, filled out and signed by the team) which relate to:

1. The relationship (the quality of relations and achievement of interpersonal relations between team members)
2. The intervention plan (setting special goals in four areas:
   (a) Symptoms
   (b) Social and family relations
   (c) Work and community activities
   (d) Accommodation
3. Prescriptions (as specified by the attendant doctor) and the taking of medication

Two cards are also filled out relating to:

"Early signs of crisis"
"Expectations and wishes in the case of crisis"

Assessments take place every 6 months (half-yearly for 2 years in total). During verification, compliance with procedures and achievement of pre-agreed goals set by the team are evaluated. Where goals are not met, they are redefined so that they continue to be individualised, flexible and realistically achievable (Papakonstantinou et al. 2008; Papadaki et al. 2012).

The development, implementation and constant reassessment of the individualised care plan is monitored at weekly one-to-one meetings between members and their contact person. At those meetings, the member will agree to participate in all or part of the daily treatment plan depending on his needs, preferences and goals, recorded during the assessment and intervention planning stages. Client needs are assessed using the Client's Assessment of Strengths, Interests and Goals (CASIG) scale. At the start of the intervention and while it is underway, psychometric tools are used to monitor psychopathology, quality of life and family burden (PANSS, WHOQOL, Family Habits and Family Burden Scale).

The contact person also collaborates with the client's families, to reduce the family burden, modify dysfunctional behavioural patterns and provide the necessary support as the client moves towards recovery. Patients, suffering from schizophrenia in families with high levels of criticism, hostility or over-involvement, have higher levels of relapse compared to those whose families express emotion less frequently. Special psychosocial interventions can reduce the emotion expressed and modify the course of the illness. Interventions take place at the daycare centre or in cooperation with the Association of Families and Friends for Mental Health. A recent meta-analysis argues that family intervention can reduce the frequency of relapses and admissions to hospital and can encourage the taking of medication but does not affect the tendency of the individual and family to terminate contact with services. Family intervention also appears to improve social dysfunction and levels of emotion expressed within the family (Pharoah et al. 2010).

The daycare centre's daily treatment plan includes the following groups/activities:

Social skill training	Documentaries/videos
Art	Gardening
News	Cooking/day-to-day life skills
Group psychotherapy	Computers
Exercise	Board games
Self-care and health promotion	Empowerment, rights and claims
Industrial therapy	Client meetings – organising oneself
Storytelling	General meeting/community
Photography	Social outings

Involvement in daily programme groups as part of the individualised care plan serves many general and special goals. The programme includes groups for training, psychotherapy, managing the illness and medication, leisure/free time activities, skills training, cognitive rehabilitation, empowerment and so on.

For Example

The client meetings – organising oneself group and the general meeting/community group, attended by all clients and staff – promote the assumption of adult roles, initiative, cooperation and empowerment in the spirit of the recovery model, the principles of the therapeutic community and the tradition of the social club model. Along the same lines, the empowerment and rights group helps clients seek out the necessary social resources and rights of clients as equal citizens participating in society.

The exercise, self-care and health promotion groups highlight the issue of the physical health of individuals with serious mental disorders which is frequently neglected, seek to modify dysfunctional behaviours and promote the adoption of a healthy lifestyle. Obesity, smoking, lack of physical exercise and metabolic syndrome, which is frequently associated with the taking of antipsychotics, are some of the risk factors that appear to contribute to the early onset of cardiovascular disease and a 20–30 % reduction in the life expectancy of individuals with serious mental disorders (Casagrande et al. 2010; Saiga et al. 2013; O'Brien et al. 2014; Casey et al. 2011).

The cooking/day-to-day life skills groups aim to improve skills essential for living on one's own. Money management, housework, personal hygiene and use of public transport are all skills which daycare centre clients may need to be trained in and practise under protected, real-life conditions (the social outings group) in order to achieve a better quality of life. The most effective way to acquire these skills has not been confirmed by research (Tungpunkom et al. 2012).

Social skills training (Vyskocilova and Prasko 2012), cognitive remediation (McGurk et al. 2007) and CBT along with psychoeducational interventions for family and relatives, referred to above, appear from the literature review to show strong signs to being effective psychological therapies alongside the use of medication (Pfammatter et al. 2006).

Psychiatric Diagnosis and Follow-Up

The Franco Basaglia Daycare Centre provides psychiatric follow-up and prescriptions without any time limitations. Emphasis is placed on posthospital follow-up of patients with serious and persistent disorders in cooperation with the psychiatric clinic of the fifth Psychiatric Region General Hospital and specialist psychiatric hospitals. The multidisciplinary team meetings make it easier to provide comprehensive care based on the biopsychosocial model. The service is frequently offered in conjunction with interventions by the psychotherapy team, the psychosocial rehabilitation unit or the ACT team as part of an integrated care plan that meets the patient's needs.

Psychotherapy Service

The psychotherapy service has to meet the community's needs in the fifth Psychiatric Region, given the very limited availability of public psychotherapy services for "ordinary" mental health problems. Over recent years the socioeconomic crisis has in all likelihood contributed to the rise in referrals to the service of cases of stress-related and depressive disorders and has highlighted the complex, multifactorial nature of the problems. Under current conditions, what is needed is a flexible, pluralistic perspective, both during and in the theoretical orientation of psychotherapy practice in the community, in order to respond to the diverse, increased needs.

The service provides one-to-one psychoanalytical, CBT and cognitive analytical psychotherapy as well as one-to-one and group art, family and systematic psychotherapy. Psychotherapy is short term lasting 15–52 sessions, depending on the client's needs and the theoretical approach chosen as the most appropriate. At present, 31 % of new referrals to the daycare centre receive one-to-one psychotherapy and 13 % group psychotherapy. The majority of cases dealt with by the service are diagnosed as having mood (affective) disorders (F30–39).

Outcomes are assessed using the CORE-10 tool, a questionnaire which is filled out by the client before and after therapy which explores stress, depression, trauma, physical symptoms, functionality and risk.

A detailed description of short-term psychodynamic psychotherapy in the community is provided in the relevant chapter.

Social Club

The social club serves around 70 clients with serious mental disorders who live on their own or in sheltered accommodation. It is run by professionals and supported by volunteers and clients. It runs in the evening and includes training, entertainment and treatment groups. At present the groups on offer relate to:

English lessons
Empowerment and rights
Self-care/how to organise one's free time
Music, dance, theatre
Board games
Film club

The social club's aim is to raise awareness, provide training and mobilise volunteers and users of services to create a network of similar structures which they organise themselves, which are separate from mental health services.

Assertive Community Treatment (ACT)

The Franco Basaglia Daycare Centre's Assertive Community Treatment (ACT) team is aimed at patients with severe, mainly psychotic, mental disorders which are in an acute phase of the illness, especially those with a history of multiple relapses and repeated hospitalisations. It is also aimed at individuals with chronic, persistent psychopathology with greater need of psychosocial rehabilitation in relation to medication, psychotherapy, housing and work.

The team's main aim is to reduce hospitalisations and to prevent relapses, while also accompanying the individuals through the recovery process. The team consists of a psychiatrist, psychologist, social worker and nurse (see the chapter of Assertive Community Treatment – Home intervention in psychiatric events).

Networking, Promoting Mental Health

As part of community mental health practice, we can identify three levels of networks, as we saw in relation to how case management is implemented: the primary, secondary and tertiary levels, each with their own functions, typology, relations and content.

Mental health interventions are defined as "network interventions" when the professional does not approach the sufferer as a unit cut-off from the whole but considers the individual's problem to be tied into a network of relationships and interactions. Viewed from this perspective, networking is a way of thinking and acting for any professional and not the task of a specific service at the daycare centre. However, the lack of a statutorily mandated, generally accepted philosophy on how mental health services should operate in networks means a co-ordinated effort is required to set up, expand, bolster and firmly establish the use of networks (Stylianidis and Chondros 2007).

Statutorily mandated communication with health services, the involvement of the local authorities, ties between users of the services, participation of the local community in solving specific problems, the involvement of volunteers at an individual and collective level and empowerment of existing local networks are all goals which the service has.

12.9 Networking at the Daycare Centre

The aim of community actions is also to educate and promote mental health, to provide information about the daycare centre, how it works and what it does, to train professionals about mental health issues and to interface with primary healthcare, social bodies and local government authorities. These activities can include workshops, open events to provide information about mental health and talks at associations, to specific population groups like the elderly, school pupils and parents, individuals with physical conditions or disabilities and so on. Activities are also arranged to provide briefings to and train specific professionals in the community: teacher groups, training for policemen about how to handle difficult cases in the Public Prosecutor issued orders, and priest groups to provide information about basic mental health issues. Promoting mental health and social cohesion can also be done by setting up self-help groups for families and volunteers.

As part of the networking initiative and attempt to mobilise community resources and expand job opportunities for clients, the Franco Basaglia Daycare Centre supports the Association of Families and Friends for Mental Health, the Heliotrope Social Cooperative and self-help groups dealing with depression and suicide prevention.

The aim of the Association of Families and Friends for Mental Health is to engage in extensive dialogue about mental health and mental illness, to share experiences with other families coping with similar problems and to open a door to life because often difficulties in talking to someone about mental disorders can lead to a loss of social ties, to isolation and to the refusal of help. The 129 registered members are relatives, caregivers (parents, spouses, etc.) (61), users of mental health services (12), friends (of the family or aware citizens) (29) and mental health professionals (27).

Social cooperatives are statutorily mandated social enterprises that operate in the context of solidarity-based social entrepreneurship. They promote socioeconomic integration and the reinclusion of individuals who have suffered from mental illnesses in the labour market and seek to provide high-quality services and products in a competitive environment. They function as mental health units which contribute to improved levels of autonomy for employees/persons with mental problems and to improving the social and individual skills of those persons to ensure they integrate into the socioeconomic fabric of society and the labour market and also function as businesses providing high-quality services and products in a competitive environment.

The Heliotrope Social Cooperative in the fifth Psychiatric Region was founded in July 2008 on the initiative of mental health professionals and agencies in NE Attica. It cooperates with public and private sector bodies, local government authorities and mental health bodies in the fifth Mental Health Region. The Heliotrope Social Cooperative became operational in October 2010, in partnership with the Municipality of Melissia and school committees, cleaning school playgrounds in the Melissia area. Individuals who have completed the relevant psychosocial rehabilitation programmes are involved in these activities. The cooperative also collaborates with the Ministry of Labour and Social Security to allow its employees to clean the Ministry's offices and communal areas. A canteen and restaurant are expected to open soon in the Marousi area, where light meals will be prepared and distributed.

The public care system's inability to deal with the constantly increasing number of cases, and the complex psychopathology that the crisis has allowed to emerge, makes it vital to set up a protective net for the general population based on intervention on multiple levels, whose goal is to prevent depression and, by extension suicide, to encourage treatment interventions in the community. The depression

Table 12.3 Evaluation indicators

Structure	Procedure	Outcome
Funding	Average waiting time	Severity of symptoms
Funding rate	% of users per type of treatment	Quality of life
No. of staff per area of specialisation	No. of treatments	Satisfaction with services
Max. no. of service users	Active cases	Functionality
Accessibility	Dropout rate	Hospitalisations

This entire process is under way at present in cooperation with the Istituto Mario Negri in Milano

self-help groups are a particularly important means for dealing with depressive symptoms since they promote increased social participation, life satisfaction and reduced stigma (Bologna and Pulice 2011), while it has also been observed that in people to take on such a role, their psychiatric symptoms reduce and their interpersonal relations and skills improve (Moran et al. 2012). Introducing these interventions is a priority since the report on the review of the PSCYHARGOS III Programme (2011–2020) (MHSS 2012) stated that, "in Greece there are very few self-help groups due to the stigma attached to mental illness and the short tradition of involvement in such endeavours, and also non-involvement by services in such endeavours (with few exceptions)". In cooperation with the Hellenic Society of Mood Affective Disorders (MAZI), the Athens Archdiocese and the Salten Psychiatric Centre (in Bodo, Norway), the Regional Development and Mental Health Association undertook to implement an innovative action called "Self-Help, Networking and Therapeutic Support in dealing with depression in urban and island areas" which was financed as part of the "We are all Citizens" programme, which is part of the EEA Financial Mechanism for Greece. The programme seeks to empower and bolster civic society in Greece and is being implemented by the Bodossaki Foundation in cooperation with the EEA's Financial Mechanism Office (http://www.weareallcitizens.gr).

Research, Evaluation and Documentation

Evaluation of the clinical effectiveness and regular documentation and presentation of daycare centre services are integral to its operations. The evaluation of services is done at local and individual levels in relation to structure, procedures and the outcomes of treatments, using the Matrix Model. Emphasis is placed on the opinion of the users of services. Table 12.3 shows three aspects of the evaluation indicators (Thornicroft and Tansella 2010).

12.10 Discussion

Documentation, Research and Evaluation

The documentation of the effectiveness of the daycare centre as a structured set of psychosocial rehabilitation interventions is not adequate at present. Even though individual interventions have been documented, a recent systematic review did not manage to identify randomised controlled studies relating to the overall operation of such a structure, which in the research is defined as a non-medical sector daycare centre (social welfare structures and not-for-profit organisations (Catty et al. 2007). Note that the major diversity of services provided makes research difficult. Research, ongoing evaluation and documentation of services require resources but are necessary and a condition for establishing, disseminating and developing best practices. The limitation on available resources in general, and especially those available for research, the possible objections from professionals to the study of measurable outcomes, the downgrading of empirical studies and the disproportionately low interest in narratives and the viewpoint of patients are major risks for the future of quality psychosocial rehabilitation services in Greece's mental health system.

A Change of Paradigm

The focus of rehabilitation services on the recovery model determines the services' philosophy and practice, redefines their relationships with users of services and opens the path for development. The recovery model does not justify a cutback in services but a transformation. It is reasonable to suppose that the path to recovery includes a gradual reduction in the contact users of services have with mental health services and increasingly greater use of community resources. The daycare centre operates as a locus in the wider community network, giving form and structure to care, combining different services in an attempt to respond to the individual's complex needs at that specific point in time and the needs of the community the individual belongs to.

The transformation of daycare centres requires that in organisational terms they be included in a sectorised network of community mental health services. The proper running of such a structure requires a culture of enquiry and for one to constantly call into doubt established practices. Main considers that ideas expressed in the ego of a generation shift to the superego in the next and acquire a ritual character, thereby losing their creative urge (Campling 2001). Rotelli (1988) talked about a perpetual process of renewal, deconstruction and reconstruction of new institutions in the community as an ideological and scientific framework for limiting the neo-institutionalist culture.

The Risk of Chronicity Outside the Asylum's Walls and Neo-institutionalist Phenomena

Neo-institutionalism, meaning the transfer of the asylum's functions and chronicity to community structures like daycare centres, is a constant threat and has been a reason for the criticism they have received about their role in a network of services and even about their necessity and very existence. Every psychiatric care institution need not necessarily be considered a therapeutic institution a priori. Even after the spread of the social psychiatry movement and the deinstitutionalisation movement, modern history teaches us that an initial intention to treat patients or an ideology that seeks to overturn traditional practices can gradually slip back into a rigid, stereotypical anti-treatment, asylum-like way of working even outside the asylum's walls. P.C. Racamier (1992) points out that "care organisations have a tendency to adjust to psychopathology and to treat it. When that adjustment is very good, then they retain it and reproduce it in perpetuity".

According to J. Hochmann, identifying, understanding, processing and giving meaning to the chronicity which arises from the illness, from the viewpoint of psychocognition, can contribute to defence against the phenomenon of chronicity and fatal repetition. The dialectic of "dependence-autonomy" at the core of the individualised care plan requires persistent work by both the treatment team and also by the patient, so that their relationship is not an end in itself and simply a means of reproducing complete dependence or assimilation, but is a tool for change. The relationship sits within an institutional, organisational and mental setting that can favour the autonomy of the subject. The way in which the multidisciplinary team operates, coupled with external supervision, treatment agreements with a clear start, middle and end, as well as case management which is recorded and re-evaluated at regular intervals in the presence of a third-party guarantor, are just some of the institutional, organisational and psychocognitive attempts being made to overcome the assimilating dualist relationship and achronicity which leads to phenomena of institutionalisation. Therapeutic or rehabilitative activism, the constant search for action far from the needs and preferences of the users of services, may well be the diametrical opposite of what we have been describing, a maniacal defence of the institution in relation to chronicity, which also removes the assignation of meaning and consequently proves to be equally futile and a dead end (Stylianidis 2002).

Optimum Use of Resources or Limitations on Costs and Care

The tendency to limit the development of services and the dramatic reduction in economic costs through the recent adoption of "managed care" by the Greek Ministry of Health, as a part of liberal policy in the health sector, could lead to the degradation of services and a widening gap between the level of treated and untreated morbidity in the general population. The recurring finding that psychosocial treatments are being used less is worrying. The long-term impact of managed care and the clinical and social effects on patients with schizophrenia still need to be fully assessed. It is likely to increase the gap between needs and the services provided (Mojtabai et al. 2009). The unquestioning transfer of epidemiological and management data from some other country to the Greek context would be arbitrary but does add another dimension to the complex problem that exists. The almost total lack of epidemiological data about mental health services in Greece, except for recent studies about the crisis, makes it harder to assess the situation and plan actions.

Towards a New Paradigm?

The complete transformation of the traditional biomedical model of care into a comprehensive network of community mental health services focused on recovery is a complicated process, in both historical and social terms, whose outcome depends on numerous factors and parameters. One of those is the adoption of innovative, documented best practices in how daycare centres can be run so as to avoid phenomena of neo-institutionalism in the community and to promote the empowerment of users of services and the networking of services.

Acknowledgements The authors would like to thank K. Papakonstantinou (scientific officer of the Franco Basaglia Daycare Centre 2007–2012) for his important contribution to developing the daycare centre and transforming it and would also like to thank clinical psychologist K. Papadaki.

Many thanks to the present and past employees and volunteers of the Franco Basaglia Daycare Centre who seek out stories and meaning via the multidisciplinary team.

Bibliography

Anthony WA (2000) A recovery-oriented service system: setting some system standards. Psychiatr Rehabil J 24(2):159–168

Anthony WA, Farkas MD (2009) A primer on the psychiatric rehabilitation process. Center for Psychiatric Rehabilitation, Sargent College of Health and Rehabilitation Sciences, Boston University, Boston

Association of Therapeutic Communities (1999) The need for an NHS policy on developing the role of therapeutic communities in the treatment of 'Personality Disorder'. ATC, London

Barnard RI, Robbins LL, Tetzlaff FM (1952) The day hospital as an extension of psychiatric treatment. Bull Menn Clin 16(2):50–56

Beck A, Rector N, Stolar N, Grant P (2009) Schizophrenia: cognitive theory, research, and therapy. Guilford Press, New York

Biasi S, D'Avanzo B, De Stefani R (2006) Percorsi di cura condivisi; Uno strumento per la condivisione reale e verificabile dei Percorsi di cura. Azienda Provinciale per i Servizi Sanitari, Trento, Available at http://www.fareassieme.it/wp-content/uploads/2011/08/02-APSS-Percorsi-INTRO-epta.pdf, Accessed on 20.8.2014

Bierer J (1948) Social therapeutic clubs. HK Lewis, London

Bion WR (1955) Language and the schizophrenic. In: Klein M, Heimann P, Money-Kyrle R (eds) New directions in psychoanalysis. Tavistock Publication, London, pp 220–239

Bleandonu G, Despinoy M (1974) Hôpitaux de jour et psychiatrie dans la communauté: étude documentaire, institutionnelle et critique. Payot, Paris

Bologna MJ, Pulice RT (2011) Evaluation of a peer-run hospital diversion program: a descriptive study. Am J Psychiatr Rehabil 14(4):272–286

Bonsack C et al (2013) Le case management de transition. Arcos, Lausanne

Briscoe J, McCabe R, Priebe S, Kallert T (2004) A national survey of psychiatric day hospitals. Psychiatr Bull 28(5):160–163

Burns T (2004) Community mental health teams: a guide to current practices. Oxford University Press, Oxford

Byrne M (2005) Community mental health team functioning: a review of the literature. Ir Psychol 21(12):347–350

Cameron DE (1947) The day hospital; an experimental form of hospitalization for psychiatric patients. Mod Hosp 69(3):60–62

Campling P (2001) Therapeutic communities. Adv Psychiatr Treat 7(5):365–372

Carrier J, Kendall I (1995) Professionalism and interprofessionalism in health and community care; some theoretical issues. In: Owens P, Carrier J, Horder J (eds) Interprofessional issues in community and primary health care. Macmillan, London, pp 9–36

Carson J, Bartlett H, Croucher P (1991) Stress in community psychiatric nursing: a preliminary investigation. Community Psychiatr Nurs J 11(8):12

Casagrande SS, Jerome GJ, Dalcin AT, Dickerson FB, Anderson CA, Appel LJ, Charleston J, Crum RM, Young DR, Guallar E, Frick KD, Goldberg RW, Oefinger M, Finkelstein J, Gennusa JV 3rd, Fred-Omojole O, Campbell LM, Wang NY, Daumit GL (2010) Randomised trial of achieving healthy lifestyles in psychiatric rehabilitation: the ACHIEVE trial. BMC Psychiatry 10(1):108

Casey DA, Rodriguez M, Northcott C, Vickar G, Shihabuddin L (2011) Schizophrenia: medical illness, mortality, and aging. Int J Psychiatry Med 41(3):245–251

Catty J, Goddard K, Burns T (2005) Social services day-care and health services day-care in mental health: do they differ? Int J Soc Psychiatry 51(2):151–161

Catty JS, Bunstead Z, Burns T, Comas A (2007) Day centres for severe mental illness. Cochrane Database Syst Rev (1):CD001710

Chevallier-Fougas S (2009) Mise en perspective de deux conceptions du soin psychiatrique adulte: La psychothérapie institutionnelle et la réhabilitation psycho-sociale. Diplôme d'état de docteur en médecine. Université d'Angers, Angers

Deegan E (1988) Recovery: the lived experience of rehabilitation. Psychosoc Rehabil J 11:11–19

Dickey B, Ware NC (2008) Therapeutic communities and mental health system reform. Psychiatr Rehabil J 32(2):105–109

Edward C (1994) The clubhouse model of psychosocial rehabilitation and the development of an evening and weekend recreation program. Glob Ther Recreat III 140–145

Farkas MD, Jansen M, Penk W (2007) Psychosocial rehabilitation: approach of choice for those with serious mental illnesses. J Rehabil Res Dev 44(6):801–812

Guide for organising and running day-care support and follow-up centres/Psychargos Phase II, 2005, Athens, June 2005 (in Greek)

Gunderson JG (1978) Defining the therapeutic processes in psychiatric milieus. Psychiatry J Study Interpersonal Process 41(4):327–335

Haigh R (1999) The quintessence of a therapeutic community. In: Campling P, Haigh R (eds) Therapeutic communities: past, present and future. Jessica Kingsley Publishers, London, pp 246–257

Handa K, Grace J, Trigoboff E, Olympia JL, Annalett D, Watson T, Poulose MC, Muzaffar T, Noyes FL, Kabatt A, Cushman S, Antonelli M, Baxter-Banks G, Newcomer D (2009) Continuing day treatment programs promote recovery in schizophrenia: a case-based study. Psychiatry (Edgmont) 6(4):32

Hannigan B (1999) Joint working in community mental health: prospects and challenges. Health Soc Care Community 7(1):25–31

Hatzistavrakis G, Sakellaropoulos P (2010) Psychoanalysis and psychosis: a difficult but necessary relationship. In: Fitsiou P (ed) The emotional bond between the patient and therapist as the foundation of psychiatry. Papazisis Press, Athens (in Greek)

Hochmann, J. (2003a). The psychomental institution: the psychomental institution. The role of mental care theory within the framework of de-institutionalisation. In: Sakellaropoulos P (Ed.) De-institutionalization and its relation to primary health care. Papazisis Publications: Athens

Hochmann J (2003b) Psychoanalytical theory of psychiatric care of psychoses. In: Damigos D (ed) Deinstitutionalisation and its relationship with primary care. Papazisis Press, Athens, p 452 (in Greek)

Holloway F (1991) Day-care in an inner city. II. Quality of the services. Br J Psychiatry 158(6):810–816

Hornby S (1993) Collaborative care: interprofessional interagency and interpersonal. Blackwell Scientific Publications, Oxford

Hoult J (1986) Community care of the acute mentally ill. Br J Psychiatry 149:137–144

Ives GA (1975) Psychiatric day-care. Can Fam Physician 21(10):61–63

Jauhar S, McKenna PJ, Radua J, Fung E, Salvador R, Laws KR (2014) Cognitive-behavioural therapy for the symptoms of schizophrenia: systematic review and meta-analysis with examination of potential bias. Br J Psychiatry 204(1):20–29

Jeffries N, Chan KK (2004) Multidisciplinary team working: is it both hostile and effective? Int J Gynaecol Cancer 14(2):210–211

Jones C, Hacker D, Cormac I, Meaden A, Irving CB (2012) Cognitive behavioural therapy versus other psychosocial treatments for schizophrenia. Cochrane Database of Systematic Reviews 2012, Issue 4. Art. No.: CD008712. DOI: 10.1002/14651858.CD008712.pub2

Knapp M, Beecham J, Koutsgeorgopoulou V et al (1994) Service use and costs of home-based versus hospital based care for people with serious mental illness. Br J Psychiatry 165:195–203

Liberman R (2008) Recovery from disability: manual of psychiatric rehabilitation. American Psychiatric Publishing Incorporated, Washington, DC

Lieberman J, Drake R, Sederer L, Belger A, Keefe R, Perkins D, Stroup S (2008) Science and recovery in schizophrenia. Psychiatr Serv 59(5):487–496

Madianos M (2005) Psychiatry and rehabilitation. Kastaniotis Press, Athens (in Greek)

Madianos M (2010) Social psychiatric and community mental health, 7th edn. Kastaniotis Press, Athens, in Greek

Mak KY (1994) The changing roles of psychiatric day hospitals in Hong Kong. J Hong Kong Coll Psychiatrists 4:29–34

Mantonakis I, Gyra E, Katan K, Theochari K, Gianakou V, Xagorari E, Stefanis K (1994) Day Hospitals as a multi-faceted therapeutic reconstructive experience. In: Christodoulou GN, Kontaxakis VP (eds) Issues in preventative psychiatry, vol II. Mental Health Centre, Athens, p 433, in Greek

Marshall M, Crowther R, Almaraz-Serrano AM, Tyrer P (2001) Day hospital versus out-patient care for psychiatric disorders. Cochrane Database Syst Rev. 2001;(3):CD003240

Mbaya P, Creed F, Tomenson B (1998) The different uses of day hospitals. Acta Psychiatr Scand 98(4):283–287

McGurk S, Twamley E, Sitzer D, McHugo G, Mueser K (2007) A meta-analysis of cognitive remediation in schizophrenia. Am J Psychiatr 164(12):1791–1802

Ministry of Health & Social Solidarity (2012) Report of the working group to revise the PSYCHARGOS Programme – PSYCHARGOS III National Action Plan (2011–2020). Ministry of Health and Social Security, Athens, Available at: http://www.psychargos.gov.gr/Documents2/%CE%9D%CE%95%CE%91/%CE%A8%CE%A5%CE%A7%CE%91%CE%A1%CE%93%CE%A9%CE%A3%20%CE%93'%20(2011-2020).pdf, accessed on 31.7.2014

Mojtabai R, Fochtmann L, Chang SW, Kotov R, Craig TJ, Bromet E (2009) Unmet need for mental health care in schizophrenia: an overview of literature and new data from a first-admission study. Schizophr Bull 35(4):679–695

Moran GS, Russinova Z, Gidugu V, Yim JY, Sprague C (2012) Benefits and mechanisms of recovery among peer providers with psychiatric illnesses. Qual Health Res 22(3):304–319

Morrison A (2008) Cognitive-behavioural therapy. In: Mueser KT, Jeste DV (eds) Clinical handbook of schizophrenia. Guilford Press, New York, pp 226–238

Norman IJ, Peck E (1999) Working together in adult community mental health services: An inter-professional dialogue. J Ment Health 8:217–230

Novotny PM (2011) Psychiatric rehabilitation and Adult Rehabilitative Mental Health Services (ARMHS): the development of an ARMHS Documentation Training Manual (Doctoral dissertation, University of Saint Thomas)

O'Brien C, Gardner Sood P, Corlett SK, Ismail K, Smith S, Atakan Z, Greenwood K, Joseph C, Gaughran F (2014) Provision of health promotion programmes to people with serious mental illness: a mapping exercise of four South London boroughs. J Psychiatr Ment Health Nurs 21(2):121–127

Onyett S, Ford R (1996) Multidisciplinary community teams: Where is the wreckage? J Ment Health 5:47–55

Onyett S, Smith H (1998) The structure and organisation of community mental health teams. In: Brooker C, Repper J (eds) Serious mental health problems in the community policy, practice and research. Balliere Tindall, London, pp 62–86

Onyett S, Pillinger T, Muijen M (1995) Making community mental health teams work. Sainsbury Centre for Mental Health, London

Onyett S, Pillinger T, Muijen M (1997) Job satisfaction and burnout among members of community mental health teams. J Ment Health 6(1):55–66

Ovretveit J (1993) Co-ordinating community care: multidisciplinary teams and care management. McGraw-Hill International, New York

Papadaki K, Papakonstantinou K, Stylianidis S (2012) Joint management of psychosocial rehabilitation pathways/programmes on the Percorsi di Cura Condivisi model. Presentation of an innovative action for empowerment and recovery of chronic mental patients at the day-care centre run by the Regional Development and Mental Health Association. Synapsis J 25(8):54–59 (in Greek)

Papakonstnatinou K, Papadaki K, Stylianidis S (2008) A day-care centre for psychotic patients. Psychiatriki J 20:255–261 (in Greek)

Parsons T (1977) Social systems and the evolution of action theory, vol 62. Free Press, New York

Peck E, Norman IJ (1999) Working together in adult community mental health services: exploring inter-professional role relations. J Ment Health 8(3):231–243

Pfammatter M, Junghan UM, Brenner HD (2006) Efficacy of psychological therapy in schizophrenia: conclusions from meta-analyses. Schizophr Bull 32(Suppl 1):S64–S80

Pharoah F, Mari J, Rathbone J, Wong W (2010) Family intervention for schizophrenia. Cochrane Database Syst Rev (12):CD000088

Pratt CW, Gill KJ, Barrett NM, Roberts MM (2007) Psychiatric rehabilitation, 2nd edn. Academic, San Diego

Racamier PC (1992) Le génie des origines: psychanalyse et psychoses. Payot, France

Raeburn T, Halcomb E, Walter G, Cleary M (2013) An overview of the clubhouse model of psychiatric rehabilitation. Australas Psychiatry 21(4):376–378

Rössler W (2006) Psychiatric rehabilitation today: an overview. World Psychiatry 5(3):151

Rotelli F (1988) L'istituzione inventata. Per la salute mentale/for mental health, Rivista Centro Regionale Studi e Ricerche sulla Salute Mentale (1)

Sadock BJ, Sadock VA (2008) Kaplan & Sadock's concise textbook of clinical psychiatry. Lippincott Williams & Wilkins, Philadelphia

Saiga M, Watanabe T, Yoshioka SI (2013) Physical and mental factors associated with obesity in individuals with mental disorders attending psychiatric day-care facilities. Yonago Acta Med 56(1):1

Shorter E (2006) A historical dictionary of psychiatry. Oxford University Press, New York, p. 247

Stylianidis S (2002) Institutions, foundations and the psychoanalytic approach to the psychotherapy of psychoses. In: Tzavaras N, Ploumpidis D, Stylianidis S (eds) Schizophrenia: a phenomenological and psychoanalytical approach. Kastaniotis Press, Athens, in Greek

Stylianidis S, Chondros P (2007) Reference points in the running of local mental health networks. Greek Med Arch 24(3):216–223 (in Greek)

Stylianidis S, Lavdas M, Markou K, Belekou P (2013) The concept of recovery from serious mental illness in modern psychiatric care: from concept to implementation in day-to-day practice. Synapsis J 31(9):55–64 (in Greek)

Substance Abuse and Mental Health Services Administration (2012) Mental health, United States, 2010. HHS Publication No. (SMA) 12-4681. Substance Abuse and Mental Health Services Administration, Rockville

Thornicroft G, Tansella M (2010) Για μία καλύτερη φροντίδα της ψυχικής υγείας: Ηθική και δεοντολογία, τεκμήρια και εμπειρία. Αθήνα: Εκδόσεις Τόπος

Torrey EF, Fisher D (1998) Left behind: the seriously mentally ill in the managed care era. Interview by Robin Dorman. Behav Healthc Mag 7(6):12

Tungpunkom P, Maayan N, Soares-Weiser K (2012) Life skills programmes for chronic mental illnesses. Cochrane Database Syst Rev (1):CD000381

Tyrer P, Evans K, Gandhi N, Lamont A, Harrison-Read P, Johnson T (1998) Randomised controlled trial of two models of care for discharged psychiatric patients. BMJ 316(7125):106–109

Vyskocilova J, Prasko J (2012) Social skills training in psychiatry. Act Nerv Super Rediviva 54(4):159–170

Warner R (2006) The diffusion of two successful rehabilitation models. World Psychiatry 5(3):160

Washburn S, Conrad M (1979) Organisation of the therapeutic milieu in the partial hospital. In: Luber RF (ed) Partial hospitalisation. A current perspective. Plenum Press, New York, pp 47–70

Wilson K (2008) The changing face of day hospitals for older people with mental illness. Royal College of Psychiatrists, London

World Health Organisation (WHO) (1996) Psychosocial rehabilitation: a consensus statement, GENEVA. World Health Organisation, Geneva, Retrieved from http://www.who.int/iris/handle/10665/60630 #sthash.oaMaaMeA.dpuf

13

Assertive Community Treatment: Home Intervention for People with Severe and Enduring Mental Health Problems: Designing the Greek Model

Alex Krokidas, Xenia Varvaressou, and Stelios Stylianidis

Abstract

Home intervention for people with severe and enduring mental health problems – assertive community treatment (ACT) – is an intensive intervention programme in the community for people with severe mental illnesses. In the 35 years since the introduction of this specific model, numerous intervention teams were established worldwide, while the criticism directed at the model on the matter of methodology (intervention techniques and targeting) as well as the cost-effectiveness of similar programmes is interesting. Hereinafter, the authors examine the attempts made to form similar teams in Greece, while focusing on the particular socioeconomic conditions and legal/institutional framework in which such attempts were made.

Finally, they present the EPAPSY Day Centre Home Intervention Team and, at the same time, raise the question concerning the manner in which such teams will be supported and framed.

"Tonight we Improvise" (Questa Sera si Recita a Soggeto)

(Luigi Pirandello, 1929)

A. Krokidas
Service Manager, EPAPSY Recovery and Rehabilitation Day Centre, Athens, Greece
e-mail: alexkrokidas@btinternet.com

X. Varvaressou
Home Intervention Team Manager, EPAPSY Recovery and Rehabilitation Day Centre, Athens, Greece

S. Stylianidis (✉)
Department of Psychology, Panteion University, Athens, Greece
e-mail: stylianidis.st@gmail.com

13.1 Introduction

Home intervention – (Assertive Community Treatment, ACT) – is an intensive intervention programme in the community for people with serious mental illnesses (usually schizophrenia or psychotic disorders). As a community intervention model, it has been in operation over the last 35 years. It was developed initially as a pilot programme in the USA by a team of psychiatrists who concluded that traditional psychiatric services did not offer targeted patients' continuity of care. Emphasis was placed on the intensive and methodical use of community resources towards improving social skills and quality of life, without offering any specific medical-oriented approach focusing on pharmacotherapy and the reduction of symptoms.

An ACT team is called to deal with an "abnormal" condition. Abnormality is defined on the basis of a fundamental and necessary conceptual clarification: the distinction between an *emergency* and a crisis.

An emergency psychiatric event is a series of conditions where (Stylianidis et al. 2006):

1. The condition and behaviour of an individual is deemed by someone – and not the individual himself – likely to have a *rapid* catastrophic effect on the individual or another person.
2. The resources available at the time the emergency psychiatric event occurs are not sufficient to cope with it.

Consequently, a crisis situation may include some and/or the above characteristics, but evolve at a slower pace, the effect is not immediate and care for the situation may be delayed for a short period of time.

The aim was to address every patient need (Drukker et al. 2014), such as housing, food and clothing (basic subsistence needs) and develop skills to enable them to manage the needs of a normal social life, particularly for people who, because of repeated admissions, were deprived of the continuity of a normal life in the community. Another significant goal was the possibility of employment (sheltered and/or competitive) and to support a patient self-empowerment system free from dependence relationships (Nordén et al. 2012). Parallel goals were how to teach patients to approach diversity (Leete 1989), marginalisation and stigmatisation. Finally, a significant part of intervention involved educating significant others in the life of the patients (Mavreas et al. 1992) and/or how to reconnect with these significant others so as to enable the extended family system to function relatively smoothly (Tschoop et al. 2001; van Vugt et al. 2012; Watts and Priebe 2002).

In the 35 years since the introduction of this specific model, numerous intervention teams were established worldwide, while the criticism directed at the model on the matter of methodology (intervention techniques and targeting) as well as the cost-effectiveness of similar programmes is interesting.

The concept of "coercion" has been from the outset a structural dimension of the Community Living Programme as well as a high point of the criticism directed at the model. This specific dimension is subject to many interpretations because of the close and assertive therapeutic relationship developed between the therapist and the patient. The dimension of "coercion" and the "strategies" designed to commit the patient to the programme raise both moral issues and ontological and epistemological issues concerning the application of the ACT model.

A key point of criticism refers to the paternalistic practices for which the ACT model has been accused of using. More precisely, it is aimed at patients who show increased resistance to any therapeutic intervention and, therefore, reproached as one of the most "directed" approaches which seems to be contrary to the basic principles of the recovery practice advocating a patient's freedom of choice, the gradual process of empowerment and dynamic presence, autonomy, participation and co-decision in therapy and recovery (Stylianidies et al. 2013; Deegan 1988; Dubuis et al. 2006; Amering and Schmolke 2009; Farkas 2007; Kidd et al. 2010).

An interesting point is that the founders of the model argued that an ACT programme should not be applied to this end and that it should, conversely, through its application aim to allow patients to live freely in the community and improving their quality of life and the convergence of the ACT model and the recovery model (Salyers et al. 2009, 2013; Salyers and Tsemberis 2007). According to the founders of the model, ACT teams operating through coercion or patient "compliance" mechanisms must radically change their practices to the extent that such operation is contrary to the philosophy of the model.

13.2 Structural Features of the Model

An Assertive Community Treatment programme is intended for patients suffering from severe psychopathological illnesses (psychosis, major depressive episodes with suicidal tendencies) who are in an acute phase of the disease, show increased symptoms (highly active symptoms or suicidal tendencies) and a poor track record of relapses and admissions (Rosen et al. 2007).

The target population of this model are, among others, homeless people with a manifest mental disorder, people with dual diagnosis (history of use/abuse of substances and mental disorder) and people facing problems with justice. Issues associated with mental illness are organic health problems (hepatitis, diabetes) and there is an almost complete absence of a social network that could provide support and benefit the patient. A structural feature which serves as a common denominator is that ACT programmes are intended for people who show a high degree of non-functionality in daily autonomous life issues.

A basic, "traditionally" structural feature in the workings of an ACT programme tending to limit the extent of application of the model which is an additional point of criticism is its *purely clinical orientation*. More specifically, a primary objective for patients who enter the ACT programme, which also spearheads the clinical orientation of the model, is to stabilise the symptoms, avoid relapses and admissions and the regular receipt of medication. The key difference from an inpatient therapy model with a clinical orientation is that the ACT team and the way it operates must be assertive, directed *at the* patient with a view to "keep" him/her in therapy and provide stability in the treatment effort, as well as continuity in the provision of services (Stanhope and Matejkowski 2010; Phillips et al. 2001).

Basic Characteristics of an ACT Team

Multidisciplinary medical team: The responsibility for treatment, support and rehabilitation is shared among the members of the team. There are certain distinct roles (such as the team co-ordinator and the psychiatrist); however, responsibility is shared among the members of the team.

Continuity in the provision of services by the entire ACT team.

Team approach techniques: The Assertive Community Treatment model has been criticised for the level of pressure/"coercion" exercised on patient with the aim to commit them to the treatment.

Low patient-therapist ratio; usually each member of the team is responsible for about 10–15 patients.

Any intervention by the team takes place where the problem is located each time, i.e. in the community (in vivo).

Management of medication.

Focus on the management of daily life issues.

The services are provided 24 h a day.

An individual treatment plan is always designed for each patient.

There is no time limit as to the duration of each intervention.

The team operates assertively with respect to the commitment of patients to the treatment and supervises their progress.

13.3 Alternative Community-Based Services: From the Mental Hospital to the Community

The USA

In the 1970s, at the Mendota Institute of Mental Health (Madison, Wisconsin, USA), the psychiatrists Arnold Marx, Mary Ann Test and Leonard Stein (Dixon 2000) established that inpatient services could only provide a temporary adjustment of their medication and a temporary remission of symptoms to specific patients diagnosed with schizophrenia who very frequently used their psychiatric services because of repeated relapses and compulsory admissions. The provision of limited and repeated services to this specific patient group led to the *revolving door patient* effect without any possibility of consistent therapy and rehabilitation. The patients not only failed to show any improvement but also showed, subsequently, a high risk of relapses. At the same time, the specific characteristics of these patients, such as the inability to cope with stressful situations in the community and their "dependence" on the services provided by the mental health system, were serious indications of the failure of the traditional psychiatric model and, inevitably, their referral to the community for care.

With a view to reverse this established "traditional" treatment of patients with schizophrenia, Leonard Stein and his team designed a pilot programme called *Training in community living*. The purpose of this programme was to work within the community with patients with a poor psychiatric track record and the development and improvement of social skills and living skills to enable them to regain the ability for social integration. The philosophy consisted of an assertive move "towards the patient", in their natural living environment and a clear – initially – clinical orientation of the intervention. At the same time, the objective was also the smooth transition of the patient from the mental hospital to the community, helping the patient adapt to the community after a prolonged hospitalisation and the need to provide continuous care rather than the usual fragmentation of mental health services observed in the community.

In an attempt to conduct a "field test" of the new community intervention model, Stein set up two main groups with common characteristics based on importance but also on the qualitative characteristics of the disease, specifically, an "experimental" group consisting of patients participating in the programme and two control groups consisting of patients receiving inpatient services. This test seeks, among other things, to respond to the criticism directed at the emerging model regarding its effectiveness and implementation cost (Drake et al. 2009).

Overall, the findings showed that the services provided in the community helped significantly these specific patients, by mitigating the development and intensity of symptoms, relapses and mandatory admission. In addition, they helped in the development of qualitative of daily living aspects associated with reacquired social skills and living skills.

The pilot phase (*community treatment group*) of this first form of intervention in the community for patients with schizophrenia during the acute phase of the disease was renamed *Community Treatment Program* and, subsequently, *Assertive Community Treatment* or *Program of Assertive Community Treatment* (*PACT*).

Starting with the Mendota Institute of Mental Health, the new community intervention programme was adopted by a number of Centres for Psychosocial Rehabilitation in many states. A significant historical reference is the programme implemented by the Thresholds Centre for Psychosocial Rehabilitation in Chicago. In this Centre, ACT teams were set up since the late 1980s for people with severe mental health problems who are deaf, people with dual diagnosis (mental illness and drug/alcohol abuse) and people with a mental illness who had committed a punishable act (Salyers et al. 2003).

Similar ACT teams were set up in many English-speaking countries, indicatively, (based on the Thresholds Centre for Psychosocial Rehabilitation) in Canada, Australia, Italy (following the Trieste "example"), France and the UK.

The UK

In contrast with the American model, ACT in England was introduced within an already integrated (despite all its serious institutional and organisational problems) community mental health services framework, with the most important structure being the Community Mental Health Team. The process of deinstitutionalisation and transfer of care to the community was, generally and essentially, "completed" when the pilot Assertive Outreach Teams (AOT) were launched in the UK in the 1990s.

To be precise, when we refer to the "completion" of the process, we don't mean that the care in the community system functioned effectively and free of problems. Indeed, the purpose underlying the establishment of the first AOTs in the UK was precisely to solve problems, such as dealing with "difficult" patients, i.e. patients who were unable (or refused) to cooperate with the existing services (difficult to engage), or patients with multiple admissions (revolving door patients). We simply mean that Victorian asylums were permanently closed and the last "chronic" patients were transferred to the community. The fact that the institutional framework and the various host structures were unable, as it turned out, to respond effectively on a treatment/rehabilitation/organisational level to the psychosocial need of a particularly vulnerable population does not mean a framework did not exist. Furthermore, from the outset, the manner in which the asylums were closed without adequate community care structures in place was criticised (Chapman et al. 1991; Langan 1990; Webb and Wistow 1987).

The decision to shut down the most emblematic Victorian asylum, the Colney Hatch Lunatic Asylum, renamed later Friern Hospital (the largest in nineteenth-century Europe), was taken in 1989, and the building was finally sold in 1993 (together with 165 ha of land). The closure of Friern Barnet marked the end of the asylum era. The fact that the building was converted into luxury flats was perhaps, also symbolic of an era indelibly marked by the neoliberal ideology and politics of Margaret Thatcher's government. The fact that, although the vision of care in the community existed since the 1950s, Care in the Community was officially adopted as a policy by Thatcher's government in the early 1980s should not escape our historical attention.

It is not our intention here to position ourselves ideologically vis-à-vis Thatcher's and her successor John Major's neoliberalism but to at least adumbrate the general guiding parameters within which Care in the Community was built and further developed at that particular historical juncture.

Briefly, these were the introduction of a mixed economy of care and the creation of an internal market in the field of care services and the introduction of legislative frameworks such as, for example, Compulsory Competitive Tendering which promoted competition between service providers principally based on cost and with a view to reducing drastically local government expenses.

So, the official intended purpose for the deinstitutionalisation policy and the transfer of care to the community, other than for romantic and humanitarian reasons, was to reduce costs and government expenditure in the mental health domain. Whether this objective was finally achieved remains to this day an open question.

The Establishment of Assertive Outreach Teams

To comprehend the particularity of the ACT approach as implemented in the UK, we must carry out a comparative analysis between Assertive Outreach Teams and "traditional" CMHTs.

CMHT, as mentioned above, was the central community structure for the provision of mental health services until 3–4 years ago, when the system changed. Specifically, and in somewhat simple terms, the system of services may be divided into four categories: (1) community based outreach teams, i.e. primarily CMHTs, as other teams were established later, as we shall see below; (2) inpatient services; (3) day services, i.e. day centres; and (4) housing and rehabilitation structures.

Before examining the home intervention teams, it would be useful to have a general picture of the other three service categories, since such teams do not operate in a vacuum but are developed along with other parts of the system.

Inpatient services. Following the closure of asylums, psychiatric wards were mainly relocated in general hospitals. The involuntary admission process is governed by the 1983 Mental Health Act (amended in 2007). At this point, it is important to state that, contrary to Greece where patients are transferred to mental hospitals by police without the presence of any other person in pursuance of a court order, in the UK involuntary admissions are not permitted without the presence of at least one approved social worker and, after 2007, an approved mental health professional and two psychiatrists (and in special cases, only one). Theoretically, planning for the discharge of patients begins on the first day of admission. Where necessary, the patient is referred to a CMHT or any other team which will be responsible for his/her care in the community. Both parties have an institutional obligation to cooperate so as not to prolong hospitalisation only because a support programme in the community has not been established.

Daycare structures include mainly day centres and recovery centres. On an institutional level, the difference between the two is that the first operates independently from the NHS mental health structures and is managed by non-profit organisations, e.g. MIND, while the latter are from the NHS facilities. As a result, recovery centres (called day hospitals up to a few years ago) also provide psychiatric monitoring and prescription services, while classic day centres don't. Both are governed by the psychosocial rehabilitation philosophy and strive to operate under the recovery model. The programme offered by recovery centres is, in principle, more intensive and short term, usually up to 2 month, whereas the day centre programme is more long term. Until recently, i.e. about 5 years ago, day centres were not subject to time limitations, i.e. patients could stay in day centres for as long as they wished. In recent years, this has changed for many reasons. A significant concern was the development of a transmuted form of institutionalisation and chronicity, where day centres operated as "ghettos" sustaining and encouraging patient reinstitutonalisation, with a "protection" logic consistent with that of earlier asylum structures. The message to day centres was clear-cut: "You may not operate as final destinations, but as stepping stones in a patient's journey, a practice intended to ensure the maximum possible level of patient independence. If you are unable to contribute substantially to the social rehabilitation of patients, you are of no further use". The message was not rhetorical since it was translated into financing mechanisms leading to radical cuts in funding and the closure of many day centres.

Housing structures cover a wide range of needs and are generally divided into those providing a relatively short stay (up to 2 years) and those providing a long stay for individuals who are assessed as very difficult to move to independent residential accommodation. However, even structures designed for long-term patient stay are subject to the institutional requirement of re-evaluating at regular intervals the progress of each patient and documenting in detail the medical and rehabilitation interventions carried out with a view to encouraging each patient to acquire the appropriate skills that would allow him to move to short-term stay structures and, finally, to sheltered or independent residential accommodation with the support of home intervention teams. Whether such structures are satisfactory and compliant is a major subject for empirical research. The risk, as already mentioned in the bibliography, is the development of a new form of institutionalisation or re-institutionalisation in the community. A long stay in structures is one aspect of this phenomenon (Priebe 2004).

Getting back to the home intervention teams, the basic structure of the system on the level of referrals (again on a somewhat simplified basis) over the last 30 or so years (significant changes were made over the last 3–4 years) operated with the CMHTs accepting mainly, but not exclusively, referrals from primary healthcare professionals (GPs, i.e. general practitioners) following an assessment process, or undertaking to care for patients in the community, or referring them to other services, or both.

A typical CMHT has the following characteristics (Burns and Guest 1999):

This is an interprofessional/multidisciplinary team consisting of specialised mental health professionals, psychiatrist(s), social workers, nurses (community psychiatric nurses), occupational therapists and psychologists. Each team has its own secretarial support. It is also customary, although not required by law, for the teams to include a welfare rights specialist and, sometimes, an occupational therapist who provides occupational rehabilitation.

The multidisciplinary nature of the team is not random and reflects the institutionally established multidisciplinary and comprehensive provision of mental health services in the community to individuals with severe and persistent psychosocial issues. The terms "*severe*" and "*persistent*" are used to translate the established terminology "severe and enduring". How one defines traditionally the term "severe and enduring" is an interesting question raised somewhat arbitrarily in the daily life of CMHTs. Arbitrarily, in the sense that up to at least the introduction of the HoNOS system a few years ago, the evaluation of cases referred to CMHTs and the decision as to whether such cases were appropriate was not based on a common scale, such as, e.g. PANSS, BPRS, although these were used rather ad hoc (Bond and Salyers 2004).

It should be noted that, historically, CMHTs provided services to individuals across a broad diagnostic spectrum. So, they did not exclude individuals with depression, personality disorders, obsessive-compulsive disorders and related disorders, so long as they fell within the category of "severe and enduring mental illness".

Detailed Description of the Services Provided by a CMHT

Any member of the team, whatever their specialty, may carry out a comprehensive needs assessment. A common practice is that the assessment is carried by two members from different disciplines, e.g. a psychiatrist and a social worker. However, this varies from team to team. This assessment includes:

An examination of the current mental state (CMS) and psychiatric history
Personal and family history
Potential impact/burden on family and dependents
Support networks
Use of substances and/or alcohol
Risk to self and/or others
Forensic history
Other health issues (physical health)
History of previous contact with mental health services
Skills and competencies (strengths)
Social background, including housing, financial situation, benefits, etc.

Following this assessment and if it is decided that the team will take over the care of the patient, a care co-ordinator or case manager is assigned. This is followed by the planning stage of an individualised care plan (formulation of care plan). When this is agreed, it is recorded and signed by the patient, the case manager and others involved in the plan.

But what is the exact meaning of *case management*? It is quite simply the organisational and therapeutic principle of any individualised care plan for each beneficiary. In theory, it's the principle on which the care plan designed for each patient is based on an assessment of his/her needs, expectations and competencies. This may sound obvious but, actually, it is not that simple. All we have to do is remember the different "asylum logic" or Ervin Goffman's (1968) "total institutions" models. The asylum/institution logic does not ask: "Why are you here, where did you come from, where do you want to go, how can I help you reach this goal?" It provides an a priori answer to a question that was never asked, saying: "You are here with the others and, since you are here, this is your role and these are the rules, and the same role and rules apply to all".

An individualised care plan may not by definition be formulated before any assessment of the needs of the individual contacting the mental health services system. Hereat lies perhaps the likelihood of a conceptual confusion. An individualised plan does not exclude the central planning of services to meet the needs of specific population groups. Indeed, the success of the former is directly related to the success of the latter.

On a practical/organisational level, the model works with each individualised plan co-ordinator being responsible for the co-ordination of the various interventions mutually agreed as necessary on a case-by-case basis. However, the co-ordinator is not just an intermediary (broker). Building a therapeutic relationship initially between the co-ordinator and the user is an integral part of this approach. This, however, is the greatest challenge as this relationship does not follow the rules and methodology of a specific psychotherapeutic model, although, naturally, it may and usually does draw on various models and approaches depending on the preferences and training of the mental health professional. And this is the particularity of this type of therapeutic relationship which is developed and evolves not on the couch or in some practitioner's clinic or office but "out there", at home, in a café, in the street or such other place where the mental health profession must go to meet the patient. A relationship which, naturally, does not stop however much it is tested when the patient is hospitalised.

In practice, the care co-ordinator/case manager is responsible for a specific number of "cases". At this point, it should be pointed out that the rather unfortunate English term "caseload" may refer to the burden or workload assigned to each co-ordinator. Of course, when the number of cases assigned to members of the team places is heavy, the term is rather apt.

Contact with the patient takes place mainly at home. This is a fundamental principle of the care in the community approach. The frequency of visits is subject to negotiation and agreement but in fact they rarely take place more than once a week. If the need arises for more intensive support in order to avert a crisis which could lead to an admission, then the crisis team which is able to offer daily support for a short time period intervenes.

Such interventions may include the administration of medication, psychological treatment and support, family support, psychoeducation, support and advocacy and support in matters relating to benefits, housing, rights, support in the development of social networks, employment, education, cooperation and interconnection with other service structures. In summary, they cater to a broad range of needs related to psychosocial rehabilitation. The fact that such interventions are not limited to administering medication is an important and key component of the psychosocial rehabilitation philosophy and approach.

The progress of any individualised plan is monitored/assessed at regular intervals and provided for under the institutional/legislative framework [at least since 1990 with the introduction of the Care Programme Approach (CPA)]. The teams operate within strictly specified geographical boundaries (sectorisation), while in terms of caseload, staff and composition of the teams, the relevant guide of the Ministry of Health [Mental Health Policy Implementation Guide (PIG) for CMHTs, Department of Health, 2002a] recommends the following:

Each team can handle a population of 10,000–60,000 persons, depending on local morbidity levels and distances travelled by the members of the team when they visit patients.

13 Assertive Community Treatment

Each team, according to the guide, should be composed by eight full-time care coordinators, each being responsible for a maximum 35 cases, as well as 1 consultant psychiatrist, 1-1,5 clinical psychologist(s), 1-3 support staff, 1-1,5 other medical staff and 1-1,5 secretarial support staff.

An indicative estimate is 4½ CMHTs for a population of 250,000 persons (Boardman and Parsonage 2007). The recommended number of staff (WTO = whole time equivalent) per team and cumulatively is set out in detail in the table below.

Requisite full time staff for a population of 250,000 persons – Community Mental Health Teams (CMHTs)

Staff	Full time ratio per team	Total number of staff for a population of 250,000 persons (i.e. for 4,5 teams)
For continuous care	Total = 9,5	Total = 42,75
Community psychiatric nurses	5	22,5
Social workers	2,8	12,6
Occupational therapists	1,7	7,65
For assessment of needs	Total = 5	Total = 22,5
Community psychiatric nurses	3	13,5
Social workers	2	9
Other professionals	Total = 8,5	Total = 38,25
Psychiatrists (consultants)	1	4,5
Other medical staff	2	9
Clinical psychologists	1	4,5
Team supervisors	1	4,5
Pharmacists	0,5	2,25
Professionals for dual diagnosis	1	4,5
Professionals for mental disability	1	4,5
Supervisors for work rehabilitation	1	4,5
Non-professional staff	Total = 7,44	Total = 33,5
Pharmacy technicians	0,44	2,0
Trainee psychologists	1	4,5
Support staff	Not taken into consideration	
Qualified vocational rehabilitation staff	1	4,5
Staff for ethnic minorities	1	4,5
Secretarial support	4	18,0
Total staff	30,44	137,0

So, what are the differences introduced in the ACT model and Assertive Outreach Teams? Initially, the assumption/promise put forward was that, with the reduction of admissions as the primary indicator, these would be more efficient and cost-effective. However, how can one justify the emergence of specialised AOT teams in the UK scene, insofar as both their structure and their operation are actually similar, if not identical, to that of CMHTs? One difference was that, by design, AOTs would have a significantly smaller clinical work volume (caseloads), 12–15 per team member, compared to 35 per each CMHT member. It was deemed almost axiomatic that the smaller caseloads would translate into more intensive work with each patient and, therefore, better outcomes. The answer at this juncture, i.e. after years of parallel and supplementary operation to the CMHTs, and following a number of surveys, is that there were no changes, or at least no radical changes (Burns 2010; Stull et al. 2010).

The initial assumption/promise did not come to pass, as established by Burns (2010): "The small volume of cases and specific ACT team staffing model did not result in any difference in term of outcomes. The organisational structure of habitual/traditional CMHTs is mainly similar to that of ACT's and indications are that they provide identical outcomes with much fewer resources. Consequently, the value of any investment on resources to create highly conforming ACTs can only be called into question".

The reply to the legitimate question why, therefore, do they still exist and operate today in the UK could perhaps be given to some extent using systemic terms. The evolutionary tendency of the mental health services system over the last 25 years or so followed the direction of an ever-increasing specialisation of structures and services. Traditional CMHTs have ceased to exist as such (and, furthermore, the name has ceased to exist) or were transformed into specialised teams serving patients who are categorised and regrouped on the basis of a complex methodology which includes diagnosis, needs, functionality and type of intervention. This is the famous HoNOS, the pivotal tool of the PbR or Payment by Result system implemented in the UK National Health System in recent years.

The following are a few examples of the specialised teams which have emerged and introduced in an increasingly complex structured system:

Assessment and Brief Treatment or Referral Teams. Multidisciplinary teams specialising in new cases entering the system. To a large extent, referrals originate from primary healthcare, i.e. the GPs. Depending on the assessment, they either refer the patient to other teams or provide brief support and treatment (up to 6 months) and refer the patient back to primary healthcare.

Recovery and Rehabilitation Teams. Perhaps the closest offspring of traditional CMHTs. These are multidisciplinary teams providing support and rehabilitation services only to individuals with psychosis. They operate with approximately 40 cases per care co-ordinator. They, as all other teams, follow the classic individual care plan methodology and approach, as institutionally established within the CPA (Care Programme Approach) framework. As of the introduction of the

Payment by Result system 2–4 years ago and the HoNOS patients clustering tool, such patients are exclusively those who fall under the clusters 13, 14 and 15.

Crisis Teams, or as they are now called *Crisis Resolution and Home Treatment Teams*. Institutionally, the gatekeepers of involuntary admissions. They intervene when patients who are under the care of other teams experience a severe relapse and face the risk of being hospitalised. For example, they provide intensive, daily and brief (up to 2 weeks) home support and treatment in order to prevent hospitalisation. They operate 24/7, 365 days a year (at least, theoretically, but in practice they rarely visit patients after 10 pm but there is always a member of the team on call).

Emergency Duty Teams or *Out of Hours Teams*. They operate from 5 pm to 8 am and their role is to intervene in emergency cases, wherever they come from. If necessary, they arrange admission in hospital.

Early Intervention Psychosis Teams. Multidisciplinary teams providing services exclusively to individuals experiencing their first psychotic episode. The main theoretical operational principal is the DUP (duration of untreated psychosis) which is defined as the time between the manifestation of the first psychotic symptom and the initiation of drug treatment. The shorter the time, the better the outcome. This is, in simplified terms, the concept of such teams. Initially, the model was similar to the AOT model, at least with respect to the number of cases per team member, about 12 to 1, i.e. small caseloads and intensive intervention. However, gradually, caseloads rose to the level of 30 to1. In addition, the age limits were 18–35, but very recently the age limit of 35 was eliminated and only a minimum limit persists, since all cases under 18 are taken care by child psychiatric services.

Assertive Outreach Teams. These are, of course, multidisciplinary teams based on the US ACT model, which we have already mentioned. These teams target a specific patient population who refuse or are unable to contact mental health services (difficult to engage patients) with multiple involuntary admissions (revolving door patients). The theoretical model calls for small caseloads, approximately 12 to 1, and is based on team approach, i.e. although a care coordinator is assigned, he/she is not the only one visiting the patient but all the members of the team (not at the same time). It was deemed almost axiomatic that smaller caseloads would translate into more intensive work with each patient and, therefore, better outcomes and, at least, a reduction in duration and frequency of admissions. Studies do not appear to confirm this initial assumption/promise.

Fixated Threat Assessment Teams. A very particular English "innovation". The sole purpose of such teams is to assess and respond to incidents where members of the royal family, politicians and celebrities are threatened. A relevant study showed that 83 % of those likely to threaten, in one way or another, members of the royal family suffered from psychosis (James et al. 2009).

Forensic Mental Health Teams. Multidisciplinary teams for individuals who have committed criminal offences in a setting of mental illness. Likewise, they operate according to the classic individual care plan methodology and approach, with a clear emphasis on preventing the further involvement of patients in punishable criminal acts.

Homeless Outreach Teams. Multidisciplinary teams specialising in psychosocial interventions intended for homeless people with mental illnesses. They operate with the same philosophy based on the individual care plan. Clear emphasis is placed on helping users find suitable accommodation

One can easily guess the patients' path from team to team, through a complex referral system, which is by no means unusual in the way the system operates in the UK.

Our objective, as already mentioned above, was not to carry out an overall assessment and evaluation of the mental health system in the UK. We simply tried to outline a single category of the mental health services system, the home intervention teams. It is unavoidably an imperfect and incomplete picture since we did not examine how such teams are structurally integrated into the overall system which includes inpatient treatment services, daily services and accommodation structures. Historically and gradually, the centre of gravity may have shifted from hospital/asylum structures; however, this does not naturally mean that hospital admissions have disappeared. In fact, recently and, despite all the specialised services provided in the community, we observe an increase in involuntary admissions in the UK, an increase of 12 % over the last 5 years, where 17,000 individuals are "detained" under the Mental Health Act according to the annual Quality Care Commission 2012/2013 report.

Greece

In Greece, in the late 1960s, a team of psychiatrists at the Aiginiteio Hospital led by Professor P. Sakellaropoulos promoted care in the community for individuals with psychoses in an effort to avoid relapses and mandatory admissions. This was a first pilot project confined to the geographical limits of Attica.

The purpose of the first core teams established under the acronym "PCHP" (Psychiatric Care at the Home of the Patient) was to intervene in a crisis and keep the patient at home and in the community. Even though the teams providing psychiatric care at the home of the patient operated for many years targeting individuals with psychosis in an acute phase of the disease through interventions for the purpose of managing any relapses and to keep the patient at home and in the community, they subsequently also provided care to individuals with psychomotor problems (e.g. CNS problems) who developed an associated mental disorder and individuals who, for various reasons, were unable to contact the community and request the provision of mental health services.

However, a key finding was that due to the relative cumbersome nature of psychiatric reforms in Greece, home intervention teams with the structural characteristics of such intervention teams have not yet been established in Greece. With the exception, for specific methodological reasons, of mobile mental health units operating in many Greek regions, the provision of home intervention services to individuals with severe psychopathologies is limited largely to visits by mental health professionals (social workers and carers) from the local municipalities. However, this approach does not provide a methodologically integrated care plan and is often inconsistent in the continuity of care.

Mobile mental health units are community intervention teams with a structural characteristic which differentiates them from PCHP teams and ACT teams. Such mobile mental health units provide their services to both children and adults (see relevant chapters). Their key objective is to intervene on a primary prevention level mainly in geographically remote areas and provide a broad range of psychosocial rehabilitation and psychiatric care services to patients and their families.

A targeted and methodical cooperation is required between all available health services, such as health centres, hospitals, rural clinics and local authorities in order to achieve the above objectives.

The Assertive Community Treatment Team of the "Franco Basaglia" Psychosocial Intervention Centre of the Association for Regional Development and Mental Health (EPAPSY)

In January 2013, the first Assertive Community Treatment team was founded with a view to reinforce the already existing day centre of the Association for Regional Development and for the purpose of providing services in the fifth ToPSY (psychiatric sector in terms of sectorisation) which includes the following municipalities in Attica:

326.000 κάτοικοι.

Agios Stefanos, *Amaroussio*, Anoixi, Afidnes, Varnavas, *Vrilissia*, Grammatico, Polydendrio, Dionyssos, Drossia, Ekali, Kalamos, Kapandritis, Avlona, *Kifissia*, Kouvaras, Kryoneri, Lykovryssi, Malakassa, Marathonas, Markopoulo, Melissia, Nea Erythraia, *Nea Makri*, Nea Palatia, Nea Penteli, Pefki, Pikermi, *Rafina*, Rodopolis, Oropos, Spata, *Artemida*, Stamata, Sykaminos.

The team was staffed by two psychologists, one psychiatric nurse and one social worker.

According to the Mental Health Policy Implementation Guide (PIG) for Community Mental Health Teams in the UK (Boardman and Parsonage 2007), a home intervention team covers an area with a population of 10,000–60,000 inhabitants, and this is dependent on local mortality rates and distances travelled by the members of the team to carry out such visits. In light of the above, we propose to establish a team consisting of eight full-time members. We propose that each member of the team be assigned a load of 35 clinical cases of a total of about 300–350 cases. More specifically, the team shall consist of the following:

Three to four community psychiatric nurses
Two to three social workers
1-1,5 occupational therapists
1-1,5 clinical psychologists
One psychiatrist
1-1,5 other medical disciplines
One to three support workers
1-1,5 secretaries
Receptionists

At first glance it is clear that the day centre ACT is trying to cover an area with a quintuple population with no community mental health services provided other than by the psychiatric department of the general hospital which operates as a satellite hospital for this specific area and with one fifth of the necessary personnel. Another paradox affecting the ontological aspect of this team is that the Ministry of Health does not officially recognise this specific service as a home intervention unit, at least until the time of writing this document, although it does recognise the services provided.

Therefore, in an effort to design the characteristics of a model taking into consideration the socioeconomic conditions in our country (Stylianidis 2003), we were influenced mainly by the English model with the following specificities: the model being formulated combines elements from various specialised teams outlined above. More specifically, it operates up to a certain extent as a crisis intervention team, intensifying its interventions in the event of a serious threat of relapse and hospitalisation or other serious risks. It responds, as necessary, on the same day to cases where the threat is assessed as immediate, e.g. someone calls and reports suicidal thoughts – within 20 min from the call two members of the team depart and visit the caller. In this specific case, and after investing many hours in exploring and assessing the situation, they avert the crisis and evaluate the need to take on the case or to refer it to a more appropriate service, reinforcing thereby a process of interconnection and ongoing treatment for the patient.

Then, the Day Center ACT team integrates elements of *early interventioning psychosis*, in cooperation with the Adolescent Psychiatry Services and intervening in cases of early occurrence of the disease, either on a secondary prevention level (when the patient has already been hospitalised) or even on a primary level (see relevant vignette at the end of this chapter). In such cases, the services provided include medication support and psychiatric monitoring, psychoeducation and family therapy.

Another operational aspect of the Day Center ACT team includes intervention to revolving door patients, individuals with many admissions and great difficulty to commit to any form of therapy.

Services Provided

The services provided by the ACT team are as follows:

Access to mental and general health services
Psychological support
Resolution of practical and social issues, claims for benefits and pensions
Settlement of bills and outstanding financial obligations
Intervention to improve residential premises
Development of daily living and socialisation skills
Psychoeducation
Family counselling and family therapy
Prescription of medication
Psychiatric monitoring

Other than designing individual plans, the team develops demand conditions, which is something new in the current referral system, by appealing to mental hospitals and general hospital psychiatric departments and trying to educate mental health professionals to refer individuals who could receive the services of an ACT team in a timely manner.

The methodological tools used are:

PANSS (Positive and Negative Syndrome Scale): the results for each patient will allow us to identify each patient's position on the quality of symptoms axis and, consequently, the type of intervention required according to the ACT programme. This scale is administered during the first meeting with the patient (intake), if feasible, and then again 6 months later.
GAF (Global Assessment of Functioning): the aim is to explore the overall functionality of an individual, in terms of life in the community.
Comprehensive individual care plan with re-evaluation of needs and objectives every 6 months.

Certain initial outcome indices concern the *reduction of the number of admissions* and the *avoidance of relapses* for individuals receiving the services of the ACT team during the period of commitment to the programme and compared – based on their track record – against the previous number of relapses/admissions. Specifically:

Vignette of ACT Team Case
Siblings D.P. and I.P.

I. Referral
   D.P. and I.P. are two 55- and 53-year-old siblings, respectively. They were referred to us by the social services department of their municipality of residence in the Northern Suburbs. The reason for this referral was twofold: first, D. had caused serious problems to all the services of the municipality as he was aggressive and offensive towards all employees and the local community over the last 10 years and was stigmatised as the region's "madman". Second, the

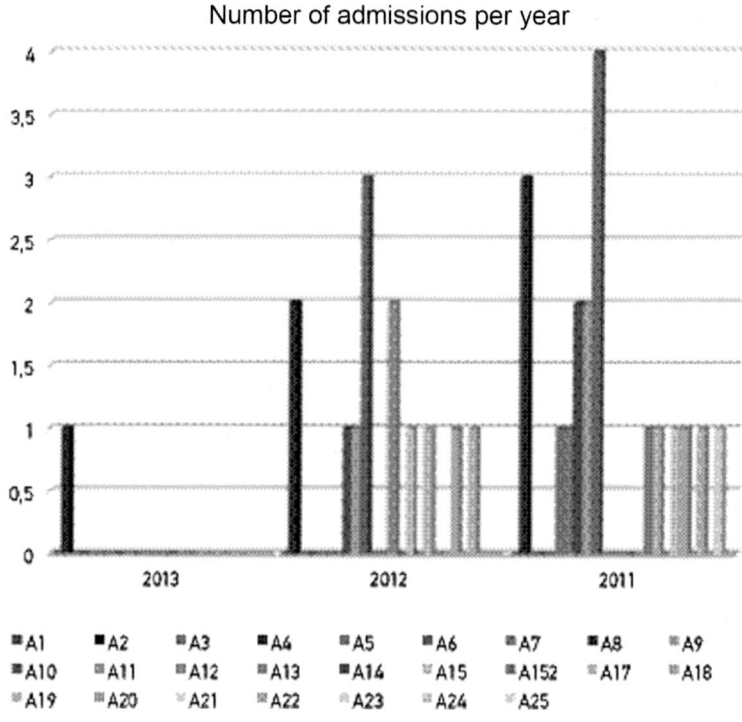

Αριθμός νοσηλειών ανά έτος = Number of admissions per year

lack of any municipal specialised mental health professional staff did not facilitate the provision of ongoing care.

II. Psychosocial history

D. mentions domestic violence during their childhood from a very stern and overbearing father, who worked as a builder and an alcohol abuser. The mother is depicted as a passive and busy housewife. The first signs of the disease appeared around the age of 19 when he was involuntarily hospitalised for the first time. At the same time, he began taking on occasional jobs but stopped at the age of 27 and received a disability pension because of his health problems and recurrent hospitalisations. He describes his hospitalisations as traumatic and abusive experiences. On the average, over the last 30 years, he has been involuntarily hospitalised twice every year.

I. attended high school up to the last grade. She managed to complete a hairdresser course and worked for 2–3 years as a hairdresser, but because of the deterioration of her condition she stopped working. The onset of the disease occurred at the age of 19. Since then, she has been hospitalised about ten times. She very often talks about her unfortunate engagement and her wish to marry and have a family, a wish which is very often a structural component of an erotic delirium. The information provided by colleagues from the municipal social services is that, perhaps, the two siblings have a sexual relationship.

The father passed away in 1983 and the mother in 2009. For several years, the mother was bedridden due to serious health problems. The first serious complaints from the neighbourhood received by the municipality referred to the inadequate care provided to the elderly mother by the siblings and the likelihood that she was being physically and verbally abused. However, after the death of her husband, D. and I. were placed under her guardianship.

III. Clinical picture

D. has been diagnosed on the axis as F30-39 – bipolar disorder with psychotic features (ideas of grandeur, auditory and visual hallucinations). In 2009, D. attempted to commit suicide. He has not provided any information on any other attempt. His sister I. has been diagnosed with F20 schizophrenia.

For a period of 3–4 months since the team's intervention, D. and I. have no insight. D. speaks mainly of his "sufferings", referring to his hospitalisations as "the will of God", who will "elevate" him. I. wonders what's wrong with them which leads to their hospitalisation. A working assumption for both siblings is that this is a case of a folie a deux (shared psychosis), where D. exhibits a prevalent delirium. It is typical that for several months they spoke roughly at the same time about what has happened to them using much the same common experiences, with D. leading I., permitting her to talk or not. After several months of intervention they talk about their "small problem" and about experiencing "great stress".

IV. ACT team intervention

The ACT team took charge of the two siblings at the end of August 2013. Their living conditions were appalling. They lived in a house with the bare necessities, inadequate water supply because the plumbing network was damaged, full of animal faeces, piles of dirty clothes scattered on the floor, many broken appliances and lots of junk, mouldy dishes and food in the sink and their many debts and unpaid bills (electricity and water supply, taxes, etc.) and virtually without heat. They got their meals from the municipal soup kitchen and, at the same time, they spent both their pensions to buy ready meals.

During the first meeting, D. was suspicious, irritable and resented our presence in his home. He felt that the neighbours would suspect he was being visited by mental health professionals and that he would be stigmatised, even though the neighbourhood was already aware of him. He also said that he was ashamed of the conditions in his house.

Three days after our first meeting, he visited the offices of the municipality in a frantic condition and verbally attacked the employees. The municipality initiated immediately the process for his involuntary admission and D. was admitted to a psychiatric clinic. It should be noted that at that time he had not been taking his medication for 3 months.

We started treating D. at the hospital and I. at home. In the hospital, D. complained about the conditions, was worried about his sister and was anxiously waiting to be discharged. We began discussing and preparing a care and support plan. It should be noted that he expressed his gratitude regarding our visit during his stay at the hospital. This was the first time any service such as ours was involved in the difficult *transition* from the hospital to the community.

During the first 2 months after being discharged from the hospital, the discussion regarding his medication plan and the preparation of a care plan were completed. The siblings are visited at home twice a week mainly by the psychologist, the nurse and the psychiatrist and, in addition, there was frequent telephone contact. D. showed signs of a relapse, given his refusal to take his medication for a long period. Visits were intensified. The main medical objective was to convince D. to commit to a minimum medication regimen in order to avoid a new relapse and prevent the likelihood of a new admission, something which was achieved and resulted in avoiding a new involuntary admission. During this 10-month intervention, D. and I. have not been hospitalised.

V. Main axes of work

During this 10-month intervention by the team, the two siblings have joined a personal care plan.

The following objectives were achieved under the main axes of work undertaken by the ACT team:

1. *Frequency of visits*

    The visits were scheduled to once a week and there is also frequent telephone contact with the case manager.

2. *Practical help with daily life skills activities*

    (a) A money management plan was set in place, given that both siblings receive pensions which are sufficient to cover their needs.

    (b) The house was cleaned by members of the team as well as with the help of both siblings. A member of the team is responsible for the weekly visit to the house during which daily chores (home care, preparation of meals, etc.) are carried out according to a specific plan. All home supplies are also purchased once a week, with the cooperation of D. and I. In addition, we contacted voluntary charity organisations which offered furniture and kitchen utensils.

3. *Medication regimen*

    The ACT team has also undertaken to provide both siblings their injectable medication. At the same time, the team has undertaken to accompany the siblings during medical visits (pathologist, endocrinologist, dentist). Finally, the team psychiatrist has undertaken the psychiatric follow-up care and the prescription of medication.

4. *Help with social welfare benefits and financial aid*

    The team has tried to accumulate the siblings' debts and make arrangements with public authorities as well as settle any outstanding bills. Actions were taken to integrate them as vulnerable people into the social residential tariff of the power supplier in order to secure a significant reduction in power consumption and claim all the rights and benefits to which they are entitled to as disabled persons.

5. *Interconnection of services*

    Throughout the intervention, the team maintains an interconnection with all the municipal services and the welfare department in order to ensure a greater flow of resources from the community to the two siblings as well as to monitor the case in the best possible way.

6. *Accommodation and rehabilitation of accommodation facilities*

For D., rehabilitation will be achieved – as he himself says – through the settlement of his debts and improved living conditions. Therefore, in strict recovery terms, through the beneficiary's perspective, this is now being achieved.

Concerning the house where the two siblings live, efforts have been made to repair damages and secure new electrical appliances and furniture.

7. *Work with the family*

This is a rather difficult part of the job considering the previously strained relations with the family as well as D.'s disdain mainly for his relatives. However, as they refer frequently to one to three relatives (cousins) with whom they would like to reconnect, the team has tried to locate them and establish a new relationship with them. An interesting fact is D's now diminished insight relating to his "behaviour issues" – as he says – that led relatives to keep their distance.

8. *Commitment*

A structural element of the work of the ACT team with the siblings on which all the aforementioned axes of intervention are based is the sibling's extent of commitment to the treatment plan and cooperation with the team.

Two key elements contributed to this effect: first, our visits at the hospital when D. was admitted when we began working with him. He felt, as he himself says, the "companionship" offered by the members of the team during one of his many admissions and that someone cared for him. Second is the fact that the members of the team were not judgmental about his living conditions. This intervention was established on the basis of a fine and fragile line between a specific methodological approach by the professionals and dealing with the siblings under their own "terms": the permission to enter their home as well as accept their hospitality terms – sit with them on dirty furniture and accept their treats and the acceptance of their diversity and their different living conditions.

Outcomes (D)

Tools
GAF on the first intake: 15
GAF – currently (10 months later): 35

PANNS on the first intake:
Positive: 34
Negative: 30
Overall: 75

PANNS – currently (10 months later):
Positive: 26
Negative: 23
Overall: 60

ACT Team Case Vignette
Y.L.

I. Psychosocial background facts

Y is a young 24-year-old man, the son of a family of four. He has a brother who is 3 years older. His father is a retired civil servant and his mother a hairdresser. He lives with his family in a privately owned house in the North Suburbs.

II. Clinical facts

Y's parents visited us in January 2014. They described the change in their son's condition over the last months. About a year before our meeting with the parents, Y was a particularly sociable young man, with many friends, who very went out often during the week to have fun with his friends and was meticulous about his appearance.

Since Christmas 2012, Y began withdrawing, had no telephone contact with his friends and avoids meeting them. The parents refer to a period when he often went to the bathroom and they worried that he suffered from some kind of renal disease.

He is described as a bad student and quite highly strung, irritable. A year ago he was quite a drinker. Now he doesn't drink or smoke. Over the last few months he refuses to cut his hair, shave or take a bath and does so only after being encouraged by his mother and, then, only once every 3 weeks.

His parents described in detail Y's rituals. He spends a long time in the bathroom (approximately 50 min every time and as frequently as two to three times a day) and cleans it meticulously. Because there is only one bathroom in the house, if any other member of the family needs to use it, Y agrees to come out with some difficulty but goes back in to "finish" what he was doing. He doesn't drink water, only juices. He washes his face thoroughly, refuses to use the toilet soap and prefers to use the kitchen soap.

Other rituals include the use of objects such as, for example, opening and closing his mobile phone, counting coins and stacking them up and placing them in a particular way. All these activities may last for about an hour. After some months, he refused to sleep in his bed and instead sleeps sitting up on the sofa.

Y began quarrelling with his parents who were unable to understand the "meaning" of all these rituals. The only thing giving the impression that he is relatively able to function as a healthy person is his work. He works with his brothers in a technical company which manufactures signs and unfailingly asks his mother every day to wake him up to go to work.

In autumn 2013, the parents tried to bring Y into contact with a private psychiatrist, who after one session prescribed an antidepressant. Y refused to take it. The quarrels at home persisted, there was no follow up from the psychiatrist and the parents decided to contact another practitioner in parallel with our own intervention.

A key factor of the intervention is that the parents are seeking a specific medication solution for Y, even if he is unaware of this (covert administration of medication), while the ACT team intervention moves in a completely opposite direction. The private psychiatrist prescribed risperidone in liquid form and advised them to administer it covertly in water or juice. The parents employed this "method" for a week; however, the ACT team's intervention includes two points which convinced them to stop:

> First, Y must first understand through our meetings what is happening to him, trust the members of the team and build a therapeutic relationship with us. The covert administration of medication and the resulting recession of the symptoms would not help him in the process of understanding, gaining insight and taking responsibility for his health condition and treatment.
>
> Second, morally, the covert administration of medication violates Y's rights as a patient.

III. Interventions

We started seeing Y in February 2014. He showed up about 50 min late as he first had to complete his rituals. He was guarded, aloof and wary. The first meetings were of a psychoeducational nature for him and his parents in an effort to alleviate their anxiety and Y's wariness as to who we are. The first two to three times he asked us to not visit him again. At that time and while Y's verbal abuse of his parents increased, his father informed us that he had initiated the process of involuntary admission (by court order). We urged him to "freeze" the process and return to the team and work with Y. Along with the meetings and a psychoeducational process to inform Y on the use of medication, their potential adverse effects as well as how this medication could help him, the team psychiatrist prescribed overtly risperidone in liquid form. Y was convinced and has ever since been taking his medication and is monitored on regular basis by the psychiatrist. Y's diagnosis moves along the F20–29 axis with an estimation of initial occurrence of the disease.

At the same time, we initiated a structured family therapy intervention by family therapists at the day centre in which Y now participates. In addition, the psychiatric monitoring takes place in the day centre during meetings which Y attends unfailingly.

IV. Axes of work

The following objectives were achieved under the main axes of work in cooperation with the ACT team:

1. *Frequency of visits*

    The visits are scheduled to once a week in the form of socialisation outings and there is also frequent telephone contact with the case manager. Y is now open to outings and also plans activities outside the home without the members of the team.

2. *Practical help with daily life skills activities*

    Support in self-care to which Y responds very successfully (he showers often, cuts his hair and shaves regularly).

3. *Medication*

    He now takes his medication on his own. His clinical picture shows some signs of depression. This is an expected outcome given that Y is now gaining insight, is becoming connected with his history, started giving again thought to his health condition and identifying problems in his relations with others.

At the same time, a significant reduction in active symptoms and rituals has been observed while he no longer sleeps on the sofa.

4. *Help with social welfare benefits and financial aid*

Y communicated his desire to change his job and work voluntarily in various activities. The team supports him in these areas.

5. *Accommodation and rehabilitation of accommodation facilities*

He expressed the need to live alone at some point and this is a significant item in his personal care plan and assertive recovery process.

6. *Work with the family*

The family therapy sessions where all participate are ongoing. Y is thinking of reuniting with his old friends and the team is encouraging him in this effort.

7. *Commitment*

During this 4-month intervention, Y and the other members of the family participate actively in setting up and implementing his personal care plan.

Outcomes

Tools
GAF: on the first intake, 42
GAF: currently (four months later), 61

PANNS: on the first intake:
Positive: 23
Negative: 36
Overall: 67

PANNS – currently (4 months later):
Positive: 16
Negative: 24
Overall: 44

In Lieu of Conclusion: Findings, Outlook and Concerns

As we have already indicated, any efforts to establish home intervention teams in Greece have never been included in the strategic plan for psychiatric reform. Any individual efforts which may have been pockets of good practice, though never assessed, remained just that, i.e. pockets within an institutional framework that did not envisage and still does not envisage the establishment of such teams and their systemic integration with other mental health services structures. The national action plan at this stage of psychiatric reform in Greece leaves little doubt about this. The mobile units are a special case only for remote areas.

The question is why reform in Greece bypasses what is possibly the quintessential psychosocial rehabilitation community structure which is the home intervention teams. We use intentionally the designation "quintessential", in the sense that the interventions by home intervention teams are not provided within any structures (pre-)designed by mental health professionals but at the users' home, i.e. in a space that does not belong to and was not designed by mental health professionals. Contrary to this, all community services (other than the limited liability social cooperative [LLSC – KoiSPE] and, of course, the mobile units) are patient "reception" structures, e.g. day centres, mental health centres, residential units, boarding houses, sheltered residential accommodation, etc. Of course, we are not suggesting that such structures are less useful, but we are just highlighting, at least in our opinion, one interesting difference with symbolic, moral as well as therapeutic/rehabilitation aspects and consequences.

Our initial question remains unanswered but let's not rush to engage in worn-out and off-the-shelf criticisms "against any person responsible". We choose to put it forward as an issue for further discussion and analysis, not only for Greece but also for other countries. Moreover, as regards the home intervention model in particular, Greece does not fall short compared to other countries. The World Health Organisation report (2008), *Policies and Practices for Mental Health in Europe: Meeting the challenges*, states indicatively that only in the UK (England and Wales but not Scotland) all patients with chronic and serious mental illnesses have access to Assertive Outreach Teams. In 16 of the 42 countries covered by the report, e.g. a percentage of 38 %, do not have access to such services (WHO 2008). For example, in Italy the percentage of patients with access is between 1 % and 20 %, in Germany 51–80 % and in Switzerland 1–20 % (Table 6.12). In terms of home intervention teams for the treatment of a first psychotic episode (early intervention psychosis), 80–100 % have access to such services in three countries only (Germany, UK and Luxembourg). In Italy and Switzerland the percentage is between 51 % and 80 % (Table 6.14).

We could say then, by way of a provisional conclusion, that, Greece is not exactly an exception as regards the existence and operation of home intervention teams. Of course, this doesn't mean that we must accept this situation as is. The subject of psychiatric reform remains open.

Bibliography

Amering M, Schmolke M (2009) Recovery in mental health: reshaping scientific and clinical responsibilities. Wiley, West Sussex

Boardman J, Parsonage M (2007) Delivering the government's mental health policies. SCMH, London

Bond GR, Salyers MP (2004) Prediction of outcome from the Dartmouth assertive community treatment fidelity scale. CNS Spectr 9(12):937–942

Burns T (2010) The rise and fall of assertive community treatment? Int Rev Psychiatry 22(2):130–137

Burns T, Guest L (1999) Running an assertive community treatment team. Adv Psychiatr Treat 5(5):348–356

Chapman T, Goodwin S, Hennely R (1991) A new deal for the mentally ill: progress for propaganda? Crit Soc Policy 11(32):5–20

Deegan PE (1988) Recovery: the lived experience of rehabilitation. Psychosoc Rehabil J 11(4):11–19

Dixon L (2000) Assertive community treatment: twenty-five years of gold. Psychiatr Serv 51(6):759–765

Drake RE, Bond GR, Essock SM (2009) Implementing evidence-based practice for people with schizophrenia. Schizophr Bull 35(4):704–713

Drukker M, Laan W, Dreef F, Driessen G, Smeets H, Van Os J (2014) Can assertive community treatment remedy patients dropping out of treatment due to fragmented services? Community Ment Health J 50(4):454–459

Dubuis J, Stylianidis S, Harnois GP (2006) La réhabilitation: une problématique mondiale. Inf Psychiatr 82(4):321–330

Farkas M (2007) The vision of recovery today: what it is and what it means for services. World Psychiatry 6(2):68

Goffman E (1968) Asylums: essays on the social situation of mental patients and other inmates. Aldine Transaction, Chicago

James DV, Mullen PE, Pathé MT, Meloy JR, Preston LF, Darnley B, Farnham FR (2009) Stalkers and harassers of royalty: the role of mental illness and motivation. Psychol Med 39(09):1479–1490

Kidd S, George L, O' Connell M, Sylvestre J, Kirkpatrick H, Browne G, Thabane L (2010) Fidelity and recovery – orientation in assertive community treatment. Community Ment Health J 46(4):342–350

Langan M (1990) Community care in the 1990's. Crit Soc Policy 29:58–70

Leete E (1989) How I perceive and manage my illness. Schizophr Bull 15(2):197

Mavreas VG, Tomaras V, Karydi V, Economou M, Stefanis CN (1992) Expressed emotion in families of chronic schizophrenics and its association with clinical measures. Soc Psychiatry Psychiatr Epidemiol 27(1):4–9

Nordén T, Malm U, Norlander T (2012) Resource Group Assertive Community Treatment (RAct) as a tool of empowerment for clients with severe mental illness: a meta-analysis. Clin Pract Epidemiol Mental Health: CP & EMH 8:144–151

Phillips SD, Burns BJ, Edgar ER, Mueser KT, Linkins KW, Rosenheck RA, Herr ECM (2001) Moving assertive community treatment into standard practice. Psychiatr Serv 52(6):771–779

Priebe S (2004) Institutionalization revisited–with and without walls. Acta Psychiatr Scand 110(2):81–82

Rosen A, Mueser KT, Teesson M (2007) Assertive community treatment-issues from scientific and clinical literature with implications for practice. J Rehabil Res Dev 44(6):813

Salyers MP, Tsemberis S (2007) ACT and recovery: integrating evidence-based practice and recovery orientation on assertive community treatment teams. Community Ment Health J 43(6):619–641

Salyers MP, Bond GR, Teague GB, Cox JF, Smith ME, Hicks ML, Koop JI (2003) Is it ACT yet? Real-world examples of evaluating the degree of implementation for assertive community treatment. J Behav Health Serv Res 30(3):304–320

Salyers M, Hichks L, McGuire A, Banmgandner H, Ring K, Hea-Won K (2009) A pilot to enhance the recovery orientation of ACT through per-provided illness management and recovery. Am J Psychiatr Rehabil 12(3):191–204

Salyers MP, Stull LG, Rollins AL, McGrew JH, Hicks LJ, Thomas D, Strieter D (2013) Measuring the recovery orientation of assertive community treatment. J Am Psychiatr Nurses Assoc 19(3):117–128

Stanhope V, Matejkowski J (2010) Understanding the role of individual consumer–provider relationships within assertive community treatment. Community Ment Health J 46(4):309–318

Stull L, McGrew J, Salyers M (2010) Staff and consumer perspectives on defining treatment success and failure in assertive community treatment. Psychiatr Serv 61(9):929–932

Stylianidies S, Lavdas N, Markou K, Belekou P (2013) The concept of recovery from a serious psychiatric illness in modern psychiatric care: from the conceptual approach to its implementation in daily practice. Synapsis 24(1):55–64

Stylianidis S (2003) Assertive community treatment: investigation of its application in Greek psychiatry. Arch Hell Med 20(3):243–250

Stylianidis S, Gionakis N, Pantelidou S (2006) Guide for the organisation of crisis and emergency services. Ministry of Health and Social Solidarity, Operational Plan "Health – Welfare 2000-2006", Athens

Tschoop M, Berren N, Bong C (2001) Consumer perceptions of ACT interventions. Community Ment Health J 47:408–414 van Vugt MD, Kroon H, Delespaul PA, Mulder CL (2012) Consumer-providers in assertive community treatment programs: associations with client outcomes. Psychiatr Serv 63(5):477–481

Watts J, Priebe S (2002) A phenomenological account of users' experiences of assertive community treatment. Bioethics 16(5):439–454

Webb AL, Wistow G (1987) Social work, social care and social planning: the personal social services since seebohm. Longman, London

World Health Organization (WHO) Regional Office for Europe (2008) Policies and practices for mental health in Europe: meeting the challenges. WHO Regional Office Europe. http://www.euro.who.int/__data/assets/pdf_file/0006/96450/E91732.pdf

Brief Psychotherapy in a Community Framework

14

Marina Skourteli and Stelios Stylianidis

Abstract

This chapter addresses the need to integrate brief psychotherapy as the most appropriate model for the provision of psychotherapeutic intervention in a public or community framework. The discussion begins with a historical overview of the development of brief psychotherapy starting from psychoanalysis and goes on to point out the key principles highlighting the differences between brief psychotherapy and open psychoanalytic treatment, particularly within the context the modern socioeconomic challenges governing the provision of mental health. It also addresses the psychodynamic approach in brief psychotherapy and presents research findings with regard to its effectiveness. Common factors with regard to the effectiveness of brief psychotherapy are highlighted with the main focus on the therapeutic alliance and the therapist's role; these are shown through a clinical example of brief psychotherapy in the community. Finally, the pressing need is highlighted for intensive training and supervision for psychotherapists working in a intensive, brief therapeutic framework.

M. Skourteli (✉)
CPsychol Specialising in Psychotherapy, DPsych., AFBPsS, HCPC Reg.,
Head of Psychotherapy Service, 'Franco Basaglia' Day Centre, EPAPSY, Athens, Greece
e-mail: marina.skourteli@gmail.com

S. Stylianidis
Department of Psychology, Panteion University, Athens, Greece
e-mail: stylianidis.st@gmail.com

14.1 Introduction

This chapter tries to point out the necessity of integrating and utilising brief psychotherapy in a public mental health framework, in particular that of the reality in Greece, given the socioeconomic crisis conditions. Although the authors are trained in psychodynamics/psychoanalysis, they make a conscious choice to adapt psychodynamic/psychoanalytical principles, approaches and techniques into a public mental health framework. In a public system with its accompanying socioeconomic challenges, the target of this standpoint is not the full understanding of the patient's unconscious outside the boundaries of time, but the recognition of a limit that ensures the immediate therapeutic benefit of both the patient and the therapist, meeting in a public framework of mental health provision (Gillieron 1994, 1997; Despland et al. 2010). The work begins with a historical overview of brief psychotherapy development from Freud and his followers extending to the current socio-economic background and the contemporary challenges surrounding their implementation in public mental health frameworks. The significance of the initial case estimates during the first interview is set out as an integral part of the therapeutic process in brief psychotherapy, followed by the basic therapeutic principles governing the practice of brief psychotherapy, which are radically different to those of "open" psychotherapy. Due to the limited space, the chapter addresses only the psychodynamic approach to brief psychotherapy, which is supported by research regarding its effectiveness relative to corresponding "open" psychotherapy treatments. In conclusion, the importance of the therapeutic alliance and the therapist's role in brief psychotherapy is showcased, as well as the imperative need for intensive training and supervision of the therapists working in a fast-paced, brief therapeutic framework. Finally, the Greek example of brief psychotherapy in a public framework is put forth as well as a clinical vignette from the Psychosocial Intervention Day Centre of EPAPSY.

14.2 Historical Overview

According to many, it was Freud who first used brief psychotherapy. According to Freud, the patient's symptoms were due to unconscious, traumatic but regressed memories, which, once recalled, together with their emotional foundation, and made conscious, led to symptom elimination (Symington 1986; Mander 2000; Coren 2001). Recognising, however, that not all patients were eligible for hypnosis, the classic method used to recall regressed memories from the unconscious, Freud, during the pre-analytical period, developed the "cathartic" method, a process whereby the patient lays on the divan bed and, with the help of the analyst, who applied gentle pressure on the patient's forehead and actively encouraged him to remember, the regressed memories were recalled and the conflicting emotions were experienced, resulting in the restoration of mental health. Despite the fact that these early therapeutic approaches and techniques were experimental and were later modified (e.g. after this first technique of the cathartic method, Freud went on to the free association method), they were in essence brief, specific symptom oriented and significantly based on the therapist's active participation (Freud 1893, 1895, 1905). In that sense, these first psychoanalytical approaches were the same or similar to contemporary brief psychotherapeutic approaches, where the clarity, the active therapeutic attitude and the focus on a specific therapeutic planning are important elements (Mander 2000; Coren 2001).

During this early period, the analyst maintained an active or even guiding attitude, whereby he often encouraged the recall of regressed memories from the unconscious, while supporting as well as updating the patient regarding the process and course of analysis, through an active therapeutic practice. Later, especially in the context of his disputes with his followers, Freud abandoned this position, in order to defend the clarity of psychoanalysis as an inclusive model for the deeper and fuller understanding of the individual's psycho-cognitive function (Freud 1917, 1920, 1923). Even so, the early psychoanalytical attitude made the patient more of a collaborator that is a passive recipient of the analyst's interpretations. Here, it is worth mentioning that transference became the central and most important element of psychoanalysis much later. Freud initially believed that psychoanalysis was not indicated for people with major pathology and that, on the contrary, it was appropriate for the lighter cases. It is interesting that today, many psychoanalysts, as well as some researchers, maintain the exact opposite, namely, that psychoanalysis is also indicated for major psychopathology cases (Mander 2000; Coren 2001; de Maat et al. 2009).

The first treatments Freud gave were exceptionally brief and lasted just a few weeks or months. For example, Gustav Mahler and Katharina's analysis (Jones 1956; Kuehn 1965) was conducted over the duration of a walk, while Bruno Walter and Lucy R.'s analyses lasted six sessions and 9 weeks respectively (Freud 1893; Walter 1947; Sterba 1951; Coren 2001). As we said before, and particularly within the context of Freud's attempt to ensure the clarity of psychoanalysis as a robust therapeutic model for the in-depth understanding of the individual's psycho-cognitive system, the cathartic method was finally replaced by that of free association, which required therapeutic neutrality, and correspondingly increased the possibility of the patient's regression from the therapeutic process. The concepts of resistance, defence, character analysis and the in-depth working through as well as the issue of the end of therapy may be considered as the natural aftermath of this new technique, which inevitably made treatment duration a lot longer. At the same time, analysts became less active, supportive or "challenging" in their attitude, while the interpretation (mainly of patient transference) became the tool for analysis and therapeutic change. Gradually, treatments lost the boundaries of time and acquired a quality of timelessness. Consequently, the need to focus on specific therapeutic targets or symptomatic relief ceased to be a therapeutic priority (Coren 2001).

Freud's theory was actually based on a purely intrapsychic, solitary supposition of the psyche that paid scant attention to the role or participation of others. Also in the context of therapy, the analyst remains a distant observer to the therapeutic process. Many of Freud's followers, such as Otto Rank, Sandor Ferenczi and later Alexander and French, Michael Balint and David Malan, adopted a critical stance to the scientific positions and clinical applications of the theory of psychoanalysis and proposed instead clinical approaches based on an intersubjective background that continue to influence the development of brief psychotherapy to this day. For Rank (1929), for example, therapy (much as life) must have an end, and issues such as separation, dependence and differentiation emerge in each therapy session. Acceptance of the reality of the end, according to Rank (1929), can be seen as the dominant characteristic of any "successful" treatment, while the determination of a clear end date and the investigation of the reactions relating to it would make it a therapeutic priority. Rank's theory on brief psychotherapy (the ideal duration was considered to be a period of 7–9 months, symbolic of the gestation period) is what led to the final rupture of his relationship with Freud in 1926 (Lieberman et al. 2012).

Just like Rank, Ferenczi (Ferenczi and Rank 1925) was also concerned with the increasing inactivity, passivity and a tendency to intellectualise (he thought that psychoanalysis became a chiefly academic exercise that benefited the analyst more than the patient), as well as the lack of emotional reciprocity between the analyst and the patient. Ferenczi believed that by emphasising the most important dimension of the therapeutic relationship, namely, the emotional interaction between patient and analyst, the duration of therapy would become briefer. He also questioned the axiom of therapeutic neutrality, as he believed that a scientific, objective interpretation did not help vulnerable patients as much as a supportive therapeutic attitude. Many of the therapeutic interventions suggested by Ferenczi (e.g. hugging his patients for comfort, or his attempts at "mutual" analysis) were particularly controversial, and his name never recovered in psychoanalytical circles. Even so, something worth retaining from his theory is the emphasis and weight attributed to the dynamics of the therapeutic relationship and the need for flexibility and adaptation of the therapeutic framework to the needs of the patient (Symington 1986;·Stanton 1990;·Mander 2000;·Coren 2001).

Alexander and French (1946) considered their work a natural extension of the early relational models introduced by Rank and Ferenczi. According to Alexander and French, the purpose of therapy was not so much the recall of regressed memories, the historical reconstruction and correctness of interpretations, but the direct emotional experience of the patient within the session, which had to be brief and intense in order to be transformative. The "corrective emotional experience" actually referred to a new iteration of an old conflict; the tendency of the patient to repeat past trauma in the context of analysis had to be dealt with a new, different therapeutic response, and it was this "discrepancy" that was considered restorative. Again, Alexander and French identify the concept of therapeutic flexibility as key; they maintained that the analyst ought to adapt the therapeutic framework to the patient's needs and not the reverse. Recognising the risk of dependence of vulnerable patients from analysis, Alexander and French (1946) believed that breaks and short separations during therapy (such as extraordinary absence due to illness or scheduled vacations) helped rather than disrupting the analytical process, thus suggesting that therapy was not just limited to the context of the session but rather extended between sessions too.

Alexander and French (1946) were particularly criticised with regard to the concept of "corrective emotional experience", which was characterised as a manipulation of transference. Their assistance, however, as well as that of Rank and Ferenczi, contributed significantly to the implementation of psychoanalytical concepts in treatments of shorter duration and in the differentiation of psychoanalysis as a separate therapeutic approach, as well as the term "psychoanalytical" as a concept that may enrich different theoretical frameworks (Lemma 2014; Gillieron 1991, 1994). Even more significant is the fact that these new trends propelled the move from a solitary, biological view of the psyche to a modern object-oriented relational theory taking the therapeutic relation to a dynamic process, where the one side affects and is affected by the other (Mander 2000; Coren 2001; Mitchell 1988, 2000).

14.3 The Socioeconomic Framework of Brief Psychotherapy

Besides the theoretical and clinical factors governing the principles of brief psychotherapy, the discussion of its development as a separate therapeutic model would be incomplete if it didn't also establish the role of the wider socioeconomic framework of the provision of mental health. Particularly within the past two decades there is wide, international recognition of the financial cost, mainly of "common" mental disorders, such as anxiety and depression (Murray and Lopez 1997; Laylard 2006; WHO 2008). Although these common disorders are not as serious compared to chronic disorders, such as schizophrenia, their total cost with regard to "disability" and the economic burden they cause is clearly bigger (Andrews and Henderson 2000; Gillieron 1994; Gask et al. 2009a, b; Sartorius 2009).

For many years, the impact of mental disorders at public health level was extremely difficult to quantify, as most international research used mortality as a comparative indicator between various medical disorders. The World Bank introduced a new methodology for calculating "disability" resulting from the various disorders. It is calculated that neuropsychiatric disorders are responsible for 8 % of the total economic burden, measured by the number of work years lost due to the disability they cause. Specifically, in ages between 15 and 44, mental disorders are responsible for 12 % of the total economic burden, while if we include self-destructive behaviours (e.g. the use of alcohol as self-medication), this rate rises to 15.1 % for women and 16.1 % for men. On the basis of the above, it is forecast that by 2020, mental disorders will be responsible for 15 % of the total economic burden, while depression will come second after ischemic heart disease, regarding the cost of the disability it causes. These rates of disability (from the point of view of diminished capability to work) may be even higher if we include the phenomenon of somatisation or medically unexplainable symptoms, whereby patients present physical problems that have no organic aetiology (Thomas and Lewis 2009).

One economic analysis in Great Britain (Laylard 2006) maintains that the new "psychological technologies" have the capability of resolving long-term unemployment due to a mental disorder, for example, through the implementation of a small number of sessions of cognitive-behavioural therapy, which may actually be administered with the help of a computer or by untrained "psychological therapists". These suppositions are particularly problematic not just from a scientific and ethical viewpoint but also because they include the risk of poorly thought-out neoliberal policies, where each attempt to shorten therapy may be seen as a managed care technique and the provision of brief psychotherapy in a public context as a consumable product. On the other hand, full understanding of the patient, unhindered by the limits of time, cannot be ensured within the context of a public system and under the conditions of a socioeconomic crisis. Although these phenomena indicate the socioeconomic parameters of public psychiatric treatment and the risks they pose, it is important to point out the need for increased availability and accessibility of brief psychological treatment for "common" mental health problems in a community or primary context (Stylianidis 1995).

14.4 Initial Assessment of the Case in Brief Psychotherapy

Initial assessment with regard to patient eligibility for brief psychotherapy during the first interview differs significantly from that of "open" psychotherapies. At first, the development of the object-oriented relationship led to identification of the duality governing the therapeutic relationship, while the emergence of intersubjectivity as a scientific framework (Mitchell 1988, 2000) respectively places the issue of the initial assessment in a more interactive, bidirectional and flexible framework of reciprocity (Symington 1986; Mander 2000; Coren 2001). Gillieron (1994) points out the significance of the patient's initial assessment during the first session even within the context of a treatment of four sessions' duration.

The meaning of the initial assessment during the first interview consists of three main fields: purpose, target and procedure. As these priorities may often differ between patient and therapist, an important element during the assessment process is the establishment of a therapeutic cooperation (or alliance), which, on the one hand, is an integral part of any effective treatment and, on the other, facilitates taking the patient's history, which in turn allows the psychological expression of his difficulties and the selection of the brief therapy model (Dewan et al. 2009; Leichsenring 2009). A key question of the initial assessment is "why now" – the reason why the patient is seeking psychotherapeutic assistance at this precise time forms the specific framework. Often, the need to seek assistance at a specific time is motivated by an external factor, indirectly related to the patient's history, as in the example that follows:

> Anna, survivor of a particularly aggressive form of breast cancer that necessitated a double mastectomy, presented with major symptoms of depression, when a colleague was diagnosed with breast cancer two years later.

Upon the initial assessment, it is a good idea for the patient to receive some basic information about the treatment he will follow, particularly regarding its structure, purpose and method, in order to ensure transparency and convergence but also a particular therapeutic contract that specifies mutual expectations and obligations.

This is of use mainly for patients from different cultural backgrounds that may have a different concept and expectations with regard to what constitutes psychotherapy. This attitude of participation and cooperation is a key difference between brief and open psychotherapy, as the latter argues that the clarification of the therapeutic framework may affect patient transference and by extension compromise treatment quality (Mander 2000; Coren 2001).

Careful clinical listening of the patient regarding the difficulties he is facing (not only what is being said but also what is not being said) is an extremely important element of the assessment, as the narrative style and the emerging repeated interpersonal motifs (e.g. "I'm not making myself understood") are directly linked to the therapeutic framework.

> Peter, 36 years old, with chronic depression, difficulty in forming interpersonal relations and intense schizoid elements, arrives at the assessment session and states during his narration that 'he doesn't get on well with women'. The therapist, pointing out her gender, wonders what this means to Peter and how it can affect their possible cooperation.

This way, the patient gets a first taste of therapy, while the therapist assesses the form that the therapy may take (Tantum 1995; Dewan et al. 2009). Any form of assessment ought to include the current problem; the presence of possible co-morbidity (especially behaviours used as self-medicating means, such as eating disorders, substance or alcohol abuse); history of significant interpersonal relationships, including therapeutic ones; and existence of physical or mental diseases, as well as expectations, previous experiences or fears with regard to therapy and the therapist (pre-transference is an equally important assessment element to the content of the initial assessment). The therapist ought to remember that the initial assessment is not a monodimensional, static, diagnostic position of observation and collection of information, but a dynamic, developing process, directly related to the therapeutic one (Mander 2000; Coren 2001; Dewan et al. 2009). The initial assessment procedure on the one hand needs to be based on scientifically documented criteria and on the other to remain flexible and sensitive to new data as this emerges in the course of treatment.

Although the selection criteria differ depending on the theoretical approach, in general terms, brief psychotherapy is indicated for persons with specific problems, sufficient motivation, the capability to form interpersonal relations and containment of impulses and frustrations, while also establishing intrapsychic, physical and social aspects of the human experience. Vaslamatzis and Verveniotis (1985) mention that patients who stayed and completed a course of brief psychodynamic psychotherapy in a psychiatric hospital psychotherapy department were highly motivated, brought a specific problem and were in "crisis". Correspondingly, part of the literature maintains that brief therapy is contraindicated for patients with difficulty in dealing with separation, intense acting-out and excessive use of early defence mechanisms (Coren 2001; Dewan et al. 2009). In all this, however, there is extensive literature maintaining that even the most difficult, borderline patients may benefit from brief psychotherapeutic intervention [e.g. the synthetic approaches of mentalisation-based treatment, rational-emotive therapy and dialectical-behaviour therapy are mentioned (Fonagy 1991; Allen and Fonagy 2006; Ryle 1998; Koerner and Linehan 2003; Gabbard 2009)]. Even within a brief psychotherapeutic framework, the earliest the trauma is developmentally, the longer-term therapy is indicated.

The focus of brief psychotherapy is not so much the patient's behavioural "correction" as the investigation of peripheral difficulties or problems, which are directly linked to his behavioural structure. We point out again that the "ideal" and "clarity" of full and in-depth understanding of the individual's psycho-cognitive instrument, as it emerges through psychoanalysis, are not feasible or advisable in the context of brief psychotherapy, particularly when the provision of the latter is carried out in a public framework. Due to the limits in time and the focused therapeutic approach, the priority of the initial assessment includes the establishment of the therapeutic alliance from the first session and the immediate identification of possible negative emotions to therapy (Leichsenring 2009), and those two elements are connected with a more active therapeutic position. The issue of initial assessment during the first interview has less to do with treatment duration or number of sessions (e.g. a therapeutic intervention of 1 year is considered brief if its end has been determined from the outset) and more with the most appropriate type of therapy (interpretative, investigative, supportive, oriented towards the resolution of specific difficulties/symptoms, etc.). The attitude of the therapist as to brief psychotherapy, including the capability of frustration containment and the management of frequent and multiple separations, is also a significant criterion in the provision of brief psychotherapy (Messer and Warren 1995; Vaslamatzis et al. 1986, 1989; Gillieron 1994).

14.5 Therapeutic Principles in Brief Psychotherapy

In brief psychotherapy, the establishment of a specific therapeutic target is the most important element from the point of view of technique. As to the technique, the ensuing fields are the therapeutic focus, the therapist's attitude and the end of the psychotherapy.

The Therapeutic Focus

Contrary to "open" psychotherapeutic approaches, where the entire clinical material the patient brings is addressed as important and directly linked to current symptomatology, brief psychotherapy requires the identification of one core target. In this sense, the clinical material produced by the patient is addressed as more or less relevant to the core target, while clinical listening requires a stance of selective neglect of the material. Identification of the core target in brief psychotherapy serves to maintain narrative cohesion and continuity, which interweaves sessions and organises the therapeutic process, while also reducing the risk of "pointless wandering" in fields that do not comprise therapeutic priority within the limited time frame. In psychodynamic approach and brief psychotherapy in particular (but not exclusively), the core target refers to repeated interpersonal or relational motifs, which occur again and again in various aspects of the patient's life (Mander 2000; Coren 2001; Dewan et al. 2009; Leichsenring 2009). Identification of the core target is a mutual process while the target of the therapy must remain flexible, more as a guide than a destination, and expedient to the patient's actual, latent needs. Expressing the core target requires on the part of the therapist the attitude of a conscious observer, with full knowledge of theory and, more importantly, creativity and freedom from traditional ways of thinking, where the patient has to "fit" into predetermined diagnostic categories and by extension to be treated with stereotyped therapeutic interventions (Balint et al. 1972; Coren 2001).

The Therapist's Attitude

The concept of therapeutic activity is contrary to the image of the more neutral, less active analytical stance that dominates open psychotherapies. In brief psychotherapy, the therapeutic activity serves to maintain the core target, the ideal levels of the patient's thymic stimulation during therapy (Fonagy et al. 2008; Dewan et al. 2009), but also to avoid the patient's dependence from the therapist. The therapist's attitude differs significantly in brief psychotherapy. The concept of therapeutic neutrality and detachment (which possibly reflect the need of psychoanalysis to be as distant as possible from the early methods of catharsis and hypnosis) has been questioned mainly by Mitchell (1997), who believes that even analytical neutrality is, in essence, a kind of participation (Gill 1994). From this intersubjective viewpoint, the analyst's silence is potentially as harmful as activity, especially when addressed without thinking and with a lack of reflection regarding its effects in the therapeutic process. In order to showcase the problem of analytical neutrality, Mitchell gives the following clinical example:

> A psychotherapist adopts a strictly silent attitude in therapy, but her chair creaks (as the patient finds out) each time she refers to a specific clinical material. The patient senses that the creak in the chair communicates some sort of malaise on the therapist's part, but despite this eminently significant material, namely the therapist's participation in the dynamic process and the (non-) response to it by the patient, it is never mentioned and analysed. (Mitchell 1997, p. 13, in Coren 2001)

In brief psychotherapy, the therapist's attitude becomes the objective of reflection always in reference to the patient's core conflict and the therapeutic focus. In the context of the time limitations governing brief psychotherapy, the therapist's neutrality or silence includes the risk of increasing the patient's anxiety to a degree threatening the therapeutic alliance, particularly in patients with more serious psychopathology. The attitude of therapeutic neutrality as well as that of activity must be addressed in relation to how much they contribute to the service of therapeutic focus or in respect to the patient's relational difficulties (Mander 2000; Coren 2001; Dewan et al. 2009).

Here we should clarify that the therapeutic activity is not tantamount to the provision of advice or directivity. The concept of activity refers to the direct shift in focus from the "out there" to the "here and now" of therapy. Direct identification and investigation of the patient's negative emotions of resistance from as early as the first session seem to cement the therapeutic alliance. In the research of Vaslamatzis and Verveniotis (1985), the processing of translatif reactions of patients towards their therapist early in treatment increased the probability that they might remain and complete their brief psychodynamic therapy and not leave early. The active therapeutic attitude in brief psychotherapy communicates the openness of the therapeutic framework to acquit and contain difficult emotions of diversity or ambivalence, probably contrary to other relationships that the patient experiences (Mander 2000; Coren 2001; Gabbard 2009).

The End of Psychotherapy

The core dilemma governing brief psychotherapy is the question of the end: specifically whether the end of the treatment must be determined precisely prior to its start or whether the clinical contract may allow supplementary or follow-up sessions after the end of the treatment. In any case, what must be avoided and is clearly a bad practice in the context of brief therapy is an unclear stance with regard to the end, which results in an unstable, uncertain and noninclusive therapeutic framework. The availability of supplementary sessions includes the risk of denial of the reality of the end as a general concept (e.g. as a symbolism of death) and is generally considered to be unhelpful, as the ambivalent management of the end may cancel the effectiveness of therapy in its entirety (Mann 1973; Coren 2001). Furthermore, the availability of supplementary sessions (which may communicate difficulties with regard to the end both on the part of the therapist and that of the patient) may unconsciously reflect a therapeutic doubt or uncertainty related to the patient's readiness to stop (making him seem fragile or dependent). Management of the end, besides being real, is also symbolic and reflects the patient's psychic representation and containment by the therapist. The end (in its physical as well as symbolic dimension) is the most important element of brief psychotherapy and must be set from the start of treatment. The thematic of end, loss and separation must be interwoven with the therapy's narrative fabric from the start and throughout its duration and not investigated when treatment is approaching its end. The end of psychotherapy brings to the forefront issues of loss, separation or mourning (Holmes 2001), while the manner in which the patient is related to the end reflects motifs of forming and ending interpersonal relations:

> Vicky, an intergenerationally traumatised patient (her father was a war veteran and suffered with PTSD) comes to therapy with depression and a history of self-injury. Although the therapeutic contract provides from the start 20 sessions and despite all references to the end of treatment throughout its duration, Vicky "forgets" the end, consequently experiencing it violently and angrily as a traumatic abandonment. The interpretation of Vicky's repeated unconscious tendency to (re-)injure herself, avoiding or "forgetting" the mental processing of the end, relieves the patient and allows her to contain and reflect on the feelings of loss and anger related to the end of treatment.

It appears that the patient's transference with regard to the non-infinite dimension of time is directly linked to his relational history and core focus, so the time constraints set by the institutional framework, the patient's mental function and his acting-out in the transference/countertransference dynamic meet in the "here and now" of treatment with regard to the theme of its end (Gillieron 1991, 1994). Also, the therapist's history related to loss and separation appears to be activated and become involved in the therapeutic dyad dynamic with regard to the end (Vaslamatzis et al. 1986; Boyer and Hoffman 1993). Vaslamatzis et al. (1989) state that the less certain therapists declared they were regarding the end of brief psychodynamic psychotherapy management, the more probable it became for patients to withdraw from the treatment prematurely. One can get a taste of the end of psychotherapy by observing how each patient manages the end of each therapeutic session. Some patients are punctual as to the start and end of sessions, while others find separation hard and try to avoid the end, presenting important material during the last minutes of the session. The end of the therapy session reflects a microcosm of the end of treatment reminding the significance of separation in therapy on a weekly basis (Mander 2000; Coren 2001; Holmes 2001).

Although the issues of therapeutic focus, therapeutic activity and the end of therapy comprise basic characteristics of all brief psychotherapies, the individual fields that therapy focuses on differ depending in the therapist's theoretical model. Therefore, the target may be set relative to the symptomatology or some specific problem, or it can focus on the patient's structural or behavioural details. The therapeutic view should also include a developmental aspect as to the patient's issues, as the same event or symptom may have a different meaning or significance when occurring at a different age or stage of his life. Due to the limited space, this chapter addresses only the psychodynamic approach in brief psychotherapy, while it provides suggested literature references for other, equally important brief therapeutic approaches widely applied in a public framework (Gabbard 2009).

14.6 The Psychodynamic School in Brief Psychotherapy

The term "psychodynamic" suggests that psychism is not a static field; on the contrary, it includes powers that seek expression, release or satisfaction. According to Freud, the impulse refers to a dynamic process and to a "push" that forces the individual to abolish this internal status of intensity and physical stimulation through an object (LaPlanche and Pontalis 1986). With the development of the school of object-oriented relations, the concept of the impulse acquires an interpersonal existence and interpretation, where this intrapsychic intensity is the need of the subject to relate to the object rather than being just a biological function of release. The activity of psychism is not limited only to external relations but essentially to relations between objects. The concept of the self as an observer of internal processes suggests that the dynamic psychic activity takes place both intra-psychically and inter-personally (Symington 1986; Jacobs 2001; Nelson-Jones 2001; Maroda 2010). The psychodynamic theories say that the first years in the life of an infant and its relationship with its mother and father have a determining effect on personality and mental health development in adult life (Slade 2008; Cassidy and Shaver 2008). The psychodynamic school believes that the real, repeated interpersonal interactions between mother and infant are introjected and become psycho-cognitive representations [in a process where the interpersonal becomes intrapsychic (Maroda 2010; Gabbard 2009)]. These representations or internal work models describe the relations between different aspects or dimensions of the self, while they are directly involved in thymic stimulation and regulation (Goldberg 2000), defence mechanisms (Holmes 1997; Bifulco 2002; Hesse 2008; Gabbard 2009), memory and attention processes (Coan 2008), cognitive structures (Lopez and Brennan 2000; Holmes 2001) and the function of reflection (Main 1991, 1993; Fonagy 2004; Allen and Fonagy 2006; Schore 1994, 2003; Coan 2008) of the adult. The latest research from the field of neuropsychology showcases the role of early bonds and trauma in the formation of the brain, particularly with regard to impulse control, empathy, thymic stimulation and self-regulation (Schore 1994, 2003; Fonagy et al. 2008; Greene 2011).

Psychic representations created in childhood are maintained with relative stability in adulthood, where they contribute significantly in psychopathology adaptation and development (Mallinckrodt 2000; Feeney and Collins 2001; Bateman and Fonagy 2004; Mikulincer and Shaver 2008; Dozier et al. 2008). Psychic representations are activated particularly in the context of interpersonal relations including the therapeutic relationship. Just like a parent, the therapist provides availability, responsiveness, stability and security, thymic regulation and relief, a basis of containment and reflection from where the patient can investigate internal and external reality and "play" on his own, in the presence of the therapist (Farber et al. 1995; Holmes 1997, 1999; Mander 2000; Wallin 2007). Accordingly, the manner in which the therapist is being experienced, his perception, the cognitive and emotional response towards him (the transference) are influenced by the patient's unconscious, early psychic representations, often irrespectively of the therapist's behaviour (Mallinckrodt et al. 1995; Mallinckrodt 2000; Malan 2001; Westen and Gabbard 2002; Slade 2008; Mallinckrodt and Jeong 2015), often irrespectively of the therapist's behaviour (Goldman and Anderson 2007).

Malan (1979, 2001) linked the elements of psychic representations and relational motifs formed during early life, to the patient's interpersonal relationships in adulthood and transference with the "here and now" of therapy. The "triangle of insight" suggested by Malan (1979, 2001) shapes the threefold connection between transference, the patient's current relationships outside of therapy and the relationships with significant others in the past. The triangle of insight is connected with another psychoanalytic triangle, the triangle of conflict, which consists of the secret emotion or impulse, the patient's defences and the problem or symptom he presents. The therapist works methodically with the objective of linking the two triangles, pointing out the coherence between the points within but also between the triangles (e.g. how transference, defences, core conflict, as they emerge in the therapeutic relationship, re-emerge in the patient's current and past relationships) (Malan 1976, 1979, 2001; Coren 2001; Dewan et al. 2009). With regard to transference, the technique in brief therapy differs radically from that in open therapies; emphasis is given less in the achievement of transference awareness on the part of the patient and more on how transference is used actively in relation to core focus. The manner in which the patient is related to the interpretation reveals significant information on the repeated relational motifs, the thymic background of interactions as well as the attempts to deregulate the thymic stimulation that therapy may possibly activate (Mander 2000; Coren 2001). For example, if a pertinent or misguided interpretation causes anger, how does the patient manage this conflict: Does he fight with the therapist, withdraw emotionally and act out passively and aggressively through self-destructive behaviours? Does he begin to miss or cancel sessions? And finally, how does this information relate to the patient's other relationships outside of therapy?

Malan's technique, although arising from psychoanalysis, effectively adapts to brief psychodynamic psychotherapy in relation to the core target and the patient's relational motifs, in particular with regard to ending and separation (Coren 2001). Once more, we point out that Malan's (1979, 2001) technique does not aspire to fully understand the patient's unconscious in its entirety outside the boundaries of time, but aims at an in-depth understanding of current issues that he brings and their composition within the immediate, intersubjective as well as institutional framework of psychotherapy.

Randomised control trials (RCTs) have shown brief psychodynamic psychotherapy to be effective for patients with major depression, emotional and stress disorders (Knekt et al. 2008, 2011), somatisation disorders, psychogenetic bulimia and cluster C personality disorders (Leichsenring 2009; Vinnars et al. 2005), while its effectiveness is increased in combination with pharmacotherapy (Kay 2009). Synthetic representations of brief psychoanalytical psychotherapy with a good and documented basis as to its effectiveness are the mentalisation-based treatment (Bateman and Fonagy 2004; Allen and Fonagy 2006; Fonagy et al. 2008) and the dynamic interpersonal psychotherapy (Lemma et al. 2011).

14.7 The Effectiveness of Brief Psychotherapy

In the past, the relationship between psychotherapy and psychiatry has been tense. Research development in the fields of neuroscience, genetics and psychopharmacology (Gabbard 2009) emphasises the use of pharmacology and fast solutions to the detriment of traditional psychological treatments. Within this biomedical field of knowledge, Kandel (1998) has noted the plasticity of synaptic connectivity in the brain, which can be modified through good psychotherapeutic practice. In fact, Goldapple and his associates (2004) have begun mapping the areas of the brain that are modified as a result of psychotherapy (anterior cingulate και hippocampus), in contrast to the ones that are modified through medication (prefrontal cortex). The combination of neuroscience with psychotherapy is one of the fastest developing and exciting fields of research, as it finally appears to be bridging the void between psychological treatment and biological function.

In general terms, psychotherapy has been proven effective with positive results for various theoretical approaches and technical interventions (Lambert et al. 1986; Smith et al. 1980; Andrews and Harvey 1981; Shapiro and Shapiro 1982; Lambert and Bergin 1994). Specifically, at the end of treatment, the average patient makes up to 80 % improvement compared to the control groups that do not receive psychotherapy. The effectiveness of psychotherapy is comparable with that of pharmacotherapy, while in many cases their combination promotes the effectiveness of the treatment (Friedman and Thase 2009; Kay 2009). The extent of the effect produced by psychotherapy is commensurate or higher in duration or depth to that produced by the administration of psychoactive substances (Andrews 1982, 1983; Lambert 2003; Friedman and Thase 2009; Kay 2009). The increased recognition of the neuroscientific existence of psychotherapy in conjunction with the long-term absence of a substantial empirical basis makes the need for the systematic evaluation imperative with regard to the effectiveness and efficiency of psychotherapy.

As to the effectiveness of brief psychotherapy compared to that of the open alternative approaches that are not time limited (and given the small empirical basis with regard to the latter), it is argued that short-term, brief psychotherapy is just as effective with the longer-term approaches (Garfield 1998; Coren 2001; Leichsenring et al. 2004; Lewis et al. 2008). A new research trend regarding the effectiveness of brief psychodynamic therapy also supports its efficiency in the long term, after the end of treatment (Gelso and Johnson 1983; Lemma et al. 2011; Lemma 2014). Vinnars and his associates (2005) compared the effectiveness of an open, nonstructured psychodynamic psychotherapy with that of a brief structured psychodynamic psychotherapy [based on the protocol of Crits-Christoph et al. (1988, 1991) that focuses on the immediate interpretation of translatif, core interpersonal motifs] for 156 patients with personality disorder. The differences between open and brief interventions with regard to their effectiveness (reduced personality disorder characteristics, psychiatric symptoms, improved general interpersonal function and reduced requests for help by the mental health services) are reported as minimal after 1 year of treatment, when both interventions are provided by experienced, well-qualified therapists (Vinnars et al. 2005). Also, Knekt and his associates (2011) compared the effectiveness of brief and open psychodynamic psychotherapies and psychoanalysis for 326 patients with anxiety and affective disorders. All psychotherapeutic approaches were effective in reducing the patients' psychiatric symptoms and general functioning 5 years after the start of treatment. During the first year, brief psychotherapies were more effective than psychoanalysis, while open psychodynamic psychotherapies were more effective after 3 years. Psychoanalysis seemed to be more effective after 5 years of therapy. The authors conclude that while psychotherapies of brief and middle duration produced faster results than psychoanalysis, the latter appeared to produce more established and long-term benefits (Knekt et al. 2008, 2011; de Maat et al. 2009). Cumulatively, it seems that although the effectiveness of open psychodynamic psychotherapies produces longer-term benefits through structural, behavioural changes, the effectiveness of the corresponding brief approaches is more direct and therefore implementable in a public or community framework; these findings place open and brief psychotherapies in a complementarity range that can be exploited depending on the patient's needs and the capabilities of the institutional framework (Leichsenring 2009). On the other hand, the belief that the therapeutic depth is achieved only in a long-term context is not empirically supported; on the contrary, research proves that the patient's core interpersonal motifs emerge very soon in treatment (Crits-Christoph et al. 1988; Luborsky and Crits-Cristoph 1998; Mallinckrodt 2000), supporting in this sense Winnicott's view that the depth of therapy is not related to intensity or duration.

Extensive literature reviews and research efficiency post-analyses bring out a plethora of therapeutic and para-therapeutic variables in psychotherapy patient improvement. These include factors outside of therapy (the patient's behavioural characteristics, the quality of his support network, accessibility to self-help sources, disorder chronicity, gravity and complexity, etc.) that correspond to 40 % of the improvement as well as the effect of the patient's expectations with regard to the help he expects from treatment (placebo effect), corresponding to 15 % of the improvement (Lambert and Barley 2002; Garfield 2003; Lambert 2003; Papadopoulos 2007). In an important research comparing cognitive-behavioural treatment and interpersonal psychotherapy (IPT) to a control group only taking imipramine, the slight superiority highlighting the interpersonal approach for the more disturbed patients disappeared when factors outside of therapy and the patients' expectations were checked with regard to the effectiveness of treatment (both psychotherapeutic and pharmaceutical) (Elkin et al. 1989; Ahn and Wampold 2001; Arnkoff et al. 2002). A plethora of factors common to all psychotherapies irrespective of theoretical approach have been flagged as being involved in 30 % of the improvement; these include, among others, empathy, the therapist's respect and authenticity towards the patient and therapeutic allegiance quality that favours the patient's integration and signification difficulties as a start for the exploration of internal and external conflicts (Lambert 2003; Norcross 2002; Holmes 2001; Wallin 2007; Rosenfeld 2009).

The common factors for therapeutic change refer in theory at least to the necessary and sufficient conditions introduced by Rogers (1957). Although the literature is unanimous as to the necessity of these conditions being present in any therapeutic relationship (even between psychiatrist and patient, in order to maximise the latter's response to adherence to the pharmaceutical treatment), the different theoretical schools disagree with regard to their sufficiency as unique factors of change. For example, Miller et al. (1980) note the significance of the therapist's empathy even in uniquely behavioural treatments. Correspondingly, Lafferty et al. (1991) and Elliott et al. (1991) point out the central role of empathy in the effectiveness of psychotherapy, with the less effective therapists in their sample being characterised by the lowest levels of empathy and understanding with regard to the patient. At the same time, therapist evaluation with regard to the effectiveness of treatment does not seem to correspond (it is systematically lower) with the patient's subjective evaluation (Cooley and LaJoy 1980).

Despite this, newer research from the field of neuroscience demonstrates that empathy, although necessary as a condition, is not sufficient for the therapeutic change. Comparing purely personality-centred treatments with synthetic approaches that harmonise basic Rogerian conditions with Gestalt experiential techniques, Greenberg and Watson (1998) point out that the most "energetic" approaches were effective faster in patients with major depression, especially with regard to interpersonal difficulties and the levels of anguish related to the end of psychotherapy. Correspondingly, in their extensive research with regard to mentalisation treatment, Fonagy et al. (2004) and neuroscientist Schore (1994, 2003) mention that empathy alone is not sufficient for therapeutic change, as the solidifying of insight requires a ground of ideal thymic stimulation levels from the patient, something that results from the therapist's active attitude. The significance of the therapist's active and lively attitude in brief psychotherapy is noted also by Roth and Fonagy (2005), who point out that non-specific, unclear approaches (from a theoretical and technical aspect) are less effective in more serious pathologies.

Conventional evaluation methods that compare different theoretical psychotherapeutic approaches in the wide range of emotional and interpersonal disorders have not culminated in clear conclusions showcasing a specific school as superior to another. The absence of essential differences with regard to the effectiveness further supports the effect of common factors in psychotherapy (Lambert 2003; Luborsky et al. 1975; Bergin and Lambert 1978; Elkin et al. 1989; Lambert and Barley 2002; Meltzoff and Kornreich 1970), while the small differences distinguished for certain techniques implemented in specific diagnostic categories and symptomatologies beg the question "What works for whom in psychotherapy?" (Quality Assurance Project 1983; Robinson et al. 1990; Norcross 2002; Lambert 2003; Lewis et al. 2008; Rosenfeld 2009; Gabbard 2009). In this sense, the theoretical and clinical field of knowledge with regard to the effectiveness of different approaches is shown to be localised and not global. The methodological limitations often involved in the "artificial" status of the findings with regard to the effectiveness of different theoretical approaches in brief psychotherapy point out the need for careful and critical implementation in clinical practice (Allen et al. 2008).

In any case, the general finding of non-difference with regard to effectiveness refers to the conclusion that the different theoretical approaches conquer similar targets through different procedures or methods and through the presence of therapeutic factors, common to all psychotherapies, dominated by the therapeutic alliance (Lambert 2003; Lambert and Barley 2002).

14.8 The Therapeutic Alliance

The concept of the therapeutic alliance has attracted particular interest with regard to its role in the effectiveness of psychotherapy, although it is accepted that the alliance is only one aspect of the therapeutic relationship (Clarkson 2003). It is widely accepted that the alliance includes both the therapist's and the patient's variables and consists of the characteristics of the therapeutic purpose, the targets and the bond between therapist and client. The therapist's contribution to the alliance includes the capability to provide the aforementioned code conditions, the ability to resolve conflict within the alliance and mutual cooperation with regard to the purpose and the target of the treatment (Hovarth and Bedi 2002; Lambert and Barley 2002; Gabbard 2009). The patient's contribution to the alliance refers to his ability to create an emotional bond with the therapist and to be able to participate in the treatment with purpose (Luborsky and Luborsky 2006; Gabbard 2009). The contribution of the therapeutic alliance in the effectiveness of treatment is transtheoretically recognised, as its components (both the patient's and the therapist's characteristics) are common in all psychotherapies, irrespective of theoretical approach (Horvath 2005; Horvath and Luborsky 1993; Norcross and Goldfried 2003). Research in the therapeutic alliance put it forth as a factor that is not just ahead of therapeutic change but is also an active ingredient of psychotherapy. For example, Safran και Wallner (1991) say that mutual evaluation of the alliance (by the therapist and the patient) already after the third brief cognitive psychotherapy session forecasts its effectiveness after its completion; other research supports these findings (Martin et al. 2000; Horvath 2005). Also, Gaston et al. (2002) mention that the contribution of the alliance accounted for 36–57 % of patient improvement in their research irrespective of the theoretical or technical approach. Castonguay and his associates (1996) compared the role of the alliance in two groups of patients with major depression, who were following brief cognitive therapy or its combination with pharmacotherapy. In their attempt to minimise the contribution of therapist characteristics, the therapists followed a strict protocol in the provision of treatment, while the alliance evaluation was conducted by the patients and independent judges. The two variables related to therapy effectiveness and the patients' symptom improvement were the therapeutic alliance and the therapist's emotional participation in the therapeutic relationship. Finally, in the big research of the NIMH, Krupnick and his associates (1996) showed the role of the therapeutic alliance in the effectiveness if treatment for patients with major depression is an active common factor in psychotherapeutic, pharmaceutical and pseudo-pharmaceutical interventions.

In general terms, what emerges from the literature is that some therapists are better than others in the provision of the interpersonal conditions that forecast the improvement of the patient's symptoms and the effectiveness of the treatment. The therapist's characteristics as variables clearly involved in the effectiveness of the treatment have attracted particular research interest, especially from the aspect of the attachment theory, as can be seen below.

14.9 The Therapist's Role

The attempts to evaluate effectiveness communicate an ethical, professional attitude to show that psychotherapy is a worthwhile, empirically documented and reliable therapeutic method, which supplements biomedical approaches in mental health. A significant limitation of existing literature is that the therapist is illustrated as a depersonalised sponsor of standardised therapeutic interventions. In its implementation, effectiveness and efficiency research appears to systematically attempt to minimise or isolate the personality of the therapist as a core change factor and the interpersonal dimension of psychotherapy as one of deeply restorative process (Coren 2001). However, a number of converging instances of research show that the therapist is a therapeutic factor directly linked to the effectiveness of brief psychotherapy. Luborsky and his associates (1986) mention that the differences due to the therapist's personality significantly exceeded those that were due to specific technical interventions. These results have been confirmed recently by Crits-Christoph et al. (1991), Wampold (2001), Huppert et al. (2001) and Project MATCH Research Group (1998). It is strange then that while the literature points to the significance of the therapeutic relationship, there are few clear instructions given with regard to the therapist's attitude. Instead, all instructions accompanying clinical practice with no exception refer to purely diagnostic categories (DSM-V 2014).

Although specific techniques have been proven effective for specific disorders (Lambert 2003; Lilienfield 2005; Rosenfeld 2009; Allen et al. 2008), the question that emerges is to what extent do psychological treatments adapt to the patient's person, the stage of change and his behavioural characteristics and not exclusively to his diagnosis. Clinical practice shows that different patients respond better to different approaches, while recent research (especially in the areas of the therapist's countertransference and attachment) brings up the issue of client-therapist match (Norcross 2002). For example, Hayes (1995) and Rosenberg and Hayes (2002) developed a structural theory of countertransference that includes notions of origins, triggers, manifestations, effects and management. According to it, the therapist's relational characteristics or conflicts are activated by the client's characteristics or behaviours and are manifested with emotional, cognitive and behavioural reactions, which affect not only therapeutic interaction quality but also the outcome and effectiveness of treatment (Vaslamatzis et al. 1986).

The systematic research into countertransference allows a deeper understanding of the dynamic, the therapeutic "use" of self by the therapist and what comprises "corrective emotional experience" (Friedman and Gelso 2000; Bernier and Dozier 2002; Bridges 2006). For example, Hardy and his associates (1999) say that psychodynamic therapists working in a brief 16-week framework tended to respond with "mirroring" and an inclusive attitude to anxious-"preoccupied" patients and with interpretive interventions to more avoidant patients. Rubino and his associates (2000) report that therapists with insecure attachment respond with less empathy and depth to patients with similar attachment characteristics to their own; similar findings are also reported by Mohr et al. (2005). In an important research, Dozier et al. (1994) investigated the therapist's attachment role in his therapeutic interventions towards patients with serious psychiatric disorders. It is said that therapists with more secure attachment tended to trace the deeper, less distinguishable (unconscious) patient needs while less secure therapists, the more obvious, conscious patient needs, thus showcasing the role of the therapists' intrapsychic characteristics in the choice of their therapeutic interventions. The concept of asymmetry or dissimilarity between the therapist-client relational structures was also investigated by Tyrell and his associates (1999), who report that the relational structure disparity in the therapeutic dyad was related to higher evaluations (on the part of the clients) of the treatment effectiveness with regard to their mental, social and professional functioning; the therapist-client matching appears to help the therapeutic process "revising" the patient's internal working models (Tyrell et al. 1999). In total, these findings showcase the interaction of the therapist-client relational structures in the dynamic and by extension the effectiveness of the therapeutic relationship, thus underlining the therapist's role (Gelso and Hayes 2007; Vaslamatzis et al. 1986).

14.10 Training and Supervision in Brief Psychotherapy

One of the problems with brief psychotherapy is that it is mistakenly thought of as a condensed form of psychoanalysis; although its theoretical basis results from psychoanalytical thinking, its clinical implementation requires specialised training, therapeutic flexibility and pluralism and does not seek full understanding of the unconscious in its timeless entirety. Despite its documented effectiveness for specific clinical populations and symptomatologies, brief psychotherapy is often addressed as a lesser psychotherapeutic alternative solution, which is necessary in view of a lack of long-term or open therapy availability in a community or primary context. During their first interview, many patients react with doubt or disbelief to the "brevity" of the offered treatment (although the time frame of brief psychotherapy differs depending on the institutional framework: treatment predetermining its end from the start, with an average duration of 4–6 months, is considered brief in literature). At the same time, many therapists working within a brief framework also agree with the belief or fear that brief psychotherapy is no more that the "poor relation" of "pure bred" open psychotherapies (Coren 2001).

The therapist's attitude, values and beliefs with regard to the brevity of the framework significantly affect the therapeutic relationship's dynamics, while it is possible that it may bring forth personal and professional issues for the therapist, such as guilt and frustration regarding the patient's treatment or abandonment, anger against the system that does not allow more sessions or a feeling of professional inadequacy, a "not good enough therapist" (Vaslamatzis et al. 1989). Such therapeutic reactions include the risk of the patient as well as the therapist acting out this ambivalence. Many therapists deal with brief therapy as an introduction to a longer-term treatment rather than a stand-alone area of knowledge with essential and sufficient existence. The therapist's occupation with the possibility of future treatment distracts focus from the therapeutic core and the "here and now", something that may reflect a defensive denial of the end on the therapist's part (Mander 2000; Coren 2001; Gelso and Hayes 2007).

The non-timeless time frame of brief approaches is psychically and mentally demanding for therapists. Clinical work includes the frequent alternation of starting and ending therapeutic relationships, a large number of patients per week and the need for awareness, focus and activation with regard to the therapeutic target. Due to these conditions, therapists may become vulnerable to professional exhaustion syndrome, which is manifested with loss of empathy or psychic co-ordination with the patient or with raised emphasis in technique or theory and, at the same time, loss in reflective function on clinical practice (Coren 2001; Hawkins and Shohet 2006).

These issues bring to the forefront the need for regular supervision and personal analysis for therapists (both trainees and experienced professionals) who work in the fast-paced and demanding brief psychotherapy framework. Supervision offers a context for reflection, a safe basis from where the therapist may deconstruct and investigate aspects of the therapeutic process, identify blind spots or conflicts, remain clinically aware and ensure an ethical practice (Hawkins and Shohet 2006). Perhaps, the most significant aspect of supervision is the reflexive function conditioning, namely, the capability of objectifying and observing the dynamics in therapy and the therapist's intrapsychic processes, for the purpose of better understanding the clinical material and the flexible maintenance of the "ideal" emotional therapeutic distance, depending on the patient's needs (Symington 1986; Casement 1991; Meszaros 2004; Allen and Fonagy 2006; Gelso and Hayes 2007; Mander 2000). The institutional framework and its capability to respond to the challenges of brief therapy also affect the therapeutic process and the dynamics among the staff. The administration of institutions implementing brief therapy should recognise the pressure weighing on therapists, who see more and more cases, as well as the risk of professional exhaustion, by providing support and regular supervision for the entire cross-sector group (Coren 2001; Hawkins and Shohet 2006).

14.11 A Greek Experience: The EPAPSY Day Centre

This discussion should not exclude the significant contribution of Greek scientists, who have tried to implement and utilise the theoretical and clinical knowledge regarding the provision of brief psychotherapy in a public framework. In Greece, from as early as the 1980s, the Psychotherapy Department of the Eginitio Hospital has integrated brief psychodynamic psychotherapy [specifically the approach by Malan (1979) and Sifneos (1979) in the services it provides] and has produced a wealth of research material with regard to both the client and the therapist's parameters contributing to its effectiveness (Vaslamatzis and Verveniotis 1985; Vaslamatzis et al. 1986, 1989). As well, the Fokis and Evia Mobile Mental Health Units have been providing brief psychotherapy services since 1990, responding to the population's increased need and demand for realistic and accessible mental healthcare in the community (Stylianidis 1995).

The Psychosocial Intervention Day Centre in the "Franco Basaglia" community is a "hybrid", atypical mental health structure, among the first in Greece, which combines elements of day hospital and mental health centre in an attempt to bridge the gap between secondary care and (non-existent in our country) organised primary care. The day centre consists of a cross-sector group of psychiatrists, psychologists, social workers and psychiatric nurses and provides, among others, psychiatric monitoring and prescription, brief individual and group psychotherapy, home intervention and psychosocial rehabilitation services.

The psychotherapy service is staffed by psychologists-therapists from various approaches (three psychodynamic-psychoanalytical psychotherapists, one cognitive-behavioural psychotherapist, one cognitive-analytical psychotherapist and five art therapists working under the supervision of more experienced therapists), while it responds to a wide range of psychic disorders, such as emotional disorders (50 %), personality disorders (25 %), psychotic disorders (5 %) and neurotic and somatoform disorders (20 %). Fifteen percent of referrals for the psychotherapy service come from general psychiatric hospitals, 41 % from mental health centres and 44 % corresponds to self-referrals or referrals from private individuals. The psychotherapy service is evaluated with regard to its effectiveness, while the theoretical approach option is evaluated on the basis of patient needs. The average duration of psychotherapy varies from 15 to 24 sessions, while for major pathologies the duration is extended to 52 sessions. The day centre splits the psychotherapeutic and pharmaceutical care it provided to psychotherapy patients (split treatment) (namely, the two are provided by different professionals), in order to protect the therapeutic boundaries, to generate "pure" translatif reactions towards the psychotherapist and to prevent the patient from dedicating the session to pharmacology issues to the detriment of psychological issues. The pros and cons of split and combined care are put forth by Kay (2009). The psychotherapy group attends group supervision twice a week as well as a monthly psychoanalytical approach supervision with an external supervisor. The following clinical vignette is set out as an example of implementation of 9-month brief psychotherapy at the day centre.

> Dimosthenis is a 45-year old single man, who has been diagnosed with bipolar disorder with psychotic elements. He comes to therapy with a persistent depression complaint, at the prompting of his private psychiatrist after a suicide attempt a few months earlier. His medication regimen includes an anticonvulsant factor, two mood adjusters (one of them lithium), two antidepressants (SSRI and SSNRI), two antipsychotics (one typical and one atypical and, from time to time, a sedative. Dimosthenis arrives punctually at the initial evaluation, is neat and clean, but his monotonous voice and expressionless face project a mournful and heavy quality. During the first session, Dimosthenis appears particularly cautious, passive as well as aggressive as to his expectations (pre-transference) and challenges the therapist asking her how she can believe that "someone in his condition" can be helped by psychotherapy. Dimosthenis identifies in particular with his bipolar diagnosis and refers to his "disease" in a riveting and unwavering manner. He has a history of three previous attempts at psychotherapy (two instances of cognitive-behavioural therapy and one of psychoanalysis) about which he says that despite his therapists well-meaning motivation, were not particularly helpful. The therapist directly realises Dimosthenis's challenge to prove and defend the value of the "objective" (the treatment) she will offer and makes a mental note of her counter-transference) defensive position, rejection anxiety but also empathy for his fear) as a significant element of the patient's transference and his interpersonal motifs in the "here and now" as well as in other relationships. The psychotherapist wonders if Dimosthenis believes he can be helped and what moves him to seek help this time, given the disappointment that accompanies the previous psychotherapeutic attempts.
>
> Dimosthenis comes from a well-to-do family and has an older brother, with whom he describes his relationship as one of conflict. His father was a successful businessman, a perfectionist, strict and frugal with his emotions. Dimosthenis's mother died of cancer when the patient was 17 years old, three years after her diagnosis; Dimosthenis has very few memories from his childhood (which he describes as "foggy") and describes his

mother as a saint, a feature that attributes to her the quality of an idealised, elusive, unreachable and frustrating object. In general terms, the patient's family background stressed power, success, conquest and strongly rejected any semblance of vulnerability, fear or anguish. As a child, Dimosthenis was an excellent student, and a perfectionist in all his occupations. He remembers himself as independent and unconnected and as not having particular need of connection, despite being popular at school. The start and diagnosis of the disorder at the age of 17 coincides with the mother's death; the family does not seem to have processed mourning and while the father and the brother went on with their career, Dimosthenis broke down, almost as though permitting the others to continue. Despite Dimosthenis's attempts to go on with his studies and succeed his father in business (like his brother), none of his efforts bore fruit and Dimosthenis has been unemployed for the last 10 years. Upon referral, Dimosthenis shows he has a reduced support network; he has very few friends whom he believes he is a burden to and has had one love affair at the age of 18.

The first concern of the treatment is to establish a strong therapeutic alliance, a safe basis from which Dimosthenis can explore aspects of his psyche. The end of the treatment is set from the beginning, but Dimosthenis minimises its significance, saying it is still too far off for him to be concerned about it (largely as he has minimised the effect of his mother's death on him). During the first sessions, the therapist realises and "hosts" Dimosthenis's need for psychic distance and the therapeutic relationship develops slowly but steadily; when nearness becomes threatening for Dimosthenis, he cancels sessions, which is interpreted right away as a distance-nearness regulator. Dimosthenis's ego strength at the start of treatment appears vulnerable in containing internal conflict and the defences he uses include splitting, projective identification and primary projection, denial, emotional isolation, repression and intellectualisation. These principally early defences indicate a pre-Oedipal trauma, which deteriorates with the loss of the mother at a vulnerable age. Dimosthenis's object oriented relationships are played out through his repeated interpersonal motifs and transference towards the therapist; one of these is that he is a burden and is undesirable to his friends as well as her. During a specific session, Dimosthenis arrives very frightened and tells the therapist that during his last visit to his psychiatrist, she warned him against psychotherapy, telling him that raking up the past will not help him. The immediate counter-transference felt by the therapist was intense anxiety that the treatment was "hurting" the patient and would lead him to a relapse. The institutional supervision helps the therapist to contain this excessive, almost paranoid anxiety and explain it as an attempt at splitting between the two professionals involved in the patient's care. During the next session, after divulging to the therapist some innermost, persisting paranoid thoughts, Dimosthenis confides to her that now, he is very worried about her; that he is putting her at risk and may have "harmed" her. Looking into these two events together with Dimosthenis, a second interpersonal model begins to appear in the opposing pair "I harm others – others harm me," which appears to be related to his unconscious, core conflict. Dimosthenis's childhood wish to "conquer" and connect with his elusive mother is futile, forbidden, dirty, bad, causes shame and rage and is thus suppressed; her death causes her further idealisation and even sainthood. Denial and splitting allow Dimosthenis to insulate the "bad" emotions of shame and anger, so that they will not infect the idealised ones, while projection and projective identification (which includes the therapist's psychic "preparedness" to receive his projection) allows him to unload them on those around him. The treatment is organised around Malan's two triangles; interpretation and signification of these defences related to chronic depression with paranoid elements and the core conflict improves the dynamics of the therapeutic relationship. Dimosthenis's therapy is in progress, while 5 months of treatment still remain; in the latest session, Dimosthenis was able to say that the treatment is important to him and that he feels closer to this therapist. Particular attention is given to the end of the treatment so the motif of avoiding the end is not repeated resulting in the patient not speaking of his emotions as to the loss of the therapeutic relationship.

14.12 In Conclusion

Brief psychotherapy appears to comprise a significant part of applied psychiatric care globally in a primary and community framework (Gabbard 2009; Gask et al. 2009a, b; Sartorius 2009). This tendency projects both the capability of developing new ethical and scientific positions and significant challenges with regard to their implementation. On the one hand, generalised and vague, idiosyncratic or unstructured clinical estimations without the will to make assessments no longer seem to have a place in the clinical environment. On the other, this new reality includes the risk of making psychotherapy one more product for consumption, by losing its intersubjective background (Stylianidis 1995; Coren 2001). Placing emphasis upon standardised, undifferentiated techniques, treatment contains the risk of clinical and professional alienation, denial of the complexity of mental anguish and restriction of therapeutic freedom, whilst the significance of the reflexive, exploratory and personal aspects of treatment may be sacrificed in the name of functionality and strategy; institutional and economic pressure for fast and effective treatment must be the objective of reflection of the cross-sector group. Brief psychotherapy is not a panacea for all patients. On the contrary, it must be part of a wide range of provision of mental health services, including long-term treatment, critically implemented depending on each patient's needs. This chapter attempted to showcase the significance of brief psychotherapy with regard to its accessibility and effectiveness in a public framework, in full awareness of this choice and its limitations. The therapist working in a short-term framework must have achieved a sound, long psychodynamic/psychoanalytical education (supplementary to the briefness of the treatment he provides), which will integrate and also differentiate elements of the brief and the open approach in psychotherapy. The need for a pluralistic approach is therefore pointed out that may listen to and respond more to the patient's rather than the therapist's needs or those of the institutional framework that provides mental health services in a public framework (Stylianidis 1995; Coren 2001; Norcross and Goldfried 2003; Lemma 2014).

Bibliography

Ahn H, Wampold BE (2001) Where oh where are the specific ingredients? A meta-analysis of component studies in counselling and psychotherapy. J Couns Psychol 48:251–257

Alexander F, French TM (1946) Psychodynamic therapy. Ronald Press, New York

Allen JC, Fonagy P (eds) (2006) Handbook of mentalisation-based treatment. Wiley, Chichester

Allen JC, Fonagy P, Bateman AW (2008) Mentalising in clinical practice. American Psychoatric Publishing, Arlington

American Psychiatric Association (2013) The diagnostic and statistical manual of mental disorders: DSM 5. bookpointUS, Arlington

Andrews G (1982) A methodology for preparing ideal treatment outlines in psychiatry. Aust N Z J Psychiatry 16:153–158

Andrews G (1983) A treatment outline for depressive disorders. Aust N Z J Psychiatry 17:129–146

Andrews G, Harvey R (1981) Does psychotherapy benefit neurotic patients? A re-analysis of the Smith, Glass & Miller data. Arch Gen Psychiatry 38:1203–1208

Andrews G, Henderson S (eds) (2000) Unmet need in psychiatry. Cambridge University Press, Cambridge

Andrews G, Slade T, Issakidis C (2002) Deconstructing co-morbidity: data from the Australian National Survey of Mental Health and Wellbeing. Br J Psychiatry 181:306–314

Arnkoff DB, Glass CR, Shapiro SJ (2002) Expectations and preferences. In: Norcross JC (ed) Psychotherapy relationships that work- therapist contributions and responsiveness to patients. Oxford University Press, New York

Balint M, Ornstein P, Balint E (1972) Focal psychotherapy: an example of applied psychoanalysis. Tavistock, London

Bateman AW, Fonagy P (2004) Psychotherapy for borderline personality disorder: mentalisation-based treatment. Oxford Medical Publications, Oxford University Press, Oxford

Bergin AE, Lambert MJ (1978) The evaluation of outcomes in psychotherapy. In: Garfield SL, Bergin (eds) Handbook of psychotherapy and behaviour change: an empirical analysis. Wiley, New York

Bernier A, Dozier M (2002) The client- counsellor match and the corrective emotional experience: evidence from interpersonal and attachment research. Psychother Theory Res Pract Train 39(1):32–43

Bifulco A (2002) Attachment style measurement: a clinical and epistemological perspective. Attach Hum Dev 4(2):180–188

Boyer SP, Hoffman MA (1993) Therapists' affective reactions to termination: impact of therapist loss history and client sensitivity to loss. J Couns Psychol 40:271–277

Brent DA, Kolko DJ, Birmaher B, Baugher M, Bridge J, Roth C, Holder D (1998) Predictors of treatment efficacy in a clinical trial of three psychosocial treatments for adolescent depression. J Am Acad Child Adolesc Psychiatry 37(9):906–914

Bridges MR (2006) Activating the corrective emotional experience. J Clin Psychol 62(5):551–568

Casement PJ (1991) Learning from the patient. The Guildford Press, New York

Cassidy J, Shaver PR (eds) (2008) Handbook of attachment-theory, research and clinical applications. The Guildford Press, New York

Castonguay LG, Goldfried MR, Wiser S, Raue PJ, Hayes AM (1996) Predicting the effect of cognitive therapy for depression: a study of unique and common factors. J Consult Clin Psychol 64:497–504

Clarkson P (2003) The therapeutic relationship, 2nd edn. Whurr Publishers, London

Coan J (2008) Toward a neuroscience of attachment. In: Cassidy J, Shaver PR (eds) Handbook of attachment- theory, research and clinical applications. The Guildford Press, New York

Cooley EJ, LaJoy R (1980) Therapeutic relationship and improvement as perceived by clients and therapists. J Clin Psychol 36:562–570

Coren A (2001) Short-term psychotherapy: a psychodynamic approach. Palgrave, Basinstoke

Crits-Christoph P, Luborsky L, Dahl L, Popp C, Mellon J, Mark D (1988) Clinicians can agree in assessing relationship patterns in psychotherapy. Arch Gen Psychiatry 45:1001–1004

Crits-Christoph P, Baranackie K, Kurcias J, Beck A, Carroll K, Perry K, Zitrin C (1991) Meta-analysis of therapist effects in psychotherapy outcome studies. Psychother Res 1(2):81–91

de Maat S, de Jonghe F, Schoevers R, Dekker J (2009) The effectiveness of long-term psychoanalytic therapy: a systematic review of empirical studies. Harv Rev Psychiatry 17(1):1–23

Despland J-M, Luc M, de Roten Y (2010) Intervention psychodynamique brève. Elsevier Masson, Paris

Dewan M, Weerasekera P, Stormon L (2009) Techniques of brief psychodynamic psychotherapy. In: Gabbard GO (ed) Textbook of psychotherapeutic treatments. American Psychiatric Publishing, London

Dozier M, Cue KL, Barrett L (1994) Clinicians as caregivers: the role of attachment organization in treatment. J Consult Clin Psychol 62(4):793–800

Dozier M, Chase Stovall-McClough K, Albus KE (2008) Attachment and psychopathology in adulthood. In: Cassidy J, Shaver PR (eds) Handbook of attachment- theory, research and clinical applications. The Guildford Press, New York

DSM-V (2014) Diagnostic and Statistical Manual of Mental Disorders, Fifth Edition: American Psychiatric Association

Elkin I, Shea MT, Watkins JT, Imber SD, Sotsky SM, Collins JF, Parloff MB (1989) National Institute of Mental Health treatment of depression collaborative research program: general effectiveness of treatments. Arch Gen Psychiatry 46(11):971–982

Elliott R, Clark C, Kemery V (1991) Analysing clients' post-session accounts of significant therapy events. Paper presented at the Society for Psychotherapy Research. Lyon

Farber BA, Lippert RA, Nevas DB (1995) The therapist as an attachment figure. Psychotherapy 32(2):204–212

Feeney BC, Collins NL (2001) Predictors of caregiving in adult intimate relationships: an attachment theoretical perspective. J Pers Soc Psychol 80(6):972–994

Ferenczi S, Rank O (1925) The development of psychoanalysis. International University Press, Madison

Fonagy P (1991) Thinking about thinking: some clinical and theoretical considerations in the treatment of a borderline patient. Int J Psychoanal 72:639–656

Fonagy P (2004) Psychotherapy meets neuroscience: a more focused future for psychotherapy research. Psychiatr Bull 28:357–359

Fonagy P, Gergely G, Jurist EL, Target M (2004) Affect regulation, mentalisation and the development of the self. Karnac, London

Fonagy P, Gergely G, Target M (2008) Psychoanalytic constructs and attachment theory and research. In: Cassidy J, Shaver PR (eds) Handbook of attachment- theory, research and clinical applications. The Guildford Press, New York

Freud S (1893 [1955]) Miss Lucy R, case histories from studies on hysteria. The standard edition of the complete psychological works of Sigmund Freud. vol. 2 (1893–1895): studies on hysteria. Hogarth Press, London

Freud S (1893 [1955]) New introductory lectures on psychoanalysis (Lectures XXIX–XXXV). The standard edition of the complete psychological works of Sigmund Freud. vol. 22. Hogarth Press, London

Freud S (1895 [1955]) Case histories from studies on hysteria. The standard edition of the complete psychological works of Sigmund Freud. vol. 2 (1893–1895): studies on hysteria. Hogarth Press, London

Freud S (1905 [1955]) Fragment of an analysis of a case of hysteria. The standard edition of the complete psychological works of Sigmund Freud. vol. 5. Hogarth Press, London

Freud S (1917 [1955]) Introductory lectures on psychoanalysis, part III: general theory of the neuroses. The standard edition of the complete psychological works of Sigmund Freud. vol. 16. Hogarth Press, London

Freud S (1920 [1955]) Beyond the pleasure. The standard edition of the complete psychological works of Sigmund Freud. vol. 5. Hogarth Press, London

Freud S (1923 [1955]) The ego and the id. The standard edition of the complete psychological works of Sigmund Freud. vol. 19. Hogarth Press, London

Friedman S, Gelso CJ (2000) The development of the inventory of countertransference behaviour. J Clin Psychol 56:1221–1235

Friedman ES, Thase ME (2009) Combining cognitive-behavioural therapy with medication. In: Gabbard GO (ed) Textbook of psychotherapeutic treatments. American Psychiatric Publishing, London

Gabbard GO (2009) Textbook of psychotherapeutic treatments. American Psychiatric Publishing, London

Garfield S (1998) The practice of brief psychotherapy. Wiley, Chichester

Garfield SL (2003) Eclectic psychotherapy: a common factors approach. In: Norcross JC, Goldfried MR (eds) Handbook of psychotherapy integration. Oxford University Press, New York

Gask L, Lester H, Kendrick T, Peveler R (2009a) What is primary care mental health? In: Gask L, Lester H, Kendrick T, Peveler R (eds) Primary care mental health. The Royal College of Psychiatrists Publications, London

Gask L, Dowrick C, Klinkman M, Gureje O (2009b) Diagnosis and classification of mental illness: a view from primary care. In: Gask L, Lester H, Kendrick T, Peveler R (eds) Primary care mental health. The Royal College of Psychiatrists Publications, London

Gaston L, Marmar CR, Thompson LW, Gallagher D (2002) The importance of the alliance in psychotherapy of elderly depressed patients. J Gerontol Psychol Sci 16:383–411

Gelso CJ, Hayes JA (2007) Countertransference and the therapist's inner experience-perils and possibilities. Lawrence Erlbaum Associates, NJ

Gelso CJ, Johnson DH (1983) Explorations in time-limited counselling and psychotherapy. Teachers College Press, New York

Gill M (1994) Psychoanalysis in transition. Analytic Press, Hillsdale

Gillieron E (1991) Βραχείες ψυχοθεραπείες και ψυχανάλυση (Les psychotherapies breves). Αθήνα: Εκδόσεις Εστία

Gillieron E (1994) Le premier entretien en psychothérapie. Dunod, Paris

Gillieron E (1997) Les psychothérapies brèves. PUF, Paris

Goldapple K, Segal Z, Garson C, Lau M, Bieling P, Kennedy S, Mayberg H (2004) Modulation of cortical-limbic pathways in major depression: treatment-specific effects of cognitive behavior therapy. Arch Gen Psychiatry 61(1):34–41

Goldberg S (2000) Attachment and development. Arnold, London

Goldman GA, Anderson T (2007) Quality of object relations and security of attachment as predictors of early therapeutic alliance. J Couns Psychol 54:111–117

Greenberg LS, Watson J (1998) Experiential therapy for depression: differential effects of client-centred relationship conditions and process experiential interventions. Psychother Res 8:210–224

Greene V (2011) Emotional development in psychoanalysis, attachment theory and neuroscience: creating connections. Routledge, Hove

Hardy GE, Aldridge J, Davidson C, Rowe C, Reilly S, Shapiro DA (1999) Therapist responsiveness to patient attachment styles and issues observed in patient-identified significant events in psychodynamic-interpersonal psychotherapy. Psychother Res 9:36–53

Hawkins P, Shohet R (2006) Supervision in the helping professions, 3rd edn. Open University Press, New York

Hayes JA (1995) Countertransference in group psychotherapy: waking a sleeping dog. Int J Group Psychother 45:521–535

Hesse E (2008) The adult attachment interview: protocol, method of analysis and empirical studies. In: Cassidy J, Shaver PR (eds) Handbook of attachment- theory, research and clinical applications. The Guildford Press, New York

Holmes J (1997) Attachment, autonomy, intimacy: some implications of attachment theory. Br J Med Psychol 70:231–248

Holmes J (1999) Ghosts in the consulting room: an attachment perspective on intergenerational transmission. Attach Hum Dev 1(1):115–131

Holmes J (2001) The search for the secure base: attachment theory and psychotherapy. Routledge, Hove

Horvath AO (2005) The therapeutic relationship: research and theory. Psychother Res 15(1–2):3–7

Horvath AO, Luborsky L (1993) The role of the therapeutic alliance in psychotherapy. J Consult Clin Psychol 61:561–573

Hovarth AO, Bedi RB (2002) The alliance. In: Norcross JC (ed) Psychotherapy relationships that work- therapist contributions and responsiveness to patients. Oxford University Press, New York

Huppert JD, Bufka LF, Barlow DH, Gorman JM, Shear MK, Woods SW (2001) Therapists, therapist variables and cognitive-behaviour therapy outcome in a multicentre trial for panic disorder. J Consult Clin Psychol 69:747–755

Jacobs M (2001) Psychodynamic counselling in action, 3rd edn. Sage, London

Jones E (1956) Sigmund Freud: life and work, vol 1. Hogarth Press, London
Kandel E (1998) A new intellectual framework for psychiatry. Am J Psychiatry 155:457–469
Kay J (2009) Combining psychodynamic psychotherapy with medication. In: Gabbard GO (ed) Textbook of psychotherapeutic treatments. American Psychiatric Publishing, London
Knekt P, Lindfors O, Härkänen T, Välikoski M, Virtala E, Laaksonen MA ... Renlund C (2008) Randomized trial on the effectiveness of long-and short-term psychodynamic psychotherapy and solution-focused therapy on psychiatric symptoms during a 3-year follow-up. Psychol Med 38(05):689–703
Knekt P, Lindfors O, Laaksonen MA, Renlund C, Haaramo P, Härkänen T, Virtala E (2011) Quasi-experimental study on the effectiveness of psychoanalysis, long-term and short-term psychotherapy on psychiatric symptoms, work ability and functional capacity during a 5-year follow-up. J Affect Disord 132(1):37–47
Koerner K, Linehan MM (2003) Integrative therapy for borderline personality disorder: dialectical behavior therapy. In: Norcross JC, Goldfried MR (eds) Handbook of psychotherapy integration. Oxford University Press, New York
Krupnick JL, Sotsky SM, Simmens S, Moyer J, Elkin I, Watkins J, Pilkonis PA (1996) The role of the therapeutic alliance in psychotherapy and pharmacotherapy. J Consult Clin Psychol 64:532–539
Kuehn JL (1965) Encounter at Leyden: Gustav Mahler consults Sigmund Freud. Psychoanal Rev 52:345–364
Lafferty P, Beutler LE, Crago M (1991) Differences between more and less effective psychotherapists: a study of select therapist variables. J Consult Clin Psychol 57:76–80
Lambert MJ (2003) Psychotherapy outcome research: implications for integrative and eclectic therapists. In: Norcross JC, Goldfried MR (eds) Handbook of psychotherapy integration. Oxford University Press, New York
Lambert MJ, Barley DE (2002) Research summary on the therapeutic relationship and psychotherapy outcome. In: Norcross JC (ed) Psychotherapy relationships that work- therapist contributions and responsiveness to patients. Oxford University Press, New York
Lambert MJ, Bergin AE (1994) The effectiveness of psychotherapy. In: Bergin AE, Garfield SL (eds) Handbook of psychotherapy and behaviour change, 4th edn. Wiley, New York
Lambert MJ, Ogles BM (2002) The efficacy and effectiveness of psychotherapy. In: Lambert MJ (ed) Handbook of psychotherapy and behaviour change, 5th edn. Wiley, New York
LaPlanche J, Pontalis JB (1986) Λεξιλόγιο της ψυχανάλυσης (5η έκδοση). Αθήνα: Εκδόσεις Κέδρος
Laylard R (2006) The case for psychological treatment centres. Br Med J 332:1030–1032
Leichsenring F (2009) Applications of psychodynamic psychotherapy to specific disorders: efficacy and indications. In: Gabbard GO (ed) Textbook of psychotherapeutic treatments. American Psychiatric Publishing, London
Leichsenring F, Rabung S, Leibing E (2004) The efficacy of short-term psychodynamic psychotherapy in specific psychiatric disorders: a meta-analysis. Arch Gen Psychiatry 61:1208–1216
Lemma A (2014) In praise of pluralism. Ther Today 24(10):38–40
Lemma A, Target M, Fonagy P (2011) Brief dynamic interpersonal therapy: a clinician's guide. Oxford University Press, Oxford
Lewis AJ, Dennerstein M, Gibbs PM (2008) Short-term psychodynamic psychotherapy: review of recent process and outcome studies. Aust N Z J Psychiatry 42:445–455
Lieberman EJ, Kramer R, Richter GC (2012) The letters of Sigmund Freud and Otto Rank: inside psychoanalysis. The John Hopkins University Press, Baltimore
Lilienfield S (2005) Scientifically unsupported and supported interventions for childhood psychopathology: a summary. Pediatrics 115(3):761–764
Lopez FG, Brennan KA (2000) Dynamic processes underlying adult attachment organisation: towards an attachment theoretical perspective on the healthy and effective self. J Couns Psychol 47(3):283–300
Luborsky L, Crits-Cristoph P (1998) Understanding transference: the core conflictual relationship theme method. American Psychological Association, Washington, DC

Luborsky L, Luborsky E (2006) Research and psychotherapy: the vital link. Rowman & Littlefield, New York

Luborsky L, Singer B, Luborsky L (1975) Comparative studies of psychotherapies: is it true that everybody has won and all must have prizes? Arch Gen Psychiatry 32:995–1008

Luborsky L, Crits-Christoph P, McLellan AT, Woody G, Piper W, Liberman B, Pilkonis P (1986) Do therapists vary much in their success? Findings from four outcome studies. Am J Orthopsychiatry 56(4):501

Luborsky L, Diguer L, Seligman DA, Rosenthal R, Krause ED, Johnson S, Schweizer E (1999) The researcher's own therapy allegiances: a "wild card" in comparisons of treatment efficacy. Clin Psychol Sci Pract 6(1):95–106

Luborsky L, Rosenthal R, Diguer L, Andrusyna TP, Berman JS, Levitt JT, Krause ED (2002) The dodo bird verdict is alive and well-mostly. Clin Psychol Sci Pract 9(1):2–12

Main M (1991) Metacognitive knowledge, metacognitive monitoring and singular (coherent) versus multiple (incoherent) models of attachment: findings and directions for future research. In: Parkes CM, Stevenson-Hinde J, Marris P (eds) Attachment across the life-cycle. Routledge, London

Main M (1993) Discourse, prediction and recent studies in attachment: implications for psychoanalysis. J Am Psychoanal Assoc 41:209–245

Malan DH (1976) The frontier of brief psychotherapy: an example of the convergence of research and clinical practice. Plenum, New York

Malan DH (1979) Individual psychotherapy and the science of psychodynamics. Butterworth, London

Malan DH (2001) Individual psychotherapy and the science of psychodynamics. Hodder Arnold, London

Mallinckrodt B (2000) Attachment, social competencies, social support and interpersonal processes in psychotherapy. Psychother Res 10(3):239–266

Mallinckrodt B, Gantt DL, Coble HM (1995) Attachment patterns in the psychotherapy relationship: development of the Client Attachment to Therapist Scale. J Couns Psychol 42(3):307–317

Mallinckrodt B, Jeong J (2015) Meta-analysis of client attachment to therapist: associations with working alliance and client pretherapy attachment. Psychotherapy 52(1):134–139

Mander G (2000) A psychodynamic approach to brief therapy. Sage, London

Mann J (1973) Time-limited psychotherapy. Harvard University Press, Cambridge, MA

Maroda KJ (2010) Psychodynamic techniques: working with emotion in the therapeutic relationship. The Guildford Press, New York

Martin DJ, Garske JP, Davis MK (2000) Relation of therapeutic alliance with outcome and other variables: a meta-analytic review. J Consult Clin Psychol 68:438–450

Meltzoff J, Kornreich M (1970) Research in psychotherapy. Atherton, New York

Messer SB, Wampold BE (2002) Let's face facts: common factors are more potent than specific therapy ingredients. Clin Psychol Sci Pract 9(1):18–22

Messer SB, Warren SW (1995) Models of brief psychodynamic therapy: a comparative approach. Guidford Press, New York

Meszaros J (2004) Psychoanalysis is a two-way street. Int Forum Psychoanal 13:105–113

Mikulincer M, Shaver PR (2008) Adult attachment and affect regulation. In: Cassidy J, Shaver PR (eds) Handbook of attachment- theory, research and clinical applications. The Guildford Press, New York

Miller WR, Taylor CA, West JC (1980) Focused versus broad-spectrum behaviour therapy for problem drinkers. J Consult Clin Psychol 48:590–601

Mitchell SA (1988) Relational concepts in psychoanalysis: an integration. Harvard University Press, Massachusetts

Mitchell SA (1997) Influence and autonomy in psychoanalysis. Analytic Press, Hillsdale

Mitchell SA (2000) Relationality: from attachment to intersubjectivity. Routledge, London

Mohr JJ, Gelso CJ, Hill CE (2005) Client and counsellor trainees' attachment as predictors of session evaluation and countertransference behaviour in first counselling sessions. J Couns Psychol 52(3):298–309

Murray CJ, Lopez AD (1997) Alternative projections of mortality and disability by cause 1990–2020: Global Burden of Disease Study. Lancet 349:1436–1442

Nelson-Jones R (2001) Theory and practice of counselling and therapy, 3rd edn. Sage, London

Norcross JC (2002) Psychotherapy relationships that work- therapist contributions and responsiveness to patients. Oxford University Press, New York

Norcross JC, Goldfried MR (2003) Handbook of psychotherapy integration. Oxford University Press, New York

Papadopoulos RK (2007) Refugees, trauma and adversity-activated development. Eur J Psychother Couns 9(3):301–312

Project MATCH Research Group (1998) Therapist effects in three treatments for alcohol problems. Psychother Res 8(4):455–474

Rank O (1929) The trauma of birth. Harper & Row, New York

Robinson LA, Berman JS, Neimeyer RA (1990) Psychotherapy for the treatment of depression: a comprehensive review of controlled outcome research. Psychol Bull 108:30–49

Rogers CR (1957) The necessary and sufficient conditions of therapeutic personality change. J Consult Psychol 22:95–103

Rosenberg EW, Hayes JA (2002) Origins, consequences and management of countertransference: a case study. J Couns Psychol 49(2):221–232

Rosenfeld GW (2009) Beyond evidence-based psychotherapy: fostering the eight sources of change in child and adolescent treatment. Routledge, New York

Roth A, Fonagy P (2005) What works for whom? A critical review of psychotherapy research. The Guildford Press, New York

Rubino G, Barker C, Roth T, Fearon P (2000) Therapist empathy and depth of interpretation in response to potential alliance ruptures: the role of therapist and patient attachment styles. Psychother Res 10(4):408–420

Ryle A (1998) Cognitive analytic therapy and borderline personality disorder: the model and the method. Wiley, Chichester

Safran JD, Wallner LK (1991) The relative predictive validity of two therapeutic alliance measures in cognitive therapy. Psychol Assess: J Consult Clin Psychol 3:188–195

Sartorius N (2009) Mental health and primary health care: an international policy perspective. In: Gask L, Lester H, Kendrick T, Peveler R (eds) Primary care mental health. RCPsych Publications, Glasgow

Schore AN (1994) Affect regulation and the development of the self: the neurobiology of emotional development. Lawrence Erlbaum Associates, NJ

Schore AN (2003) Affect regulation and the repair of the self. W.W. Norton & Company, New York

Shapiro DA, Shapiro D (1982) Meta-analysis of comparative therapy outcome studies: a replication and refinement. Psychol Bull 92:581–604

Sifneos P (1979) Short-term dynamic psychotherapy. Plenum Press, New York

Slade A (2008) The implications of attachment theory and research for adult psychotherapy: research and clinical perspectives. In: Cassidy J, Shaver PR (eds) Handbook of attachment-theory, research and clinical applications. The Guildford Press, New York

Smith ML, Glass GV, Miller TI (1980) The benefits of psychotherapy. John Hopkins University Press, Baltimore

Spielmans GI, Pasek LF, McFall JP (2007) What are the active ingredients in cognitive and behavioural therapy for anxious and depressed children? A meta-analytic review. Clin Psychol Rev 27(5):642–654

Stanton M (1990) Sandor Ferenczi-reconsidering active intervention. Free Association Books, London

Stylianidis S (1995) Brief psychoanalytic psychotherapies in the context of public health, Doctoral Dissertation, Dimokreitio University of Thrace, Alexandroupoli

Sterba R (1951) A case of brief psychotherapy by Sigmund Freud. Psychoanal Rev 38:75–80

Symington N (1986) The analytic experience: lectures from the Tavistock. Free Assosiation Books, London

Tantum D (1995) Why assess? In: Mace C (ed) The art and science of assessment in psychotherapy. Routledge, London

Thomas L, Lewis G (2009) The epidemiology of mental illness. In: Gask L, Lester H, Kendrick T, Peveler R (eds) Primary care mental health. The Royal College of Psychiatrists Publications, London

Tyrell CL, Dozier M, Teague GB, Fallot RD (1999) Effective treatment relationships for persons with serious psychiatric disorders: the importance of attachment states of mind. J Consult Clin Psychol 67:725–733

Van Lerberghe W (2008) The world health report 2008: primary health care: now more than ever. World Health Organization, Geneva

Vaslamatzis G, Verveniotis S (1985) Early dropouts in brief dynamic psychotherapy. Psychother Psychosom 44:205–210

Vaslamatzis G, Kanellos P, Tserpe V, Verveniotis S (1986) Countertransference responses in short-term dynamic psychotherapy. Psychother Psychosom 46:105–109

Vaslamatzis G, Markidis M, Katsouyanni K (1989) Study of the patients' difficulties in ending brief psychoanalytic psychotherapy. Psychother Psychosom 52:173–178

Vinnars B, Barber JP, Noren K, Gallop R, Weinryb RM (2005) Manualised supportive-expressive psychotherapy versus non-manualised community-delivered psychodynamic therapy for patients with personality disorders: bridging efficacy and effectiveness. Am J Psychiatry 162:1933–1940

Wallin DJ (2007) Attachment in psychotherapy. The Guildford Press, New York

Walter B (1947) Theme and variations. Hamish Hamilton, London

Wampold B (2001) The great psychotherapy debate: models, methods and findings. Erlbaum, NJ

Wampold B, Minami E, Bastin TW, Tierney SC (2002) A meta-(re)analysis of the effects of cognitive therapy versus 'other therapies' for depression. J Affect Disord 68:159–165

Weisz JR, McCarty CA, Valeri SM (2006) Effects of psychotherapy for depression in children and adolescents: a meta-analysis. Psychol Bull 132(1):132–149

Westen D, Gabbard GO (2002) Developments in cognitive neuroscience II: implications for theories of transference. J Am Psychoanal Assoc 50:99–134

Westen D, Morrison K (2001) A multidimensional meta-analysis of treatments for depression, panic and generalised anxiety disorder: an empirical examination of the status of empirically supported therapies. J Consult Clin Psychol 69(6):875–899

Wittchen HU, Nelson CB, Lachner G (1998) Prevalence of mental disorders and psychosocial impairments in adolescents and young adults. Psychol Med 28(01):109–126

World Health Organization (WHO) (2008) The World Health Report 2008. Primary Health Care: now more than ever. WHO Press, Switzerland

Στυλιανίδης Σ (1995) Οι βραχείες ψυχαναλυτικές ψυχοθεραπείες στα πλαίσια της δημόσιας περίθαλψης (Διδακτορική Διατριβή). Δημοκρίτειο Πανεπιστήμιο Θράκης, Αλεξανδρούπολη

Προτεινόμενη βιβλιογραφία

Beck AT, Freeman A (1990) Cognitive therapy for personality disorders. Guildford, New York

Beck AT, Rush AJ, Shaw BF, Emery G (1979) Cognitive therapy of depression. Guilford, New York

Beitman BD, Manring J (2009) Theory and practice of psychotherapy integration. In: Gabbard GO (ed) Textbook of psychotherapeutic treatments. American Psychiatric Publishing, London

Clark DA, Hollifield M, Leahy R, Beck J (2009) Theory of cognitive therapy. In: Gabbard GO (ed) Textbook of psychotherapeutic treatments. American Psychiatric Publishing, London

Ellis A (1973) Humanistic psychotherapy: a rational-emotive approach. McGraw Hill, New York

Epp AM, Dobson KS, Cottraux J (2009) Applications of individual cognitive-behavioural therapy to specific disorders: efficacy and indications. In: Gabbard GO (ed) Textbook of psychotherapeutic treatments. American Psychiatric Publishing, London

Norcross JC, Newman CF (2003) Psychotherapy integration: setting the context. In: Norcross JC, Goldfried MR (eds) Handbook of psychotherapy integration. Oxford University Press, New York

Wheelis J (2009) Theory and practice of dialectical behavioural therapy. In: Gabbard GO (ed) Textbook of psychotherapeutic treatments. American Psychiatric Publishing, London

Young JE (1994) Cognitive therapy for personality disorders: a schema-focused approach. Personal Resource Exchange, Sarasota

Community Mental Healthcare for Migrants

15

Nikos Gionakis and Stelios Stylianidis

Abstract

This chapter discusses the relationship between migration and mental health, as it is illustrated in the way trends are formulated, in the field of relevant research on the one hand and, on the other, in the recommendations offered for the mental health of migrants on the other. The second part deals with the basic organisational and operational aspects of a mental health unit for migrants, the Babel Day Centre (Athens, Greece), and presents the challenges that its multidisciplinary team faces along with the ways it attempts to manage them. Upon completion of this chapter, the reader will have received ample stimuli for reflection on the important issue of service provision to migrants.

15.1 Introduction

The period from the middle of the twentieth century to date has been defined as the age of migration (Watters 2007). In fact, humans have always been on the move (the history of humanity is a history of peoples' movements and the meeting between

---

"χαῖρε, ξεῖνε, παρ' ἄμμι φιλήσεαι· αὐτὰρ ἔπειτα δείπνου πασσάμενος μυθήσεαι ὅττεό σε χρή."
("Greetings, stranger. You are welcome here.
After you've had dinner, you can tell us what you need".)
(Homer, Odyssey, A, 123–124, English translation by S. Lombardo)

N. Gionakis (✉)
Psychlogist, Scientific Responsible, Day Centre Babel, Athens, Greece
e-mail: nikosgionakis@gmail.com

S. Stylianidis
Department of Psychology, Panteion University, Athens, Greece
e-mail: stylianidis.st@gmail.com

© Springer International Publishing Switzerland 2016
S. Stylianidis (ed.), *Social and Community Psychiatry: Towards a Critical, Patient-Oriented Approach*, DOI 10.1007/978-3-319-28616-7_15

them); however the migratory flows of our time, in terms of scale, globalisation and social/economic consequences, have no precedent.

Migration is defined as a process of social change during which an individual moves from one cultural framework to another for the purpose of settling – permanently or temporarily (Bhugra and Jones 2001). This change may be due to different reasons, usually social/economic, political, educational and environmental (idem). Travel duration to the country of settlement varies and depends upon different factors; movement may be conducted individually or in groups (factors such as the reason for departure play an important role in this), while, after settlement in a country, a significant number of the migrants will form ethnic minorities.

In the last 40 years, migratory flows have doubled compared to the past; recently the number of people forced to abandon their countries of origin for another country (refugees), or their homes for other regions within their country (internally displaced), has risen dramatically. According to UNHCR, in 2013 the number of refugees internally displaced throughout the world was calculated at 51,2 million, 86 % of which have sought refuge in developing countries (http://unhcr.org/trends2013/). It is expected that by 2050, 150,000,000 people will have migrated, not because of economic reasons but because of the climate changes observed on the planet.

The presence of migrants in a country triggers phenomena related to the social and individual changes emerging from coexistence with the natives [see, e.g. acculturation, namely, the mutual changes arising when individuals or groups from different cultural backgrounds come into direct and constant contact], creating the need for integration policies, namely, relevant to the migrants exercising their rights in the country of settlement.

Featuring highly among these rights is access to health and mental health services. Health is a fundamental human and social right. It also is, at the same time, an important factor in the life of migrants, directly linked to integration: "Migrants whose health condition is poor or who cannot move due to health problems, are obstructed in the efforts for integration. […] Disease accentuates marginalisation and marginalisation accentuates disease, creating the conditions for a gradual decline. At the same time, integration is a prerequisite for the provision of effective health care, which is often impeded by inadequate accessibility. Access to effective health care must be viewed as equally important as housing and education for living and by extension the migrants' integration" (Ingleby et al. 2005).

15.2 Migration and Mental Health

The relation between migration and mental health has been the objective of study since the 1930s. Ødegaard's (1932) paper on the prevalence of schizophrenia among Norwegian migrants in the USA is known; the paper was the start of a series of research efforts, the objective of which was the effect of migration on mental health and the reverse. In this section, we will present some findings as they have been described in published meta-analyses.

According to Kirmayer and his associates (2011), the prevalence of common mental disorders among migrants is initially lower than in the general population and increases with the passage of time until it becomes equal to that of the general population. As to the refugees, those among them that have been exposed to violence often suffer from higher rates of disorders related to trauma, including post-traumatic stress disorder (PTSD) and chronic pain or other physical syndromes. In Fazel's and his associates' meta-analysis, about 1 in 10 adult refugees in high-income Western countries suffers from PTSD, 1 in 20 from major depression and approximately 1 in 25 from general anxiety disorder. In many cases these disorders coexist. With regard to children, the same meta-analysis has shown that approximately one in ten children presented with PTSD (Fazel et al. 2005).

The research questions changed in 1960. Instead of seeking *why* the migrants had higher (or lower) rates of mental disorders, researchers began wondering *under what conditions* migrants present higher rates of disease (Murphy 1977).

The overview by Zissi (2006) concludes with the finding that the studies and the research trying to associate the migration condition with bad mental health have given varied, often conflicting, results, while there are more than a few ensuing methodological difficulties (most of the overviews have reached the same findings). Therefore, the requirement is to study the factors that make migration a negative experience causing an adverse impact on mental health, as well as the factors that are protective for migrants against the new challenges and requirements in the receiving country. According to the author, it is therefore possible to arrive at the identification of three groups of factors, the presence of which may play a protective role in the migration process, while their absence may be related to a negative impact. These factors refer to:

(a) *The migrant's personal characteristics*, whether these are premigration ones (gender, age, education level) or they emerge during migration (internal resources, search skills, acculturation tactics).
(b) *Social interaction characteristics*, in the migrant's immediate environment (e.g. family) as well as that of the community where he belongs (e.g. diaspora community, neighbourhood, school). Networks consisting of relatives that ensure positive reciprocity, exchange of information and practical support favourably influence the migrant's psychosocial adjustment, while, on the contrary, the dense, traditional orientation networks of relatives have a negative impact, especially on women migrants.
(c) *Characteristics of the receiving country's wider political and socioeconomic framework*, such as multiculturalism, unemployment levels and the implementation of migration policy measures, intercultural education programmes and health services recognising cultural peculiarities. According to Zissis, empirical findings show that migrant rejection by native residents, unemployment, high levels of bureaucracy and the lack of culturally sensitive policy implementation constitute threatening conditions for their adjustment. The author, however, ascertains that this group of factors has been studied less in social sciences, and therefore, our knowledge regarding the role they play in the migrants' individual biographies is not enriched.

Specialists draw attention to the need of looking into the conditions that pertain to the mental health of special groups among migrants, such as minors and, in particular, unaccompanied minors, victims of trafficking, the elderly, refugees, survivors of torture and abuse, heads of single-parent families and different sexual orientation individuals. For example, it has been found that exposure to violence is linked to the appearance of post-traumatic stress disorder, that the adverse experiences children live through during the trip or after arrival at the receiving country play a significant role in the manifestation of psychic disorder symptoms and also that children separated very young from their parents due to migration run a greater risk of presenting with such symptoms (Bhugra et al. 2011).

Discussion has recently begun on the consequences of migration in the reception areas of health system, as well as the consequences of the lack of accessibility to the health system (mental health, in our case) on migrants. The relevant questions mainly pertain (1) to the level of which health and mental health policy is formulated (by governments, healthcare authorities or individual service provision) and (2) the level of service provision (by health professionals and services). The aim is that health and mental health professionals may be informed with regard to the migrants' special needs and may be trained so that they can offer more effective care. It is necessary to pay particular attention to these and other similar questions as it is now clear that even if the "healthy migrant phenomenon" is valid at the time of arrival, most migrants will obtain a lower socioeconomic position in the receiving country, which alone will undermine the possibility of their maintaining a positive health status. We should recall that relating migrants to "special health problems" refers to long-gone eras and in particular to the time of the colonies, when the migrant was seen as "inappropriate" or "exotic". In fact, the health problems for which migrants often seek help are common, usual diseases that anyone could suffer from (Ingleby 2008).

Further issues concerning the specialists pertain to (a) the effect of conditions prevailing in the transit countries and the receiving countries on the mental health of migrants and (b) the way that the receiving countries' agencies should be organised in order to provide the appropriate answers on the migrants' mental health problems. As to the first question, researchers usually refer to conditions such as confinement and the threat of extradition, limited access to employment, housing, education and social benefits as well as the consequences of boredom, isolation and discrimination. In these cases, more and more researchers are documenting the manifestation of post-migration stress and the weight it adds on pre-existing disorders (Silove et al. 2000). As to the second question, it is interesting to examine the extended directives and recommendations as well as the characteristics that good practices should have in the context of migration and refugee mental healthcare. Directives have been issued by the World Psychiatric Association (Bhugra et al. 2011) and the European Office of the World Health Organisation (Gionakis 2009), while on the matter of good practices, the points made by Watters and Ingleby (2004) and Watters (2010) are interesting.

The common point in all the aforementioned is identifying the need to (a) take measures to ensure migrant access to the appropriate, integrated and culturally sensitive agencies equipped with sufficient resources; (b) pay particular attention to extroversion and the mobility of community resources, as well as the promotion of migrant participation in management/administration of such agencies; (c) achieve agency co-ordination and cooperation with them to ensure care continuity; (d) retain awareness of the political dimension of the agencies and have professionals engage in their activities accordingly (see advocacy) and have clear relevant policies taking into consideration the migrants', refugees' and asylum seekers' human rights; (e) operate continuous training programmes, so that human resources can be supported in order to acquire cultural adequacy and apply it to daily practice and also to develop knowledge and training networks for the identification and dissemination of good practices; and (f) to organise registration and monitoring systems for the agencies' control and evaluation.

15.3 Mental Health Agencies for Migrants Internationally: Theoretical and Practical Approaches

In some countries, such as France, Italy, Spain, the United Kingdom and Australia, there has been a notable development of organising and providing specialised services to migrants and, in several cases, to special categories of individuals, such as, for example, survivors of torture, trafficking victims, children and adolescents, etc. Some of these agencies are the Centre Minkowska in Paris, continuing the French tradition in ethnopsychiatry; the Centro Franz Fanon in Turin; the Transcultural Psychiatry Unit in Victoria, Australia; the Freedom from Torture Foundation in London, which specialises in the rehabilitation of survivors of torture, as does the Dignity Institute in Copenhagen; the Psychopathological and Psychosocial Support Service for Immigrants and Refugees (SAPPIR) in the Sant Pere Claver Hospital in Barcelona; and others. Each team follows its own approach, both on theoretical and practical-operational level. We could say that, irrespective of the approach each of them has adopted, they are all facing similar challenges which they try to manage utilising specific – and appropriately adapted – tools and strategies. Here we will examine the main among these challenges.

Cultural Competence

Culture affects the way in which "people relate to disease, manifest symptoms, organise search for help behaviour, make decisions on who is normal or not, approach therapists (and therapists clients) and understand ethics and the changing stages of conscience" (Ridley et al. 1998).

Particular emphasis has been given in recent years to the demands of clinical work with people from different ethnocultural origins. Cultural sensitivity, cultural awareness, cultural adequacy and cultural proficiency are abilities that a health/mental health agency must have, among others, in order to competently receive and respond to requests from migrants, namely, from clients who differ by ethnoculture and language.

Cultural competence is defined by the US Department of Health and Human Services as "a set of cultural behaviours, attitudes and policies within a system that enables its professionals to work effectively in cross cultural situations". The term refers to the professional's capability to honour and respect the beliefs, the language, the manners of interpersonal communication and the behaviours of individuals and families receiving the services as well as the staff providing these services. Another common definition widely used in mental health considers cultural skill as "a set of congruent behaviors, attitudes, and policies that come together in a system, agency, or among professionals that enable them to work effectively in cross-cultural situations" (Cross et al. 1989).

In this sense, the health practitioner must, among other things, respect the different language, the values and customs of a social group, know the main points of the individual's cultural framework and have the will to explore his/her own beliefs and prejudices. She/he must also integrate the individual's culture in health provision and be open to the various ways that the patient participates in his/her treatment.

Cultural competence allows the professional (better yet the multidisciplinary team and the institution in its totality) to conduct assessments of the migrants' psychosocial needs. Doing this takes into consideration their triple "diversity": cultural background, migration condition and mental (ill) health. In addition, it facilitates the professional's approach to the individual in such a way as to make the assessment of his/her needs be the result of a process. In such a process, needs are not determined by the professional alone but are conjointly identified. In this sense, meeting the needs is the result of negotiation between the individual (who then is raised to a subject) and the agency or rather the network of agencies. Through this process, unique for each person, the network becomes a set of places and moments that receives them as subjects with respect and dignity, without conditions and prerequisites.

The establishment of an effective relationship with the beneficiary implies a negotiation process between the two sides. This will lead to the development of culturally appropriate management and treatment plans. The professional should become aware of the explanatory model the beneficiary uses in order to manage his/her disease. This negotiation will include the following steps (Seah et al. 2002, p. 30–31):

1. "Eliciting the client's explanatory model
2. Outlining the practitioner's explanatory model
3. Comparing the models
4. Conceptually translating and negotiating an understanding and acceptance of one model with the other
5. Developing a mutually acceptable treatment plan"

In some cases it may be feasible to utilise different methods, such as "Western" drug treatment, cultural mediation and other traditional therapeutic means.

Cultural Mediation

The major issue during communication between people with different ethnocultural origins is to ensure that what one person says coincides with what the other is hearing. It is also important to take into consideration that communication consists both of verbal and nonverbal transfer of valuable information and that – as a rule – more than one message is communicated at the same time.

In many cultures, terms such as "mental" "mood", "anxiety", etc. have different meanings or do not exist at all in different cultures than the Western one. Moreover, the request for assistance follows different routes, the provision of help has specific codes and daily living routine unfolds differently. The role of the *mediator* is critical in order to bridge these and other differences.

The language/cultural mediator helps by explaining to the professional how to address problems that are presented during the session in the context of the patient's culture of origin. She/he does not just explain the context of the specific culture; she/he discusses it with the health professional. In other approaches, the mediator is a regular member of the team receiving the request and manages the case therapeutically. The mediator will participate in the creation of a common language in the team, a language that keeps the team together. The mediator is therefore not a neutral "tool" facilitating the comprehension of the language's precoded meanings but rather a determining factor in building a common ground for communication.

The role of the mediator is not limited in facilitating the therapist to approach the patient but also to assist the patient in finding his/her way in the new living environment. Thus, it is important to accompany the migrant patient to the various agencies that offer him/her support so that she/he may learn to use them effectively.

Ethnopsychiatry and Moving Population Care in the Community: Querying an Example

According to Stylianidis and Bagourdis (2008), the definitions that have been used from time to time to determine the trend promoting the enrichment if the psychiatric view with cultural elements (cultural relativism) vary depending with each researcher's research and scientific interests.

The term *transcultural psychiatry* is controversial. Whether it is appropriate or not is questioned by many experts, as besides *transcultural psychiatry*, other terms such as *comparative, ecological, prescientific, ethnopsychiatry* or just *cultural psychiatry* are used as well. It is possible that the different approaches of the term showcase the multifaceted nature of the researched objective, as anthropology, medical history, psychology, sociology and social work as well as nursing are used besides psychiatry and medicine.

Kraepelin (1904) used the term *comparative psychiatry*. The same term was used by Yap (1974) and Murphy (1982), subsequently (Litllewood 1990). In the USA, psychiatrists began using the term transcultural psychiatry introduced by Wittkower in the 1950s. Wittkower clarifies that the concept of transcultural psychiatry is determined by five targets: (1) exploring the similarities and differences in the manifestation of mental disease in different countries, (2) identifying the cultural factors indicating a predisposition for mental disease and mental health, (3) assessing the effect of cultural factors in the prevalence of mental disorders and the nature of mental disease, (4) studying the kind of interventions preferred to be used in different cultural frameworks and (5) comparing the different attitudes against mental disease in different civilisations and cultures (Wittkower 1966, p. 228). Okpaku (1998) proceeded along the same lines. In 1988, Kleinman introduced the term "new transcultural psychiatry", in order to determine the new trend prevailing at the time in the USA, which then became more widely known as "cultural psychiatry" or the "psychiatry of culture" (Favazza and Oman 1978).

The massive scale and complexity of the migration phenomenon places the field of ethnopsychiatry into radical restructuring, at least in the way this had been defined by colonial psychiatry. Theoretical examples that emerged from the 1960s *despite* the increasing number of ethnopsychiatric studies remain anchored to date in their majority on old stereotypes and antiquated interpretation models of the relationship between culture and mental disorder: these stereotypes are characterised by strong prejudice, a vague definition of culture and mainly by a constant interest for classification of Western psychiatry in the emergence of new clinical categories, techniques and knowledge, which, however, did not show the required careful and in-depth analysis of the political and social framework where these psychopathologies flourished (Beneduce 2007). In other words, psychiatry that meant to consider the patients' "culture" or the different forms of social or family structure as parameters to be taken into consideration in the diagnostic and therapeutic process remained inaccessible, not comprehending the economic contrast that causes migration, the correlation of forces between the involved parties, the moral conflict, as well as the set of consequences that the daily actual and symbolic violence causes to the populations of the colonies.

The examples in literature on this type of violence on populations that, according to Balandier (1955) acquired a form of social surgery, are numerous and indicative of this positivistic trend in psychiatry (Cartwright 1851 – drapetomania or pathological indifference "dysaesthesia aethiopica" (Vaughan 1991; Morrison 1988; Garrigues 2003).

Bourdieu (2003) spoke of "symbolic violence", of a "sweet and invisible" violence, wishing to determine specific relations in the area of pedagogy, sexism and racism. This formulation by Bourdieu could reliably define the type of relationships that were established between colonising and local populations and to a great extent "dressed up the correlation of power". The symbolic power is the power of acting on the world, by acting on the representation of this world (Bourdieu and Wacquant 1992).

The challenge of the meeting and therapy with the other, when the other is part of an increasing number of moving populations in the world, is a complex scientific, political and cultural problem. How could we consider the role of cultural identity in clinical narratives of foreign citizens who cannot accept what we as Western societies call "social integration"? What kind of dialogue can be conducted with therapeutic techniques that are formed within completely different fields and horizons, where the interpretation of effectiveness is completely different to that of traditional Western psychiatry? Perhaps the time has come to explore not just the function of the symbols originating from a different cultural framework or their effectiveness (Levi-Strauss 1978) but also their power to cause disease or even death. Recent social anthropology, ethnology and critical psychiatry literature underline the scientific fragility of ethnopsychiatry or transcultural psychiatry: terms such as "invention of culture", "mixed identities" (métis), "construction of authenticity" and "invention of tradition" are serious indications of the scientific identity of other terms, such as ethnos (a people), culture, tradition or identity, and underline the risks deriving from the attempt of objectification, according to the classification of Western tradition or their political manipulation.

Therefore, the challenge of meeting and caring for moving populations requires us to redetermine the basic concepts that had supported the scientific edifice of ethnopsychiatry. As Hannerz (1998) says: "each complex culture must be seen as a moving set of connections. The connections we see are those between signifiers and forms that transport them, but at the same time, connections between individuals are established through the social organisation of the signifier".

The reception, understanding, meeting and mental healthcare of the other lead us to look differently at the "cultural identity" in the current context of globalisation. In this multifaceted meeting with "the other", there cannot exist mutually acceptable lines of interpretation of the unconscious in individuals or groups, irrespective of the framework in which they live, exist and relate to others.

The recent genocides, the responsibility of the West in feeding and reproducing pre-existing ethnic tension differences and the conflict to conquer wealth-producing resources of developing countries in the geopolitical sphere give us the general context and cause to reflect first on our own clinical view and our own ambivalence in view of the complexity of these individuals' requests and needs.

If anthropology is the search between individual freedom and social meaning (Augé 2009), ethnopsychiatry of moving populations must be referred to the understanding of this fluidity, these tensions and our own structural ambivalence in the context of our meeting with them.

15.4 One Example of Organising Migrants' Mental Healthcare in the Community: Babel Day Centre in Athens

Let us begin with three stories:

> When she arrived in Greece from Sierra Leone, Georgetta was impressed to find people who were in their 40s and their parents were still alive. She had lost hers in the civil war; she didn't even have time to bury them. It weighs on her; not burying your parents is a grave sin. She can't sleep at night; the spirits keep her awake, reminding her of her duty.
>
> Nazrul did not want to leave his country, Bangladesh. He wanted to stay there, study business administration and find a job in that field. But he was the one, together with his

brother, selected by the family to immigrate and help the rest of them survive. Shortly after arriving in Greece (where he found a tailor's job and worked for twelve hours a day) he started seeing things that others did not see, he began wandering, fearing for his life.

The family of 13-year old Faroul was forced to leave Afghanistan because of her father's political beliefs. Before they were able to leave, Faroul and her sister were kidnapped. The kidnappers demanded ransom. The family collected the money with help from others, but not the full amount. The uncle who went to the negotiation (to hand the money over and get the children back) was murdered by the kidnappers because he didn't have the full ransom amount. Faroul has trouble sleeping at night and has difficulty remembering. As does her mother...

The Babel Day Centre started its operation in November 2007 in Kypseli, a multicultural Athenian district. It is a mental health unit that provides services to migrants. Priority is given to those who have difficulty accessing or are banned from mental health services, either because they are illegal aliens or they have yet to achieve adequate knowledge of Greek, so that they may communicate with the professionals in mainstream mental health agencies. However, since Babel operates in the context of public mental health and there is no other unit like in throughout Athens, it has no exclusion criteria for requests addressed to it. Each request receives an answer, even if it is a referral to another unit (only people with substance and alcohol abuse/addiction are not taken in charge; instead, they are referred to specialised units).

An extensive information campaign was implemented for organisations addressing migrants' (a) mental health needs, (b) physical health needs and (c) social needs and mainstream organisations where migrants could apply, in order to make Babel known and build a cooperation and referral network. Through this ongoing campaign, it has been possible to inform a wide range of organisations about Babel, the services it provides and the ways in which someone may apply to it. Also, a media campaign was designed, mainly for the migration mass media, in order to make its operation directly known to potential interested parties; an effort has been made to approach representatives of the so-called migration communities.

Babel receives requests from anyone irrespective of age, gender, ethnicity, religion and residence status (legal or not) in our country. It also receives requests pertaining to couples and families. Since January 2008, when the clinical work began, till December 2013, Babel had received 2,210 requests of which 1,256 were undertaken as "cases". These people came from 74 different countries. Of the "cases", 55.4 % did not understand Greek, while 18.75 % had problems with legal stay in Greece.

Access to Babel is not subject to specific rules. Anyone can apply in the most expedient way to them: by phone, in person or through another professional. The request is received by a member of the multidisciplinary team and the first clinical meeting is then scheduled. Both on reception of the request and on the first clinical meeting, the aim is for the applicant to establish a contact with the unit. In order to achieve this aim, an attempt is made to help the applicant understand that at Babel there is someone available to listen to him/her. This is made possible as there are no formalities upon reception, communication is done in his/her own language and the staff allows the expression of the challenges she/he is facing in his daily living.

Many migrants find it hard to trust easily. In most cases they are referred to Babel without an explanation as to the reason, or the kind of provided services and what to expect from them, making contact even more difficult.

Starting from the premise that migrants and refugees with mental health issues and/or mental disorders (namely, ones that can also be distinguished by their triple otherness: the migration condition, different ethnic-cultural origins, mental disorder experience) are in particularly vulnerable positions while they also have sufficient reserves of mental resilience, the overall goal of Babel is to provide the appropriate care and support services to underpin their resilience. In order to achieve this, an attempt is made to create a *home* (see below) able to actively listen, understand and support any person (individual, couple, family, group) addressing a request to Babel related to mental health. In this space, besides having the mental disorder symptoms treated, it is possible for the applicant to establish the meaning of the loss of country has for them as well as the expectations of a new life on an individual, family and social/cultural level. Emphasis is given to the *individualised approach*, while the *individual care plan* prepared and implemented is the result of *negotiation* between the framework and the person to whom the service is provided. This means that there is no previously set "service menu"; depending on the negotiation and the needs that will emerge, services may be "invented" that have not been offered to another applicant before and may not be offered to anyone in the future, as they are appropriate to the specific person, the specific family and so on.

As mental health is favourably or adversely affected by a multitude of factors (risk and protection), the Babel multidisciplinary team tries to maintain its readiness in order to trace (in the context of the "assessment") the existence of such factors and take action (by applying the principles of promoting mental health). So to make the assessment, it is of essential significance to acquire information regarding the applicant's quality of life and the degree of his integration (particularly if he wishes to remain in the country). This information pertains to the status and capability of caring for physical health, covering basic needs (housing, clothing, nutrition), employment, the existence of a support network, knowledge of Greek, legal or not residence in the country, integration into education (for children and adolescents) and similar "non-clinical variables". Addressing the needs linked to these variables is a priority for the Babel team, and to this end, a *client-centred network* is convened each time to undertake the planning and implementation/assessment of the individual treatment and rehabilitation. This includes interventions on all aspects of an individual's or a family's life (by the end of 2013, Babel had developed cooperations with more than 200 entities – state, local government, non-profit, volunteer, as well as informal active citizen networks). The cooperation is necessary to address the needs of the beneficiaries in terms of health and mental health, social care, employment, education, recreation, culture, legal aid, etc. As a result, the beneficiary becomes a "client" of a network and not of a unit, and each unit has to operate as an "open system" in constant communication with the community. In such a way, the unit makes an effort to "correct" its own imperfections by making use of resources available in other institutions. In order for the network (or rather for the multiple networks) to operate successfully, constant communication is necessary between the professionals of the participating organisations. This communication takes place using any possible form (face-to-face meetings, telephone contact, teleconference, e-mail, etc.). Communication is effective and cooperation becomes efficient under certain preconditions. For example, the cultivation of a common language between professionals, compliance to specific and mutually acceptable principles and the will to cooperate (therefore also to compromise and everything else that cooperation involves) can contribute to this end.

Clinical Approach

Clinical work at Babel is based in many respects on the theoretical approach of R. K. Papadopoulos (see Papadopoulos 1997, 2000, 2001, 2002, 2007, 2011), director of the Essex University Centre for Trauma, Asylum and Refugees, concerning refugees who constitute the majority of Babel beneficiaries (such approach can be also used with other migrants, adapted accordingly). Central concept to Papadopoulos' theoretical approach is that of *psycho-ecological settledness* (more recently, the "psycho-" component has been replaced by "onto-"). *Psycho-ecological settledness* is the product of a unique combination of the "tangible" and "intangible" elements of our identity: "tangible" elements include gender, age, physical and psychological characteristics, profession, family status, political and ideological affiliation, religious beliefs, activities and hobbies, culture, nationality, family, body, etc., while the "intangible" elements (the term "intangible elements" signifies the sensory data related to home and the sense of "belonging") comprise the basis on which we build the tangible elements. According to Papadopoulos this set of "intangible" elements of our identity form a *mosaic substrate of identity* because "each element on its own may not be of relevance but in combination with the others, much like a mosaic, form a coherent pattern, a design that accommodates all the elements which are part of our identity but which we become aware of usually when they are absent, when we lose them" (Papadopoulos 2011, p. 20). He proposes that involuntary loss of home refugees experience is not only about the conscious loss of the family home with all its material, sentimental and psychological values, but it creates a more fundamental psychological disturbance of their whole sense of "psycho-ecological settledness"; this, in turn, activates a *nostalgic disorientation* (the term refers to the unique psychological experience of migrants and refugees in particular, which is not a psychiatric disorder; actually, all those who have lost – refugees against their will – their hearth, namely, their home with all its dimensions, share a deep sense of nostalgic longing to restore this type of loss) which is a much more fundamental and primary disturbance than the sense of losing tangible possessions or social positions – "it is a loss that affects refugees deeply yet in an way that is difficult to grasp clearly its nature" (ibidem).

Those who lose their home involuntarily and are dislocated, says Papadopoulos, experience the effects of a multidimensional, deep and permanent loss and feel disoriented because they have a hard time accurately identifying the source and exact nature of loss of home. The loss creates a void that makes migrants – and even more so refugees, people who left their homes because they were in danger – feel that they have no space, that they do not belong and that nothing contains them (with regard to this, Losi (2000) says that migrants are balancing between two worlds, unable to feel that they belong to either one).

Also central to Papadopoulos' approach is the view that, paradoxically, despite their adverse nature, the devastating events linked to the migration condition (irrespective of the degree of their toughness and the adversity of their consequences, as in the case of refugees) can also help people reorganise their life, to regroup it and give it new meaning. Exposure to adversity can (a) lead to negative consequences (mental disorder), (b) have no effect on the person's resilience and (c) have positive consequences, namely, cause new skills to be born that the person did not have previously, precisely because of their exposure to adversity (adversity-activated development).

The assessment of the status of a person appealing or being referred to Babel adopts the guidelines that are born from the aforementioned theoretical approaches. Although in their first iteration they pertain to asylum seekers, with small adjustments they may be used for the different migrant categories. According to them, the assessment process looks for (a) the positions where an individual is vulnerable and those where he appears to have maintained his resilience, (b) the factors responsible for this situation (individual, familial, environmental, contextual) and (c) the missing information necessary for the completion of as full and dynamic image as possible of the individual and his interactions.

The process suggested by the specific methodology tends to avoid turning the migration experience into "pathology" and instead valorises its positive characteristics. Following Papadopoulos' theoretical approach, the assessment (which is not separate from the therapeutic intervention) investigates the adverse consequences of the migration experience, the neutral ones (namely, the individual's characteristics that remained untouched after the migration experience) and the positive (in which positive characteristics that the individual did not possess previously were activated due to his exposure to the specific adversity).

The explored indicators are the following:

(A) *External circumstances*: Adverse and facilitative circumstances pertaining to the categories below. It is of essential significance to check if the migrant enjoys the benefit of basic rights: (a) physical safety, (b) financial security to enable at least survival (benefits/employment), (c) education, (d) housing and (e) avoidance of exposure to discrimination (gender, racial, ethnic, religious, sexual orientation, etc.).
(B) *Family constellation*: Adverse and facilitative circumstances regarding the following categories: (a) age, (b) gender, (c) family composition (e.g. divorced, reconstituted, active links with the extended family) and (d) family role (e.g. single mother, single head of a household, unaccompanied minor, isolated elderly person, etc.).
(C) *Physical health*: Adverse and facilitative conditions (e.g. good health, medical problems, disability, etc.).

(D) *Psychological/psychiatric state*: Adverse and facilitative circumstances and responses to adversity: negative (mental disorder, distressful psychological reactions), resilience functions and adversity-activated development functions.
(E) *Links with the community*: Participation and/or isolation relevant to their preferred community with regard to the following categories: (a) ethnic, (b) racial, (c) political, (d) religious, (e) ideological, (f) cultural, (g) local (geographical), etc.

  Isolation may be due either to the actual absence of the specific category in the receiving country or to their inability to have access to it for any reason.
(F) *Links with the wider society*: Participation and/or isolation with regard to the wider society.
(G) *Degree of difference*: Difference between home and receiving country with regard to the following categories: (a) language, (b) educational system (in relation to functioning in the current context, e.g. not just the education level attained but also whether one's qualifications are recognised in the receiving country), (c) cultural norms and practices, (d) urban/rural living context and (e) general life style.

  This dimension does not correspond only to the actual degree of difference but also to the extent to which the applicant is capable of handling these differences. Category: "duration of stay at the receiving country" is of particular significance as to this point.
(H) *Type of journey*: Degree of hardship endured in reaching the receiving country and/or positive experiences gained along the journey. For example, were they smuggled, trafficked, followed a long and arduous journey through many other countries or did they arrive directly and with fewer hardships?
(I) *Legal position*: Degree of current legal complications. Is their legal case simple or is it complicated by specific factors?
(J) *Daily routine*: The degree to which the migrant is able to engage in life and lead a fulfilling life with a daily routine that reflects his active involvement, e.g. visiting friends, attending classes, engaging in sport activities, etc. (Papadopoulos 2011, p. 51).

The reception process, the assessment with the active participation of the beneficiary and the activation of resources in the community which address an individual's or a family's basic needs, all these components contribute to the creation of a "home". This is where the beneficiary can feel safe and protected. Such feelings are considered necessary for the beginning of the therapeutic process. B. Cyrulnik states that "psycho-traumatic experiences are almost the same, no matter the cultural context… Each culture, however, provides the expression capability of the trauma in the post-traumatic phase that either allows re-processing leading to resilience or it impedes it" (Cyrulnik 2011, p. 16). So, "home" plays precisely this role: it provides the possibility to express the trauma, hence permitting its reprocessing that will lead to a new resilience state. It also uses all the skills and other positive elements that were activated by the adversity. This is a process that requires time, patience, endurance and respect of one's pace. Disbelief, cautiousness, the experience of abuse in the receiving country, racist behaviours and the obstacles placed before access to rights and the feeling of unfairness and disappointment, all those are factors impeding the therapeutic process. The latter is frequently challenged as it collides against obstacles related to new adversities faced by the beneficiary in his daily, "ordinary" life.

The Challenges of Clinical Work with Migrant Populations

Migrants' mental healthcare constitutes a challenge for mental health professionals and services (Gionakis 2013). The following factors contribute to this:

- *Identity*. In one of the first scenes of Costa-Gavras' film *Eden à l' Ouest*, (*Paradise in the West*), the migrants, who are in a boat, are asked to get rid of their identity cards and passports, when a boat makes its appearance. They tear them apart and throw them in the sea. A gesture showing that entrance into Europe requires the denial of one's own identity. The loss of one's country, the separation from one's family, the length of the journey and the payment of the smugglers, all have preceded this. Subsequently, without identity, like Pirandello's Mattia Pascal, they discover that at least in the Western World, entry in an *actual* reality is a prerequisite so that someone can exist.
- Who are the migrants? Some of them went to a country as tourists, liked it and stayed. Others are migrant workers. Some of them are EU nationals who move in other EU states, others originate from countries that until recently were not (but now are) EU members and others come from "third countries" (outside the EU). Many are seeking asylum and have been waiting (for years) for their request to be examined. Among them there are people with specific features needing particular attention (unaccompanied minors, survivors of torture, victims of trafficking and so on). Others were identified as refugees or granted with humanitarian protection status. Many wish to request asylum, but not in the country they have arrived in; for this reason they do not apply for it and therefore remain in the country illegally. Some are not refugees, but as there are no other ways for them to obtain legal residence status, they claim that they are. Many have arrived to stay and others, perhaps the majority, to leave but are unable to do so. As a result, they continue their journey illegally as they do not possess the necessary travel documents. Finally, some have arrived and are willing to stay, but they soon discover that things are not as they expected them to be and realise they must either go back or proceed to another destination.
- *The therapeutic alliance*. The therapeutic approach implies challenges too. The beneficiary is confronted to a different language, a different culture, a different world view and a different signification system. Furthermore, the reception and living conditions in the country create frustration, thus leading to the feeling of disbelief and, often, to hostility. Many of the beneficiaries may not agree with the way Westerners perceive and live their life. On the contrary, they may regard psychological, social, political and physical issues as an integral whole that

cannot be separated in different components (i.e., "inside/outside", "mental/somatic", "political/social", cfr. Ingleby and Watters, 2005). As a result, they may not recognise the problems "within" the individual or have a different view as to what is the priority or the best intervention to carry out. As per Arthur Kleinman's idea, the "explanatory models" of the person seeking assistance may not match those of the professional they meet (Kleinman 1980).
- Much has been written about the features of the professional's "cultural sensitivity", "cultural awareness" and "cultural competency" (Seah et al. op.cit; Saldaña 2001). The personal history of each individual, the acculturation strategy she/he adopts and one's own expectations are elements shaping the uniqueness of the "suffering subject". To approach this uniqueness, the mental health staff is helped by his/her own culture and world view, his/her own technical training and his/her own availability. Staff should accept that cultural sensitivity, awareness, competency and proficiency pertain to diversity in all its representations and forms and not just to the ethno-cultural one.
- *Access to rights.* In many countries there is a significant gap between the legal recognition of rights and the possibility to practice them in a concrete way. Such conditions permit the ascertainment of an "as if" function of the institutions. Especially regarding people coming from different countries, cultures and backgrounds, the manifest or underlying racism has the function of a meta-context. The latter undermines any attempt to establish a relationship of trust and create a safe framework between the service personnel and the "beneficiaries", namely, a framework that will permit (and will be facilitated by) the exercise of such rights. Discrimination is the ground for the lack of access to rights. This is the case of people who are "different", such as those with a mental disorder. The institutional history of psychiatric care in many countries is full of examples of violations of rights. This occurs despite lawmakers' efforts, such as the ones regarding involuntary care, which are not applied.
- *Inadequacy of Resources.* There is a lack of resources that discourages professionals to meet the complex and multiple needs of migrants with mental disorders. The lack of resources does not just affect migrants, but in their case this lack creates unsustainable situations. A simple example related to service accessibility arises from the need to make communication possible with the patients. In the case of people who do not speak the local language, the cooperation with language or cultural mediators is a prerequisite in order to facilitate communication. Indeed, the appropriate training (of the people taking on the role of the mediator as well as of the mental health professionals working with the aliens) is necessary in the cooperation. Despite that fact, such resources are lacking in the psychiatric care system in many countries and in many cases are considered to be an unnecessary luxury. To the insufficiency of resources, one must also add the insufficiency of rehabilitation initiatives (such as, for instance, the case of vocational rehabilitation, which is almost prohibitive in some categories – see asylum seekers – integration in the education system, which is not supported, etc.). It is obvious that the relevant conditions (to the context of life) raise significant obstacles to a person's attempts for social and economic integration.

- *The risk of victimisation.* As it has become almost a stereotype, it is very easy for someone to fall into the trap of seeing a person traumatised by the adverse condition they have lived through in every migrant, especially in the case of refugees. In reality, as repeatedly discussed in this chapter, many do not just survive intact to a significant extent despite all they have experienced under inhuman and tough conditions; they are empowered further from their exposure to adversity, finding a meaning in their pain and are in a position to turn their experiences into positive ones, drawing new strength and experiencing a transformative renewal (Papadopoulos 2007). This means that a mental health service must take seriously into consideration this position and act accordingly. The modern approaches, post-traumatic growth (Calhoun and Tedeschi 2006) and positive transformation following trauma (Herold et al. 2008) (just like everything discussed in this chapter on adversity-activated development), could possibly contribute to the formulation of this position.

In order to address these challenges, a mental health unit should benefit from the professional knowledge and skills of the multidisciplinary team, as well as continuous training and supervision. It can also depend on the resources outside the unit, namely, the network of cooperating bodies, institutions and volunteers. All of these together – and not separately – stand out as requirements for feasible effectiveness of the clinical services.

Other Aspects of the Work of Babel

Clinical work is the main activity that Babel chiefly engages in. However, the unit is also active in other areas, the most important of which are:

- *Networking.* Babel's networking with other institutions (state, local government and non-profit sector units) allows the achievement of a critical range of targets linked to the centre's mission. These targets include the efforts to plan and implement integrated interventions in the community, raising awareness/training professionals and the community, agreeing on joint political action (advocating in favour of integration and anti-discriminatory policies, etc.) and, last but not least, participating in peer consultations.
- *Education.* Education and continuous training are components of the operation of Babel. This includes organising internal training programmes for Babel staff, interns and volunteers; initial/continuous training of professionals, the main job objective of whom is either working with migrants (security forces, holding centres, hosting units, health institutions, asylum seeker support organisations) or coming into contact with migrants in the course of their work (teachers, civil servants, others); pre- and post-degree level education (through participation in courses and internships) for domestic and foreign students; training package preparation (the training packages compiled by Babel pertain to areas such as effective cooperation with interpreters, integration of foreign pupils at school,

migrant mental healthcare); and publications aiming at continuous improvement of the skills of professionals in the field. An important field of education is the one pertaining to the training of language facilitators on the basis of specific guidelines (Miletic et al. 2006).
- *Volunteering.* A large part of the activities of Babel is carried out by people offering their services voluntarily. In most cases they are mental health professionals who wish to contribute to the work done by Babel, and they operate on humanitarian, political and social motivations. Their work is varied; they conduct specialised individual and group therapeutic or rehabilitation activities, accompany, provide training and address the needs of everyday life of the beneficiaries. The volunteer work is contracted through an individual agreement for the provision of services, which describes the purpose, duration, frequency and other commitments by Babel volunteers.

In conclusion, one could say that Babel does not operate as a "traditional" day centre, in order to provide effective mental healthcare to migrants. "Provision of effective mental health services" in this case means taking into account the complexity of these peoples' situation, the vulnerable positions they may be in, as well as the resilience they have developed, the need to actively approach them supporting the potential of communication in a language they understand, through the creation of a framework they can perceive as familiar and within which they can gradually feel safety and trust. This framework must direct its (manifold) activities not just towards migrants but also towards a wide range of stakeholders, who participate – each from his/her own vantage point – in the formulation of facilitative or adverse integration conditions.

15.5 In Conclusion

The migration condition is closely related to the history of humans. The history of humans is a history of movements, meetings and encounters. There is a plethora of different reasons for these movements; they can be coercive or mass movements (as in the case of refugees). The migration condition comprises a reality of particular complexity; therefore, the approach that will explore and intervene must be of corresponding complexity. The migrants themselves create categories that are internally very different, and it would be extremely risky to voice general and generalised determinations on their behalf. As stated elsewhere, not identifying these peculiarities has turned ineffective many of the interventions designed for this purpose, resulting in totally controversial results, far from what had been expected (Gionakis 2008).

The situation becomes even more complex when the attempt is related to exploring the relationship between migration and mental health. It appears, at least insofar as what is currently acceptable, that it is important to identify the consequences of the conditions under which migrants live in the countries where they settle on mental health and not just those related to what they "bring along" from their countries of origin. In this sense, emphasis is given to the principles and the manner of organising the framework of mental health in the countries of settlement, so that it may be in a position to provide the appropriate services.

The framework that will receive and support migrants with mental health problems and mental disorders must have the capability to negotiate with the person the creation of a new "home" within which it will be possible to lay the foundations to develop a relationship of trust. This will allow the person's *subjectification*, namely, the capability for them and others to recognise oneself as the producer of significance, a significance which, to begin with, can be expressed within a hospitable framework of services, so that he may then seek a connection with others, "attempt emotional and material transactions, learn to interact" (Saraceno 2010). This, continues Saraceno, "requires mutual adjustments between the subject and the environment: more capable subjects and more tolerant environments". Of course, the necessary condition is the availability of services that accept to play this role, to experiment with new ways of approaching the potential beneficiaries, to "open up" to other services, to question themselves, to seek new intervention objectives and to accept the complexity of reality and that of mental suffering, namely, in terms of social psychiatry, to become deinstitutionalised.

Bibliography

Augé M (2009) Pour une anthropologie de la mobilité. Payot, Paris
Balandier G (1955) Sociologie Actuelle de l'Afrique noire: dynamique der changements sociaux un Afrique Centrale. PUF, Paris
Beneduce R (2007) Etnopsichiatria: sofferenza mentale e alterità fra storia, dominio e cultura. Carocci, Roma
Bhugra D, Jones P (2001) Migration and mental illness. Adv Psychiatr Treat 7(3):216–222
Bhugra D, Gupta S, Bhui K, Craig T, Dogra N, Ingleby JD, Kirkbride J, Moussaoui D, Nazroo J, Qureshi A, Stompe T, Tribe R (2011) WPA guidance on mental health and mental health care in migrants. World Psychiatry 10(1):2–10
Bourdieu P (2003) Firing back: against the tyranny of the market 2, vol 2. Verso, New York
Bourdieu P, Wacquant LJ (1992) Réponses: pour une anthropologie réflexive. Seuil, Paris, p 129
Calhoun LG, Tedeschi RG (eds) (2006) Handbook of post-traumatic growth: research and practice. Erlbaum, Mahwah
Cartwright SA (1851) How to save the republic, and the position of the south in the union. University of Michigan: Humanities Text Initiative, Michigan
Cross T et al (1989) Towards a culturally competent system of care, with the assistance of the Portland research and training center for improved services to severely emotionally handicapped children and their families. CASSP Technical Assistance Center, Georgetown University Development Center, Washington, DC
Cyrulnik B (2011) Autobiography of a scarecrow. Kelefthos Publications, Athens, p 16
Favazza AR, Oman NM (1978) Foundations of cultural psychiatry. Am J Psychiatry 135:293–303
Fazel M, Wheeler J, Danesh J (2005) Prevalence of serious mental disorder in 7000 refugees resettled in western countries: a systematic review. Lancet 365(9467):1309–1314
Garrigues E (2003) Les villages noirs en France et en Europe ou le zoo humain d'après la collection de Gerard Levy. In: L'Ethnographie. L'Entretemps éditions, Paris, pp 13–51
Gionakis N (2008) Introduction. In: Gionakis N (ed) Crossing borders: trauma perpetuation or care? "Babel" Day Care Centre Publication, Athens, pp 13–18

Gionakis N (2009) The care of migrant mental health in Greece. In: Sakellis I (ed) Psychiatric reform in Greece. Sakoulas Publications, Athens, pp 129–133

Gionakis N (2013) When rights seem a luxury: migrant mental health care. Synapsis 27:42–45

Hannerz U (1998) Transnational research. In: Bernard HR (ed) Handbook of methods in cultural anthropology. AltaMira Press, London, pp 235–256

Herold DM, Fedor DB, Caldwell S, Liu Y (2008) The effects of transformational and change leadership on employees' commitment to a change: a multilevel study. J Appl Psychol 93(2):346

Ingleby D (2008) European research on migration and health – AMAC research programme background article – assisting migrants and communities, Accessed 15.7.14

Ingleby D, Watters C (2005) Mental health and social care for asylum seekers and refugees: a comparative study. In: Ingleby D (ed) Forced migration and mental health: rethinking the care of refugees and displaced persons. Springer, New York, pp 193–212

Ingleby D, Chimienti M, Ormond M, de Freitas C (2005) The role of health in integration. In: Fonseca ML, Malheiros J (eds) Social integration and mobility: education, housing and health. Centro de Estudos Geográficos, Lisbon, pp 88–119

Kirmayer LJ, Narasiah L, Munoz M, Rashid M, Ryder AG, Guzder J, Hassan G, Rousseau C, Pottie K (2011) Common mental health problems in migrants and refugees: general approach in primary care. Can Med Assoc J 183(12):E959–E967

Kleinman A (1980) Patients and healers in the context of culture: an exploration of the borderland between anthropology, medicine, and psychiatry. University of California Press, Berkeley

Kraepelin E (1904) Vergleichende Psychiatrie (Comparative psychiatry). Zbl Nervenheilkunde Psychiatr 27(1904):433–437 (in German)

Levi-Strauss CM (1978) Myth and meaning. Schocken, New York

Littlewood R (1990) From categories to contexts: a decade of the "new cross-cultural psychiatry". Br J Psychiatry 156:308–327

Losi N (2000) Vite altrove. Migrazione e disagio psichico. Feltrinelli, Milano

Miletic T, Piu M, Minas H, Stankovska M, Stolk Y, Klimidis S (2006) Guidelines for working effectively with interpreters in mental health settings. Victorian Transcultural Psychiatry Unit (VTPU)

Morrison T (1988) Amatissima. Frassinelli, Piacenza

Murphy HBM (1977) Migration, culture and mental health. Psychol Med 7(04):677–684

Murphy HBM (1982) Comparative psychiatry. Springer, Berlin

Ødegaard Ø (1932) Emigration and insanity: a study of mental disease among the Norwegianborn population of Minnesota. Acta Psychiatr Scand 7(4):1–206

Okpaku SO (1998) Clinical methods in transcultural psychiatry. American Psychiatric Press, Washington, DC

Papadopoulos RK (1997) Individual identity and collective narratives of conflict. Harvest: J Jungian Stud 43(2):7–26

Papadopoulos RK (2000) A matter of shades: trauma and psychosocial work in Kosovo. In: Losi N (ed) Psychosocial and trauma response in war-torn societies: the case of Kosovo. IOM, Geneva

Papadopoulos RK (2001) Refugee families: issues of systemic supervision. J Fam Ther 23(4):405–422

Papadopoulos RK (2002) Refugees, home and trauma. In: Papadopoulos RK (ed) Therapeutic care for refugees. No place like home. Karnac. Tavistock Clinic Series, London

Papadopoulos RK (2007) Refugees, trauma and adversity-activated development. Eur J Psychother Couns 9(3):301–312

Papadopoulos RK (2011) Enhancing vulnerable asylum seekers protection – trainer's manual, International Organization of Migration. Accessed 16.7.14

Ridley CR, Li LC, Hill CL (1998) Multicultural assessment: reexamination, reconceptualization, and practical application. Couns Psychol 26(6):827–910

Saldaña D (2001) Cultural competency: a practical guide for mental health service providers. Hogg Foundation for Mental Health. University Of Texas at Austin

Saraceno B (2010) Il paradigma della sofferenza urbana. Accessed 15.7.14
Seah E, Tilbury F, Wright B, Rooney R, Jayasuriya P (2002) Cultural awareness tool. West Australian Transcultural Mental Health Centre, The Royal Australian College of General Practitioners WA Research Unit, Commonwealth Department of Health and Ageing and Multicultural Mental Health Australia, http://www.mhima.org.au/pdts/Cultural_aware_tool.pdf. Accessed 16.7.14
Silove D, Steel Z, Watters C (2000) Policies of deterrence and the mental health of asylum seekers. JAMA 284(5):604–611
Stylianidis S, Bagourdi E (2008) Social psychiatry and culture. In: Stylianidis S, Stylianoudi M (eds) Community and psychiatric reform: the Evia experience 1988–2008. Motivo-Topos Publications, Athens, pp 49–83
Vaughan AT (1991) Curing their ills. Colonial power and African illness. Polity Press, Cambridge
Watters C (2007) The mental health care of asylum seekers and refugees. In: Knapp M, McDaid D, Mossialos E, Thornikroft G (eds) Mental health policy and practice through Europe. Milton Keynes. Open University Press, Berkshire, pp 356–373
Watters C (2010) Migrants, refugees and mental health care in Europe. Hell J Psychol 7:21–37
Watters C, Ingleby D (2004) Locations of care: meeting the mental health and social care needs of refugees in Europe. Int J Law Psychiatry 27:549–570
Wittkower E (1966) Perspectives of transcultural psychiatry. In: Proceedings of the IV World Congress of Psychiatry. Madrid, 5–11 Sept, pp 228–234
Yap PM (1974) Comparative psychiatry: a theoretical framework. University of Toronto Press, Toronto
Zissi A (2006) Migration and mental health: empirical finding review. Psychology 13(3):95–108

Modern Technologies and Applications and Community Psychiatry

16

Orestis Giotakos

Abstract

The provision of remote psychological support services was initiated in the 1970s with the psychological support helplines. Such services are a continuously growing field of mental healthcare, given that many mental healthcare units are located in remote areas and unable to provide immediate psychological and counselling services in response to crisis situations. Other support services, such as online counselling and teleconferencing services in a telepsychiatry context, may also contribute significantly in an integrated crisis intervention system aiming to prevent the effects of psychological trauma and regain an individual's functionality. Online support is provided in the form of information guides and self-help groups or online counselling services, as the process involving two persons has been defined, the therapist and the client, in verbal or written communication via an Internet connection. The benefits of this specific practice, such as accessibility, comfort, anonymity, facilitation of face-to-face psychotherapy and low cost, make, in specific cases, online counselling the therapy of choice. Although the use of the Internet seems promising for the treatment of psychiatric disorders, specialists disagree on the ethical practice of psychotherapy in an interactive, digital environment. Issues such as know-how and the management of technical problems, difficulties in the diagnostic process, verbal and nonverbal cues, crisis management, preservation of therapeutic alliance, protection of personal information, age limitations and respect of boundaries in terms of space, time and the dynamics of the therapeutic relationship and, finally, the training and supervisory process of online therapists are some of the issues to be addressed.

O. Giotakos, MD, MSc, PhD
Director, Psychiatric Department, 414 Army Hospital, Athens, Greece

2 Erifilis, 11634 Athens, Greece
e-mail: info@obrela.gr

16.1 Introduction

The spread of the use of the telephone and the Internet has led to the potential to provide additional health services and information. The term "e-mental health" comprises a wide range of interactions, such relationships between service users and scientists (via email, live online counselling and searching for information) or specialist-to-specialist or specialist-to-trainee communication (supervision, evaluation of subordinates, specialised counselling-diagnosis, assessment of information, ongoing training through two-way systems). E-mental health includes the following general counselling services: information (information transmitted over the Internet or by electronic means, client records and advice), recommendation and advocacy (through referral to other service providers and the establishment of relationships [in the form of documents forwarded to mail lists and chat groups]) and direct relationships between consultants and clients (by e-mail or live chat). The benefits of online counselling, such as accessibility, commuting, comfort, anonymity, facilitation of face-to-face psychotherapy and low cost, may make, in certain cases, online counselling the main therapy of choice (APA 1997; Giotakos 2008).

16.2 Psychological Support Over the Phone

Objectives, Promotion and Assessment

The objective of a support helpline varies according to the type of services provided. All policies, procedures and objectives must be written and disclosed to both the helpline workers and the general public. The manner in which a helpline is promoted should accurately reflect its purpose so that it is clear for whom it is intended and the type of requests the specialists working at the helpline are able to handle. In addition, a clear staff selection and training plan should be in place and available to the supervisory committee or anyone assuming the overall responsibility for the management of the helpline. The methods used to select, train, supervise and support the helpline staff are monitored, reviewed, modified and improved through designated meetings between helpline supervisors and workers. The recording and compilation of call statistics are considered useful for the better and more efficient management of the helpline. Monitoring the manner in which such services are provided, recording the number of calls and classifying them according to type of request and intervention determine the needs that the helpline staff is called to meet, the requirements of the population for which it is intended and any likely shortcomings and deficiencies of the service. The promotion of a psychological support helpline must be clear as to the type of help offered and the subjects covered as well as how callers may contact them, i.e. helpline operating hours, address, e-mail or website. This enables the public to use the helpline by whatever means they prefer and are available to them. The impact and effectiveness of the promotion must be frequently reassessed (Giotakos and Triantafyllou 2006; Sanders 1993).

Many terms, such as review, monitoring, determination, assessment, evaluation, performance indices, qualitative and quantitative measurements, procedures, conclusions and impact, are used in the appraisal process of the services provided by the psychological support helpline. This appraisal may be internal or external. A self-appraisal is an internal organisational procedure which enables a concise review of any action on a personal or organisational level. Some psychological support helplines employ external appraisers. This appraisal is linked to accreditation. Any accreditation process must include an external organisation, acknowledged for the quality of its services, to carry out the appraisal based on specific criteria. The necessary information to be collected regarding the effectiveness of the helpline varies according to its purpose. The appraisal of a psychiatric support helpline aiming to provide information or advice differs and may often be carried out more easily than the appraisal of helplines focusing on emotional support. On the whole, however, the key information for each appraisal includes quantitative information about incoming calls, unanswered calls and information about the quality of responses to such calls.

Type of Services Provided

Counselling Over-the-phone counselling may be defined as a service during which a trainee consultant works with a client or a group of clients, over the phone, to enable the client (service user) to explore and process personal situations, problems or crises in a single session, a short-term or long-term therapeutic relationship. In the latter two cases, a type of contract is established between the client and the consultant and this may also include a financial relationship between the two parties.

Information During this individual function of the service, specific information is provided in response to specific requests and the reported circumstances. Although a friendly tone of voice is deemed useful and advantageous, an in-depth discussion is not mandatory unless further clarification is needed on the issue concerned. The person answering the phone must be able to provide immediate information on the issue. In this context, issues relating to social welfare may also be resolved.

Support Insight is a prerequisite skill on the part of the consultant for over-the-phone support. This skill is inherent in some people and whether it may be acquired and effective in a counselling context is disputed by many.

Management of Call by a Person in Crisis

Every call to the psychiatric support helpline is expected to have a specific structure. The same rules, certainly, apply to all tele-applications, such as teleconferencing in the context of telepsychiatry. Such contacts always have a beginning, a middle and an end as well as the following distinct stages (Giotakos and Triantafyllou 2006; Sanders 1993).

Establishment of the relationship The helpline must be located in an environment which allows the consultant to focus on the reason of the call. This requires an environment free of any likely and unnecessary distraction, such as background noise. If this is feasible, it would be advisable for the consultant to let the phone ring two or three times so that he/she may focus on the caller and give him/her time to prepare. For many callers, the manner of answering their call will define whether they will stay on the line. The caller's greeting must be in line with the policy of the helpline.

Exploration of content This stage covers the main part of the call. The consultant needs to be particularly careful so as to "follow" rather than lead or guide the caller. While dialling the number, many callers have not yet organised their thoughts about what they actually want to say. They may, perhaps, need to be listened to more attentively so that they may understand what is happening to them and what is their actual requirement from the helpline. The consultant must continue listening and responding in a way that helps the caller explain their situation and needs as well as their feelings with respect to the situation and assure them about their emotional support and insight for their needs, i.e. their willingness to see things from their side and stand by them through this hardship. Therefore, a consultant's basic training should include the development of active listening as well as the development of call handling skills.

Clarification of basic issues This stage may not be necessary but could, however, become more relevant if one of the most important objectives of the helpline is emotional support. Consultants should be sensitive to the reactions of the callers so that they can "read" when they need to move in this or that direction and, at the same time, "perceive" the feelings of the callers and avoid pressuring them to continue beyond their point of endurance at this stage.

Closure Each call must certainly come to an end and the manner in which it will come to an end often determines whether the caller will feel comfortable to use the support or information offered to them. It may also affect their feelings and prompt them to call again. A "good closure" may include a summary or a recap of the call by the consultant which includes acceptance and acknowledgement of the caller's feelings.

After the call This is an important part of the call, just as important as the actual communication with caller. Time should be dedicated to review how the call was handled. There is no such thing as a "perfect" call and depending on how willing someone is to assess their performance and accept their colleagues' support and feedback, the more effective they will be in the future. It is advisable for the workers to take the opportunity to review the last call and "recover" before proceeding to the next call. An "internal supervision" of the call by the consultant or, even better, discussing the call with a colleague could facilitate this process.

The consultant must not feel obliged to proceed to the next call, especially if they are still affected or preoccupied with their feelings for the previous caller. Also, it is preferable that they complete as soon as possible the relevant call paperwork. The more they put off this to a later time, the more difficult it will be to recollect the details of the call.

"Difficult" Calls

Many psychological support helplines receive calls which, for whatever reason, are considered "difficult". Such calls may affect the specialist answering the call and/or the entire service. In cases where the psychological support helpline consultant is affected by the caller, they must first become aware of this and then request support, supervision and, perhaps, additional training. A psychological support helpline may employ external consultants to supervise and counsel the staff.

"Difficult" calls are extremely angry calls, calls from people threatening to commit suicide, sexually inappropriate calls, hoax calls, calls by people who are intoxicated, racists, homophobes or calls of a threatening nature and repeated calls. The specialists employed by psychological support helplines must be trained in order to be able to handle such so-called "difficult" calls within the boundaries set by the service where they work. Many psychological support helplines deem it useful to incorporate a separate "suicide call" service which forms part of their confidentiality policy. Likewise, a specific way could be developed to answer calls of an abusive, sexual, racist or homophobic nature. The specialists providing psychological support services over the phone cannot be left to manage such calls on their own and without support. Certain callers, such as repeat callers, may cause problems to the entire service as they overstep the specific boundaries of the psychological support helpline. They could even cause anger. It is, therefore, necessary to develop specific ways for all the helpline workers to manage such calls, even preplanned written replies.

The following strategies have often proved to be particularly helpful in cases of "difficult" calls:

Keeping written confidential records accessible to all other helpline workers and supervisors. Such records must be checked at regular intervals.
Agreeing upon an action plan with the caller which should be added to the record. If the caller does not agree, such refusal must be recorded. The staff that will subsequently contact, directly or indirectly, the caller must be familiar with this plan and follow it.
Involving other specialists in this action plan. The counselling process must be ongoing as the plan develops.
The personal safety of the caller and any persons contacting them as well as the personal safety of all helpline workers must also be taken into consideration. In certain cases it may be necessary to involve the police or other services (Giotakos and Triantafyllou 2006; Sanders 1993).

16.3 Psychological Support via Teleconferencing (Telepsychiatry)

Determination of Needs

Telepsychiatry is defined as the application of modern telecommunication technologies to mental health services. Telepsychiatry is one of the most dynamically growing fields of telemedicine today. The capability of modern telecommunication systems to transmit audio and video provides the basic tool for remote mental health services, i.e. verbal and nonverbal communication. With the help of modern IT systems, any information of interest to any mental health services user is transmitted remotely and readily accessible to the examiner, the therapist or other specialist. Furthermore, the accelerated growth of telepsychiatry services addresses two modern trends in the field of mental health: on the one hand, the increasing need for mental health services which often exceeds the capacity of available human resources and, on the other hand, the contemporary need to provide healthcare services and psychosocial support at a regional level. Generally, we could talk about three integral parts: videoconferencing (bidirectional transmission of digital images in real time between two or more positions), the electronic psychiatric file (software used to save, edit and transfer patient information) and online services (such as e-therapy, e-learning, etc.). The clinical and other applications of such systems are able to support basic operational needs of the mental health services in our country (Rees and Stone 2005; Giotakos 2008).

Services Provided

The services provided through such telepsychiatry systems can be classified under the following categories:

Services requiring direct communication between the user and a specific scientist (psychiatrist, psychologist, social worker), i.e. interviews, sessions, application of various tests or questionnaires. Such services include the examination and monitoring of patients as well as various psychotherapies.

Services requiring cooperation between mental health professionals, such as, for example, direct consultation with a specialist in relation to cases (e.g. between psychiatrist and general practitioner), discussions between scientists from different fields to manage cases and the operation of the "therapeutic team".

User information services, such as special assistance, support and information through dedicated webpages (information on mental health, queries to specialists).

e-learning services. Particularly in the mental health field, this may include a live or recorded demonstration of an interview (via teleconferencing or online) or the direct supervision by the trainer during the session conducted by the trainee. These also include the general forms, such as online courses in the form of webinars, scientific debates and lectures via teleconferencing.

Web-based management services. Teleconferencing and the transmission of data (documents, information, etc.) allow managers to participate remotely in administrative functions. The "users" (users) of telepsychiatry services may be primary healthcare units (psychosocial care groups located in remote areas or regional clinics) and secondary healthcare units (healthcare centres lacking mental health services or various other community structures, such as day centres and/or correctional facilities). The "provider" of such services is usually the central Tertiary Mental Health Unit (psychiatric hospital or psychiatry department of any general hospital). Special applications for the provision of specialised services and training (special centres, universities, etc.) may also involve working together with other bodies.

16.4 Online Psychological Support

Determination of Needs

In 1997, the American Psychological Association and, in 2001, the British Psychological Society established rules of conduct relating to ethical practice and online counselling. The Internet offers users more than one platforms to communicate and as a means of prevention in mental health, this takes various forms. The specialist-therapist may be actively present and involved in the session with the beneficiary (*counselling* via *e-mail, teleconferencing, videoconferencing*). Individuals may also look for ways to help themselves, with online support groups or self-help literature and counselling. In this field, we come across the terms *online counselling* or *online therapy* (the corresponding terms in international bibliography are online counselling/online therapy/Internet-delivered psychotherapy/web-based therapy/cyber counselling/e-therapy). In general, this is a process involving two parties, the therapist and the client, in a verbal or written communication via an Internet connection, using a PC, or via e-mail (Andersson et al. 2009, 2011; Carlbring et al. 2005; Haberstroh et al. 2007; Moritz et al. 2011; Murphy et al. 2011; Oravec 2000; Skinner and Latchford 2006; Liebert et al. 2006; Suler 2000; Sucala et al. 2012; Titov 2011).

Services Provided

Counselling via e-mail The exchange of e-mails is considered the most common way of communication over the Internet. Counselling by e-mail is now an outdated form of support as the discussion between the therapist and the client does not occur in real time.

Counselling via live chat Counselling via live chat is a form of support occurring in real time, as the therapist and the client are able to converse by typing.

Counselling via video conferencing using a camera Video conferencing is mainly based on free software, such as Skype, which enable users to chat while maintaining visual contact. The use of a camera, which is either built in the PC or attached to it, is necessary for the visualisation of the dialogue. The ability to exchange further information for the counselling process is achieved through video recording using a camera. The specific communication platform is more complex than the above mentioned as it requires additional equipment and a faster Internet connection.

Online support groups *Online self-help/support groups* allow users to expose themselves anonymously in a group, exchange experiences with people facing the same problem and provide mutual support. Registered members post topics for discussion with other members facing the same problem and are able to reply at any time of the day, free of charge. Confidentiality in such groups is not ensured as the flow of new members entering the group and older members leaving it is ongoing.

The type of interventions used in online counselling is clearly influenced by the social learning theory and cognitive behavioural therapy. This therapy aims to reduce the reported symptoms, change dysfunctional behaviours and prevent future relapses.

The Benefits

Accessibility Direct and easy access to support services via the Internet is one of the benefits of this practice for individuals who, otherwise, would not be able to seek therapy. Individuals residing in remote areas lacking an organised framework or a mental health specialist, individuals with reduced mobility, indigent individuals without health insurance and victims of intimate partner violence who don't want to draw the attention of their partners, are able to search for assistance services via the Internet.

Anonymity Individuals from a closed social system may perhaps find it difficult to seek help from a local mental health service because they fear social stigmatisation. Furthermore, clients concerned about being criticised by the specialist seek online support to express their thoughts and feelings from a more detached position.

Low cost The cost of online counselling is much lower than that of face-to-face therapy. A videoconference session using a camera and a live teleconference is usually paid for by credit card, and payment is effected on the date of the next session. Counselling via e-mail may be free of charge or not, and such fees may correspond to an amount charged on an e-mail basis or a larger amount for an unlimited number of e-mails.

Ethical Considerations

In general, specialists disagree on the ability to provide support to any individual within the infinite environment of the World Wide Web (Welfel 2013; Lee 2010; Giotakos 2008). Other than the rules of conduct governing the practice of psychotherapy, additional ethical practice concerns are raised relating exclusively to online counselling:

Know-how and management of technical problems A therapist practising online counselling, other than being well trained, must also have practical knowledge on the use of PCs and surfing on the Internet. At the same time, it is necessary to assess whether the client is eligible for online counselling: *Does this specific client possess the necessary know-how? How experienced is he/she in the use of the Internet? How developed are his/her writing and typing skills in terms of speed, adequacy and content? From which location will the client be communicating online with the therapist? Are there any risks of disclosure of personal data?*

Initial assessment A careful assessment may reveal that someone is not eligible for this type of intervention. The problem being reported, the client's request, any prior counselling experiences, current therapy expectations and the reason for which he chose the Internet as a means should be thoroughly examined. The likelihood that the beneficiary may have an audio-visual or mobility problem, a chronic physical condition or any other particular condition should also be examined. During the first phase of the therapy and for a more qualified assessment of the needs of any individual, it is recommended to hold a face-to-face meeting or a telephone conversation and to dispatch electronically self-reference questionnaires for completion – a method which is as reliable as the completion of questionnaires in printed form.

Verbal vs. nonverbal communication A disadvantage of online counselling is the fact that nonverbal cues are not perceptible. The written word is not the same as the spoken word, either in terms of content, quantity or style. For example, sarcasm is difficult to perceive in a text, a fact which may lead to a significant misinterpretation from the part of the therapist. It is recommended that the therapist encourage the clients to mention any likely difficulties so as to minimise this possibility. Contrary to written communication, counselling via video recording allows the observation of facial expressions.

Therapeutic relationship A safe and trustful therapeutic relationship, characterised by insight, authenticity and unconditional acceptance, is a necessary condition for the psychotherapy to be effective. It is, however, possible to establish a therapeutic relationship via the Internet. Studies on the therapeutic alliance associate its existence with a positive therapeutic result, recognising its value as equivalent to that of face-to-face counselling.

Personal information When a user decides to reveal any personal information on the Internet, it is impossible to guarantee completely its secure path. A breach may be caused by a hacker or due to user error. The *password* must be codified and strictly personal and the name of the sender should be carefully verified before sending an email. Sending messages via an encrypted web page reduces the dissemination of information. Moreover, the use of a public PC, at home, in the workplace, in an Internet café or a library, could compromise the personal information of an individual. Both *e-mails* and *chat* could come into the possession of third parties. In order to protect written sessions with therapists, it is recommended that the individual delete their browsing history when using a public PC and create a new account which will not be shared. Safeguarding the therapy is equally important as protecting the client's privacy. In written session via live teleconferencing or email, there is always the possibility that a client will use the sessions' texts for legal purposes, e.g. in child custody cases. Therefore, the therapists must also be particularly careful with the content of their reports.

Age Older people may find it difficult to respond to the condition of online counselling. On the other hand, a therapist should not accept to treat minors without a signed and duly certified declaration from the parent or legal guardian of the minor.

Training of the therapist In the case of counselling only services, it is difficult to verify any training, specialisation and professional qualifications of a therapist, psychologist or psychiatrist. To enable an interested party to obtain the necessary information regarding the training of the specialist, it is proposed that their curriculum vitae be published together with certain contact details of their training bodies. Supervision, a necessary process for the ethical practice of counselling, may be carried out by a certified, well versed in online support matters, as employing a supervisor with considerable experience in online support is rather difficult.

Bibliography

Andersson G, Carlbring P, Berger T, Almlöv J, Cuijpers P (2009) What makes internet therapy work? Cogn Behav Ther 38:55–60

Andersson G, Ljotsson B, Weise C (2011) Internet-delivered treatment to promote health. Curr Opin Psychiatry 24:168–172

APA (1997) APA statement on services by telephone, teleconferencing, and internet. American Psychological Association, Washington, DC

Carlbring P, Nilsson-Ihrfelt E, Waara J, Kollenstam C, Buhrman M, Kaldo V, Soderberg M, Ekselius L, Andersson G (2005) Treatment of panic disorder: live therapy vs. self-help via the Internet. Behav Res Ther 43:1321–1333

Giotakos O (ed) (2008) Crisis intervention: emergency psychological problems. Archipelagos Publications, Athens

Giotakos O, Triantafyllou Th (ed) (2006) Psychological support over the phone. Athens: Ellinika Grammata Publications

Haberstroh S, Duffey T, Evans M, Glee R, Trepal H (2007) The experience of online counseling. J Ment Health Couns 29:269–282

Lee S (2010) Contemporary issues of ethical e-therapy. J Ethics Ment Health 5(1):1–5

Liebert T, Archer J, Munson J, York G (2006) An exploratory study of client perceptions of internet counselling and the therapeutic alliance. J Ment Health Couns 28:69–84

Moritz S, Wittekind CE, Hauschildt M, Timpano KR (2011) Do it yourself? Self-help and online therapy for people with obsessive-compulsive disorder. Curr Opin Psychiatry 24:541–548

Murphy L, Mitchell D, Hallett R (2011) A comparison of client characteristics in cyber and in-person counselling. Stud Health Technol Inform 167:149–153

Oravec IA (2000) Online counselling and the internet: perspective for mental health care supervision and education. J Ment Health 9:121–136

Rees CS, Stone S (2005) Therapeutic alliance in face-to-face versus videoconferenced. Psychother Prof Psychol: Res Pract 36:649–653

Sanders P (1993) An incomplete guide to using counselling skills on the telephone. PCCS Books, Manchester

Skinner AEG, Latchford G (2006) Attitudes to counselling via the internet: a comparison between in-person counselling clients and internet support group users. Couns Psychother Res 6:158–163

Sucala M, Schnur JB, Constantino MJ, Miller SJ, Brackman EH, Montgomery GH (2012) The therapeutic relationship in e-therapy for mental health: a systematic review. J Med Int Res 2;14(4):e110. doi: 10.2196/jmir.2084. Review

Suler J (2000) Psychotherapy in cyberspace: a 5-dimensional model of online and computer-mediated psychotherapy. Cyberpsychol Behav 3:151–160

Titov N (2011) Internet-delivered psychotherapy for depression in adults. Curr Opin Psychiatry 24:18–23

Welfel ER (2013) Ethics in counselling & psychotherapy: standards, research, and emerging issues, 4th edn. Brooks/Cole Cengage Learing, Pacific Grove, Belmont

Assessment and Management of Domestic Violence Cases Within a Community Mental Health Services Framework

17

Stella Pantelidou, Athina Vakalopoulou, and Stelios Stylianidis

Abstract

This chapter describes the phenomenon of domestic violence, its rise over recent years in Greece and abroad and its consequences, placing emphasis mainly on the way that cases of child abuse and abuse of adults are assessed and managed by community mental health services. In addition, it presents a guideline for the detection of domestic violence as well as the proposed therapeutic approaches based on existing literature. Reference is also made to the management of a child abuse case and the therapeutic plan implemented, in cooperation with all community actors, in the course of the operation of the Mental Health Mobile Unit for Northeast Cyclades. Finally, it highlights the importance of developing actions to prevent domestic violence.

17.1 Introduction

The phenomenon of domestic violence has been, and still is, for most societies a taboo subject: frequently, any reference to violence in a family on the one hand, appeared only in mythology and literature, or in police reports as to certain of its

---

S. Pantelidou (✉) • A. Vakalopoulou
Association for Regional Development and Mental Health (EPAPSY), Athens, Greece
e-mail: stpantelidou@hotmail.com

S. Stylianidis
Department of Psychology, Panteion University, Athens, Greece
e-mail: stylianidis.st@gmail.com

© Springer International Publishing Switzerland 2016
S. Stylianidis (ed.), *Social and Community Psychiatry: Towards a Critical, Patient-Oriented Approach*, DOI 10.1007/978-3-319-28616-7_17

aspects while, on the other hand, idealisation of the family, particularly in Greece, casts a veil of silent complicity and tolerance with respect to this threat against the family ideal. The first objective of this chapter is not just to explain terms and concepts theoretically but to also describe the extent of this phenomenon in our country, in Europe and the rest of the world.

The working assumption of the issues discussed is to examine violence not as something external to us but as a phenomenon growing within us and in our interpersonal relationship, within the families which may be both warm and supportive as well as dangerous and which, under the current "fluid circumstances", are threatened by extinction or radical changes.

The second objective of this chapter, building on such issues, is to develop programmes and action plans at the community level to manage domestic violence in the most effective manner possible.

However, the phenomena of unravelling social ties, the vicious cycle of lack of financial resources, social exclusion and mental disorders, cultural admixtures and migration, revolutionary progress in the health sciences through new assisted reproductive technologies, gave rise to new forms of familial organisation, and parental roles. New phenomena which could constitute sources of instability, uncertainty and risk, therefore, support the prevalence of domestic violence.

How can we manage this violence which stems from a pathologically structured family *modus operandi*, through the understanding of intrapsychic, group and intergenerational dynamics? Conflict, trauma, unexpressed, hatred, envy and neglect could result into incapacitating and dysfunctional situations, inasmuch as they are developing within an environment of social disgrace and cover-up of such catastrophic phenomena by the local society's own defensive mechanisms. The "unexpressed" grows in an insidious, slow and silent, however, often unanticipated and violent, manner. The mental health interdisciplinary team working in the community has a therapeutic, ethical and social responsibility to intervene, acting as a catalyst, and eliminate this collective denial and collective cover-up of such phenomena by the local society itself.

17.2 Definition of Concepts and Terms

Different definitions have been attributed to the term "domestic violence". It refers mainly to any form of violence (physical, sexual or psychological) exerted against a member or members of the family. The forms of power and control exercised include threats, verbal abuse, breaking objects, torture of animals, emotional abuse (humiliation, contempt), financial abuse (prohibition of work, withholding of financial resources), isolation, displays of extreme jealousy etc.

In summary, the main forms of violence include the following:

Psychological violence (verbal abuse, humiliation, threats, swearing, prohibition to leave the house, etc.)
Sexual violence (rape and attempt to rape, sexual humiliation, sexual exploitation)

Financial violence (lack of financial freedom)
Physical violence (punching, slapping, shoving, injuring etc.)
Stalking

The victims of domestic violence could be men, women and children. According to the "UN Declaration on the Elimination of Violence Against Women" (CEDAW, as adopted by the Word Conference on Human Rights in Vienna, in 1993), violence is defined as "any act of gender-based violence that results in, or is likely to result in, physical, sexual or psychological harm or suffering to women, including threats of such acts, coercion or arbitrary deprivations of liberty, whether occurring in public or in private life". The term "violence against women" may refer to physical or psychological assaults, emotional and psychological abuse, rape and sexual abuse/harassment, incest, "honour" crimes etc. Social class, gender, nationality, race and religion may affect the likelihood of someone experiencing violence.

Child Abuse

Child abuse and neglect refer to "any recent act or failure to act from the part of a parent or caretaker of a child, which results in death, serious physical or emotional harm, sexual abuse or exploitation, or an act or failure to act which presents an imminent risk of serious harm" (Child Abuse Prevention and Treatment Act, CAPTA, 93-247).

The primary types of child abuse are physical, emotional and sexual. Physical abuse of a child is defined as the deliberate use of force against a child, which results in harm to the child's health, survival, development or dignity. It includes behaviours such as beating, kicking, shaking, biting, choking, burning, poisoning and causing asphyxia. Emotional abuse includes acts or omissions on the part of the parents or caretakers of a child which have caused or could cause behavioural, cognitive, emotional or mental disorders (Covell and Howe 2009). Finally, sexual abuse refers to engaging, exploiting, soliciting, inducing, grooming, persuading or coercing a child to participate or cause others to participate in any sexual behaviour or imitation of such behaviour for the purpose of producing a visual representation of this behaviour (NCCAN 2005, p. 3).

17.3 Historical Background

The first studies on understanding the phenomenon of domestic violence were conducted in the 1960s, a period during which the extent of child abuse was initially established (Gil 1970). In 1970, mainly as a result of the feminist movement, researchers focused their interest both on spousal violence and child abuse (Gelles 1974). Abuse of elders attracted particular attention around 1980 (Steinmetz 1978). Towards the end of 1970, a rise was observed in child sexual abuse cases (Finkelhor

1979, 1984), while research data confirmed cases of beatings in spousal relationships (Russell 1982; Shields et al. 1990).

Feminist theory has undoubtedly been the cornerstone in encouraging researchers, and every society, to study the roles of both genders and the circumstances which may lead to value systems that justify sexism, the prerogatives of men against women and the socialisation of both genders (Healey et al. 1998). Such value systems appear to reflect the patriarchal structure of societies where the man is considered all-powerful (Ahmad et al. 2004). Therefore, despite its long history and prevalence in every society, domestic violence has been part of an overarching feminist stand against patriarchal structures towards the end of 1960, while in early 1970, when the feminist movement of abused women was introduced in Britain, it also assumed political dimensions resulting in the establishment of the first community support centre for battered women and their children in 1971, the *Chiswick Women's Aid*. So, gradually, domestic violence became one of the major basic human rights violation issues and a major threat to the health and integrity of the members of a family (Ellsberg and Heise 2005).

All the above resulted in raising public awareness and aroused the researchers' interest in the different forms of domestic violence and their consequences (Dobash and Dobash 1979). In the absence of any investigation of this phenomenon over the past decades, one of the major research questions raised in 1970 related to its extent.

In Greece, the changing socioeconomic circumstances together with the redistribution of roles between the two genders and the different perception as to the role of each family member resulted in mobilising international organisations and the enactment of law 3500/2006 (Government Gazette A´ 2006 Issue No. 232), entitled "On combating domestic violence and other provisions". The purpose of this law is to combat the phenomenon of domestic violence according to the principles of freedom, self-determination and human dignity and enhance the harmonious cohabitation family members. During the meeting of the UN Experts Group on 24/01/2007, the Greek Delegation presented law 3500/2006, which underlined the obligation of the state to adopt measures for gender equality, by providing protection and assistance to victims, training public stakeholders and creating a database to monitor this phenomenon. In addition, the law focused specifically on criminal mediation, according to which the rights of victims are fully protected and women are, at the same time, encouraged to seek help from public authorities (Stefanidou 2010). According to Tomaras (2008), "this new law is a significant step forward in Greek legal culture as it makes, more than sufficiently, clear that the family is not a vacuum and that its behavioural values, rules and standards must comply with those of the social hypersystem to which it belongs and with which it interacts". However, several difficulties and problems were encountered on the way forward to implementing the above law and the institution of criminal mediation.

17.4 Extent of the Phenomenon

Studies over the last decades established that the phenomenon of domestic violence is global. Comparing the frequency of cases in various countries, the transnational study conducted by the World Health Organisation (WHO) (Garcia-Moreno et al.

2005) concluded that physical and/or sexual violence varies from 15 % in Japan up to 70 % in Ethiopia and Peru. 21 % of the women interviewed in the USA reported that they have been physically or sexually assaulted and/or both by their partners, while it is estimated that 37 % of the women in maternity wards have been abused (Garcia-Moreno et al. 2005). Furthermore, 13–16 % of respondents reported that they have experienced violence at some point up to age of 49.

Almost in every country included in the survey, approximately 50 % of the women experience violence in the family and, in fact, the first incident occurs in the age group 15–24.

Studies conducted in EU countries confirm that women are the primary victims of domestic violence, in the form of physical, psychological, emotional and/or sexual violence. A study conducted by the Council of Europe (Fact Sheet, Council of Europe Campaign to Combat Violence against Women, including Domestic Violence 2012) concluded that one in four women experience such violence at least once in their life and 6–10 % of women are reported to be victims of violence during any year. However, several studies indicate that men are also victims of domestic violence, although to a lesser extent than women (one man out of ten women victims) (Walby and Myhill 2001). The research data on violence exerted by members of the family other than the husband is limited. Therefore, further research is required as regards the detection and identification of the needs of different victim types.

In Greece, research on the phenomenon of domestic violence only started in the 1990s. The majority of information as to the frequency of domestic violence cases is obtained from the General Secretariat for Gender Equality. According to data collected from women victims who contacted the counselling services in the period 2002–2005, the first incident of violence usually occurs after the marriage (56.06 %), and women, despite their spouse's violent behaviour (80 %), continue to live with them (65.22 %). The most common form of violence is psychological and emotional violence, whereas psychological violence is less frequently reported. Based on the first Panhellenic study on the extent, the nature and the aspects of violence against women in Greek families (Artinopoulou and Farsedakis 2003), 56 % of the women interviewed experienced verbal and/or psychological violence, the most common form of which was contempt (19 %), insults (16.40 %), restrictions (10.90 %), isolation from friends and family (5.5 %) and threats (4.30 %) Another study concerning a population of 1122 adults, in the 18–64 age group, residing in Greek urban areas (Tzamalouka et al. 2007), concluded that emotional violence was the most common form of violence in the family (27 %), whereas physical violence amounted to 18.7 %. Finally, a recent study on the detection of emotional and physical abuse of women after childbirth indicated that 35.6 % of the mothers interviewed had experienced spousal violence.

Recent studies associate the Greek financial crisis with the crisis in relations within the family. The new socioeconomic circumstances often lead to changes in familial role patterns, the change of balances in family structures, tensions and conflicts between family members (Anagnostopoulos and Soumaki 2011). Moreover, this new situation is likely to make it more difficult for a member of the family who is being abused to break the pattern and leave the relationship because of their financial dependency. A study conducted by the Hellenic Society for the Study of Human

Sexuality (EMAS) and the Andrology Institute with the title "Greece in the crisis and the MoU" (Kallidonis 2013) indicated that cases of violence (physical, sexual, verbal) in our country increased by 47 % over the last months, with one out of three women being beaten. The most prevalent forms of violence exerted by men are verbal violence (72 %), followed by financial blackmail (59 %), sexual humiliation (55 %), beatings (23 %) and rapes (18 %). As to the economic profile of men who exert violence against their partners, 44 % were unemployed, 39 % in poor financial situation and only 17 % were financially sound.

Traditional family norms are considered sacred and impervious to external factors which, considered in conjunction with the personal nature of the crime of violence between its members, make domestic violence "sinister" at every level (Kilpatrick 2004). Victims, mainly women, hesitate to report exactly what happened to them because they fear being re-victimised by police and judicial authorities (Panoussis 1994). A typical example of this is the fact that the first epidemiological survey conducted in our country in 2003 (Artinopoulou and Farsedakis 2003) revealed that a large proportion of women did not identify the behaviours they experience in their family environment as being tantamount to abuse and within the concept of violence. Ethnic minorities and female migrants are more likely to postpone reporting such incidents than other women, either because of the fear of deportation or because the norms of a society prohibit the disclosure of negative incidents in most cases (Farah et al. 2004). Therefore, the private nature of the phenomenon of violence in the family and the victims' predominant reluctance to self-report assaults present a challenge in mapping precisely the prevalence of this phenomenon.

The frequency of physical abuse is estimated to approximately 2 % of the child population (Akmatov 2010). According to the World Health Organisation, it is estimated that 1 in 5000–10,000 children under the age of 5 dies every year as a result of physical abuse, and 1 in 180–1000 are referred to a health or social protection service as a result of abuse. In Europe, the prevalence of physical violence is between 5 % and 50 % (Lampe 2002).

A recent study by the Directorate for Mental Health and Social Welfare of the Child Health Institute on child abuse (Petroulaki et al. 2013) indicated that one in two elementary, junior high and high school pupils in Athens, Thessaloniki and Crete has experienced physical violence, one in ten children has experienced sexual violence over the last year alone and 76 % of children reported they had fallen victim to physical violence at some point during their childhood, whereas the corresponding figure of those reporting sexual violence stands at 16.2 %.

In 2012, the Smile of the Child SOS Helpline received 366 reports of cases of abuse concerning 691 children in total (Klontza 2012). Specifically, the reports concerned the abuse of children in the 0–6 age group (43 %), while this figure for children in the 7–12 age group is 32.5 %. As to the forms of abuse, the reports for 331 children (48 %) concerned neglect or abandonment, followed immediately by physical abuse (i.e. 41 %, 283 children). This is followed by coercion to beggary (4 %), psychological abuse and sexual abuse (3 %) and, last, forced child prostitution (1 %). Compared to 2012, the reports for child abuse submitted to the organisation rose by 66 %.

17.5 Male Victims of Domestic Violence

A "silent" and not so recognisable form of domestic violence is also that exerted by women against their partners. According to a study, male victims of domestic violence usually are emotionally dependent on their partners, show a clear lack of self-confidence, consider that this violence is their own fault and don't believe that they would be better off in another relationship (Migliaccio 2002). And, in case children are involved, men worry that they will be unable to remain in contact with them and are, therefore, compelled to remain in the problematic relationship, often to protect the children, given that women who exert violence against their spouses are very likely to abuse their children too (Margolin et al. 2003; Straus 1990). Finally, a man's need to suppress pain and appear strong and in control also inhibits their ability to leave the relationship, admit they have been victimised and seek support (Fontes et al. 2003).

Violence among same-sex couples is a complex phenomenon and as frequent as violence between different-sex couples (McClennen 2005). However, the services available to deal with such cases are almost non-existent. And here too, this form of violence is to a large extent "silent" (Turell 2000).

The effects of domestic violence are summarised in Table 17.1.

Table 17.1 The effects of domestic violence

Effects of domestic violence against adults
The adverse effects of domestic violence are derived from research findings over the last decades. The basic types of this phenomenon are inextricably linked to serious (Coker et al. 2000) physical and mental health implications (Coker et al. 2000)
Physical abuse can cause injuries and persistent illnesses, such as chronic pain, irritable bowel syndrome, backaches and headaches (Ratner 1993). Female domestic violence victims may experience a greater number of unwanted pregnancies, miscarriages and premature births (Sullivan and Knutson 2000). In addition, they show high levels of sexually transmitted diseases, including AIDS (Walker 2000)
Several studies confirm that domestic violence is also linked with the onset of mental disorders, such as depression, anxiety, post-traumatic stress (Wolfe et al. 1985; McCauley et al. 1995; Houskamp and Foy 1991)
Effects of domestic violence against children
It has been found that children who have been exposed to violence in the home may show signs and symptoms of:
Low self-confidence, anxiety, post-traumatic stress, depression
Increased risk of substance-related disorders
Hyperactivity, concentration problems
Antisocial behaviour
Guilt, anger, fear
Poor school performance
Emotional instability
Behavioural problems
Passivity

Wolfe and Birt (1997), Prekaté (2008), Giotakos (2004)

17.6 Identification and Assessment of Domestic Violence Cases

It is important for mental health professional to include in their daily routine domestic violence assessment practices and to be able to identify any signs and symptoms implying abuse (Warshaw 1996; Appelt and Kaselitz 2000).

Adults may show the following:

Physical signs
Frequent physical injuries (bruises, fractures, cuts) and the explanations for how they occurred may be inconsistent or vague. Typically, they most frequently occur to the head, the face, the neck and parts of the body which they usually cover with clothes, such as the chest, breasts and abdomen.
Hearing problems.
Complications during pregnancy or gynaecological problems; any injury, inexplicable pain, mental disorder, suicide attempt and substance abuse during pregnancy may be related to violence in the family.
Psychosomatic symptoms
Signs of fear (tachycardia, hypertension, fremitus, perspiration, nausea, stomach pain, pains around the heart, breathlessness)
Signs of weakness (sense of weakness, depression, fatigue)
Signs of stress (headaches, sleep disorders, stomach pains, menstrual disorders)
Psychological symptoms
Anxiety, depression
Withdrawal/social isolation
Suicidal tendency, self-destructive behaviour
Low self-esteem
Fear
Sense of guilt and shame
Post-traumatic stress disorder symptoms
Substance abuse

In order to detect domestic violence, particularly where the victims are women and children, the scientific team participating in the implementation of the EMPOWER_W (Daphne Project) translated into Greek the handbook used by mental health services and social services in London (Barnet Multi-Agency Domestic Violence Identification Flow Chart – Bell).

By way of example, we list a few introductory questions for adults on the subject of domestic violence (Bell et al. 2007; Roberts 2002; Warshaw 1996):

Do you experience problems in your relationship with your partner? Do you sometimes disagree or fight? Do your fights ever get violent? Did you ever feel fearful? Were you ever injured?
You seem to be scared of your partner. Could you talk to us about this? Does he ever behave in a way that frightens you?
You mentioned that your husband loses his temper with the children. Could you tell us more about this? Has he ever hit or threatened you or your children?

Is your partner ever jealous? How does he react when he feels jealous?
Have your children ever been injured during violent incidents between you and your husband? Do they often witness such incidents?
Has your partner ever tried to control you by threatening to hit you or your family?
Has he ever tried to restrict your freedom, control or keep you from doing things which are important to you (such as work, see your friends or family)?
Does your partner often humiliate, insult or blame you?
Do you fear your partner? Do you feel you are in danger? Is it safe for you to go home?
Does your partner have any alcohol- or drug-related problems and/or psychological issues? How does he behave in such circumstances? Do you need specific support with respect to any such issues?

As regards the detection of child abuse, it is essential to take into account and assess any risk factors as well as any of the following signs (Prekaté and Giotakos 2005; WHO 2006):

Denial or delay in providing medical care to a child for health-related problems
Failure to provide for a child's daily needs and hygiene (clothing, food, assistance in studying at home)
Frequent accidents
Frequent absences from school
Lack of emotional support from the parents
Threats, underestimation of the child and his/her abilities
Unreasonable prohibitions and control
Social isolation of the child and the family
Marks on the body, such as bruises and burns which the child may possibly try to cover them with clothes
Stunted growth
Sexualised behaviour
Fear/reaction of the child to any physical contact

17.7 Management of Domestic Violence Cases with Adult Victims

Managing domestic violence cases with adult victims includes primarily (a) the risk assessment and development of a safety plan for the abused adult and any minor family members (if any), (b) the assessment and management of violence-related physical health problems (acute or chronic), (c) evaluation and treatment of any likely mental disorder and disorder related to the victim's or the perpetrator's drug abuse and (d) the provision of psychotherapy services including counselling, individual psychotherapy, couple and family therapy (where appropriate) and referring the perpetrator to a therapeutic programme (Table 17.2).

Table 17.2 Management of domestic violence cases

Risk assessment and safety plan
Risk assessment refers to an abused individual's perception of the dangers associated with an abusive relationship: whether remaining in the relationship or trying to leave increases or reduces the risk to the individual and perhaps the children
The specialist should help the victim recognise such behaviours and the characteristics of a perpetrator associated with such violent behaviour
A number of factors which have been acknowledged as crucial in assessing the level of risk associated with serious cases of violence are set out below (Schechter 1982):
Background of the perpetrator
Previous aggression against the victim or others
Suicide attempts or threats
Threats, attempts or ideations to commit homicide
Use of weapons in the past
History of victimisation during childhood or of witnessing violent acts against his mother or their siblings
Behaviour of the perpetrator
Substance or alcohol abuse
Stalking or persecussion behaviour
Threatening and sadistic sexual behaviour
Escalating frequency and intensity of aggressive behaviour
Physical and sexual abuse of children
Abuse during pregnancy
Personality of the perpetrator
Paranoid, jealous
Dismissive of others' feelings or lack of insight
Serious mental disorder
Possessiveness
Setting
Divorce
Availability of weapons
Losses: professional, death, illnesses
Suicide attempts on the part of the victim
Poor social support on the part of victim
Substance abuse on the part of the victim
Safety plan
Whenever someone works with domestic violence victims, it is essential to develop an action – safety plan. The specialist should discuss with the victim the following possibilities (Warshaw 1996; Roberts 2002):
A. If they leave the home
Can they stay for a while with friends or family?
Can they stay for a while in a shelter for domestic violence victims?
Can they move to another community?
Discuss matters concerning financial resources and means of transportation
Discuss the necessary documents and items they must carry with them in case they need to leave the home urgently (ID cards, passports, birth certificates, other important documents, papers, medication, money, credit cards etc.)

Table 17.2 (continued)

If they have to meet the perpetrator after leaving the home, this meeting should take place in a public place
The special conditions associated with nonurban areas (social exclusion, lack of services and lack of transportation) should be taken into consideration
B. If they remain at home
The specialist should discuss any actions and situations which have proven to be supportive in the past and reduced the risk or likelihood of injuries in time of crisis:
Mobilisation of social network for emotional and practical support
Calling the police or a neighbour who is able to recognise an emergency situation
Initiation of legal procedures when deemed necessary (reporting the incident to police, protective measures etc.)
Prepare to remove the victim and the children from the home in case of escalating violence in order to protect them
Removal of weapons
Prepare the children for any eventual removal from the home together with the victim. Explain that the children are not to blame for the situation they are experiencing
Encourage them to begin thinking of a more independent life in case the situation does not change
Encourage them to discuss the situation with people they trust so as to alleviate the sense of isolation experienced

Basic Principles of Counselling Women Who Have Suffered Domestic Violence

In principle, a professional needs to present a calm, neutral and supportive attitude. It is useful to draw the attention of the individual who has experienced a serious mental trauma that this does not rule out the possibility of returning to a normal and functional life (Roberts 2002). More specifically:

- The session must be held in a quiet place, without the presence of other parties, and always in a climate of safety and trust.
- A mental health professional must show insight, respect and understanding and reassure the domestic violence victim that the feelings they express are normal and expected due to their circumstances (Safta et al. 2010).
- Some basic information on domestic violence, the forms, the dynamics, the consequences of violent acts and the specialised bodies that provide assistance on a social, psychological and legal level should be provided.
- The specialist must help the victim understand that all forms of violence (physical, sexual, psychological) have consequences and that they should never be accepted or tolerated. Moreover, the responsibility for any violent behaviour rests with the perpetrator, and such behaviour represents a means of control and manipulation on their part.
- The safety of the victim and their charges are the most important element that a specialist must ensure during each session. This concern must be expressed openly, in a direct and clear manner (Safta et al. 2010).

The limits of confidentiality in the therapeutic relationship must be clearly defined. It is important from the outset to stress that the mental health specialist is obliged to report to the authorities any potential abuse – neglect of any minor family members.

From the outset, the main goal is to promote self-control and empowerment by:
- Stressing their character strengths, their abilities and sources of support available to them
- Stressing the victim's right to have an opinion and be the "specialist" in their own life in order to make the appropriate choices
- Identifying social support resources

The professional needs to discuss with the victim some ways to manage the situation, encourage them to propose solutions to the problem and respect any decisions (Safta et al. 2010).

It is essential to take cultural differences into account. A specialised interpreter must be present when this is required for the purpose of communication.

The community where the victim resides must also be taken into account, i.e. the differences, for example, when their permanent place of residence is a small provincial town, a small village or a large rural centre.

The professional must be aware of his own attitudes, experiences and reactions towards violence by:

- Recognising his limits in terms of time and energy.
- Recognising and managing with supervisory assistance (and personal therapy) his need to be an "omnipotent" specialist.
- Realising to the extent possible his own preconceptions and beliefs on the subject of violence.
- Accepting, without expressing any dissatisfaction, the wish of an individual to remain in an abusive relationship.
- Acknowledging that he/she is probably one of the few people in the life of the individual who has suffered domestic violence who has treated them with respect and understanding (Nelson 2002).
- Having realistic expectations as to the goals of the therapeutic intervention so as not to become controlling, stressed or disappointed.
- Always bearing in mind that they need to protect themselves. If, for some reason, they feel that their safety is threatened, the competent authorities need to be informed.

Other than the level of counselling, it is essential to help the individual who has suffered domestic violence by providing psychotherapy on a personal or group level. Psychotherapeutic interventions must be carried out by professionals with specific training in psychotherapy.

Any short-term cognitive-behavioural therapy could be useful in approaching any cognitive aspects of functionality and decision taken on financial, legal, interpersonal and training matters. Training in problem-solving techniques (D'Zurilla and Nezu 1999) can enhance their decision-making capability. With the support of the problem-solving model, the patient is empowered to maintain control over the decisions they take in their lives. Moreover, the therapy aims to develop assertiveness, enhance self-respect, manage stress and anger, improve communication etc. Geffner and Mantooth (2000) propose a psychoeducational model for individuals and couples, with a focus on the areas identified above.

Longer- or short-term psychodynamic type interventions are also recommended to facilitate processing and managing the trauma, feelings of guilt and self-blame, dysfunctional and violent interpersonal relationships and also to mitigate the impact and consequences of this fatal cycle within the family system (Despland et al. 2010).

Psychodynamic interventions in a major system crisis situation require the therapeutic team to formulate and define-submit to the family a "psychodynamic hypothesis for the crisis" and an integrated intervention plan to manage this situation.

The common overall objective of such interventions is to develop a subjectification process for each individual member of the family and as the family as a group. When the mental and, often, the physical death invades and occupies the therapeutic setting, one fundamental, clinical question remains: how can we, as therapists, gain access to this symbolic-subjective aspect, without concealing the fact that the members of the family have become actual objects of abuse by their environment?

"Every individualisation-subjectification mental process is a "betrayal": Either a "betrayal" of the individual-father, whose tyranny must cease, or of the 'body-mother' from which we must break away" (Scarfone 1999, page 108).

The therapeutic approach should ensure an intermediary space, where it is possible to imagine and process the function of the family group and its history. The multiple traumas, expectations, secrets, disagreements, complaints, violent outbursts and incestual environment, according to Racamier (1995), should be the object of new significations. The fundamental paradox lurks throughout the treatment period: "Living together kills us, but separation could be fatal" (Pozzi 1999).

Finally, it has been debated at length, with conflicting views, whether couple therapy is recommended in cases of interpersonal violence. There are criticisms, on the basis of which couple therapy is not recommended in cases of abuse of one partner by the other, as such an approach could result in the re-victimisation of the abused partner and allow the perpetrator to justify their violent acts (Avis 1992; Gondolf 1995; Kaufman 1992). On the other hand, based on various models set forth in literature, there are indications that couple therapy in cases of interpersonal violence may be effective (Bentovim 1995; Goldner 1998; Hammel 2008; Caplan 2008). An initial assessment of certain factors, such as the safety of the children and the adult who has suffered violence, the couple's motivation for therapy and coexisting problems requiring additional therapeutic interventions (e.g. substance dependence), is essential before making a decision for couple therapy. A couple therapy model, which is focused on matters relating to the relationship, dynamics and interaction between the couple, trauma management, the meaning attributed to violence by each member of the couple and in deconstructing the violent moment, is proposed by Goldner (1998). At the same time, it is based on the principle that violence, abuse and inequality are not morally acceptable in any form, highlighting the perpetrator's responsibility for such violent acts and the victim's responsibility to safeguard their safety.

Support Groups

Group therapy is effective for domestic violence victims (Tutty et al. 1993). Such groups are usually psychoeducational type groups and provide a framework in which the members can work on matters relating to the dynamics of abusive relationships, communication skills and management of emotions (Dutton 1992). While therapeutic models vary, some general objectives are common and include:

Ensuring the future safety of the woman
Processing feelings of guilt and self-blame
Enhancing self-esteem
Understanding the dynamics associated with domestic violence
Expressing anger at and bereavement for the above relationship
Developing support networks and reducing social isolation

The EU Project EMPOWER_W (www.empowerw.eu), implemented in the period 2011–2013, aimed to evaluate the impact of a number of funded interventions in the light of the EU Daphne Programme (Pantelidou et al. 2011). Specifically, women who have suffered domestic violence, but also mental health problems, participated in a psychoeducational group which sought to bolster their self-esteem and increase control over their life. A special training programme was also developed for women who had suffered domestic violence in the past so that they could, in turn, become self-help group co-ordinators. At the same time, mental health professionals had the opportunity to participate in a training programme intended to improve their ability to identify and manage cases of domestic violence. Services specialising in the management of domestic violence cases and academic institutions from the UK, Italy, Poland and Slovenia also participated in this programme. In Greece, in an attempt to address this phenomenon in the islands, where social services are underdeveloped or inexistent, and the existing problems in healthcare services often make it impossible to deal with such cases, the programme was developed and implemented by the EPAPSY Mental Health Mobile Unit for Northeast Cyclades.

The positive findings for the women who participated in the programme confirm its effectiveness: It seemed that any abuse-related emotions (anger, guilt, fear) had receded, their self-esteem was improved, they now managed stress effectively and they had developed a more assertive attitude. On the other hand, after the end of the training programme, mental health professionals expressed their satisfaction with the intervention and the need for similar interventions in the future, and it seemed that management of domestic violence skills had improved.

At the same time, in cases of domestic violence, the perpetrator should also be referred for treatment. His psychological assessment is also important so as to address any coexisting mental disorder. Various approaches based on specialised programmes including mainly psychoeducational groups have been put forward in literature (Mills 2003; Braithwaite and Strang 2002). Individual therapy models include cognitive-behavioural therapy approaches, with a focus on changing beliefs on violence, the perpetrator's responsibility, and non-acceptance of violence, the development of communication and anger and stress management skills (Dutton 2003; Babcock et al. 2004). However, models combining psychodynamic techniques in interventions are also put forward as effective (Lawson et al. 2012).

17.8 Management of Domestic Violence Cases with Minor Victims

The management of domestic violence cases with minor victims by a community mental health service includes psychosocial interventions on many levels; hence cooperation with social services, health services, legal services and other community services is essential. More generally, the role of the competent services' professionals is to provide care with a view to mitigate the impact of abuse and prevent the continued exposure of the child to abusive acts. The timely detection of abuse and immediate intervention help in reducing the long-term adverse effects for the child.

On a first level, in cases of suspected abuse or when the mental health specialist receives information regarding the possible abuse of a minor, the competent authorities, i.e. the Public Prosecutor, should be notified. Under law 3500 (article 23), in cases of suspected abuse, teachers should take the same action. Based on the information provided, the Public Prosecutor calls for a social investigation to be carried out by a social worker from the competent social services. The social investigation is carried out, and if deemed necessary, a child psychiatric expert evaluation, a medicolegal examination of the child and a psychiatric examination of the parents-guardians (where appropriate) may also be requested. Furthermore, any emergency medical situation is addressed immediately when necessary (paediatric examination and treatment). Upon completion of the social investigation and the examinations deemed necessary, the services need to cooperate to prepare a therapeutic plan for the child and the other members of the family.

It is necessary to ensure the protection of the child and to assess whether the child can remain in the family and receive support by the competent services or whether the child must be removed from the home and the person who exercised violence (and whether legal action is required). It may be necessary to admit the child to a paediatric or child psychiatric hospital until the requisite assessments have been carried out and a decision is taken as to whether the child can go back to the family environment or whether they should be placed in a child protection institution. If the child remains in the family, social support must be provided to the family and it should be supervised with regard to childcare and the non-use of violence. At the same time, psychiatric follow-up care and psychotherapy are provided to the child, and the other members of the family are monitored. In certain cases, family therapy is also recommended to manage domestic violence with child victims. This may be achieved under the following conditions (Bentovim 1995):

(a) The protection and safety of the child has been ensured and the competent services have decided that the child may remain in the family environment.
(b) The perpetrator has assumed and accepted the responsibility for the violent acts he has committed.

(c) The family has acknowledged the victim's needs and is able to make them a priority.
(d) The perpetrator has acknowledged he needs help (on a personal and family level) to deal with his psychosocial difficulties and commits to the therapeutic plan recommended (both for him and for the entire family).

Another important issue for professionals is the appropriate response when it is established that a child has been abused. Usually, children don't know how this information will be construed, whether they will be believed, supported or blamed for something. Clinical therapists stress that a negative response from the family or local society could have a detrimental effect on the child/victim and this effect could be as harmful as the abuse itself. Generally, a professional should remain calm, maintain a neutral and investigatory stance, avoid expressing strong feelings of anger/surprise/revulsion, avoid making assumptions about the perpetrator's identity, allow the child to express their feelings and reassure them saying that he must act in the interest and for the protection of the child by informing other professionals as well as the competent services (WHO 2006; Giotakos et al. 2011; Cooper and Vetere 2005).

In therapeutic work with children who have been exposed to violent behaviour, the professionals aim to (a) deal with the crushing thoughts and feelings of the children surrounding the traumatic experiences and losses they have suffered (expression of feelings, stress management, treatment of metal trauma), (b) provide the parents with support (if the child remains with the family) in terms of childcare and the non-use of violence, (c) provide social support to the child through their participation in activities which facilitate their psychosocial development and (d) cooperate with the school to provide further support to the child. At the same time, it is essential to cooperate with people who are able to provide social support to the family (friends or relatives).

Therapeutic interventions are adapted taking into account the age, mental and emotional development, difficulties and needs of the child and may include the use of various techniques. Several professionals have adapted some of the narrative treatment techniques to the particular circumstances of the children experiencing domestic violence. They develop other ways of expressing their dilemmas and skills such as, for example, letter writing, scrapbooks and painting while trying to improve the child's social support in the community (Cooper and Vetere 2005).

17.9 Example of Addressing a Case of Child Abuse by a Mental Health Community Service

In order to describe more candidly the role of mental health community services when addressing cases of child abuse, we will briefly refer to a similar case managed by the Mental Health Mobile Unit for Northeast Cyclades (Pantelidou et al. 2011; Pantelidou and Stylianidis 2010).

Following an anonymous complaint for physical violence and neglect of E., a 10-year-old minor, by her mother, the Public Prosecutor called for a social investigation to be carried out by one of the Mobile Unit social workers. E. and her mother live in a small island, in the Cyclades. This investigation revealed that the minor's 43-year-old mother has psychosocial problems (suffers from mild mental retardation, exhibits symptoms of mild depression, has financial problems and is socially isolated), which result in making it harder for her to exercise her parental role. According to information provided mainly by the school and by relatives, the child showed signs of neglect (poor hygiene, many absences from school, learning difficulties which have not been diagnosed and taken care of, spending long hours alone both at home and outside the home, numerous accidents, inadequate medical treatment of health problems she had developed over the last year). It was also established that the mother used physical violence "… when E. does not obey me", in her own words. At school, E. presented the image of an isolated child with emotional difficulties. She lives with her mother since her father passed away 4 years ago. The problems in the care of the child and the use of physical violence by the mother seem to have begun after her husband passed away.

An intervention plan based on both the child's and the mother's needs was developed in cooperation with the local authorities and services available in the community. This plan included:

The provision of psychiatric follow-up care to the child by a child psychiatrist of the Mobile Unit on a bi-weekly basis (frequency of visits of the Mobile Unit Team mental health specialists to the particular island).
The provision of psychological and counselling support to the mother by a psychiatrist of the Mobile Unit on a bi-weekly basis intended, among others, to strengthen her parental role and to cease using physical and verbal violence.
Home interventions on a weekly basis by a social worker and a nurse from the "Help at Home" programme in order to provide assistance in practical matters.
Holding regular meetings between the Mobile Unit's mental health specialists and E.'s teacher, for updates on her image at school and to draw up a common plan for the child's socialisation and support on a learning and emotional level.
The provision of support to the mother preparative to carrying out to necessary medical examinations and to address E.'s health problems.
The diagnostic assessment of learning difficulties at the Syros KEDDY (Centre for Differential Diagnosis, Diagnosis and Support) (help the mother accompany E., finding suitable accommodation for them in Syros).
Encouraging E. to participate in extracurricular activities (painting group, volleyball team).
The provision of support to the family by relatives in the island who began visiting and helping the family in practical matters.
The provision of financial support to the family (through the provision of goods) by island's Women's Association.
The systematic supervision of the family by the Mobile Unit's social worker to ensure a stable environment for the minor and to eliminate further incidents of violence and neglect. The Public Prosecutor in Syros was updated in writing on a semi-annual basis with respect to above actions and the progress of the case.

Through these interventions and the proper co-ordination of the relevant bodies and persons, E.'s psychosocial condition as well as her mother's improved significantly, and no further incidents of violence were reported.

Conclusions

Among other challenges, the current systemic socioeconomic crisis places the interdisciplinary therapeutic team working in the community before the therapeutic, legal and social responsibility to deal with ever-increasing numbers of domestic violence cases.

The implementation of interventions for the prevention and management of such complex phenomena in a community framework presents three levels of difficulty:

(a) The clinical, therapeutic and anthropological – in the sense of a deeper understanding of the community – expertise of the team to diagnose and make decisions in a relatively short time and under pressing conditions.
(b) The team's resilience as well as countertransference interactions to phenomena of abuse and violence, which is unable to comprehend and process both mentally and intellectually. Consequently, the need for constant external supervision, particularly in such cases, is a sine qua non requirement for the continuation of such strenuous, intrapsychically and socially, work.
(c) The very culture, attitude and preconception of the community vis-à-vis such phenomena, often latent and persistent, through mechanisms of suppression, tacit tolerance and denial of such phenomena when they come to light. It has been established that a simple complaint from leaders of the community involved in such incidents is not useful, if not combined with other intervention mechanisms and programmes, such as the ones described in more detail below.

The dramatic lack of specialised mental health services for children and adolescents in our country makes lobbying, together with the local communities and bodies, for the creation and consistent operation of therapeutic teams with ongoing training, supervision and material support, an absolute priority.

Therefore, it is essential to develop on national and local level actions to prevent domestic violence and violence in general. Such actions must include the following (WHO 2006, 2010):

Programmes for the prevention of violence against primary and secondary education schoolchildren; such programmes should focus on attitudes and information relating the subject of domestic violence, reducing violence tolerance and promoting non-violent ways of communication/alternative conflict resolutions techniques.

Interventions through the media: limit the presentation of violence in the media, campaigns to inform victims of the need to seek help and the support services available.

Campaigns to inform the general population on the promotion of information on the subject of abuse and overcoming stereotypes and myths surrounding violence.

Specialised interventions for migrants, based on their cultural diversities and needs, intended to help them develop nonabusive communication skills and to promote their social integration.

Systematic training of mental health and social services staff in the detection and management of domestic violence cases and development of domestic violence management protocols to be used by the services.

Teacher groups with the view to inform them on children abuse issues (identification and management at school).

Training of police officers on the management of domestic violence cases.

Preventive interventions with regard to the perpetrators (on the predisposing factors associated with violence).

Development of services offering home visits and providing social support to families.

Bibliography

Ahmad F, Riaz S, Barata P, Stewart DE (2004) Patriarchal beliefs and perceptions of abuse among South Asian immigrant women. Violence Against Women 10(3):262–282

Akmatov MK (2010) Child abuse in 28 developing and transitional countries—results from the Multiple Indicator Cluster Surveys. Int J Epidemiol 40:219–227

Anagnostopoulos DK, Soumaki E (2011) The impact of socio-economic crisis on mental health of children and adolescents. Psychiatriki 23(1):13–16

Appelt B, Kaselitz V (2000) Prevention of domestic violence against women: European survey good practice models; WAVE training programme. WAVE Office, Austrian Women's Shelter Network, Vienna

Artinopoulou V, Farsedakis J (2003) Domestic violence against women: first Panhellenic epidemiological study. Research Centre for Gender Equality (KETHI), Athens

Avis JM (1992) Where are all the family therapists? Abuse and violence within families and family therapy's response. J Marital Fam Ther 18(3):225–232

Babcock JC, Green CE, Robie C (2004) Does batterers' treatment work? A meta-analytic review of domestic violence treatment. Clin Psychol Rev 23(8):1023–1053

Bell M, Smith B, Smith R (2007) Barnet multi-agency domestic violence identification flow chart. Borough of Barnet, London

Bentovim A (1995) Trauma-organized systems: physical and sexual abuse in families. Karnac books, London

Braithwaite J, Strang H (2002) Restorative justice and family violence. Cambridge University Press, Cambridge

Caplan T (2008) Needs ABC: acquisition and behavior change-A model for group work and other psychotherapies. Forest Hill & Birch, London

Coker A, Davis KE, Arias I, Desai S, Sanderson M, Brandt H, Smith P (2000) Physical and mental health effects of intimate partner violence for men and women. Am J Prev Med 23(4): 260–268

Cooper J, Vetere A (2005) Domestic violence and family safety: a systemic approach to working with violence in families. Whurr Publishers Ltd., London

Covell K, Howe R (2009) Children, families and violence: challenges for children's rights. Jessica Kingsley Publishers, London

D'Zurilla T, Nezu A (1999) Problem-solving therapy: a social competence approach to clinical intervention, 2nd edn. Springer, New York

Despland J-M, Luc M, de Roten Y (2010) Intervention psychodynamique brève. Elsevier Masson, Paris

Dobash RE, Dobash R (1979) Violence against wives: a case against the patriarchy. Free Press, New York, pp 179–206

Domestic Violence Resource Centre (1999) Reaching out-a domestic violence resource for family and friends. G & E Printing, Australia

Dutton M (1992) Empowering and healing the battered woman. Springer, New York

Dutton D (2003) Treatment of assaultiveness. J Aggress Maltreat Trauma 7:7–28

Ellsberg M, Heise L (2005) Researching violence against women: a practical guide for researchers and activists. PATH, World Health Organization

FAct Sheet (2012) Council of Europe campaign to combat violence against women, including domestic violence

Finkelhor D (1979) Sexually victimized children. The Free Press, New York

Finkelhor D (1984) Child sexual abuse: new theory and research. Free Press, New York

Fontes M, The T, Toth G, John A, Pavo I, Jans D, Kobe B (2003) Role of flanking sequences and phosphorylation in the recognition of the simian-virus-40 large T antigen nuclear localization sequences by importin-alpha. Biochem J 15:339–349

Garcia-Moreno C, Heise L, Jansen HA, Ellsberg M, Watts C (2005) The Millennium development goals commit the 191 member states of the United Nations to sustainable, human development and recognize that equal rights and opportunities for women and men are critical for social and economic. Policy Forum; Public Health. Available at: http://www.who.int/gender/violence/who_multicountry_study/media_corner/Sciencearticle.pdf. Accessed 31.7.2014

Geffner R, Mantooth C (2000) Ending spouse/partner abuse: a psychoeducational approach for individuals and couples. Springer, New York

Gelles R (1974) The violent home. Sage, Beverly Hills

Gil DG (1970) Violence against children: physical child abuse in the United States. Harvard University Press, Cambridge, MA

Giotakos O (2004) The personality and psychiatric profile of child molesters. Tetradia Psychiatr 86:102–107

Giotakos O, Tsiliakou M, Tsitsika A (2011) Child and adolescent abuse. Period Publications, Athens

Goldner V (1998) The treatment of violence and victimization in intimate relationships. Fam Process 37:263–286

Gondolf E (1995) Alcohol abuse, wife assault and power needs. Soc Serv Rev 69(2):274–284

Hammel J (2008) Intimate partner and family abuse. A casebook of gender-inclusive therapy. Springer Publishing Company, New York

Healey KM, Smith C, O' Sullivan (1998) Batterer intervention: program approaches and criminal justice strategies. Available at: https://www.ncjrs.gov/pdffiles/168638.pdf. Accessed 5.8.2014

Houskamp BM, Foy DW (1991) The assessment of posttraumatic stress disorder in Criminal Justice. U.S. Department of Justice, National Institute of Justice. NCJ 168638, Washington, DC

Kallidonis L (2013) I have no money, I "cannot", but… I can beat up. Study by the Hellenic Society for the Study of Human Sexuality (EMAS) and the Andrology Institute. Available at: http://www.healthpress.gr/. Accessed 31.7.2014

Kaufman G (1992) The mysterious disappearance of battered women in family therapists' offices: male privilege colluding with male violence. J Marital Fam Ther 18:233–243

Kilpatrick DG (2004) What is violence against women defining and measuring the problem. J Interpers Violence 19(11):1209–1234

Klontza O (2012) Child abuse in Greece of 2012 is shocking. Newspaper *To Vima* (Athens), 20/11/2012, p 13

Knauer N (1999) Same-sex domestic violence. Temple Polit Civ Rights Law Rev 8:325–350, Available at: http://works.bepress.com/nancy_knauer/6. Accessed 31.7.2014

Lampe A (2002) Prevalence of sexual and physical abuse and emotional neglect in Europe. Z Psychosom Med 48:37–380

Lawson D, Kellam M, Quinn J, Malnar S (2012) Integrated cognitive-behavioral and psychodynamic psychotherapy for intimate partner violent men. Psychotherapy 49(2):190–201

Margolin G, Gordis EB, Medina AM, Oliver PH (2003) The co-occurrence of husband-to-wife aggression, family-of-origin aggression, and child abuse potential in a community sample implications for parenting. J Interpers Violence 18(4):413–440

McCauley J, Kern DE, Kolodner K, Dill L, Schroeder AF, De Chant HK, Ryden J, Bass EB, Derogatis LR (1995) The "battering syndrome": prevalence and clinical characteristics of domestic violence in primary care internal medicine practices. Ann Intern Med 123(10): 737–746

McClennen JC (2005) Domestic violence between same-gender partners recent findings and future research. J Interpers Violence 20(2):149–154

Migliaccio TA (2002) Abused husbands a narrative analysis. J Fam Issues 23(1):26–52

Mills L (2003) Insult to injury: rethinking our responses to intimate abuse. Princeton University Press, Princeton

National Clearinghouse on Child Abuse and Neglect (2005) Recognizing child abuse and neglect: signs and symptoms. US Department of Health and Human Services, Children's Bureau, Washington, DC

Nelson B (2002) DV resources from Academic Family Medicine Mail-list Archive-Counselling Battered Women. Available at: http://blainn.com/abuse/family/counsel.html. Accessed 5.8.2014

Pantelidou S, Stylianidis S (2010) Innovative actions, challenges and prospects of the EPAPSY Mental Health Mobile Unit for Northeast Cyclades: the example of Paros and Antiparos. In: Koulierakis G et al (eds) Clinical psychology and health psychology. Papazissis Publications, Athens, pp 309–323

Pantelidou S, Vakalopoulou A, Stylianidis S (2011) Development of special domestic violence prevention and management programmes by the EPAPSY Mental Health Mobile Unit for Northeast Cyclades. Ioannina: Minutes of the 4th Panhellenic Mobile Units Conference

Petroulaki K, Tsirigoti A, Zarokosta F, Nikolaidis G (2013) BECAN Epidemiological Survey on Child Abuse and Neglect (CAN) in Greece. Institute of Child Health, Department of Mental Health and Social Welfare, Centre for the Study and Prevention of Child Abuse and Neglect, Athens, Retrieved February 23, 2013 from http://goo.gl/LTk3y (in English) and from http://goo.gl/DatBU (in Greek)

Pozzi E (1999) Le paradigme du traître. In: P. Scarfone (sous la direction), De la trahison. PUF, Paris, p 1–33

Prekaté V (2008) Child abuse at school and in the family. Vita Publications, Athens

Prekaté V, Giotakos O (2005) Teacher and parent handbook for the identification of child abuse. Vita Publications, Athens

Racamier PC (1995) L'inceste et l'incestuel. Ed. Apsygee, Paris

Ratner PA (1993) The incidence of wife abuse and mental health status in abused wives in Edmonton, Alberta. Can J Public Health 84:246–249

Roberts A (2002) Handbook of domestic violence intervention strategies: policies, programs and legal remedies. Oxford University Press, New York

Russell DE (1982) Rape in marriage. Macmillan, New York, pp 17–24

Safta C, Stan E, Iurea C, Suditu M (2010) Counselling and assistance for women victims of domestic violence in Romania-Case Study. Procedia-Soc Behav Sci 5:2034–2041

Scarfone P (1999) De la trahison. PUF, Paris

Schechter S (1982) Women and male violence. MA South End, Boston

Shields NM, Resick PA, Hanneke CR (1990) Victims of marital rape. Treatment of family violence, John Wiley, New York, pp 165–182

Stefanidou A (2010) The concept of the family and the criminal mediation process, Series: domestic violence. Nomiki Bibliothiki Publications, Athens

Steinmetz SK (1978) Battered parents. Society 15(5):54–55

Straus MA (1990) Injury and frequency of assault and the "Representative Sample Fallacy" in measuring wife beating and child abuse. In: Straus MA, Gelles RJ (eds) Physical violence in American families: risk factors and adaptations to violence in 8,145 families. Transaction Publishing, New Brunswick, pp 75–91

Sullivan PM, Knutson JF (2000) Maltreatment and disabilities: a population based study. Child Abuse Negl 24(10):1257–1273

Tomaras V (2008) Aspects of domestic violence: law 3500/06 and the role of mental health specialists. In: Milioni F (ed) Domestic violence: outlook after law 3500/06. Sakkoulas Publications, Athens

Turell S (2000) A descriptive analysis of same-sex relationship violence for a diverse sample. J Fam Violence 15(3):281–293

Tutty LM, Bidgood BA, Rothery MA (1993) Support groups for battered women: research on their efficacy. J Fam Violence 8(4):325–343

Tzamalouka G, Parlalis S, Soultakou P, Papadakaki M, Chliaoutakis E (2007) Seeking for risk factors of Intimate Partner Violence (IPV) in a Greek national sample: the role of self-esteem. Aggress Behav J 22:354

US Dept of Health and Human Services, Admin for Children, Youth, and Families, & United States of America. Child Abuse Prevention and Treatment A.C.T. (CAPTA) of 1974 – P.L. pp 93–247

Vivilaki G, Dafermos V, Daglas M, Antoniou E, Tsopelas N, Theodorakis P, Brown J, Lionis C (2010) Identifying intimate partner violence (IPV) during the postpartum period in a Greek sample. Arch Womens Ment Health 13(6):467–476

Walby S, Myhill A (2001) Comparing the methodology of the new national surveys of violence against women. Br J Criminol 41(3):502–522

Walker LE (2000) Battered woman syndrome. Springer, New York

Warshaw C (1996) Identification, assessment and intervention with victims of domestic violence. In: Improving the health care response to domestic violence: a resource manual for health care providers. Family Violence Prevention Fund, San Francisco, pp 49–86

Wolfe VV, Birt JA (1997) Child sexual abuse. In: Mash EJ, Terdal LG (eds) Assessment of childhood disorders, 3rd edn. Guilford Press, New York, pp 569–623

Wolfe DA, Jaffe P, Wilson SK, Zak L (1985) Children of battered women: the relation of child behavior to family violence and maternal stress. J Consult Clin Psychol 53(5):657

World Health Organisation (WHO) (2006) Preventing child maltreatment: a guide to taking action and generating evidence. WHO Press, Geneva

World Health Organisation (WHO) (2010) Preventing intimate partner and sexual violence against women. Taking action and generating evidence. WHO Press, Geneva

Πανούσης Ι (1994) Βία στην Οικογένεια. Στο Ι. Πανούσης, Λ. Δημόπουλος & Β. Καρύδης (Επιμ.), *Θυματολογικά Κείμενα* (σελ. 62–63). Αθήνα: Εκδόσεις Α. Σάκκουλα

Sexuality of Patients with Serious Psychiatric Disorders in Psychosocial Rehabilitation Units

18

Stelios Stylianidis, Pepi Belecou, and Stelios Farsaliotis

Abstract

This chapter attempts a systematic theoretical and clinical study of the sexuality of psychotic patients in psychiatric institutions, in particular in those the stated objective and vision of which is to create an alternative therapeutic culture and practice. It examines the determining role and the various aspects of sexuality in the field of psychotic disorders, with particular emphasis on highlighting the role of the therapeutic team and countertransference work in psychiatric institutions, with respect to better understanding and managing the expression of sexuality of patients. This debate is highlighted through the clinical material content from a psychosocial rehabilitation unit. Commitment to thinking and hoping is a strong protection of therapeutic teams against the anxiety related to the breakdown of institutions as well as their psychosis generating and neo-institutional functioning.

For the meaning of a statement is not exhausted in what is stated. It can be disclosed only if one traces the history of its motivation and looks ahead to its implications.
Hans-Georg Gadamer

S. Stylianidis (✉)
Department of Psychology, Panteion University, Athens, Greece
e-mail: stylianidis.st@gmail.com

P. Belecou
Association for Regional Development and Mental Health (EPAPSY), Athens, Greece
e-mail: p.belecou@hotmail.com

S. Farsaliotis
Panteion University, Athens, Greece
e-mail: stylianos.farsaliotis@yahoo.fr

© Springer International Publishing Switzerland 2016
S. Stylianidis (ed.), *Social and Community Psychiatry: Towards a Critical, Patient-Oriented Approach*, DOI 10.1007/978-3-319-28616-7_18

18.1 Introduction

"Sexuality and psychiatric institutions" is a challenging subject to even attempt to define, as we consider the complexity and resilience of applying the principles of deinstitutionalisation, institutional psychotherapy (*psychothérapie institutionnelle*; Oury 1976), psychoanalytical thought in the field of psychosis and the application of the principles of *recovery* as a dynamic process of recovery-cure-empowerment of speech, life and gender, therefore a carrier of sexual drives, of the patient.

Several issues relating to the day-to-day living of subjects with a psychotic pathology in psychiatric institutions have occupied more or less systematically the minds of clinicians and specialised literature. It seems, however, that we dwell less frequently on the complex, practical, clinical, theoretical and ethical questions raised by the sexuality of the mentally ill in an institutional framework (psychiatric hospital, psychiatric departments of general hospitals, psychosocial rehabilitation housing structures). The limited number of writings on the specific topic could, in fact, be seen – at least this is our assumption – as an indication of the existence of a "pact of denial" (Kaës 2011), a form of collective repression, around these points.

What is, in general, the place of sexuality in an institution? Is human sexuality characterised by certain unique features when examined in terms of psychosis and schizophrenia in particular? What is the significance of sexuality in relation to such disorders? What about the sexuality of psychiatric patients in an institutional framework and, more specifically, the users of mental health services in psychosocial rehabilitation structures? What is the position of professionals on sexuality? In other words, what representations and practices do they have in this regard? What is the role of the therapeutic team members' position and, specifically, any countertransference work in terms of understanding and managing sexuality within the institution? What are the complex dynamics emerging between the therapist-reference person of the psychotic patient and the overall multidisciplinary therapeutic team? Certain aspects of the above-mentioned problems are set out below.

Sexuality and the interest in it did not wait for the nineteenth century or psychoanalysis to emerge. They were always present for mankind, and there have always been codes of sexual behaviour which were defined by the specific historical, social and cultural context of each community at that time (Foucault 1976–1984; Mead 1963). However, with psychoanalysis, sexuality emerged for the first time as a reflection of an entire era (Sullivan 2001), as an instrument of understanding the human world and psyche. Present in all expressions of human existence in the form of a fundamental psychic energy investment, sexuality is no longer limited to its strictly carnal, hedonistic aspect.

Prior to its psychoanalytical development of its definition, for a long time, the term "sexuality" referred almost exclusively to activities, behaviours and pleasures associated directly with the function of the genital organs. According to this strict sense of the term – which also prevails in daily speech – sexuality refers to acts and pleasures involving essentially gender, the model of which is mainly sexual intercourse. For its contemporaries, however, the advent of psychoanalysis will succeed in refuting a number of more or less established perceptions about sexuality. S. Freud and his associates will discover gradually, or rather will take a fresh look at, various previously "unknown" aspects of sexuality, as well as its key role in the human mental function.

The *Three Essays on the Theory of Sexuality* (1905), one of the cornerstones of the theory of psychoanalysis, illustrates perhaps outstandingly this effort to put forward a new approach and a wider definition of sexuality. In this paper, Freud examines infantile sexuality as the first stage of the dual-phase human sexuality development and identifies its presence from the very first moments of life. As to the adult sexual activity, due to the complex mental processes it involves, it is manifested more as a conquest of the subject and not as a given: procreation is the happy result of the progressive transformation of infantile sexuality, which it replaces and covers to a smaller or larger extent. We will also discuss in passing that in the heart of this view of psychosexual development is the concept of drive (Freud 1915a; Laplanche 2008), indissolubly linked to the object, which – although partly generated by it – is always the condition of its disclosure, as aptly highlighted by A. Green (1993).

Now, in the course of time and the vulgarisations of certain psychoanalytical discoveries, the *Three Essays scandal* seems to have lost something of its original subversive dimension. Still, the new representations of resistance manifested in the modern social and cultural landscape (Schaeffer 2008) are a reminder of the fact that the forms of repression are, in fact, unlimited, as are the faces of sexuality (McDougall 1995). In the sexual revolution of the current "liquid" social reality (Bauman 2003), together with the impressive rise of narcissism in the area of ethics (De Gaulejac 1996), the diversity of sexual practices appears to be at consensual level and transient arousal increasingly becomes a substitute of the subject's emotional and mental life. Together with N. Zaltzman (2011), we could wonder at this point, to what extent would the mass cultural spread of psychoanalysis in the modern work have contributed to modifications between the ego and the unconscious mind, affecting the psychic institutions of censorship and transferring repressions? Be it as it may, the Freudian discovery of the sexual foundations of our psychic life permits us first and foremost to understand and approach mental diseases therapeutically – at the end of the day – as sexuality disorders.

18.2 Sexuality and Psychotic Disorders

In order to better process the multiple questions on the sexuality of subjects afflicted with a mental disorder within an institutional framework, we must first turn to the significance and specific aspects of sexuality in the area of psychoses, from a psychopathological view.

Psychoanalytical literature has a wealth of tradition with regard to the quest of a cause in the area of psychoses and the attempt to present a significance, a reasoning even in the strangest among their symptomatic derivatives. This meaning – today we would say to be found and to be created – is closely related to the subject's history and in particular to its psychosexual history. Early fixations, cancellation of latent homosexual desire sublimations, narcissistic regression, delusional reconstruction and externalisation of instinctual danger through mass projections – these are, in summary, the most important points of the schema "mined" by Freud (1911) from his reading of Schreber's memoirs (Denkwürdigkeiten eines Nervenkranken) in his first systematic study of psychosis. Significant contribution from M. Klein, her students and other analysts, who dedicated a large part of their efforts in treating psychotic patients, extended in their turn the capability to approach certain archaic parts of mental life. According to the most traditional belief, the common denominator of various psychoses can be identified in a primary disorder of the libidinal relationship with reality, a disorder that may be compensated on a secondary level by creating a neo-reality (delusion as an attempt at recovery; Freud 1911, 1914; Laplanche and Pontalis 1967).

In an attempt to understand what happens with sexuality in the field of psychotic disorders, we will focus at this point on the mental processes that take place in schizophrenia and in particular at its beginning. We will use schizophrenia as principal, clinical reference, taking it as a psychotic function model. As we know, schizophrenia is a disease either gradually and softly established or manifested from the start with extremely noisy delusional symptoms, usually during adolescence and up to the first years of adult life. This extremely costly solution for the ego is a psychopathological eventuality more frequent during this period of life compared to other ages. Indeed, schizophrenia is considered specifically a disease of adolescence – provided that we accept the nosographic distinction between schizophrenia and chronic systematic psychoses (Ey et al. 1960). Acknowledging the above, however, gives us a significant premise with regard to the place of sexuality within the explanatory understanding of schizophrenia, as well as a lot of information to reflect on for its treatment.

More specifically, schizophrenia expresses a difficulty in accessing procreation, namely, an adult sexuality structured on the primacy of the genitality erogenous zones, which takes into consideration the difference and complementarity of the two sexes, for the purpose of the sexual contact. Although on the cognitive level, the anatomical difference between the two sexes seems more or less obvious, on a psychological level, sexuality as well as the wider sense of the world is not organised on the basis of the genital distinction between male and female; instead they are based mainly on pregenital fantasising. "Man" and "woman" and "penis" and "vagina" are often caught into paradoxical forms of thought, which acknowledge and at the same time deny their difference. This significant burden within the psycho-mental function of forms of reasoning and mechanisms that belong to earlier libidinal stages related to procreation is not, however, synonymous with the total absence of the latter – as would be maintained by a structural formulation (Lacan 1956; Bergeret 1974) that would make the Oedipus complex a kind of exclusive privilege of the neurotic economy. Present, therefore, in primary, raw forms, unaccompanied by the fundamental parameters of neurosis (intrapsychic conflict between desire and prohibition, integrated superego, castration anxiety, authentic triangulation, etc.), the Oedipal and progenital components cannot function as basic organisational poles of mental life.

The role of adolescence is decisive here as gender signification, namely, the subjective appropriation of genitality is the core of the internal work that the adolescent is required to carry out. This pivotal period of development requires of everyone a multifaceted reorganisation process of the ego and sexuality, starting from the reality of the radical physical changes in puberty. Therefore, the fact that schizophrenia begins where, in theory, the psychological work of adolescence should be completed, expresses an inability to process these changes, resulting in the emergence of a serious difficulty in the formation of a solid sexual identity – male or female. In other words, the anxiety of forming an identity and the fragility of schizophrenia is closely linked to the failure of the representation integration in the self-image of a biologically mature, sexually capable body. Referring to this significant difficulty that the adolescent encounters to make his body and the metamorphosis it is going through his own, English analysts M. and E. Laufer (1984) suggest the concept of a "developmental breakdown" to describe the unconscious rejection of the adolescent body's sexual identity; however, they point out the difference between natural forms of such breakdowns as the expected passing moments of crisis in adolescence and the establishment of psychotic quagmires. In such cases, if an adolescent falls victim to this kind of pathology, it can be considered a costly outcome of the work of adolescence and its insufficiencies, while entry into psychosis marks the rupture of the subjectification process (Cahn 2002).

A significant number of clinical manifestations of the psychotic range may therefore be comprehended on the basis of the issue of sexuality and the massive negative defences it motivates in the adolescent and/or the young adult. For example, the start of the psychotic process often corresponds to a painful depersonalization experience, whereby the person is under the impression that their body does not belong to them. The subject experiences its body and sexuality as foreign and extremely alarming. The body's sexual identity turns into a persecuting object, causing intense archaic anxieties to flare up. Unable to recognise himself, the patient gradually loses the feeling of cohesion of his existence. The delusional ideas he is suffering from are presented in a painful attempt to redetermine his relationship with sexuality. They therefore refer to self-image adjustments (e.g. loss of physical integrity, uncertainty as to gender, a firm belief of pregnancy), as well to origins, cancelling the difference between sexes and generations through fantasies – non-fantasies – of self-generation (auto-engendrement) (Racamier 1978).

Despite all this, "psychosis" does not signify a break or a permanent end to the function and development of a subject. The majority of sufferers from schizophrenia, or other forms of chronic psychotic pathology, live in society, work and possibly even have a family. Clinical experience in mental healthcare institutions daily confirms that the timelier the therapeutic response and the more it takes into consideration the patient's personal characteristics and history, the better it permits him to unfold his resources and his hidden capabilities and invest in hope, in order to address effectively his difficulties. The target of institutional intervention, of course, is to soothe mental anguish and help the subject to experience a more satisfactory relationship with the world and himself; therefore also with his sexuality.

If the mission of the psychiatric institutions, in particular those that are considered places of living, is the contribution to the laborious subjectification process, it is reasonable to think that the interdisciplinary therapeutic team working in the institution is the catalyst of this subjectification process, the lost signification of the subject's life, as well as its registration in everyday social reality. However, how is institutional work to permit the subject to progressively renegotiate the issue of sexuality in a more favourable way? How ready are the therapeutic team members and the team as a "mental institution" to contain and process not just the archaic forms of psychotic patients' expression of sexuality but also their own deficits related to a subsequent developmental breakdown of their own that may transform to a fear of breakdown as per Winnicott, namely, the threat of a break in the therapist's mental function and that of the extended therapeutic team within the institution?

18.3 Therapeutic Team and Countertransference Particularities in the Work with Psychotic Patients

The Therapeutic Team

The daily life of persons with psychotic disorders within psychiatric institutions and the management of their sexuality are indissolubly linked with the capability and cohesion of the interdisciplinary therapeutic team, its dynamics as well as its resilience and creativity to implement a range of principles, tasks, positions and thoughts of community based mental healthcare, deinstitutionalisation and *recovery* (Thornicroft and Tansella 2010; Anthony 1993, 2007; Farkas 2007; Deegan 1992, 1997).

The concept of a team within an institutional framework refers to all its members, which are linked on the basis of a plan and through a network of mental and emotional codes, formal or informal. This is the theoretical assumption of J. Hochman (1982) regarding the "mental institution" (*institution mentale*), which establishes a special meeting location and composition of all the team members' mental function, capable of containing and transforming psychotic psychopathology (Stylianidis 2008).

It is a fact that there is a dual reference to this conceptual context: on the one hand, it determines the significance of these live interactions for the team's individual members with regard to the satisfaction they may draw from it; on the other hand, it formulates the outcome of the patients' treatment plan. Foulkes (1964) describes this communication and relationship network as a *"group matrix"* which defines the meaning of all events that take place. This network described by Foulkes, as it develops, also includes the nonconscious reality of the teams. D. Anzieu (1975) talks about the requirement for a team to have previously existed as a fantasy, as a collective defence system against many sources of threat. R. Kaës (2011), with the "group mental apparatus", suggests approaching the team in the light of the connection and transformation processes and also highlights (1993) the collective ideal or the "group illusion" (Anzieu, as above) that unconsciously organise the teams' functioning.

The understanding of this meeting place of the TT (therapeutic team) has been greatly aided by (Bion's 1961, 1962) contribution: the concept of "containment". This last one permits the establishment of a containing space of reflection suggested by the therapeutic teams to patients with mental disorders, in order to co-give meaning to daily mediations (Stylianidis 2008). The therapeutic actions helping the recovery-healing process are conducted within this intermediate space, liberating the therapist from the dyadic relationship which is the main reason a psychotic patient feels threatened.

While discussing the concept of framework and communication, we could not leave out the contribution of anthropologist G. Bateson and the famous Palo Alto School. Bateson worked to surmount the partition between the individual and the context, which he actually called "counterfeit" (Bateson 1972, 1979). Highlighting the concept on interdependence, he placed communication in a network of relationships that individuals and their actions create, which remains in constant flux. The messages generated gain significance due to the context, as this places them in a specific space-time and gives "instructions" for their comprehension to the users. In his description about the "double bind", where two entirely opposing and mutually exclusive things are asked of the individual and their incompatibility, the first researchers said that a situation such as this would lead thinking into a complete impasse, in a nonsolution, as occurs in schizophrenia (Navridis 2005).

The basic idea of systemic thinking relevant to the context and the principles-axioms of human communication (see Watzlawick et al. 1967) are being reread in recent decades, in the light of an intersubjective dynamic. The relational model in contemporary psychoanalysis, fundamentally alternative as to the classical drive theory (Greenberg and Mitchell 1983), invites us to comprehend the therapeutic relation as the process of co-construction of a new narrative through the emergence of a common affective and symbolic meaning between the two subjects. The meeting between individuals that always takes place in a specific historical, social and cultural setting creates a special, unique intersubjective relationship, transcending any form of preconstruced reality.

Utilising the post-modern narrative thinking (Bertrando 2000; Bruner 1986, 1990; Gergen 1982, 1985; Hoffman 1990; Watzlawick 1984; Welsch 2006), we can but speak of co-development and co-construction of meanings. It is important that the stories shared between the members of a TT within the setting of a psychosocial rehabilitation institution are included in a discussion that remains "open" (Anderson and Goolishian 1988) so that the production of new meanings towards a coherent-joint narrative may become possible. Only shared meanings make interaction and communication possible (Luhmann 1995).

The "meeting" that takes place here is twofold: on the one hand, this multilevel reading framework encounters the conceptual framework of the dynamic process of recovery from mental illness, which is what we focus and work on with the patients' histories, so that they may build meaningful lives within the community. On the other hand, a meeting takes place between contemporary systemic post-modern thinking and the contemporary trends of psychoanalysis (integration; see Evans and Gilbert 2005; Holmes and Batman 2002; Lancer 2000; Pocock 1995), where the interpersonal is a pivotal point of reference and concern.

In fact, we comprehend here the complexity and the multiple levels of communication in the TT's "relational network". Functional teams are established on a joint project with rules, boundaries and culture that formulate their identity. Due to the inability of processing their own vital function, dysfunctional teams break up and are unable to provide meaning to the contradictions and difficulties establishing a resilient network of relationships: at the end of the day, they are unable to contain the patient. Contradicting messages boost the early defence mechanisms of the patients' psychotic functioning. Elements that are not processed mentally, persistently and covertly interfere, are indirectly disseminated within the therapeutic space, hampering the growth of the TT's cohesion, effectiveness and resilience. In this case, "attraction" towards the team as a factor of cohesion is limited (Yalom 1995).

Such a team process, however, towards the quest of a cohesive discourse and practice against the chaos and archaic defence mechanisms of psychosis, forces us to address the countertransference movements of the team, the psychiatric institution, the external supervisor as well as each therapist-member of the team separately. In other words, the pressing question is how to help our colleagues, who are not and will not all become psychoanalysts (and why would they?), use their countertransference in their difficult daily work with patients afflicted with a wide range of psychotic disorders.

Countertransference Particularities in Work with Psychotic Patients

The term countertransference appears relatively late in Freud's writings, specifically in his correspondence with Jung. Jung addresses the teacher as though he were a confessor, saying that he has "sinned", succumbing to the seduction of one of his patients. Freud "absolves" him, saying that the patient's transference may generate a countertransference in the analyst, a countertransference that the latter should control to the greatest possible extent through his self-analysis.

Therefore, countertransference is considered here through a dual point of view: it is primarily an erotic move. It is also an "enemy", a "parasite", the pathological effect of which we must limit (Freud 1910, 1915b). For precisely this reason, Freud later established personal analysis as a necessary stage in the analysts' training process. Later papers will enrich the concept of countertransference, adding its aggressive dimension.

In any case, CT (countertransference) remained the enemy, a "blot" on the clarity of the psychoanalytical process. Mainly two authors lead us to a CT revision. One of them is J. Lacan with his famous phrase: "There is no transference, only countertransference", which opens the debate that, looking at the big picture, CT is a creation of the psychoanalytical process. S. Viderman (1982) is close to this co-construction, with his classic *The Construction of the Psychoanalytical Space*, as is R. Diatkine, when he says that transference is not an accurate new version of the past, but rather a construction, a radically new way of thinking that the patient experiences for the first time. In this sense, CT is not a reaction to transference; it comes before it to a certain extent, or, if we wish, it exercises a certain seduction on the patient, attracting transference like a magnet attracts metal.

The other one is M. Klein, who remains closer to the Freudian concept, in the sense that CT is a result of transference. She does, however, introduce the concept of projective identification, insisting that this is not just a defence mechanism, but also an archaic way of relating which means that the individual "places or projects" parts of his inner world in the inner world of the other. So Klein believes that CT is a direct reaction of the analyst to the integration inside him of parts from his patient that continues to have an independent life in his own inner reality. In other words, CT, in cases of individuals mentally functioning in an archaic manner, becomes a true case of taking over the therapist's space. W. Bion pushed this premise by Klein to its extreme, showing that at certain particularly intense times with psychotic patients, the therapist (or the analyst) hosts feelings, emotions and even fantasies inside him that the patient is unable to contain, rejecting all these annoying elements and projecting them on the other.

These two views, however, according to which, on the one hand, CT structures transference and on the other, whereby CT becomes a simulation of transference through the projective identification process, are not necessarily opposed. Currently, within the context of modern psychotherapy and psychiatric care of psychotic patients, we can say that the transference-CT interplay is an interrelated, complementary process, where one refers to the other and the reverse. In conclusion, we tend to view CT not as the "enemy", but as a tool of knowledge that we are obligated to process.

When working in a psychiatric institution, countertransference on the patient becomes complicated due to "lateral" countertransferences. The most important one is the CT on the team. The team can be an ally or an enemy for the therapist of the psychotic. The person of reference, the therapist of the specific psychotic patient, may have the tendency to become dispersed in the team, to refuse to be differentiated from it, to feel that he is constantly under its control and to withdraw or waive any personal responsibility, taking cover behind the team decisions, as though he had no personal presence. Conversely, he can often voice intense opposition to the team, ignore both it and the therapeutic framework and believe that he is the only one able to help the patient, becoming trapped in what Michael Woodbury once called "paranoid duo", which J. Hochman called "autism for two".

It is true that psychotic patients have a tendency to blend the space and people around them, to turn it into magma, a chaos, where information is cancelled and all individuals are smelted into an "undifferentiated space". The therapists' tendency to succumb to the pressure exerted on them and to imagine themselves completely "interchangeable" with their colleague, without their personality, also comes from this premise. Psychotic patients split the objects they invest in pieces unrelated between them; they deconstruct their world into disconnected parts, isolated from each other. Often subjected to this process of splitting, the team can develop destructive tensions among its members (including the management-therapeutic position with regard to a patient's sexuality), as certain members of it may imagine that they are committed to the "saviour syndrome" alone, standing against the thirst and the fusing demand of those patients.

The CT of the therapist's team is often involved with the entire team's CT. This is collectively trapped into the embodiment of the patient's difficult situations and is transformed into a theatre of confrontationalism, which the patient cannot process either around him or with his family. For example, if his mother or father are particularly forbidding in the expression of the patient's sexuality during his adolescence, the team may develop extreme permitting positions for his sexuality within the psychiatric institution, thus believing (or creating another illusion) that it is repairing the basic lack of care the patient did not receive when he should have. This process of splitting of the therapeutic team, within which one side embodies a good repairing object and the other an evil persecuting object, was masterfully described by P. C. Racamier.

Collateral CT can also occur in the family. For example, when conflict between the team and the psychotic patient become intense and raw, when the reference therapist becomes an object of rejection or destruction by his patient, one way for him and his team to recover the missing balance is to shift its aggression to the family and not the patient, especially if these emotions cannot be mentaly processed. Therefore the family becomes the absolute bad object, and the therapist feels unconsciously reinforced in his internalised "saviour syndrome".

Collateral CT may also occur on the framework and the theory that supports the framework's function. We may consider that it represents, to a certain extent, the balance of therapist-analyst transference on his analyst and his own analysis. What the patients make us experience reactivates this transference on the framework, to the extent that the projective identification dominates in our relationship with them. Specifically, it makes us experience mainly two painful emotions: that of emotional discharge, the emotional emptiness of any kind of meaning from our therapeutic practice, and the feeling that our inner space has been invaded.

Perhaps we may be permitted here a wider observation on how fragile the psychiatric institutions staff can become in relation to the prevailing economic, moral, cultural and political crisis: When a therapist is frustrated, deprived, abused and unfulfilled by the health system for many months, when he experiences daily an uncanny, incomprehensible and repulsive semantic, symbolic and moral void, how is it possible for him to have the mental and intellectual resilience to process the raw fragments and detritus of the derivatives of projective identification? Perhaps the most mentally economical solution he has left is to withdraw into a depressive position, to disinvest the "mental institution" that can no longer offer sufficient multiple support to his psyche, as aptly noted by R. Kaës. Otherwise, he may easily slide into the position of a persecuted person or that of the victim of vampirism from the unsatisfied voraciousness of the psychotic functioning or to feel literally emptied, immobilised by feelings of incapacity and helplessness, thus finally becoming attuned to the unconscious wish of the psychotic functioning: the destruction of social bonds and the inability to transform libidinal moves to sublimation. The psychotic subject's sexual drive then easily transforms into a simple autoerotic or alloerotic functioning of discharge.

Another CT defence may be the reaction of the team or the therapist with anti-projective moves, in response to the projective attacks it is subjected to. For example, let us reflect for a while on our reactions in times of crisis and tension; we might say to the patient or think something like the following: "Who do you think I am? What do you think you are, compared to me? A poor psychotic, a nobody compared to me, a professor, who knows what is good for you and how to treat you. You owe me your respect and thanks for everything that I am doing for you". We can easily understand that even if something like this is not said verbatim, it is important to bear in mind the extent to which thoughts of this kind can deconstruct the edifice of the therapeutic/rehabilitation work with the specific psychotic patient, if we are overwhelmed with such an experience of perverse countertransference reaction. These reactions of excessive presence and giving (*réactions de prestance*) that J. Hochman describes may take the form of a therapeutic activism on all levels: medicinal, special intensive care measures, security measures, special welfare intervention, social activism of activities, uncoordinated barrage of various psychotherapeutic interventions or even interpretative activism. This is the moment when what P.C. Racamier called "omnipotence inanitaire" occurs, namely, the schizophrenic's boundless power that can make us feel as though we are nothing, throw us in complete despair and make us a wreck. There are, however, moments when the understanding of CT, the better comprehension and explanation of these archaic mental phenomena, through supervision and theory, helps us to make progress in the difficult work of caring for psychotic patients.

Our effort to keep our capability of thinking untouched, to support the theoretical and institutional framework that surrounds us, our potential to understand afterwards the meaning of what was "performed as a play" on the mental stage, all this is our identity as professionals, therapists as well as social subjects that can withstand situations without succumbing to the temptation of therapeutic omniscience or the hypomanic defence for new, utopian therapeutic targets. The value of the framework and the containing function of the team are invaluable at those moments or periods without, however, slipping towards turning psychoanalytical theory and the therapeutic framework into a fetish. It is true we need a theory in order to treat, to understand and to care for. The mental institution that functions satisfactorily gives us the capability to emotionally and mentally invest theory, transforming the institution to a space that according to Winnicott is intermediate, transitional and on the borderline of the ego and the non-ego. This space is cathexed with libidinal and narcissistic elements that can permit us to turn the CT's *acting-out*, the experience of emotional emptiness and lack of meaning, to a new narrative with new links and opening capabilities.

When, however, for obvious defensive reasons, theory is fetishized, each theoretical construction loses its vitality and creativity and is repeated stereotypically as the one and only truth, like an autoerotic intellectual game, then it means that the psychotic processes and the expressions of archaic sexuality have also gained the ground of our own psyche and the framework in which we work. It is important to use the CT as a tool of knowledge ancillary to the care of psychotics in psychiatric institutions. The psychotic patient's disease is chronic in nature; he pushes us to consider him the object of an unwholesome process that is outside of him (neurochemical, genetic disorder, etc.). He consequently forces us to unconsciously deny him the position of subject and all the conflictuality connected to this position. If we become aware of this unconscious movement of aggression to subjectification, we may better define the boundaries and negotiate his sexuality both within and outside psychiatric institutions, understanding better at CT level our own representations and projections with regard to our own sexuality as therapists.

18.4 Clinical Cases

The Clinical Field

In an attempt to answer the questions that have been asked as well as those that arise in our daily practice as mental health professionals, we present the clinical material below; it comes from a psychosocial rehabilitation unit, a boarding house in the environs of Athens. The selection of the specific material is the result of the attempt to showcase the complexity of the issue through the viewpoint of a holistic approach.

The boarding house as a "living place" for patients with psychiatric disorders is an institution that aims at psychosocial rehabilitation, within the context of psychiatric reform (Madianos 2009; Stylianidis 2009 and Chondros 2010). The boarding house operates on the basis of the principles of community psychiatry, as an intermediate structure between the asylum and life as an independent individual in the community and is required to provide such a climate as to promote human relations that both patients and professionals will commit to (Stylianidis and Chondros 2008). The main factors ensuring the successful operation of the boarding house are the staff's team work, the complementarity of roles and the intersection of competences, going beyond traditional asylum-type mentalities.

The institutional framework in which the events took place, the specific psychosocial rehabilitation unit, was mired in an extended crisis for at least 5 years. It began its operations in 2006, within the context of the PSYCHARGOS 2nd phase for psychiatric reform. This unit in particular was licenced and operated given the continuity of discontinuity with regard to the commitments and the consistency of the Hellenic State, both vis-a-vis the EU as well as the parties involved, patients and mental health professionals. Therefore, the lack of scientific adequacy, know-how, adherence to internal regulations and conceptual framework relevant to psychosocial rehabilitation was almost self-evident.

The unit hired untrained and unmotivated staff and without internal regulations and regulatory rules, soon found itself in full confusion with regard to the employees' duties and roles. Members of the TT describe their experience like: "everyone did what they wanted" and "we did not know what to do and what was right". The constant staff turnover was unprecedented (at least 100 individuals went through the unit in the first 18 months) creating discontinuity and chaos. Staff conflict at vertical and horizontal level was intense and the unit operated with competitive polarities that kept being recycled; there was always an "enemy". In practice we have the deconstruction of the mental institution and the "creation" of a psychotogenic institution, an institution that produces "madness" at the time when it is called upon to manage the patients' psychotic manifestations as well as the chronic nature of psychosis.

My first contact with the specific context was practically "chilling", uncanny. Everything was in confusion, nothing was clear. There was always a patient that "created" a crisis every day and the staff team was absent; however the first reaction to any communication or new stimulus was determined from a paranoid position. It seemed that everyone was under an imperceptible threat and each one was "fighting" for survival. Someone had to be blamed for everything that was happening; there were no boundaries at any level, and wherever they existed, they were constantly breached. On the part of the staff, there was no difference between the individual level and the professional role (Agazarian 2004). Each one acted purely "empirically" (with whatever consequences this might entail) and on the basis of their own perceptions and prejudices. For example, there were members of the staff who spoke to the patients from their personal phones at a time when they were outside the unit.

The undifferentiated TT meets the internal "chaos" and "confusion" of the psychotic patients, with the result that these spread and "infect" (Miller and Gwynne 1972; Main 1989) the unit. The concept of "defensive care systems" (Foster and Roberts 1998) refers to the community mental healthcare systems that, through the concepts of *splitting* and projection, can become harmful/unhealthy both for employees and patients. In these ways, the TT defends itself, on the one hand against the anxiety arising from the target's difficulty and anguish, and on the other, against the strong and conflicting emotions that arise in our work with the patients. The result is that the TT members do not relate with patients as "whole individuals". This process may reduce the TT's anxiety; however, it also diminishes the signification of its therapeutic work.

I immediately saw that I had to read all these symptoms through the history of the unit and the TT dynamics.

The Story of One Couple

This is the story of Maria, a 44-year-old woman, and Costas, a 52-year-old man, whom I began to get to know when I first took over the unit's scientific responsibility. From as early as our first meeting in January of 2012, they came to the office together, both stating that they were a couple, that they are engaged. They even asked me if I wished to see the "rings" and expressly stated that they "would continue being a couple". At the end of this sentence statement, which was more pressing from the part of M., they seemed to attach an imperceptible question mark, an anxiety: would I make this legitimate? I assumed it might be coming also from their need for a clear message, about what would apply going forward.

The first reaction was "anger" with what I had to "fight". The issues that had to be resolved, to bring some order in the chaos, were too many for this to also exist, which was even more complicated. The question that kept going around in my mind was "how can this be happening in a housing structure, under what rules?" The way their identity was stated to me was also particular; it was as though they did not exist as independent subjects... On a first level, my internal dialogue focused on the institutional framework and all the difficulties that a sexual relationship might create within a community structure. Of course, a love relationship might comprise a therapeutic factor and help promote subjectification in the context of the recovery process; however, what about the history of their difficulties? It was obvious that this was a relationship that was born and was "permitted" by precisely this psychotogenic and undifferentiated function of previous years. How could future changes contain this relationship so that it might acquire a functioning existence and help it have functional elements? Things appeared even more difficult as I was experiencing a contradiction through a big countertransference function: I had been called to support the relationship product of a context that I was required to change.

Initially I agreed to leave the discussion "open", implying that it would be something we would discuss further down the road. In essence it was a first manoeuvre; this relationship seemed to be a fabrication of the "prevailing illness" and I needed time. The position of the team at the time was total acceptance of this relationship, which worried me even more. While I was trying to take in all the questions that needed to be answered, I immediately began obtaining information from various sides, in an attempt to construct my own narrative.

M. is a plump woman of medium height and with pronounced female characteristics and a strong personality. Her attitude is intensely provocative and without boundaries on all levels. She was born in Athens, is a twin and is described in her history as a special and charismatic child. She completed her schooling up to the first grade of secondary school and worked in the family business until she reached the age of 17. She then presented the first problems that were manifested with an "acute psychotic episode" – mention is made of obsessions – and she started to ask for help on her own. At the age of 25, she had a love affair; when it did not go well, M. requested admission to emergency hospitals. After 9 years, at the age of 34, she attempted suicide trying to fall under a train, due to a disappointment in love. After that came 4 years of continuous hospital admissions in psychiatric facilities. She has been a resident at the boarding house since 2006. Her current diagnosis is schizoaffective disorder with elements of hysteric personality disorder. We also know that she had relationships and sexual affairs in preadolescence and that during her hospitalisations, she had two pregnancy terminations. Upon her arrival at the unit, M. had great difficulty with boundaries and manifested uncontrollable sexual behaviour. She masturbated, also using objects to do so, and many times tried to do it in public. At the same time, she made constant attempts to have sexual relationships with male patients. The staff tried to enforce boundaries and the instructions to the team at the time were that "sexual relationships are not permitted".

Costas was born in Chios and is a graduate of the second grade of elementary school. Following that he worked in various professions to earn a living. He completed his military service normally and presented the disease at the age of 29 in Boston, where he was living with his family; he was admitted to hospital with a diagnosis of "acute psychotic episode". Immediately afterwards he returned to Greece with his mother. At the age of 46, and after beating his mother up in an attempt to "exorcise" her, he was hospitalised and then moved to the unit (2006). At the time, he was described as a "very reserved and private person". No information appears in his history regarding any previous sexual behaviour. What we know is the fusing and undifferentiated relationship with his mother, with manifestations throughout the entire time they lived together. Since the episode, his mother has been living in the USA; she does not communicate with him; his sisters say "she is afraid of him". He is experiencing it as abandonment. At the same time, he blames himself for the violent incident. His current diagnosis is residual schizophrenia.

M. and C. came to the unit within just a few months of each other. When they met, M. approached him and they started spending time together. A member of the staff said that "he began to open up more, we thought that it might be good for him, there was disagreement in the team, some said that it was good for him, others not; the psychologist continued to say that these relationships should not be permitted". Then, C's roommate told the staff that he saw them having sex in the room. The intervention from the unit's administration at the time was "they are people and they have rights, let's allow them to do what they want..." "then we tried to set the boundary that they should use the room and not have sex in the common areas". During the same period, M. also had relations with other patients; C. found out or saw it; he put up with it. They said they wanted to marry; it is not certain that it was their own decision/wish or if they heard it from the staff or if, even further, they listened to the need of the framework for meaning. The staff were divided; some were happy and the administration, encouraging them, chose to hold an engagement [gathering]. The prospect of a wedding had given everyone joy ("let's give them a wedding"). The engagement took place; the staff arranged for rings to be purchased.

However, M. also continued to try to have sexual relationships with other patients at times, mainly those who suffered from schizophrenia. She usually picked persons who were not well, who were in relapse or in extreme difficulties. She complained that C. did not satisfy her sexually. Subsequently, C. had a very serious relapse, during which he tried to strangle her in order to "exorcise" her. In the time leading up to the incident, he kept telling her she was "a sinner", she "needed God to forgive her" and various other delusional "comments" of religious content. He was admitted to hospital and as soon as he returned, a member of the team says, "the famous shifts began". There had been a patient suicide and the staff and mainly the administration were afraid of "some other bad things occurring". It is worth mentioning here that at this point almost the entire staff resigned. Following that and in the context of this monitoring, the instructions on the floor were that whenever they have sex, they should leave "the door a little open", and a member of the staff must supervise discreetly. It is also important to mention that during this hospitalisation, a new cycle of relapses began for C. in the time period that followed.

The puzzle was beginning to make sense. It was obvious that the team was unable to "contain" M., who continued to provoke with hysterical symptoms. The patient's constant *acting-out* was in continuous oscillation with the *acting-out* of the TT. Most of the team members were permanently angry with her, but were unable to get her to respect boundaries. Her sexuality was chaotic, with casual [sexual] relations and a lack of respect for any boundary and prohibition. At the same time, C. seemed to be reproducing the uncomfortable fusing relationship with his mother – where M. "is in control" – and which in the past was a factor of release of his relapses.

In a flat and "arid" landscape, where there was no vital differentiation between "in" and "out" on all levels, the function of this couple brought to the surface all of the context's contradictions. It was established through a desperate attempt of the team to hold on to some kind of live objective, in a unit that was functioning psychotogenically and where nothing was actually committed to. The TT was trying to draw pleasure, to recommit and create meaning through "interventions" that were aimless timewise, awkward, undifferentiated and partly "violent". It gave contradictory messages (permitted-not permitted, happy-angry, love-hate). Besides, its entire functioning was generating inconsistency, a stalemate in its communication with the patients that swung from "everything allowed" to "nothing permitted". The actions that the team resorted to were either therapeutic "activism" (Stylianidis 2002a, b) or intensely prohibitive, autocratic and often suppressive, as is common in asylum-type psychiatric institutions. Functioning defensively and completely denying reality, the TT acted towards them as though they were an independent couple, living within the structure, separately and self-sufficiently. Even the so-called management of C's relapse by the TT is a voyeuristic act, one more entry in the perversion of the said psychiatric institution's functioning.

Fantasies of the team members were projected on the forefront in this manner, mainly serving a process of release. The institution's *as if* (Deutsch 1942) functioning varied between a tendency for fusing with the psychotic and perverted psychopathology of the couple and the mass denial of this relationship.

Yanni's Story

Yanni is a 46-year-old man with schizophrenia range problems. He was born in Volos and has three more older siblings. His history shows that his father was an alcoholic, with an addiction to gambling, and that he was often violent in his behaviour towards his family. His mother, whom Y. loved dearly, died of cancer a few years ago. He presents himself as a very reserved and lonely child. He is an upper secondary school graduate and is single. His problems began after his military service, with an "acute psychotic episode". Repeated hospitalisations followed, mainly due to his discontinuing his medication and his alcohol use; some of the hospitalisations were by order of the public prosecutor. There are no sexual relationships mentioned in his history.

He has been in the unit since 2006. At the time he was a neglected overweight man, who seemed older than his age, although he was highly functional on day-to-day level. His current diagnosis is residual schizophrenia. From the time he arrived at the unit, he displayed an intense and frequent sexual self-gratification behaviour, previously, even with his roommate present. This became a serious problem, since the two roommates had a major disagreement and no longer wished to share a room. His roommate stated that he was unable to tolerate this behaviour. It was compulsive behaviour of discharge that was not accompanied by any sexual pleasure. He was a particularly regressed patient.

Some of the TT's narratives were "in the beginning, he would do it three to four times a day; at the time, the instruction given was not to disturb his roommate", "these discussions were taboo, they were not to be conducted with the patients", "we did not talk to them about sex because we also had the precedent, the couple" and "he didn't want to go with a woman; he always had at the back of his mind that he would recover and be able to find a partner and build a life".

Due to its distress at being unable to remodel Y's repeated masturbating behaviour towards the direction of its therapeutic ideal, the TT chose the "solution" of mass withdrawal. They left him alone in his room for a long time, to find his own discharge.

Furthermore, the team's perception or fantasy about this patient had a fundamental contradiction: on the one hand it believed Y. to be the most "functional" resident in the structure but, on the other hand, "able" to have a love affair only with a patient "from inside", namely, a woman resident of the facility. Each time a female patient was scheduled to arrive, the event received great importance. Y. was very anxious as to what she would be like, if he would like her or if he would be able to have a relationship with her. It appears that each time he, as well as the team, was disappointed. It is clearly a psychotic oscillation: The team's unconscious expectation of mating was transferred to the patient, who anxiously awaited the next arrival of female residents at the boarding house. The TT unconsciously enforced its own ideal on Y., through this collective fantasy.

Afterwards – and as the "prospective partner" was not found within the unit – it was suggested by the TT that he have sex with a prostitute, which happened twice. However, Y. did not ask for it again, saying "I used to go before, now I don't need it, women are trouble". Obviously, using the word "trouble" refers to "trouble" on all levels, as he experienced it: trouble with his psychotic experiences, trouble with the TT's chaotic functioning and trouble with the ambivalence before the female object of his desire.

18.5 Challenges

Talking about psychotics is easier than talking to psychotics. In other words, the last but not the least issue is how we can help on a practical level the teams both in the process of establishing and managing this complex network of transactions, as well as that of managing countertransference when working in psychiatric institutions and in particular insofar as pertains to the sexuality of psychotic patients.

The first principle is to understand that we have to work with the therapists we have, with the level of training and skills they have, in respect of each one's professional experience. There is no point "prescribing" *guidelines* for the management of the psychotic patients' sexuality or the professionals' *burnout* through cognitive behavioural techniques, when facing such complexity. There is also no point adopting a pseudo-analytical position and stance, whereby the therapist avoids, almost in fear, any physical or emotive and affective interaction with psychotic patients. The caricature of supposed "interpretations" or supposed "connections" hiding behind a "malignant" psychoanalytical silence of a supposed listening must be avoided at all cost.

What we must ask of the therapeutic team, besides the careful observation and listening of what the other is saying or not, is the adoption of a spontaneous and genuine position towards the patients. This position must use the therapist's truly familiar mediations towards the patient (e.g. athletic activities, narration group, music, painting, etc.), avoiding two obstacles: boring repetition and boredom and excessive stimulation of the psychotic subject's psyche. Being able to wait without denying the sexual dimension of the life of psychotic patients, but also suggesting another space or context of activities, creates a friendly, warm atmosphere that is not intrusive to the other's psyche and is of primary significance in the adequately good functioning of a unit. A good service is one that can change and adapt its principles and theoretical framework to the patients' changing needs and consequently to be surprised by and process the various aspects of their sexuality in relation to the external reality (socio-economic conditions, resources, networks, stigma, resistance, etc.).

At the same time, the team must be capable of distancing itself from what it is doing; processing psychically, mentally and emotionally what it experiences; using transference, symbolisation, communication and playing; and taking pleasure from this distance that on the one hand organises and on the other permits it to turn its experience into theory. Invoking "belonging" in community psychiatry, psychoanalysis and psychiatric reform is not capable of protecting us from the eroding psychotic function.

The ruptures, the cracks, the silences, the boredom, the occasional breaches of the framework and the rules occasioned by the management of the sexuality of patients, the small errors and the unforeseen incidents in the life of an institution are just as important objects of observation as the observations of an external supervisor. The questioning vis-a-vis the immobility of psychosis and the mechanisms of neo-institutionalisation, even in community housing structures aiming at psychosocial rehabilitation and *recovery*, cannot be implemented through the fatal idealisation of the "ideal" theory (psychoanalytical, systemic, cognitive, etc.) nor through an equally fatal social activism, as defence against psychosis. As mental health professionals, we often come face to face with this paradox: although we accept the principles of community psychiatry and the model of the recovery process respecting the individuality of the patient and his personal history, at the same time we panic before the emerging complexity, finding safe "refuge" behind a single theory.

On the opposite side of this imaginary safe "refuge" that can be misleading, and respecting the emerging complexity, we place the concept of supervision. We mention it as a "continuous relationship" between the framework and its dynamics with the supervisor, who helps the TT members develop therapeutic skills, understand the dynamics produced at all levels (patient – therapist – TT – hyper-context), resolve conflict and process what is experienced, utilising their own resources. The process of the supervision to include more than one scientific field and scientific theories is a call and a challenge, as just one point of view cannot have perceptions on everything that is happening. Experience shows that the coupling of psychoanalytical and systemic supervision within a context of connection and integration helps us understand the intrapsychic, the interaction and the family history, providing us with a safer framework of understanding and utilising information. Committing to multiple audiences strengthens the "mental institution" and opens the way to meaning and to transformation of the psychotic functioning.

Conclusions

This chapter attempted a systematic theoretical and clinical study of the sexuality of psychotic patients in psychiatric institutions, in particular in those the stated objective and vision of which is to create an alternative therapeutic culture and practice. It examined the determining role and the various aspects of sexuality in the field of psychotic disorders, with particular emphasis on highlighting the role of the therapeutic team and countertransference work in psychiatric institutions, with respect to better understanding and managing the expression of sexuality of patients. This debate is highlighted through the clinical material content from a psychosocial rehabilitation unit. Commitment to thinking and hoping is a strong protection of therapeutic teams against the anxiety related to the breakdown of institutions as well as their psychosis generating and neo-institutional functioning.

Still, the systematic theoretical and clinical processing of sexuality in psychiatric institutions, in particular in those the stated objective and vision of which is to create an alternative therapeutic culture and practice, should become the objective of future research, particularly in view of the current conditions of the fragility of links and the cohesion of therapeutic teams in the midst of the socio-economic crisis. Besides, commitment to thinking and hoping is a strong protection of TTs against the anxiety related to the breakdown of institutions as well as their psychosis generating and neo-institutional functioning. The quest for solutions in the direction of the transformation of psychotic functioning must take the form of "open" dialogues, including that of scientific theories in dialectic relationship.

Bibliography

Agazarian Y (2004) Systems-centered therapy for groups. Karnac, London
Anderson H, Goolishian AH (1988) Human systems as linguistic systems: preliminary and evolving ideas about the implications for clinical theory. Fam Process 27:371–393
Anthony WA (1993) Recovery from mental illness: the guiding vision of the mental health service system in the 1990s. Psychosoc Rehabil J 16(4):11–23
Anthony WA (2007) Toward a vision of recovery. Center for Psychiatric Rehabilitation, Boston

Anzieu D (1975) Le groupe et l'inconscient. Dunod, Paris
Bateson G (1972) Steps to an ecology of mind. University of Chicago Press, Chicago, London
Bateson G (1979) Mind and nature: a necessary unit. E.P. Dutton, New York
Bauman Z (2003) Liquid love: on the frailty of human bonds. Polity Press, Cambridge
Bergeret J (1974) La personnalité normale et pathologique. Dunod, Paris, p 1996
Bertrando P (2000) Text and context: narrative, postmodernism and cybernetics. J Fam Ther 22:83–103
Bion WR (1961) Experiences in groups. Tavistock Publications, London
Bion WR (1962) Learning from experience. Heinemann, London
Bruner J (1986) Actual minds, possible worlds. Harvard University Press, Cambridge
Bruner J (1990) Acts and meaning. Harvard University Press, Cambridge
Cahn R (2002) La fin du divan? Odile Jacob, Paris
De Gaulejac V (1996) Les sources de la honte. Desclée de Brouwer, Paris
Deegan PE (1992) The independent living movement and people with psychiatric disabilities. Taking back control over our own lives. Psychosoc Rehabil J 15:5–19
Deegan PE (1997) Recovery and empowerment for people with psychiatric disabilities. Soc Work Health Care 25(3):11–24
Deutsch H (1942) Some forms of emotional disturbance and their relationship to schizophrenia. Psychoanal Q 11:301–321
Evans KR, Gilbert MC (2005) An introduction to integrative psychotherapy. Palgrave Macmillan, New York
Ey H, Bernard P, Brisset C (1960) Manuel de psychiatrie. Masson, Paris
Farkas M (2007) The vision of recovery today: what it is and what it means for services. World Psychiatry 6(2):68–72
Foster A, Roberts ZV (1998) Managing mental health in the community: chaos & containment. Routledge, London
Foucault M (1976–1984) Histoire de la sexualité. Gallimard, Paris
Foulkes SH (1964) Therapeutic group analysis. Allen and Urwin, London
Freud S (1905) Three essais on the theory of sexuality. S E 7
Freud S (1910) The future prospects of psychoanalytic therapy. S E 11
Freud S (1911) Psycho-analytic notes on an autobiographical account of a case of paranoia. S E 12
Freud S (1914) On narcissism: an introduction. S E 14
Freud S (1915a) Instincts and their vicissitudes. S E 14
Freud S (1915b) Observations on transference-love. S E 12
Gergen K (1982) Toward transformation in social knowledge. Springer, New York
Gergen K (1985) The social constructionist movement in modern psychology. Am Psychol 40:266–275
Green A (1993) Le travail du négatif. Les Éditions de Minuit, Paris
Greenberg JR, Mitchell SA (1983) Object relations in psychoanalytic theory. Harvard University Press, Cambridge
Hochmann J (1982) L' institution mentale: du rôle de la théorie dans le soins psychiatriques désinstitutionnalisés. Inf Psychiatr 58:987–991
Hoffman L (1990) Constructing realities: an art of lenses. Fam Process 29:1–12
Holmes J, Batman A (2002) Integration in psychotherapy: models and methods. Oxford University Press, Oxford
Kaës R (1993) Le Groupe et le sujet du groupe. Dunod, Paris
Kaës R (2011) Les théories psychanalytiques du groupe. PUF, Paris
Lacan J (1956) Du rejet d'un signifiant primordial. Le séminaire. Livre III, les psychoses. Seuil, Paris, 1981
Lancer G (2000) Towards a common ground in psychoanalysis and family therapy: on knowing not to know. J Fam Ther 22:61–82
Laplanche J (2008) Nouveaux fondements pour la psychanalyse. PUF, Paris
Laplanche J, Pontalis JB (1967) Vocabulaire de la psychanalyse. PUF, Paris

Laufer M, Laufer E (1984) Adolescence and developmental breakdown. A psychoanalytic view. Yale University Press, New Haven

Luhmann N (1995) Introduction to systems theory. Sakoulas Publications, Athens

Madianos M (2009) The adventures of unfinished reform: from the case of Leros to "Psychargos". In: Sakellis G (ed) Psychiatric reform in Greece: needs – suggestions – solutions. Sakoulas Publications, Athens, pp 11–24

Main IEP (1989) The ailment and other psychoanalytic essays. Free Association Books, London

McDougall J (1995) Éros aux mille et un visages. Gallimard, Paris

Mead M (1963) Mœurs et sexualité en Océanie. Plon, Paris

Miller E, Gwynne G (1972) A life apart. Tavistock, London

Navridis K (2005) The psychology of groups. Papazisis Publications, Athens

Oury J (1976) Psychiatrie et psychothérapie institutionnelle. Payot, Paris

Pocock D (1995) Searching for a better story: harnessing modern and postmodern positions in family therapy. J Fam Ther 17:149–173

Racamier PC (1978) Les paradoxes des schizophrènes. Rev Fr Psychanal 42:877–969

Schaeffer J (2008) Cent ans après les Trois Essais, que reste-t-il des trois scandales? Rev Fr Psychanal 72:761–776

Stylianidis S (2002a) The psychoanalytical approach in the context of psychiatric care of psychoses. In: Schizophrenia, phenomenological and psychoanalytical approach. Castaniotis Publications, Athens, pp 267–308

Stylianidis S (2002b) Institutions, homes and psychoanalytical approach in the psychotherapy of psychoses. In: Schizophrenia, phenomenological and psychoanalytical approach. Castaniotis Publications, Athens, pp 309–331

Stylianidis S (2008) Therapeutic framework and therapeutic process: the process of action and thought. In: Tzavaras N, Vartzopoulos I, Stylianidis S (eds) Psychoanalytical psychotherapy of schizophrenia. Castaniotis Publications, Athens, pp 129–161

Stylianidis S (2009) The stigmatising psychiatric reform. In: Sakellis G (ed) Psychiatric reform in Greece: needs – suggestions – solutions. Sakoulas Publications, Athens, pp 43–58

Stylianidis S, Chondros P (2008) An alternative view of the concept of community and the mental health networks. In: Community and psychiatric reform. Topos Publications, Athens

Stylianidis S, Chondros P (2010) Mental health care in Greece today current data and critical parameters of political health and social policy. Synchrona Themata 111:102–108

Sullivan P (2001) Psychopathologie de l'adolescent. In Press Éditions, Paris

Thornicroft G, Tansella M (2010) Better mental health care. Topos Publications, Athens

Viderman S (1982) La construction de l'espace analytique. Gallimard, Paris

Watzlawick P (1984) The invented reality: contributions of constructivism. Basic Books, New York

Watzlawick P, Jackson DD, Beavin J (1967) Pragmatics of human communication. Norton, New York

Welsch W (2006) Unsere postmoderne Moderne. Metalogos 2:29–48

Yalom I (1995) The theory and practice of group psychotherapy. Basic Books, New York

Zaltzman N (2011) Qui est le barbare? Psyché anarchiste. Débattre avec Nathalie Zaltzman. PUF, Paris, pp 189–211

Part III

Evaluation

Evaluation of Social Psychiatry Services

19

Stelios Stylianidis, Petros Skapinakis, Venetsanos Mavreas, and Michael Lavdas

Abstract

The provision of mental health services is a field that is linked more and more with issues concerning the quality of care, its evaluation as well as its quality assurance. Linking evaluation and quality of care to mental health is directly related to the shift towards a community-oriented service system. In this chapter, we will analyse concepts related to the public mental health system in Greece, quoting contemporary literature and linking it with the main concerns of psychiatric reform and the function of a community-oriented mental health system. Following this, we will present the clinical approach with the administrative-management approach relative to the evaluation and record the basic requirements for the proper collection and use of clinical information in the health systems. Finally, we will refer to the obstacles in the implementation of evaluation in the Greek mental health system with one implementation example and will underline the significance of evaluation for the protection of the users of mental health services as the direct beneficiaries of the provided services, as well as the parties involved in mental healthcare.

S. Stylianidis (✉)
Department of Psychology, Panteion University, Athens, Greece
e-mail: stylianidis.st@gmail.com

P. Skapinakis • V. Mavreas
Department of Psychiatry, School of Medicine, University of Ioannina, Ioannina, Greece
e-mail: p.skapinakis@gmail.com; vmavreas@cc.uoi.gr

M. Lavdas
Association for Regional Development and Mental Health (EPAPSY), Athens, Greece
e-mail: ml@epapsy.gr

19.1 Introduction

The practice of evaluation involves the systematic collection of information about the activities, characteristics and outcomes of programmes, services, principles or processes to improve effectiveness and make decisions with regard to the programmes/processes for future growth (Patton 1997). Evaluation in the field of health includes two areas of implementation: the evaluation of clinical-therapeutic programmes and the evaluation of services or the extended health system. The evaluation of health services and systems is defined by Tountas and Economou (2007) as the assessment of operation of a health system or the individual health services on the basis of certain criteria, according to the standards formulated either theoretically or empirically.

Generally speaking we believe that the term "evaluation" is the common denominator for a wide range of approaches that "… include the assessment of user needs and the planning of services, national health policy directions, specialised response and programme assessment studies, methodological proposals and practices, research on the users' views and satisfaction and specialists' attitudes, ways of clinical activity documentation, expenses and, finally, the rehabilitation activity assessment" (Rossi 1994).

At this point, it is important to see that care in the area of mental health is a concept with fairly different content than that regarding physical health: The problems that mental disorders and psychoses in particular cause are more complex than those caused by physical diseases, while this difference becomes bigger and reality becomes more complex if we go from the aspect of the disease to that of the patient, the issues of mental anguish, the grid of social relationships and the quality of life (Gionakis and Stylianidis 1995). We therefore understand that mental health evaluation clearly has particular characteristics, adapted to the field's particular needs.

Continuous evaluation is an important means for the implementation of community mental health service goals and the decision-making process for intervention, organisation and improvement (Tansella and Thornicroft 2001; Thornicroft and Tansella 1999). The main areas where the evaluation activities are focused are the following:

Incident outcome at psychopathology, functionality and quality of life level
Effect of mental disorders on the family
User and family's expectations and satisfaction of the provided services
Quality of provided services on the basis of the WHO criteria
Effectiveness of community actions and actions to promote mental health
Needs and effectiveness of educational interventions in professionals' teams in the community
Staff development
Needs and effectiveness of in-house training seminars for the therapeutic team members
Administrative procedures and outcomes (effectiveness on the financial level is assessed in this context – the provision of best quality services at the lowest possible cost/cost-effectiveness)

Orley (1989) identified structure with quality of service: "Service quality refers to a more general view of all aspects and resources of the service and includes levels such as the natural environment, the service's procedures, the administrative-management systems, the care practices and personal growth".

Health economist Donabedian (1978, 1988), who has been particularly focused on the definition of quality in the provision of health services, perceives *quality* "as the component of a given healthcare provision unit, but also as a value judgement on the provision of such care that can be distinguished into two kinds, technical and interpersonal". With regard to the term technical quality, Donabedian refers to the *application of specific medical interventions that aim at maximising health benefits. The interpersonal component refers to the roles and functions of individuals participating in the care process.* According to the same author, a useful distinction in the components of the health service provision sector is the following:

(a) The system's *structural* elements, which refer to those elements of the health system that generally remain fixed and do not change dynamically
(b) The system *processes* that refer to actions and effects with a dynamic-changing character
(c) The *outcome*, namely, the final result of the actions taken previously

Saraceno and Bolongaro (1988) believe that concepts structure-process-outcome have a completely different meaning and significance in psychiatry than in other areas of health and that the attempt for an accurate distinction between them is often artificial, giving few results. McGlynn and his associates (1988) agree with this, pointing out that the structural characteristics of the spaces there psychiatric care is provided are instrumental in determining both the procedure and the outcome. They continue, saying that in psychiatry, one cannot take into consideration just the administrative aspect; insofar as the procedure and the outcome, they believe that due to the absence of any studies on the experimental effectiveness of various forms of interventions, an agreement could be adopted around practices and outcomes that are not acceptable (e.g. adverse effects from psychotropic drugs, long-term uncontrolled benzodiazepine prescribing, patient abandonment in the community, long-term hospitalisation with no plans for discharge and post-hospital care, etc.).

From the foregoing, it follows that the provision of high-quality services requires, on the one hand, creating outcome standards and indices and, on the other, assessing and monitoring their adherence on the part of the agencies, improving conditions and avoiding unwanted incidents that could occur. Instituting such criteria is usually implemented at national or regional level, while monitoring agency operation and compliance at local level. The role of international and national associations of mental health professionals in the process of establishing criteria is structured on two interlinked levels: (a) the definition of certification criteria that reflect in a specific manner the formulation of the criteria, the indices and criteria for which there is consent and that can also be used in evaluation activities, aiming at recognising the proper operational quality of hospitals or services and (b) processing guidelines relevant to the treatments that meet the need, especially significant in the psychiatric field, of arriving at agreement regarding the indications relevant to the approach for the various needs and pathologies, before even getting to the formulation of good quality criteria for each therapeutic approach. There are currently several quality assurance efforts and applications in mental health (WHO, national standards) used in several countries.

If we wish to evaluate the quality of an intervention implemented by an agency, we need to see which dimension of quality we are interested in. Saraceno and Bolongaro (1988) believe that we must distinguish three quality dimensions:

- *Social quality*, which we can measure in terms of accessibility to the provision of the services, not just from the viewpoint of work organising but also from that of the cost of the accessibility for the user: emotional, cultural and financial cost. We can also measure it in terms of acceptability of the provision, namely, the degree of user satisfaction.
- *Financial quality*, which can be defined in terms of efficiency, measurable as a correlation between the total expenditure and the kind of service provided.
- *Medical quality*, which we can measure in terms of the provided services' correctness and appropriateness (Saraceno and Bolongaro 1988).

The objective of the quality of care evaluation studies is the description of the way in which the available knowledge and resources that can be used in a specific care facility are, in fact, being used to address health problems at individual or entire community level.

Within the issues of Health Services Research, the core issue is the difference between the experimentally proven *efficacy* and the *effectiveness* in everyday practice. Researchers that belong to this group maintain that significance must be given to the efficacy epidemiology and that the relationship between efficacy and effectiveness is not one of hierarchy, because it often happens that we are not sure about the effectiveness of an intervention in practice even if its effectiveness has been verified under ideal experimental conditions (Brook and Lohr 1985).

The efficiency of a service can be measured many times in terms of figure absorption (and the absorption always has time constraints, irrespective of the service's goals, insofar as the extent of the therapeutic team maturity with the correspondence of the financial resources offered and the actual needs of the people responsible or the staff). At best, the investigation of effectiveness is exhausted in the description of programmes and the number of patients who have participated in them.

In the handbook *Better Mental Health Care*, Thornicroft and Tansella (2010) say that the improvement of mental health services must rely on an *ethical basis*, the *practice based on documentation* and the *collection of experiences* obtained through the years. In the same sense, the same researchers believe that for the mental health service development and improvement to be continuous, a charter must be established that will contribute to the formulation of the services' targets and provide guidance for the steps towards this implementation. Relying on the dimensions of place and time, they suggest using the matrix model; its goal is to contribute to the overall evaluation of the strong and weak points of the local services and to the creation of an action plan for the improvement of the services. Also, this model can indicate the interdependencies between levels and phases that do not directly communicate with each other, such as between the outcome at service level and the funding at country or region level.

The matrix model

	The dimension of time		
The dimension of place	(A) Data entry phase	(B) Procedure phase	(C) Outcome phase
(1) Country/region level	1A	1B	1C
(2) Local level	2A	2B	2C
(3) Individual level	3A	3B	3C

19.2 Evaluation of Mental Health Services in the Community: Psychiatric Reform Questions

Quality assurance of the provided services in conjunction with the establishment of assessment indices and treatment protocols comprises *a continuous evaluation mechanism, which aims at achieving optimal system performance and sensitivity in changing needs*.

Criteria are usually set out with the help of the literature, through *consensus conferences*, which are conducted in the spaces comprising the evaluation objective and, finally, with the help of recognised experts. In the second case, the criteria are *implied* as the responsibility of setting out the criteria is left to the expert(s), while in the first case, the criteria are *evident* because they are set out in writing and are acceptable to all participants in the procedure (Gionakis and Stylianidis 1995).

The main questions of psychiatric reform and operation of a mental health system are the following:

1. *Who are the services for?* The question pertains to the population of individuals with a need for psychiatric care. This information comes from epidemiological research among the general population recording both the obvious (individuals with psychiatric disorders using psychiatric services) and hidden morbidity (individuals with psychiatric problems who do not use psychiatric services). In Greece, the only countrywide general population research of this kind was conducted in 2009, and its first results have already been published (Skapinakis et al. 2013).
2. *Who provides the services?* This pertains to the bodies and institutions providing psychiatric services. They have to be standardised and codified, as do "user definitions" with the philosophy, structure, goals and the type of services

provided by the various mental health units (MHUs) and the therapeutic and administrative procedures followed by them (internal regulations), namely, the following units:
- Psychiatric hospitals
- General hospital psychiatric departments
- Community mental health centres
- Hospital outpatient clinics (psychiatric hospitals, general hospital psychiatric departments)
- Chronic mental patient rehabilitation units
- Chronic mental patient hostels and boarding houses
- Special programmes and services (special clinics, mobile units, special treatment programmes, etc.)

3. *How are the services provided?* This pertains to the available effective interventions by the MHUs. The main questions seeking answers are:
   (a) *What are the necessary interventions for mental health problems?* In this case, the answer requires the presence or establishment of clinical guidelines on the basis of indications of their effectiveness, using the documented medicine criteria.
   (b) *Which interventions are available from psychiatric services?* The necessary data pertain to information on staff training and skills, as well as the use of interventions provided by the MHUs.
   (c) *How satisfactorily are patient needs covered by the services?* The answer to this question requires the definition of the concept of "need", with regard to health problems. According to Stevens and Gabbay (1991), "need is the capability of a population to benefit from their health care". Depending on the degree of cover of needs by the service, we have:
      - Needs that are not covered: These are needs for which there are effective interventions, but that the MHU is unable to cover for various reasons (lack of training, specialised staff, lack of time, etc.).
      - Needs that are covered: These are the needs that the service covers satisfactorily, either in full or in part. In the case of a need covered in part, the ensuing questions pertain to the capability of full cover and the reasons and shortcomings on which the part cover is due.
      - Needs that are covered in excess: These are needs that do not exist, but may have existed in the past and which the MHU continues to provide cover for, whereas it should have either discontinued or stopped the provision (e.g. maintaining the administration of a high neuroleptic medication dosage for patients over long time periods without due reason, providing housing to individuals who can be accepted back into the family home, etc.).

4. *How effectively are the services provided?* This pertains to the evaluation of services and interventions. The question above refers to the regular maintenance of information about the patient and the therapeutic interventions. Such information includes:
   - *Personal details* (personal and family history, history of the disease, psychopathology and functionality)

- *Socio-demographic details*
- *Basic details* on the patient's treatment or intervention and follow-up
5. *What is the quality of the provided services?* The question pertains to the services' quality assurance. As there are no criteria pertaining to conditions in Greece, a study needs to be made of the international criteria, which can be adapted to the reality in Greece with the appropriate methodology.
6. *How satisfactorily are the services provided?* This pertains to the satisfaction of users and their families as well as adherence to the stipulated therapeutic, administrative and legal processes. Research on matters of satisfaction of the users and their families with regard to the services is a parameter that is often overlooked in the evaluation of services; it is, however, significant for the reason that it illustrates how acceptable the service is by the directly involved parties, while it is very important at this point in time, when their participation in the planning and decision-making is viewed as essential and necessary. With regard to compliance with legal procedures, the evaluation pertains to the security and confidentiality of files and records, in protecting the rights of the mentally ill and adhering to the procedures related to involuntary hospitalisation.
7. *What is the position of the population about the services?* Investigation of the greater community's positions is deemed necessary as the success of the mental health system depends on them, as well as its acceptability by the general public, and it gives important information with regard to the planning of community treatment interventions.
8. *How economically are the services being provided?* This pertains to the so-called financial evaluation that is related to the efficiency of the service (or the health system). Efficiency is the quotient of the theoretically minimum expenses required to achieve the objectives by those that were actually spent and includes:
   (a) *Net cost analysis*: Cost is calculated in the monetary units that a disease or group of diseases (e.g. mental diseases) has for society. Direct costs (public or individual), loss of resources (for the society, the individual and the family) and the transfer of resources from other sectors are also taken into account.
   (b) *Cost/benefit analysis*: It is the systematic comparison in monetary units of all costs and the benefit of suggested alternative schemas, with a final investigation – first, of the degree to which this combination of schemas will achieve their set targets with a set financial investment and, second, the extent of the benefit that arises from the schemas (programmes, services, treatments) requiring a minimum investment.
   (c) *Cost/effectiveness analysis*: It is the same as the one above, except it measures the benefit in achieved results (e.g. days of work in rehabilitation programme, days of stay in the community without hospitalisation, etc.).

Questions on the Mental Health System Evaluation

The questions that arise from evaluating the mental health system are not independent from epidemiology and the conditions it studies, as we have discussed above.

Questions related to the evaluation of the system both on local and on national level are the following:

1. *How frequent is the problem?* The question pertains to the information resulting from the descriptive epidemiological research. In particular, the sub-questions are:
   - Description of "at-risk" population
   - Prevalence and consequences of mental disorders
   - Assessment of risk factors related to mental disorders, namely:
     – Relative risk
     – Attributable risk
   - Determination of cases and syndromes in the community (study of the representativeness of observed cases)
2. *How serious is the problem?* This pertains to the consequences and the aftermath of the problem on the individual and the micro-social and macro-social environment. More specifically, the questions pertain to:
   - The "objective" classification and assessment of the problem's seriousness
   - The "subjective" assessment of malaise and quality of life caused by the health problem
   - The effect of the problem on the immediate family and other relatives of the patient
   - The socioeconomic aspects of the problem
3. *Are the interventions acceptable (to the patients, the population, the other state agencies)?* The answers to these questions may be given by collecting information on a local level (qualitative and quantitative) or by accumulating data collected by local services.
4. *Does the problem seem to be increasing, stabilising or reducing?* Monitoring epidemiological trends, with repetitions of the epidemiological research at regular periods (at least every 10 years or even better every five), can yield data with regard to how the system corresponds to changing needs.

Evaluation of the health services is based on collection and use of valid and reliable information. Evaluation is an administrative process, the goal of which is to check the system's operation as to the set purposes and the intended results from it. As far as the clinician is concerned, the (clinical) information is important for the following reasons: (a) the reminder of the diagnosis and differential diagnosis criteria (use of uniform classification system such as ICD-10 and DSM-IV, use of standardised psychiatric interviews and psychiatric questionnaires), (b) the reminder of the appropriate treatments (clinical and therapeutic instructions) and (c) assessment of the outcome (symptomatology and disability before and after the intervention, indications of effectiveness of the treatment and the service, scales and questionnaires). For completely different reasons, and in the case of the administration of health services, the evaluation is based on the collection of information in the field, namely, during the provision of services to the patient. However, the evaluation process follows the opposite course to that of clinical work insofar as the collection and use of information, even though this information comes from it. According to Wing (1994), this course is as follows:

Clinical approach (bottom-top)	Administrative approach (top-bottom)
1. Clinical work with patients	1. Data collection from the clinical units
2. Clinical audit: problem assessment, treatment, audit, outcome assessment, re-evaluation	2. Epidemiology of use of the services (mental health units) by the population
3. Clinical audit of files	3. Assessment of the population's needs
4. Mental health clinical data and information system	4. Planning, staff hiring, new services creation, resource management
5. History and file confidentiality and security	5. Measuring the progress of health services and outcome
6. Data collection for the administration of health services	6. Public health policy
	7. Collection of data on the health of the entire population

The basic requirements for the proper collection and use of clinical information in the health systems are the following:

To be based on the unit-individual: The collection of detailed information on every patient in touch with the MHUs is necessary to gather the data illustrating the socio-demographic profile of the services' users, the diagnosis and psychopathology, their personal and family history, their functionality, the interventions conducted and their result, as well as patient follow-up by the mental health service system.

To be entered only once: This means that there should be a unique, uniform record of the patient in the mental health system that will be updated by the different MHUs that the individual visits during his care by the mental health sector of the mental health system. Past difficulties that existed in the maintenance of such records as well as their use by the various MHUs, which created multiple problems of communication and data collection, may be easily overcome today with the development of software applications (patient electronic file).

To come from the MHU clinical staff: Gathering the regularly collected clinical data is among the duties of the units' clinical staff. Information about special questions may come from special research in the context of the system, where both clinical and non-clinical (trained) staff may be used.

To ensure the collected data security and confidentiality: The laws pertaining to personal data collection and use must be respected. Therefore, the data collected by the staff of the units must be usable in clinical practice, with the breach of their secrecy fully prohibited, while the cumulative data must not show patient names, or show information in a way that may permit their identification. Furthermore, full security and protection of the record systems (electronic or not) must be ensured from potential outside interventions.

To use common standards permitting communication within the framework of the health system: Their reliability and validity requires their classification and codification and the generation of "user definitions" that are acceptable and can be used by all the staff.

To provide information to the following potential users:
- Mental health service users
- Mental health professionals
- Administrative services

Of course, the type and nature of the information may vary depending on the user and the purposes of use of the information.

They have to be usable for both clinical and administrative and research purposes.

In summary, the main research questions on evaluation investigations regarding mental health are as follows, as determined by Wing (1972):

How many individuals are in touch with existing services? How did they obtain contact? What kind of use of services do they conduct? What sort of changes in time is observed?

What are the needs of these individuals and their relatives?

Do current services meet needs effectively and economically?

How many of those who are not in touch with the services have needs? Are those different to the needs of individuals who are in touch with the services?

What new services or current service modifications are required to cover needs that are not currently covered?

Can imported innovations really help in need reduction?

The commonly used variables in the evaluation investigation are the following:

Volume of use (individuals, admissions, episodes, visits)

Patient (or consumer/client/user of the services) clinical and socio-demographic data

Treatment or control methods used

Treatment/hospitalisation/follow-up duration

Outcome measurements (e.g. frequency of relapses/hospitalisations during follow-up)

"New" morbidity during the service's operation

Mortality

Effects of the service on families, the staff and other services

Use of the staff and training and use of time by the staff

Patient, family and staff satisfaction

Penetration measurement of the service in the community and other bodies

Monetary and nonmonetary cost

It is also necessary to be able to achieve consent through creative dialogue – at least for "sentinel events" – so that we may further develop services that truly meet the needs of mental health. Sentinel events in psychiatry are events that should be avoided [sentinel events have been described (Morosini and Veltro 1991): new patient with more than one episode per year, a patient who does not leave his house for more than a determined period of time, patient follow-up abandoned, patient incarceration, patient suicide, etc.].

Obstacles in Evaluation Implementation in the Greek Mental Health System

Significant obstacles in evaluation implementation in the Greek mental health system are the following shortcomings:

Lack of sectorisation and reference population of the mental health system in still significant parts of the country
Lack of community involvement principles of the services
The fact that evaluation is not a system element
Lack of a common system of record keeping
Lack of common outcome criteria
Lack of therapeutic intervention standardisation

Pubic Mental Health System Evaluation Implementation Example

Systematisation of the internal pubic mental health system evaluation begins with an ex post evaluation (2009–2010) (Ministry of Health and Social Solidarity 2010), which was ongoing at the time of psychiatric reform (2011–2015) (Ministry of Health and Social Solidarity 2013).

Indicatively, we show the SWOT analysis below that was published in the report following quantitative and qualitative evaluation methods:

Capabilities	Weaknesses
1. Turn in the provision of mental health services towards a contemporary model of community psychiatric care	1. Fragmented, non-co-ordinated system that often results in the wrong provision of services
2. Contraction of the number of beds in psychiatric hospitals	2. Unequal geographic distribution of services
3. Closure of 5 psychiatric hospitals	3. Significant gaps in mental health services for children and adolescents and long waiting lists
4. Gradual acceptance of individuals with mental disorders by local communities	4. Significant gaps in mental health services for the elderly and dementia patients

Capabilities	Weaknesses
5. Raising awareness, information and promotion of mental health with the support of the media	5. Significant gaps in specialised mental health services (individuals with the autistic range of disorders, mental retardation, eating disorders)
6. Significant improvements in the context of performance of psychiatric and children's psychiatric speciality and increase in the relevant jobs	6. Significant shortfall in judiciary psychiatric services and antiquated institutional framework
	7. Inability to implement procedures and quality assurance standards in the operations of mental health services
	8. Lack of epidemiological studies on mental health
	9. Shortages of staff in supporting and ancillary roles
	10. Large number of involuntary hospitalisations
	11. Serious issues with regard to the protection of the rights of service users
	12. Limited involvement by the users of mental health services (RMHS) and advocacy
	13. Delays in the development of psychiatric departments in general hospitals
	14. Absence of self-help groups, training and support for dementia and mental health patient carers
	15. Inability of scheduling and funding of education, training and vocational rehabilitation programmes for RMHS
	16. Inadequate sectorisation implementation
	17. Excessively centralised administration model of the mental health system
	18. Lack of a clear business plan for policy implementation, with policy priorities, costing and funding

Threats	Opportunities
1. Risk of mental health system collapse/ unsustainability if the issue of its funding from the state budget is not resolved	1. Integration of existing subsystems and services
2. Existing structure issues may lead to higher fragmentation and cause a threat to the system's sustainability	2. Corrective actions for system co-ordination with clear structures and competences in the context of the PSYCHARGOS 3 proposal revision
3. Pending issues with regard to compliance with Spidla accord requirements	3. Utilisation of the National Strategic Reference Framework 2007–2013

Threats	Opportunities
4. Further burden on the system from new and emerging needs due to the consequences of the financial crisis to mental health (suicide rate, homelessness, migratory flows, etc.)	4. Development of new plan for the next stage of the reform
5. Significant resistance from the staff with regard to changes in the system	5. Transfer of know-how capability from the EU and the WHO
6. Staff reductions in legal persons governed by public law due to retirement and new hiring restrictions	6. Utilisation of public sector property to house mental health services
7. The transfer of psychiatric departments to general hospitals is likely to deprive mental health from resources that would be used for the benefit of services pertaining to general-physical health	7. Funding improvement for structures of legal persons governed by private law through the funding capability of the NSRF
8. Significant delay in NSRF available resources absorption	8. Function of the National Organisation for Healthcare Benefit Provision (EOPYY)
9. Current socioeconomic conditions	9. Integration of mental health services in primary healthcare
	10. Maturity of the institutional framework with regard to social economy

19.3 Evaluation and Human Rights

Evaluation and improvement of quality and the status of human rights, in both outpatient and hospital units, are of critical significance. An overall evaluation of the services helps trace problems within the existing healthcare practises, while it contributes to the development of effective ways to ensure that the services are of good quality and respect human rights, so that they may meet the requirements of users and promote their independence, their dignity and their right to self-determination/self-identification. Evaluation is important not just for reframing old neglect and abuse incidents but also to ensure the development of efficient and effective services in the future. Furthermore, results and recommendations from quality and human rights evaluation may be invaluable for enriching the planning of a future reform policy, scheduling and legislating as well as ensuring that these will be conducted respectfully and will promote human rights.

In conclusion, we would like to point out that the goal of a service's evaluation (and self-evaluation) process is to change its practice. The purpose of quality evaluation is not to add to the knowledge of one aspect of reality but to optimise interventions, gradually granting users and others involved in the provision of mental health services the right to express views for the continuous improvement of the services and their effectiveness (Table 19.1).

Table 19.1 Evaluation types and areas of questions and definitions relevant to good practices in the provision of services (Hollander et al. 2010)

Evaluation types and areas of questions	Definitions – description
Model planning and application	
1. Appropriateness of planning (evaluation of theoretical inclusiveness and model structure)	This relates to whether the model is well documented and is planned in such a way as to meet the programme's original goals and purposes, while remaining consistent with the criteria of good practice in the field. The reasoning of the model, its basic characteristics and structure are included and assessed in this field
2. Efficiency and effectiveness of the model's application (application evaluation)	This field examines the model's consistency to its original planning and the extent to which it was adopted in the way it was planned by the staff of the institution implementing it or any other key persons
Model functionality (evaluation of the procedure)	
3. Appropriate provision of care	Refers to the evaluation of whether the staff is adequate or not for the provision of the care. The provision of care is conducted on the basis of specific principles and procedures. The model is "functional" if the procedure of providing care services is followed
4. Care continuity and care co-ordination	Ensuring care continuity and co-ordination throughout the range of required services in this field
5. Staff skills	This field refers to the professional qualifications and skills of the individuals in the administration, management or the provision of services
Model effectiveness (outcome evaluation)	
6. Service accessibility	The degree of accessibility by the beneficiaries is evaluated, while parameters such as the following are examined: answers to questions, operating hours, easy access to services
7. Service quality	The quality of provided services is linked to the satisfaction of service users, the members of their families and the persons involved with the provision of care
8. Cost-effectiveness	The institution's value for money is evaluated and is directly linked to cost and outcome
9. Effect on health	The effect of provided services on the population's health in general
10. Model transfer and generalisation capability	The relevance of the model with other frameworks of care or provision of services is evaluated. It pertains to the extent to which the model can be adopted throughout the country and the extent to which it can be adopted by various services, institutions and frameworks. The capability of transferring innovation is evaluated
11. Sustainability	Sustainability examines how well the model can continue to function through time with alternative resources for its support

Bibliography

Brook RH, Lohr KN (1985) Efficacy, effectiveness, variations and quality: boundary-crossing research. Med Care 23:5

Donabedian A (1978) The quality of medical care. Science 200:856–864

Donabedian A (1988) Quality assessment and assurance: unity of purpose, diversity of means. Inquiry 25:173–192

Gionakis N, Stylianidis S (1995) Evaluation of quality of care in mental health: methodological observations. Psychiatry Workbooks 49:22–35

Hollander MJ, Miller JA, Kadlec H (2010) Asking the right questions to develop new policy and program-relevant knowledge for decision-making. Healthc Q 24(4):40–47

McGlynn EA, Norquist GS, Wells KB, Sullivan G, Liberman RP (1988) Quality of care research in mental health: responding to challenge. Inquiry 25:157–170

Ministry of Health and Social Solidarity (YYKA) (2010) Evaluation report of the implementation intervention of Psychiatric Reform for 2000–2009. http://www.psychargos.gov.gr/Documents2/Ypostirixi%20Forewn/Ypostirixi%20EPISTHMONIKH/Ex%20Post%20%CE%A0%CE%91%CE%A1%CE%91%CE%94%CE%9F%CE%A4%CE%95%CE%9F%202%20Teliko.pdf, προσπελάστηκε 20.7.2014

Ministry of Health and Social Solidarity (YYKA) (2013) Evaluation report of the implementation intervention of Psychiatric Reform for 2012. http://www.psychargos.gov.gr/Documents2/ON-%20GOING/%CE%A0%CE%921.2.pdf, προσπελάστηκε 20.7.2014

Morosini PL, Veltro F (1991) Process or outcome approach in the evaluation of psychiatric services. In: Freeman H, Henderson J (eds) Evaluation of comprehensive care of mentally ill. Gaskel, London

Orley J (1989) Quality assurance in mental health. Introduction to the "Evaluation of comprehensive care of the mentally ill" workshop, organised by the European Communities committee, 1–3 Dec 1989 (unpublished internal paper)

Patton M (1997) Utilization-focused evaluation, 3rd edn. Sage, Thousand Oaks

Rossi E (1994) La valutazione in psichiatria: i principali indirizzi tra pratica e ricerca. Lettera XVII:138–174

Saraceno B, Bolongaro G (1988) Questioni di valutazione nei servizi di salute mentale. Prospettive Psicoanalitiche Nel Lavoro Istituzionale 6(1):44–53

Skapinakis P, Bellos S, Koupidis S, Grammatikopoulos I, Theodorakis PN, Mavreas V (2013) Prevalence and sociodemographic associations of common mental disorders in a nationally representative sample of the general population of Greece. BMC Psychiatry 13(1):163

Stevens A, Gabbay J (1991) Needs assessment needs assessment.... Health Trends 23(1):20–23

Tansella M, Thornicroft G (eds) (2001) Mental health outcome measures. RCPsych Publications, London

Thornicroft G, Tansella M (1999) Translating ethical principles into outcome measures for mental health service research. Psychol Med 29(04):761–767

Thornicroft G, Tansella M (2010) In: Stylianidis S (ed) Better mental health care: ethics, documentation and experience. Topos Publications, Athens, Original Work Published, 2009

Tountas G, Oikonomou NA (2007) Evaluation of health services and systems. Hell Med Arch 24(1):7–21

Wing J (1972) Principles of evaluation. In: Wing JK, Hailey AM (eds) Evaluating a community psychiatric service. Oxford University Press, Oxford

Wing JK (1994) A strategy for mental health informatics. In: Andrews G, Dilling H, Ustun TB, Briscoe H (eds) Computers for mental health. Longman, St Andrews, pp 9–15

Implications of the Socioeconomic Crisis for Staff in Community PSR Units: The Case of an NGO

20

Stelios Stylianidis, Klimis Navridis, and Anna Christopoulou

Abstract

Financial strain, high unemployment rates, institutional inconstancy and job insecurity in the context of the socioeconomic crisis in Greece affect the workforce at various levels. This situation in conjunction with the austerity policies implemented for more than 5 years in the mental health field along with incomplete psychiatric reform has multilevel consequences, including severe deterioration in the quality of medical, psychiatric and social services. For these reasons, we conducted a qualitative research study, in residential units of a Greek NGO, in order to investigate the subjective experience of weakening in personnel, on the institutional group levels in association with the defence mechanisms mobilised in response to the patients' complex psychological attitudes that personnel have to manage. Suggestions for further institutional initiatives and for new themes of future research are also presented.

20.1 Introduction

In the context of the socioeconomic crisis in Greece, the underfunding of the units of an already malfunctioning "welfare state" (Sakellis 2012), especially the mental health services network, amplified the systemic structural problems (Loukidou et al. 2012; MHSS 2010, 2012, 2013) in a way that puts in question its survival ("ARGO" – Network for Psychosocial Rehabilitation and Mental Health 2012; Stylianidis

S. Stylianidis (✉)
Department of Psychology, Panteion University, Athens, Greece
e-mail: stylianidis.st@gmail.com

K. Navridis • A. Christopoulou
National and Kapodistrian University of Athens, Athens, Greece
e-mail: knav-lpp@otenet.gr; annachr@otenet.gr

2012). The obvious "paradox" experienced by all parties involved (patients, families, administrators, mental health professionals, the community) is the government's dismantling of the already malfunctioning network of mental health services, despite the significant increase in requests for psychiatric care, prevention and early therapeutic intervention in the general population, especially vulnerable social groups,

This high degree of institutional and professional insecurity causes a series of chain reactions in all operating levels of mental health services, such as residential care, family and community intervention, as well as in personnel responsible for the scientific, administrative and ethical functioning of the units, who are working to avoid the return of patients to asylums.

20.2 The Contradictions and Incomprehensible Nature of Social and Psychic Suffering in Mental Health Community Units

The theory and practice of deinstitutionalisation and the questioning of the psychiatric biomedical paradigm began in Western Europe in the 1960s and after five decades of reform efforts now stand – at least in terms of stated positions and targets – as the new example of good and evidence-based practice worldwide (Thornicroft and Tansella 2010; Basaglia et al. 2000).

One of the key questions, however, which in part concerns us in the analysis of the interview material of this research, is to what extent such institutional and organisational change succeeded in radically altering key features of the old culture such as "total institution" (Goffman 1968) and institutionalisation processes (Basaglia et al. 2000) within the new mental health facilities.

Is it possible to argue, without deforming reality through "ideological glasses", that the new "institution mentale" (Hochmann 1982), as it is or should be established, is a solid container allowing the working through of destructive group dynamics, particularly in the present circumstances? If not, then why have we left the safety of asylum, perceived through the perspective of the ancient function of shelter and protection?

According to Hinshelwood (2001), following the triumphant illusions of the anti-asylum movement, wide scepticism prevailed after we noticed serious phenomena of institutionalisation even in small community units. However, these external and internal factors, leading to a recurrence of such institutionalisation mechanisms, have not yet been adequately studied in the literature (Racamier 1973; Bion 1952; Hochmann 1982; Searles 1965; Benedetti and Andreoli 1991; Rosenfeld 2003).

20.3 Research

This qualitative research focused on the impact of the crisis for more than 5 years on the field of mental health in our country, and in particular, given the already incomplete and fragile psychiatric reform process, on the personnel of residential units of a

Greek NGO (Stylianidis and Chondros 2011). The research examined the way the personnel experiences and addresses – subjectively but also intersubjectively – the phenomena of weakening, i.e. the external devaluation of their profession, role and individual status and hence the violent attacks:

- On a personal and psychological level (professional identity and narcissism)
- At the group level (risk of decomposition and disappearance)
- At the institutional level (risk of elimination, death anxiety)

20.4 Method

The method used in this case was that of the clinical psychosocial survey (Revault d'Allonnes et al. 1989; Blanchet 1989; Trognon 1987). In the first stage, three 90 min focus group interviews were conducted with the scientific coordinators of the various units of the NGO (Banks 1957; Giami 1985; Trakas 2008) in order to identify potential main subjects. Then, 17 personal interviews followed with members of the staff and the scientific coordinators from units of the major area of Athens and the countryside. The criteria for choosing the staff members included in the sample (except for Athens vs. countryside) were (a) specialisation/position/duties and (b) age (<35, >40)/years of service in the organisation (<5, >10).

This was followed by the analysis of the empirical material. The method used was a clinical type of *interpretative content analysis*, which permits investigation of the subjective experience of the sample in greater depth (Enriquez et al. 1993). This specific approach highlights the significance of the relationship between researcher and respondent, requiring post hoc simultaneous evaluation of *hearing or reading* the notes and the transcribed interviews *later* on the one hand and the element of *intersubjective construction*, therefore the co-construction of the empirical material on the other hand, in other words, the transference of the sample participants and the researcher's countertransference (Devereux 1980).

Thus, the interviewer addresses the narrative in three ways: by selecting the theme and topics, by ordering the questions and by phrasing questions in his or her language (Bauer 1996).

This approach is consistent with the emphasis on reflexivity in the interview, exploring and combining the psychoanalytic and social aims of this study. It involves comprehension of people's subjectivities in the context of the weakening process and events of external reality which they bring to mind and convey in the intersubjective context of the interview.

All interviews, individual and group, were carried out by one of the two co-researchers in a specially designated room at the headquarters of the NGO. After each group interview, the interviewer kept detailed notes from memory. Personal interviews, each one lasting between 30 and 50 min, were recorded with the consent of the individuals.

The steps of analysing, verifying and reporting followed the seven stages of an interview inquiry (Kvale and Brinkmann 2009).

This was followed by analysis of the transcribed material.

Findings

The material from the interviews has multiple levels, involving issues of personal survival and psychological processing of breakdown anxiety as well as themes arising from the intersubjective dynamic between the members of the groups and between the group's and the organisation's management.

The subjects frequently switch from singular to the plural form (Kaës 2009), from "I" to "we", not only as an invocation for the group's support or as reference in a collective synergy regarding professional duties that are particularly demanding and difficult but very probably as obfuscation and the intervention of a subjective insecurity regarding the framework (of the job and the interview itself).

A first observation regarding underfunding or irregularity in state payment of the specific NGO and the psychological impact on employees is that these phenomena are not exclusively connected to the time period of this crisis but had also appeared in the past. Let us see what the participants in the study have to say about this:

> This problem always existed. It is not new. Because of the Ministry. Now it's more. (Lambros, General Duties in a Residential Unit, 2 years in the job)

> It is not something that started recently. For these units […] it started in 2005. That is more than six-seven years […]. The first time that the staff was not paid was in 2008 […]. From 2008 and onwards, as well as earlier, late 2007 I would say, delays began. In fact then, in 2008, we reached a six-month period without pay. (Nikos, Child psychiatrist, Scientific Coordinator at a Hostel (13 years in the job))

Thus, ever since, as many mentioned, each time that a person was to be hired, he was asked during the interview if someone from his environment could support him financially when his payment was late:

> When I was interviewed, the first thing they told me was that, you know, you will be paid every six months. You won't lose your money, you'll get it. But you will get it every six months. This didn't bother us at first. (Marina, 51, General Duties in a Hostel)

During the current circumstances, however, the major problem for the NGO's staff does not appear to be, as we will go on to see, the possibility of delay in payment continuing or increasing, but the fact that the employees can no longer predict when they will or how much they will be paid each time, as well as – the worst thing – how long they will continue to be paid:

> […]There were cutbacks and so on, but at least the employee's salary was coming in. (Nikos)

> […] and the six months that we go unpaid and the like, they will give us, I don't know, 2 monthly salaries, 1 salary. (Marina)

You don't know what will happen, when you'll get paid, if they will fire you, we don't know anything, if the structures will close, we didn't know anything. (Martha 50, General Duties at a Residential Unit)

With the workers of the NGO, survival anxiety is expressed in correlation with parameters such as age, locality (the distance between work and place of residence), the employee's previous experience of similar crises due to underfunding, their family status (existence of children or other family obligations), as well as their management method by the organisation. In particular, the greatest problem for the younger ones appears to be their extended dependence on the paternal family, due to the employment circumstances of the financial crisis, and subsequently the obstruction of their personal development towards adult life:

Basically, my brother is helping who is in the USA..

It is very hard as young people, because my partner is 26 and I am 28, so we young people are experiencing it and we are feeling it a great deal... I feel a burden that I cannot start a family. (Stefania, 28, Nurse in a Residential Unit)

I am from the countryside [...]. I have rented a house and certainly now in these circumstances I have found it very difficult to meet my obligations. How will I pay the rent. Of course, OK, my parents are helping me.... They are sending me money.. as if I were still a student.. (Kyriakos, 29, Social Worker in a Residential Unit & Mobile Unit)

On the other hand, older employees appear to experience feelings of loneliness and abandonment by the organisation and the state. These feelings are frequently transformed into a sense of personal and professional devaluation, expressed together with the patients' survival anxiety regarding their future outcome and the now existent possibility of abandonment or mental death as a result of potentially returning to the asylum. Let's see what they say themselves:

Recently, to tell you the truth, I am afraid of being unemployed. I am not afraid of anything else from the crisis. Because if I am unemployed, I cannot make ends meet. (Sotiria, Nurse, 6 years in a Hostel)

[...] when you have something else in the background, you are a bit optimistic. At first I was worried, but then I got over it. (Martha, 50, General Duties in a Residential Unit)

Things are getting tighter [...] Without any help from nowhere [...]So I look at what I can do with my hours, with my shifts, what I can decrease in my budget, what can be left aside, and what priorities there are, which are first and which are second, to be able to make ends meet. (Eleni, 42, General Duties in a Residential Unit)

The employees who are parents of young children are naturally experiencing great anxiety due to their inability to appropriately care for them. Eleni, for example, (see above) mentions:

> My children are 15 and 13 years old. Boys.. OK, things are difficult. I cannot potentially provide what we would possibly have in other circumstances and without an economic crisis. To offer as a mother. I am offering nothing to them. I am offering a roof, food, support. I cannot offer them supplies. So all this, make me feel that I am now an incompetent mother. (Eleni)

However, in older people, personal experience from past similarly pressing circumstances can operate protectively at present:

> Financial problems are not something new for me. I have experienced in the past such situations, even worse. (Gianna, 55, Psychologist)

She is referring to the crisis her family faced when her husband's business went bankrupt.

Defence Mechanisms

Consequently, the choice to explore inner unconscious movements and defence mechanisms is based on the assumption that either the subject and/or the group defend themselves against anxiety and other archaic fantasies. This psychic process significantly influences people's actions, lives, relationships and their perception of the future.

What, however, are the psychological and intersubjective phenomena that emerge through this multilevel crisis? Many interdependent psychological defence mechanisms are mobilised. In summary, we will refer to:

(a) The ***idealisation in terms of*** "family" *of the structure and the NGO* as a shield protecting against the external enemy and the paralysing uncertainty, as well as the intolerable emotions caused by the traumatic memory of a childhood deprived of affection, parental support and security or against guilt due to subjective inadequacy in fulfilling their parental role

Eleni, in the above excerpt, clearly views herself as an inadequate and incompetent mother. By contrast, she is overly active and hyper-efficient with the "tenants" of the residential unit: "Vicky can do anything", the patients say calling her, as she mentions, by the name of a famous heroine of 1821. The identification with the *Ego ideal* (Chasseguet-Smirgel 1973) in this case appears as a last defence against mental pain, fear of breakdown and rage because of the unfairness and lack of care in the work, personal and family environments. An incompetent mother in her family, Eleni is transformed into a superhuman "good" mother in her symbolic family, the residential unit, while, altruism, a result of idealisation, becomes an inexhaustible source of narcissistic satisfaction for her. Eleni's *professional identity* supports her, simultaneously keeping her psychologically alive. Moreover her professional identification with an ideal family is a substitute of her deficient maternal function.

She says:

> No one ever paid any attention to me. No one ever took care of me, not when I was five, not when I was twelve – at the age she started working - not now […] I know well what it's like not to be taken care of. No one deserves that.

Another employee mentions:

> I like this job very much. I like to come in contact with people who I really feel that they need me.. […]We are a family, this is not just the workplace.. (Marina)

(b) *In the extreme primal idealisation of the institution*:

> This job is for me a life experience. I think that I have nothing more to see than what I saw already […]. (Anna, 42, General Duties in a Residential Unit)

Or even:

> I don't have enough to get by. I can't even pay for gas for the car. But I like the job, the nature of the job, I like the subject matte (Stelios)

The person wastes away if he does not protect the work subject:

> At least I have a job, I am not unemployed and I am a step above *volunteers*. (Stelios)

What we can perhaps hear in this phrase is the echo of an unconscious protective wish which the individual assigns to his professional identity. This identity appears to be experienced as that psychological "minimum" that shields the individual in his imagination from the possibility of complete psychological and social disconnection and breakdown.

What happens, however, with the same individual's rage towards this extreme symbolic social and institutional violence that threatens his psychological integrity and survival? When the interviewer asks Stelios:

> Doesn't all this enrage you?

He replied:

> No, not at all. This has nothing to do with the job. It's not the fault of the patients. [Small pause] It's like someone who is living in a village, who has argued with the neighbour, and to get revenge he ties the neighbour's goat to his car and drags it with the rope until he kills it

Through this excerpt one recognises the brutality of Stelios' psychological experience. We are also witnessing the sequence of the psychological transformations of this experience, starting with *denial* ("No, not at all") and going through a process of displacement and *transference, idealisation, projection* and *identification*. We can also wonder about the origin of all these enigmatic internal objects and the connections between them. In other words, what could the "neighbour" and the "neighbour's goat" represent in Stelios' internal world and for what reasons? In this metaphorical scene, "the neighbour's goat" suddenly suffers a great injustice and an extreme, excessive tortuous and deadly violence. The violence of someone, who instead of addressing the "neighbour" who caused his anger and revenge, turns it against this innocent, weak little mammal, who only produces "good" milk.

> There is some friction with my colleagues – says Stelios – the younger ones sometimes do not respect the older ones.

Another transference: So who is "not respecting" Stelios? His colleagues at work or possibly the institution and the state which are literally devaluing him and his work by not paying him?

(c) *In the denial and obfuscation of all negative aspects of the work experience, with a parallel idealisation of the subject matter of the work and the projection of the hopes of the individuals into a vague and fantastical future*:

> I know that what happened to us will not last long. I am an optimist and I say that I am emotionally and financially investing in this NGO[…] Since I like the subject matter, since I want to continue, be patient, I say, as long as you last, and find something else to do on the side. (Vicky)

> […] I think that I am well in the job, I like the subject matter of the job, and I am not doing it like a … I have not reached yet such a level to say that… (pause) I will look for another job. I am fighting and I believe that at some point things will get better […]. (Jason, Nurse in a Residential Unit)

(d) *In the omnipotence with which he is invested*:

> What will happen to these people… Where would they all go? This is not simply a business that closes down, these are human souls, they are a responsibility. (Kyriakos, 32, Social Worker in Residential Unit & Mobile Unit)

Or otherwise

(e) *In moving to a paranoid position and a diffuse paranoid readiness* ("they are hiding something, they are not talking clearly to us"):

> I generally think that all NGOs that were involved with mental health are responsible. This is indirect privatization. Regardless whether it appears as a non-profit. You cannot not have profit in capitalism. You are obviously making it somewhere else. (Stefania, 29, nurse in a Residential Unit)

(f) *In the function of the **scapegoat mechanism**, **inside the structure*** (difficult patients or problematic employees):

> Most are not even wanted by their relatives.. […] I told a lady that she has to find somewhere else to go […]. (Nikos, Child Psychiatrist, Scientific Coordinator in a Hostel)

(g) *In the **fragmentation** of the function of the group*

Gianna, 55 years old, a psychologist, has been working at the day centre for the past 10 years. Throughout the day, she does many creative things with the patients: she coordinates a social club, reading groups, groups which leaf through and read newspapers and social skills training groups. But what she describes is a rather personalised care scheme, unconnected to the activities of the day centre and mainly in contrast to the fundamental principles of psychiatric reform and the declared goals of the NGO.

(h) *In overinvestment in the work subject matter* which sometimes may lead to a process of merging with the patients therefore their chronification:

> If I was working in a factory I would have protested. Here... I feel responsible for the people I am taking care of. I think that it is a serious job that is worth it [...]. (Jason, Nurse in a Residential Unit)

Gianna also refers to her job with great enthusiasm:

> I love this job a great deal. I like working with people who truly need me. It is not an inanimate object. We are a family, not only a workplace, she tells us.

Among the different groups coordinated by Gianna, there is one she calls the "parent or close relative group". The patients refer to Eleni as a "parent", despite the average age of the patients of her service being 65. In her mind, patients appear to be essentially infantilised, while she adopts an overprotective attitude towards them.

The staff's overinvestment in the patients therefore appears primarily as a defensive attitude, which expresses great difficulty in parting with patients. We could also ask whether this is to the ultimate benefit of the patients or if, on the contrary, it is included in what Racamier has described with the terms "psychotic paradoxicality". In reality, patients are permanently "trapped" in a *double bind*, according to Bateson et al. (1956), whereas the apparent aim of therapy remains for them to become as autonomous and independent as possible, the underlying goal appears nevertheless to be their maintenance in a state of almost permanent merged dependency. Eleni says:

> Time is required with psychotics. You can't hurry.

In reality, perhaps it is she who needs time to psychologically process the "other" as well as her bereavement for the time (work time? age?) that is passing.

(i) *In the projection of the origin of the breakdown anxiety to an **external enemy*** (the heartless state or the ministry which we must face united with each other and with management):

> [...] the State... doesn't care... everything is done for show. I am disappointed by the State. (Jason, Nurse in a Residential Unit)

(j) Finally, in the exceptionally adverse circumstances of this economic and sociopolitical crisis, the *scientific coordinators of the units* frequently find themselves in a difficult position: they are called upon to *intermediate between management and nursing staff*:

> The greatest difficulty for me, is to manage to achieve balance in my position. That is, between management and staff. (Natalia, 30, Psychologist, Residential Unit Scientific Coordinator)

What appears to be happening in this case is schematically the following: on the one hand, in order to maintain the organisation's cohesion and on the other for the employees to maintain their psychological cohesion, their connection to each other and to not collapse, they collectively project the "bad" object onto the state and its services and the "good" object to management, with which they identify. Thus, "it is the ministry's fault that their salaries are delayed", whereas on the other hand "management is on their side, is fighting on their behalf and is protecting their rights".

However, someone inside the organisation and at the unit level must do the "dirty job", that is, implement the policies of the NGO organisation organisationally and administratively on a daily basis, as they are formulated under pressure and the general circumstances. This person can be no other than the scientific coordinator.

The scientific coordinators, who are also personally experiencing the consequences of the crisis on a personal level, appear to be psychologically tried, constantly between two identifications: identification with the staff of the unit they are responsible for (remaining "good" with the staff but "bad" towards the management) and identification with the management and its policies (therefore appearing "good" towards the management but "bad" towards the staff).

20.5 Discussion

The findings of this qualitative research indicate that the socioeconomic crisis is consistently related to specific attitudes of personnel in residential units. In this study, reference is made to the concept of *collective mechanisms of defence*, a concept which is associated with a long-standing tradition of the clinical psychosocial orientation of organisations within the psychoanalytic framework (Jaques 1955; Menzies 1961). More recently, Hollway and Jefferson (2000), starting with their own experience using and analysing interviews in social research, refer to the same concept, acknowledging the role of *collective defence mechanisms* against anxiety, the significance of unconscious intersubjectivity in investigating the psychosocial profile of research subjects, as well as the usefulness of more flexible methods of content analysis which enable access to subjective experience and meaning.

The main collective defence mechanisms (Jaques 1955; Menzies 1961; Kernberg 1998) that they seem to mobilise in dealing with their personal and professional devaluation as well as persecutory and depressive anxiety are the idealisation of the institution and overinvestment in their job. An overprotective and dependent attitude towards the patients results as a side effect of those mechanisms and paradoxically leads to the patients' chronisation rather than empowerment and autonomy. A significant issue that arises is that the main defence mechanisms used appear related to and perhaps enhance the pre-discussed neo-institutionalisation phenomena in community mental health units.

On the other hand, it would be critical to examine in depth the function, strategy and management of the board of directors of the NGO towards the personnel in the current context of uncertainty. A first glance indicates that the administration seems to find it hard to deal with the dichotomous nature of projective identification related to the personnel (good vs. bad; good in terms of representing the collective ideal, bad in terms of a punishing mother) and to create a transitional space for cooperation and dialogue. These deficit results in the mobilisation of the defence mechanisms, which in combination with a paranoid environment, contribute to the weakening of the personnel's strength and the reinforcement of neo-institutionalisation phenomena in the community.

Conclusions

The crisis impacts negatively not only on the personal and family level of residential staff. The continual fluctuation and insecurity also debilitate the core of psychiatric reform and the new culture of care which this approach promotes. Thus, psychotherapeutic support, continual training and supervision, aimed at decreasing the negative consequences of uncertainty and internal pain, are vitally critical.

In addition the dramatic lack of funding could be dealt with through a process of empowerment-participation of staff, patients, their families and other community resources through networking in order to gain their basic rights for care.

Future planning and intervention should take into account local conditions and historical, socioeconomic and political momentum in order to apply principles of community psychiatry in order to provide mental health services given the current situation of poor resources and economic strain.

Future research is called for, using both epidemiological and qualitative methodology on a national scale, in order to further investigate and identify the psychosocial variables which contribute to the weakening of personnel. This ultimately will lead to significant improvement in the quality of patient care.

References

"ARGO" – Network for Psychosocial Rehabilitation and Mental Health (2012). Call for action from Greece re-collapse of mental health services. Retrieved from: http://mentalhealthworldwide.com/2012/11/call-for-action-from-greece/

Banks JA (1957) The group discussion as an interview technique. Sociol Rev 5(1):75–84
Basaglia F, Ongaro FB, Giannichedda MG (2000) Conferenze brasiliane. Raffaello Cortina, Milano
Bateson G, Jackson DD, Haley J, Weakland J (1956) The double bind. Behav Sci 1(4):251–254
Bauer M (1996) 'The narrative interview: comments on a technique of qualitative data collection', Papers in Social Research Methods – Qualitative Series, Vol. 1. London: London School of Economics, Methodology Institute
Benedetti G, Andreoli L (1991) Paziente e terapeuta nell'esperienza psicotica. Bollati Boringhieri, Torino
Bion WR (1952) Group dynamics: a review. Int J Psychoanal 33(2):235–247
Blanchet A (1989) L'entretien: la co-construction du sens. In: La démarche clinique en sciences humaines. Dunod, Paris, pp 18–30
Chasseguet-Smirgel J (1973) La maladie d'idéalité – Essai psychanalytique sur l'idéal du moi. L'Harmattan, Paris
Devereux G (1980) De l'angoisse a la méthode. Flammarion, Paris
Enriquez E, Houle G, Rhéaume J, Sevigny R (Dir.) (1993) L'analyse clinique dans les sciences humaines. Editions Saint-Martin, Montréal
Giami A (1985) L'entretien de groupe. In: Blanchet A et al (eds) L'entretien dans les sciences sociales. Dunod, Paris, pp 221–233
Goffman E (1968) Asylums: essays on the social situation of mental patients and other inmates. Aldine Transaction, Chicago
Hinshelwood RD (2001) Thinking about institutions. Jessica Kingsley Publishers, London
Hochmann J (1982) L'institution mentale: du rôle de la théorie dans le soins psychiatriques désinstitutionnalisés. Inf Psychiatr 58:987–991
Hollway W, Jefferson T (2000) Doing qualitative research differently: free association, narrative and the interview method. Sage, London
Jaques E (1955) Social systems as a defense against persecutory and depressive anxiety. In: Klein M, Heimann P, Money-Kyrle RE et al (eds) New directions in psychoanalysis. Basic Books, New York
Kaës R (2009) Un singulier pluriel. Dunod, Paris. Enas plithintikos enikos (trans: Diovouniotou N). Kastaniotis, Athens. (Original work published in 2007)
Kernberg OF (1998) Ideology, conflict, and leadership in groups and organizations. Yale University Press, New Haven
Kvale S, Brinkmann S (2009) Interviews: learning the craft of qualitative research interviewing. Sage, London
Loukidou E, Mastroyiannakis A, Power T, Craig T, Thornicroft G, Bouras N (2012) Greek mental health reform: views and perceptions of professionals and service users. Psychiatriki 24(1):37–44
Menzies IEP (1961) The functioning of social systems as a defence against anxiety: a report on a study of the nursing service of a general hospital. Center for Applied Social Research/Tavistock Institute of Human Relations, London
Ministry of Health and Social Solidarity (2010). Evaluation report of the activities of the Psychiatric Reform implementation for the period 2000–2009 (in Greek). http://www.psychargos.gov.gr/Documents2/Ypostirixi%20Forewn/Ypostirixi%20EPISTHMONIKH/Ex%20Post%20%CE%A0%CE%91%CE%A1%CE%91%CE%94%CE%9F%CE%A4%CE%95%CE%9F%202%20Teliko.pdf. Accessed 20 July 2014
Ministry of Health and Social Solidarity (2012). Report of the Working Group on the revision of the PSYCHARGOS – National Action Plan Psychargos C (2011–2020). Ministry of Health, Athens (in Greek). http://www.psychargos.gov.gr/Documents2/%CE%9D%CE%95%CE%91/%CE%A8%CE%A5%CE%A7%CE%91%CE%A1%CE%93%CE%A9%CE%A3%20%CE%93'%20(2011–2020).pdf. Accessed 31 July 2014
Ministry of Health and Social Solidarity (2013) Evaluation report of the activities of the Psychiatric Reform implementation year 2012 (in Greek). http://www.psychargos.gov.gr/Documents2/ON-%20GOING/%CE%A0%CE%921.2.pdf. Accessed 20 July 2014

Racamier P-C (1973) Le Psychanalyste sans divan. La psychanalyse et les institutions de soins psychiatriques. Payot, Paris

Revault d'Allonnes C, Assouly-Piquet C, Slama FB, Blanchet A, Douville O (1989) La démarche clinique en sciences humaines: documents, méthodes, problèmes. Dunod, Paris

Rosenfeld H (2003) Impasse and interpretation: therapeutic and anti-therapeutic factors in the psychoanalytic treatment of psychotic, borderline, and neurotic patients. Routledge, New York

Sakellis G (2012) Welfare state in crisis. In: Stylianidis S, Ploumpidis D (eds) Proceedings of Regional Congress for psychosocial rehabilitation. Central presentation in National Congress for Psychosocial rehabilitation: new practices for emerging needs, Athens. EPAPSY, Athens, pp 30–39

Searles H (1965 [1985]) The contribution of familial treatment to the psychotherapy of schizophrenia. In: Boszormenyi-Nagy I, Framo J (eds) Intensive family therapy: theoretical and practical aspects. Harper & Row, New York (2nd edn, Brunner/Mazel, New York)

Stylianidis S, Chondros P (2011) Crise économique, crise de la réforme psychiatrique en Grèce: indice de déficit démocratique en Europe? Inf Psychiatr 87(8):625–627

Thornicroft G, Tansella M (2010) For a better mental health care: ethics and deontology, evidence and experience. (Trans: Dermentzi M) Gia mia kaliteri frontida tis psichikis igias. Topos, Athens

Trakas D (2008) Focus groups revisited. LIT Verlag, Berlin

Trognon A (1987) Produire des donnée. In: Blanchet A, Ghiglione R, Massonnat J, Trognon A (eds) Les techniques d'enquête en sciences sociales. Dunod, Paris

Staff Evaluation and Presentation of Organisational Culture In Mental Health Structures

21

Stelios Stylianidis, Meni Koutsosimou, Nikos Symeonidis, Panagiotis Chondros, and Giorgos Chadoulis

Abstract

Staff evaluation is sub-module in the assessment of mental health services. In the present chapter, we focus on the creation of a structured staff evaluation system within the framework of mental health through the presentation of a case study in Greece and its theoretical background. Theoretical definitions are included with a focus on the concept of organisational culture. It then goes on to present how this evaluation is implemented to improve the quality of mental health services, its methodology and limitations. The establishment of criteria on the basis of which the operation of the system will be reviewed is central to this process. Consequently, the adoption or creation of indicators with good psychometric properties (validity, reliability, sensitivity to change) is a necessary investment which contributes in studying the efficiency of the system. A multifaceted methodological approach (use of multiple research tools) and simultaneous implementation of the results in educational and clinical practice are proposed. The sections on management intervention and changes focus on the following individual areas: *commitment to the goals of the organisation, participation in the work, performance, job satisfaction, psychosomatic-psychological reactions.*

S. Stylianidis
Department of Psychology, Panteion University, Athens, Greece
e-mail: stylianidis.st@gmail.com

M. Koutsosimou • N. Symeonidis • P. Chondros (✉) • G. Chadoulis
Association for Regional Development and Mental Health (EPAPSY), Athens, Greece
e-mail: pan_ch@otenet.gr

21.1 Introduction

The *assessment* of health systems and, respectively, the services provided should form an integral part of their design, organisation and administration and may be carried out at four levels: inflows (human and material resources), procedures (organisation and quality of services provided), intermediate outflows (use of services and volume of the direct results generated) and effects.

This assessment begins by identifying accurately the breadth of the system and selecting indicators (e.g. effectiveness, efficiency, equality) associated with specific performance standards.

Over time, numerous definitions of quality have been put forward. However, although there is no widely accepted definition, the various definitions put forward are quite similar. Juran, for example, defines quality as "suitability for use", which requires quality of design, quality control, availability and convenience (Berger et al. 2002). Crosby states that the quality of a product or service means compliance to standards, so that the product or service coincides with the needs of the client, while Deming defines quality as a constant improvement process, based on minimising deviations from the desired efficiency of the product (Beckford 2010). According to Feigenbaum's definition, "quality is the manner in which a company is managed so that the product meets the clients' expectations", while Ishikawa emphasises that "quality depends not only on the quality of the product but also on the staff and management, and their cooperation in solving problems (Berger et al. 2002). Finally, Taguchi considers the quality of a product as the provocation of minimal losses to society, from the moment the product is released for use (Beckford 2010).

The implementation of staff evaluation is interpreted in literature as the systematic assessment of employees, with respect to their job performance and potential for development. Historically, the act of evaluation was conceptualised after World War II, as a technique implemented in the US armed forces, and developed termwise in the period between the two World Wars (1920–1930). Today, staff evaluation is a separate sub-module in the assessment of mental health services and may, for instance, be based on daily performance data, reports, structured internal or external evaluation, self-evaluation and participation in staff meetings (work groups).

In the context of adopting the act of evaluation and its implementation in the area of mental health, its implementation as a substantial part of effective personnel management contributes in identifying the needs and opportunities for employee development and growth. Essentially, traditional performance evaluation is nothing more than a careful completion of forms. The advantage of this approach is that one gets a full picture of the situation as well as the rational views of both the evaluee and the evaluator. The *graphic rating scale* or *assessment scale*, where a sum of points is assigned to various characteristics, is a direct and secure way of presenting specific individual scores for predefined areas which are being evaluated. An inherent difficulty in any evaluation process is, of course, recognised as any valid and reliable assessment necessitates the evaluees' subjectivity. To this end, it was deemed necessary to ask the evaluees to score certain quality characteristics and to also answer open-ended questions where they would have a large amount of space to provide answers.

Over the last years, interest is focused on assessing but also in improving the efficiency of health systems. This assessment is implemented by creating comparable indicators and by measuring comparable dimensions, including quality of care, access to such care and costs (Kostagialas et al. 2008). The design of indicators ensures that control can be exercised over all factors affecting every process of a mental health service. The selection of such indicators depends on the service, its objectives and the extent of this evaluation. Such indicators do not ensure quality; however, they identify areas in need of improvement and confirm the success of the measures taken (Lazarou and Oikonomopoulou 2007).

It is true that, in recent years, there is an increasing demand for radical changes in the corporate world, aiming to reshape the working environment. In this context, it is made clear that the human factor deserves due attention, since it is the main instrument which drives and determines the dynamic growth of a company. Accordingly, the need to study how job performance, work psychology and, consequently, organisational culture and the level of job satisfaction of employees are affected has increased rapidly in recent years.

"Organisational culture refers to the working environment shared by employees within an organisation, including their shared beliefs, attitudes, values and codes of conduct", i.e. the *vehicle* which, in a clinical context, enables staff to identify circumstances and events that could contribute, for example, in improving quality, from a joint, but at the same time different, perspective (Davies 2005). The organisational climate reflects the aura of an organisation and focuses on how it operates (such as, for example, behavioural norms), while organisational culture focuses on the concept of organisational operation (e.g. shared objectives) (Schein 2004). In this respect, climate is the apparent *aspect* of culture, and for this reason it can be interpreted through the underlying levels of the latter. In general, it is difficult to distinguish the one from the other, as culture shapes the climate and the climate reflects the culture. Hence, it is difficult – if not impossible – to be aware of the climate without an in-depth approach to the culture.

There are two prevailing views-theories about what triggers *organisational behaviour*. The first, the macro-culture theory, assumes that organisational culture affects the working environment, whereas the microculture theory maintains that human attributes affect organisational culture. The organisational support theory – (Eisenberger et al. 1986; Shore and Shore 1995) seems to be a pivotal variable in understanding organisational culture. According to this theory, employees develop high levels of perception concerning the extent to which the company-organisation values their contribution and cares about their well-being. It has been established that perceived organisational support (POS) is associated with positive employee attitudes, such as increased performance, job satisfaction, commitment and reduced turnover (Rhoades and Eisenberger 2002).

The basic principles of a successful organisational culture framework, as set out below, are laid down in literature: legitimacy (partnership, orientation of acceptance), direction (strategic vision), performance (response, effectiveness and efficiency), responsibility (accountability, transparency) and fairness (equality, regulatory framework).

In daily practice, however, when staff relations lose their human character, coercion takes the place of communication and lack of enthusiasm takes the place of qualitative effort (Halligan 2006). What has now become evident from international practice and literature is that the greater part of any professional's job-related obligations cannot be stereotyped in some general fashion. It can only be promoted when self-monitoring and a climate of inspiration, creativity and readjustment prevails, while the professionals themselves do not react positively to orders and constant management monitoring, when, for example, the prevailing organisational forms are of a bureaucracy style or exclusively a "top-to-bottom" communication style.

Taking into consideration the theoretical debate above, it is not surprising that most foreign organisations which have adopted an organisational culture monitoring system have acquired an organisational conscience largely acknowledged as the *heartbeat* of the services offered. And at the level of clinical professionals groups, it is defined as the organisation/company's DNA, as it is believed to be what triggers lifelong learning and motivates employees and what also contributes in the provision of information to patients and giving them their personal *energy* and *voice*, in order to allow all of them to improve – effectively and consistently – the culture in which they coexist and interact.

Therefore, using specific definitions/questions, it is possible to capture the organisational climate or, specifically, the climate which is geared towards servicing the patient in clinical establishments, through employee perceptions, which are reflected in the patients' perceptions regarding the overall quality of the services and, ultimately, in their satisfaction with the services received. Thus, by associating the patients' perceptions with those of the employees enhances the validity of the employees' perceptions regarding the organisational development of the framework in which they work.

For the most part, however, clinical culture is disparate and inconsistent and is usually described as *differentiated* because of the different cultures coexisting within the working environment, which reflect the individual opinions and attitudes of many and diverse professional groups (Davies 2005). This results in the development, within the same organisation, of different subcultures, misconceptions and conflicts between such cultures. So, according to studies, the four prevailing subcultures are those of (a) the medical staff, (b) the nursing staff, (c) the administrative/technical staff and, finally, (d) the management.

At the same time, the factors-variables associated with the emotional intelligence of employees are another theoretical tool which could help understand organisational culture in organisations. By extension, these are the dimensions which could determine whether an employee is able to communicate with his/her colleagues, experience any job-related accomplishments and failures, establish courses of action and increase his/her performance and remain committed. Comparably, the feelings of any work group can determine those of the entire organisation. That is, any person able to express his/her feelings and control the feelings of others is also able to strengthen or weaken the group's morale and performance.

21.2 Implementation of Evaluation Towards Improving the Quality of Mental Health Services

The quality and performance of the health sector in any country and Greece in particular are increasingly drawing the attention of the state apparatus, including the citizens/patients' interest. The health sector, which in global literature is defined as the sector with the greatest range of and concentration of services in any field (clustered service) (Fitzsimmons and Fitzsimmons 2006), is about satisfying the physical, psychological and social needs of the patient. Healthcare providers in Greece are looking for new solutions to old problems, such as measuring the effectiveness of an organisation and developing alternative national funding models for the healthcare system, the quality of medical services, the adoption of new technologies (e.g. information and communication technologies or ICTs) and issues relating to patient safety.

Health service providers are increasingly confronted with a broad range of social, economic, political, regulatory and cultural changes (e.g. culture) which, compared to other humanitarian factors, lead to an increase in demand from all interested parties for greater efficiency, reduced costs and the provision of superior quality services (Tsiotras 2002).

Organisational culture is fundamental for all interested parties in the political and business world. The international community, regulatory authorities as well as several organisations have expressed views and conducted research on the best implementation of a common organisational framework in all types of organisations. Internationally, such proposals highlight the fact that the implementation of such procedures may lead to an increase in competitiveness and a better corporate image while improving the reliability of the services provided.

21.3 Presentation of Case Study

Pre-existing Situation

The division of subcultures was initially identified by the management of the Association for Regional Development and Mental Health (EPAPSY). EPAPSY was established in 1988, as part of the Leros Psychiatric Hospital deinstitutionalisation programme (www.me-psyxi.gr). It is a recognised non-governmental organisation operating in the field of psychosocial rehabilitation and mental health promotion throughout Greece. During the intervention period, and within the framework of the National Plan for Mental Health "PSYCHARGOS", it was responsible for providing *scientific and administrative support to a total of 14 units, including 2 mobile units*. More specifically, its objective is to provide a comprehensive mental healthcare model to the community and to restore the abilities of individuals with special psychosocial needs, by preparing them appropriately, on a professional and personal level, to facilitate their reintegration in daily life.

The need to highlight the challenge involved aims to ensure the smooth operation and to preserve collegiality which, in turn, lead to the creation of a work group, in order to investigate the organisational culture and identify the individual work dynamics, attitudes, perceptions and behaviours of its employees, the logic of evaluation and staff development.

Employees are useful *sources* (resources) of information for the development of a *high*-efficiency framework organisation, namely, (a) the satisfaction derived by patients through their physical and psychological contact with the employees, (b) the job satisfaction derived by the staff and (c) the organisational development and evolutionary change of the framework. The patients, on the other hand, are the most important and reliable judges.

In this particular administrative intervention, it was deemed necessary to establish sound impact indicators, since as a result of this, we were led to establish criteria on the basis of which the system's operational impact would be assessed. Consequently, the adoption or creation of indicators with good psychometric properties (validity, reliability, sensitivity to change) was a necessary investment which contributed in studying the efficiency of the system. In this context, it was decided to adopt and implement a multi-agency evaluation model for continuous quality improvement, based on the PROJECT method, i.e. a holistic action approach, considering that:

(a) A new approach to modelling the individual quality criteria is introduced (Tsirintani et al. 2010), together with assessment of the medical and nursing staff quality levels, the organisation of processes and the living conditions of patients.
(b) The manner in which the services are offered to the service users, which also shapes the final product offered, affects to a considerable extent their perception and ultimate satisfaction from the services provided (Pierrakis and Tomaras 2009).

The main objective of organisational culture evaluation is to establish a methodological continuous quality improvement (CQI) framework, in the context of "clinical governance" (CG), which is one of the most topical issues in the reorganisation and adaptation of procedures/processes, as well as all changes at the organisational culture level. The change in the existing culture is an essential precondition for the successful implementation of a uniform code of communication and operation. All employees aspire to work in an *organisation with a memory* that will provide them with lifelong learning, recognise their contribution and support their efforts to improve service quality and view mistakes as opportunities for additional learning and experience (Xyrotyri-Koufidou 2001).

Accordingly, the management of EPAPSY considers the quality of service responsiveness a key factor in promoting user satisfaction as well as the satisfaction of staff working in comparable, at the level of supply and professional competency. It has been established that acceptance of the fact that the patients/relatives' satisfaction from the care provided is related to the effectiveness of the therapy (Henderson et al. 1999), and the fact that dissatisfaction is a significant *leakage* in care continuity (Ruggeri 1994), the objective set out for this action was to ensure the best possible use of the human resources within the structures of the organisation by evaluating and retraining the existing staff.

Administrative Initiative

The change in EPAPSY's culture is a further opportunity to identify ways and possibilities to migrate professionals out of the current clinical culture *complacency zone* to a culture of *challenge* where dynamic learning prevails (Moran 2003).

The initiative taken by the administration is focused on the following:

A. Job satisfaction
B. Job involvement
C. Organisational commitment – dedication

We hope that this so-called shared culture will form part of its *defence* against any difficulties encountered, mainly owing to the complexity of the operation of the health system.

The multifaceted methodological approach (use of multiple tools) proposed, together with the ability to implement the results both in educational and clinical practice, as already proposed and supported by international literature and practice, is an *innovative element of this intervention*.

Methodology

The steps followed by the project team are described below:

A. The first phase included a review of the literature on the aforementioned fields in order to lay down in detail the theoretical framework of the research, taking into consideration the multidimensional approach of the subject matter, using the input from previous research programme analyses.
B. The second phase included the selection-combination-creation of tools to be used to identify the reference framework for the therapist staff. To enable the measurement of concepts associated with specific actions, it was necessary to record all available information in literature and any external observable behaviour, while a question/variable database was created.
C. The third phase included a survey of EPAPSY's structures which involved issuing a questionnaire to mental health professionals and patient relatives and the collection of statistical information. The staff completed five questionnaires in

total (based on quantitative and qualitative criteria) relating to socio-demographic characteristics, the needs and attitudes with respect to specific matters and policies, organisational culture, job satisfaction, mental fatigue/exhaustion, degree of responsiveness in the provision of mental health services as well as a self-evaluation. The patients' relatives also completed questionnaires relating to their satisfaction from the services provided by the organisation.

The method of reverse measurement (reverse scored) was used in some of the questions in order to prevent the mechanical completion of these questionnaires.

D. The next phase included the codification and creation of a survey data file in SPSS.
E. This was followed by the analysis of the data collected and comparative presentation of results which included individual corrections and selected modifications of the research process, based on remarks and comments on the results of the previous phase.
F. And the final phase, which included an review of the results/findings.

Results

The survey was carried out during the period March–May 2011, on all EPAPSY structures (14 residential units, 2 mobile units, 1 day centre, central administration) with 210 participants ($N=210$, 79 % women). The average age of employees participating in the survey was 35.9, of which 38 % were married and most of them (96 %) were Greek nationals. In terms of education, 36 % were primary/secondary education graduates (6–12 years of schooling), 14 % held a postgraduate academic title and 1.5 % a PhD. Half (51 %) had no prior working experience in the field of mental health prior to joining the EPAPSY. In terms of work experience, 36 % had less than 1 year, 28 % 1–4 years and 2 % over 10 years.

Subsequently, a review of any differences between the various specialisations and the views of employees as to the nature of their duties was carried out. To facilitate the analysis process and to enhance its statistical validity, the psychiatrists and psychologists were grouped in one category, SE and HE nurses in a second category and professionals in a third category which included physiotherapists, social workers and occupational therapists; a fourth category included all administrative and technical staff and, finally, a fifth category included all general clerical staff.

Escorting residents/users on outings in the community is recognised as a duty by all nurses and most of the general clerical staff as well as other mental health professionals. Most psychiatrists/psychologists and administrative/technical staff did not consider this one of their duties. Carrying out a diagnostic assessment is recognised as a duty by most psychiatrists/psychologists and approximately one out of three nurses. Employees in other work areas do not consider diagnostic assessments part of their job. The chi-square statistical verification highlighted these differences between specialties as statistically significant: $\chi^2 (4) = 72.48$, $p = 0.000$ (<0.01). Staff training did not seem to be recognised as a duty by the vast majority of the sample (82 %). The sole exception is perhaps the psychiatrists/psychologists category, where one out of two considers staff training part of their duties. The chi-square statistical verification highlighted the presence of a statistically significant interaction between this duty and their work area: χ^2 (4) =32.88, $p=0.000$ (<0.01). Training residents in independent living is recognised as one of their duties by the major part of the sample in general and the nurses and other professional and general clerical staff in particular. On the other hand, only 47 % of psychiatrists/psychologists and 2 % of administrative and technical staff consider the training of residents in independent living one of their duties. The differences identified between specialties/work areas verge on being statistically significant: χ^2 (4) =55.78, $p=0.000$ (<0.01).

As to the part that the various parameters played in the participants' decision to work for EPAPSY, the results are summarised in the table below. The highest averages reflect the highest contribution in the decision to work for EPAPSY.

Descriptive results regarding the significance of each parameter in the decision to work for EPAPSY

Reasons	Sample number	Average	Median	Standard deviation
Descent from the prefecture or the area where the structure is located	164	3.43	4	1.58
Residence in the area where the structure is located	166	3.13	3	1.56
Existence of substantial structures and specialised staff	161	2.32	2	0.98
Daily learning and development potential	164	2.07	2	0.95
Existence of an employee in the unit with a positive influence	168	3.23	3	1.48
Relaxed working conditions	160	4.13	5	1.13
Provision of services to socially vulnerable groups	165	1.83	2	0.87
Provision of services to remote areas	152	3.17	3	1.44
For income-earning purposes	163	1.87	2	0.94

The sample's most significant incentives were as follows (listed from the most significant to the less significant):

Working environment (extremely/very significant incentive for 83.6 % of the sample)
Financial rewards
Intellectual and personal development
Work experience
Recognition by the work environment
Well-organised network
Vacation
Professional development

The five areas in which the sample rated performance as high:

I give meaning to the results produced by the therapy (6, 12/7).
I establish trust relationships with the patients.
I have a good relationship with my colleagues.
I communicate smoothly with the patients.
I evaluate myself.
I provide information to patients and caregivers.
I assess the clinical needs of patients.

The five areas in which the sample rated performance as low:

1. I prepare reports on research projects (3.04/7).
2. I have access to research resources (e.g. funds, information and equipment).
3. I research the literature which is relevant to my work.
4. I undertake administrative activities.
5. I take initiatives in community work.

The factorial analysis of the organisational culture questionnaire per factor identified the following factors as significant (an explanation of their significance is provided):

Factor	Comments
Company profile	A high score is interpreted as a positive attitude towards the profile of the company
Team spirit-collegiality	A high score is interpreted as retention of confidence that collegiality/team spirit within the company/structure is at a high level
Interpersonal relations with colleagues	A high score is interpreted as reflecting the respondent's positive interpersonal relations with his/her colleagues
Interpersonal relations with colleagues	A high score is interpreted as reflecting the respondent's positive interpersonal relations with his/her superiors
Job satisfaction	A high score is interpreted as higher job satisfaction
Education-training	A high score is interpreted as retention of confidence that the respondent feels he/she has received the appropriate education and training to perform efficiently and effectively his/her duties (including the underlying weight accorded to the importance of education and training)
Recognition	A high score is interpreted as retention of confidence that EPAPSY acknowledges the efforts, initiatives and importance of the work of the staff
Evaluation mechanism	A high score is interpreted as retention of confidence that the evaluation mechanism is appropriate and relevant

21 Staff Evaluation and Presentation of Organisational Culture

Rating of structures according to their responses:

Factor	Lowest possible score (total disagreement)	Highest possible score (total agreement)	Neutral point (neither agreement nor disagreement)	Higher ranking place (median)	Lowest ranking place (median)
Company profile	14	70	42	Livadia 58	Odysseus 43
Team spirit-collegiality	7	35	21	Odysseus 34	Penteli 17
Interpersonal relations with colleagues	7	35	21	Odysseus 32.5	Lamia 13
Interpersonal relations with colleagues	8	40	24	Livadia 38	Penteli 32
Job satisfaction	4	20	12	Day Centre 20	HQ 11
Education-Training	4	20	12	Livadia 18	Ariadne 10
Recognition	3	15	9	Livadia 12	Ariadne 9
Evaluation mechanism	3	15	9	Livadia 12	HQ 9

21.4 Organisational Culture Questionnaire: Overall Score

Based on the 50 entries corresponding to 8 factors
Lowest possible score: 50 (total disagreement)
Highest possible score: 250 (total agreement)
Neutral point: 150 (neither agreement nor disagreement)

EPAPSY structure[a]	Number of respondents[b]	Median	Minimum	Maximum[c]
Livadia	15	219	181	246
Melissia DC	11	210	182	230
Eretria	15	203	170	242
Manikas – Chalkida	22	200.5	160	244
Odysseus	10	200	175	223
N.E. Cyclades	10	198.5	158	227
Lykovrissi	19	197	169	232
Thetis	15	196	139	239
Trikala	15	195	177	244
West Cyclades	10	195	167	199
Residential Unit in Chalkida	8	191.5	172	227
Penteli	17	191	161	220

EPAPSY structure[a]	Number of respondents[b]	Median	Minimum	Maximum[c]
Lamia	15	187	146	219
Ariadne	13	185	107	225
HQ	10	170	150	221

[a]The structures are set out by ranking order according to each factor score.
[b]The number of respondents does not correspond to the number of staff in the structure, but to the number of respondents in each structure whose responses were taken into account.
[c]A high score is interpreted as a positive attitude towards the organisation in general.

The qualitative analysis of the data collected was carried out based on dimensions/factors of the supportive environment found in literature, as set out below:

Emotional commitment to the company (affective organisational commitment) (Rhoades et al. 2001)
Employee expectations in terms of reward for their work (effort-reward expectancies) (Eisenberger et al. 1990)
Duration of commitment (continuance commitment) (Shore and Tetrick 1991)
Employer-employee conciliation (leader-member exchange) (Wayne et al. 1997)
Supervisor support (Kottke and Sharafinski 2008)
Equal and fair treatment (procedural justice) (Andrews and Kacmar 2001)
Job satisfaction (Aquino and Griffeth 1999)
Burnout syndrome

The review of the results focused on appraising the following points:

1. Fair treatment: refers to the quality of interpersonal treatment in the allocation of resources, as well as the provision of information to employees on the manner in which the organisation's operating procedure is monitored.
2. Supervisor support partly inefficient: wherein the selective inability of the structures to supervise their clinical work is identified, as opposed to the mobile units which indicate satisfaction.
3. Rewards-working conditions at a satisfactory level: wherein serious complaints are expressed by the entire staff, owing to delays in the flow of funding.
4. Education partly inadequate: the structures located outside the prefecture of Attica are experiencing confusion and give the impression that the organisation should take additional actions in terms of education and training, by investing in its human capital.
5. Personal characteristics: the entire staff places particular emphasis and attaches importance on behaviour between employees, team dynamics and relationships which are reflected by the patients. Relations between employees are described as satisfactory.
6. Demographic characteristics: a file was compiled with the employees' social profile, interests and needs.

Particular attention was also given to the employees' emotional capacity, since provision was made for partially completed questionnaires, in order to maintain anonymity and to ensure that the results of the survey would contribute in their self-improvement and, consequently, in improving the internal dynamics of employees.

The results identified during the analysis of qualitative data can be divided up into sets of interventions and management changes related to the following areas:

A. *Commitment to the objectives of the organisation.* On the basis of the rule of mutual cooperation, the employee is obliged to ensure the welfare of the organisation (Eisenberg and Rhoades 2006), thereby enhancing his/her own emotional commitment. At the same time, they intensify their efforts to address their social and emotional needs (Armeli et al. 1998), thereby creating a strong sense of belonging to the organisation.
B. *Participation in work.* Emphasise each employee's recognition, interest and involvement in a specific activity; the recorded lack of incentive signals; the need to motivate employees, by raising their perception of the commitment to the objectives of the organisation; and, in general, the field of mental health.
C. *Performance.* The spontaneous offer of assistance between employees, the promotion of initiatives aimed to protect the organisation against risks, as well as the development of skills which are beneficial to the organisation can improve staff performance levels.
D. *Job satisfaction.* The enhancement of positive thinking, definition of the concept of individual incentives, consideration of the needs of employees, improvement of the subjective and objective value of employees and enhancement of job retention.
E. *Psychosomatic-psychological reactions.* Practical support to the organisation for the work carried out by its employees, so as to enable them to cope with the high demands of their work. Emphasis on how to handle stress and exhaustion caused in similar fields of work.
F. Multivariable as well as exploratory factorial analysis techniques were used to analyse quantitative data.

Conclusions

According to Mair (2002), the subjective interpretation by employees of the support environment, their personal characteristics/skills and their self-efficacy beliefs account for the differences identified at the organisational culture level. For example, employees who are treated fairly by the organisation are more likely to become emotionally committed to it (Mowday et al. 1982; Meyer and Allen 1997), perform their duties, meet their obligations and respond to problems or any emerging opportunities.

In specific terms, the points of concern are outline below:

(a) Information overload: this is caused by the wealth of existing sources and the inability to assess and organise the amount of incoming information available to the organisation.
(b) Inadequate dissemination and processing of knowledge: according to initial observations, knowledge is not disseminated equally to all structures of the organisation, mainly owning to their location (topography).
(c) Obstacle-confounding phenomena in horizontal and vertical communication resulting in the distortion of the initial meaning of the mission and, more generally, the activities of the organisation.
(d) Evidence of widespread frustration relating to the inability of access of financial resources, the flow of funding and the proximity between staff and management.

Mair (2002) underlines also that staff behaviour can be analysed by incorporating the two dominant theories (macro- and microculture theory) and introducing at the same time views of the social-cognitive theory (Bandura 1997). According to this theory, behaviour and factors originating from the environment, personal and cognitive factors are interrelated. Against this background and the social and job insecurity conditions prevailing during the period in question, it is possible to interpret the fact that, despite the opportunities provided by the organisation, the employees are expressing their failure to understand this effort and, at the same time, are unable to put forward any arguments concerning their wants and needs.

Intervention Limitations

Despite the attempt to define the relationships between concepts measured for the first time using such methods, this specific intervention presents certain limitations, which do not seem to affect the validity and reliability of the results. It is initially proposed to introduce additional emotional dimensions reported in literature. Another limitation is the lack of information on alternative mechanisms through which awareness of the supportive environment affects corporate behaviour such as, for example, the feeling of obligation possibly experienced by employees which, as emphasised by Eisenberger and Rhoades (2006), mitigates this relationship.

Conclusion

The assessment of the results constitutes part of the comprehensive overview of qualitative and quantitative data in any ongoing process. At a later stage, it is proposed to conduct one-on-one interviews with the staff, as well as focus groups, in order to examine in depth the gap between the organisation's stated objectives and strategies and daily practice, particularly in residential psychosocial rehabilitation.

It is important to mention that the human factor is a company's or organisation's greatest and most lucrative asset, and it is certain that in the future, the needs to support this factor will continue to grow rapidly. In addition, live organisation should be able to process the continuous inconsistencies arising from its operation and not to rationalise them through routine or standard procedures, something which is particularly evident in the field of psychiatric reform. Furthermore, building on the research material provides a safe method of understanding the chronicity of staff work patterns and new chronicity patterns of patients, a finding documented in literature (Stylianidis et al. 2007). Finally, the *key concept* reflecting this interest in the human factor, particularly within the framework of deinstitutionalisation and psychiatric reform, is J. Hochman's *mental institution*. In order to try to understand what happens during a psychotic situation, this institution does not refer to the *hospital* but to the *ideal space* (Hochmann 2003). The multidisciplinary team protecting the system from the *spread of chaos* undertakes to create this *transitional* space, motivated by the need to help the service users (Stylianidis 2003). Our primary objective is to act accordingly in a system that generates contradictions and ambivalent feelings with apparent deficiencies and gaps in the way in which it operates (Stylianidis and Chondros 2010). The *psychomental institution* protects the operation of the therapeutic team, the user as well as their family member against the *as if* operation of the public mental health system (Stylianidis et al. 2009).

Bibliography

Andrews MC, Kacmar KM (2001) Discriminating among organizational politics, justice, and support. J Organ Behav 22:347–366
Aquino K, Griffeth R (1999) An exploration of the antecedents and consequences of perceived organizational support. J Organ Behav 22:347–366
Armeli S, Eisenberg R, Fasolo P, Lynch P (1998) POS and police performance: the moderating influence of socioemotional needs. J Appl Psychol 83:288–297
Bandura A (1997) Self-efficacy: the exercise of control. Freeman, New York
Beckford JLW (2010) Quality: a critical introduction. Routledge, New York
Berger RW, Benbow DW, Elshennawy AK, Walker FH (2002) The certified quality engineer handbook. ASK, Wisconsin
Davies H (2005) Measuring and reporting the quality of health care: issues and evidence from the international research literature. NHS Quality Improvement Scotland, Edinburgh
Eisenberger R, Rhoades L (2006) When supervisors feel supported: relationship with subordinates. Perceived supervisor support, POS and performance. J Appl Psychol 91(3):689–695
Eisenberger R, Huntington R, Hutchison S, Sowa D (1986) Perceived organizational support. J Appl Psychol 71:500–507
Eisenberger R, Fasolo PM, Davis-LaMastro V (1990) Effects of perceived organizational support on employee diligence, innovation, and commitment. J Appl Psychol 53:51–59
Fitzsimmons JA, Fitzsimmons MJ (2006) Service management: operations, strategy, and information technology. McGraw-Hill/Irwin, New York
Halligan A (2006) Clinical governance: assuring the sacred duty of trust to patients. Clin Gov Int J 11(1):5–7

Hochmann J (2003) The psychomental institution: the psychomental institution. The role of mental care theory within the framework of de-institutionalisation. In: Sakellaropoulos P (ed) De-institutionalization and its relation to primary health care. Papazisis Publications, Athens

Kostagiolas P, Kaitelidou D, Chatzopoulou M (2008) Improving the quality of health services. Papasotiriou Publications, Athens

Kottke JL, Sharafinski CE (2008) Measuring supervisory and organizational support. Educ Psychol Meas 48:1075–1079

Lazarou P, Oikonomopoulou C (2007) Mental health quality assessment indicators. International facts and Greek reality. Nossileftiki 46(2):199–214

Mair J (2002) Entrepreneurial behavior in a large traditional firm: exploring key drivers. IESE Department of Strategy INsEAd: Fontainebleau, Barcelona

Meyer LD, Allen NJ (1997) Commitment in the workplace: theory, research and application. Sage, Thousand Oaks

Moran R (2003) There's no time to learn… like the present. Clin Gov Int J 8(1):46–56

Mowday T, Porter W, Steers M (1982) Organizational linkages: the psychology of commitment, absenteeism and turnover. Academic, San Diego

Pierrakis G, Tomaras P (2009) The role of patient satisfaction in the development of health care services marketing. Nossileftiki 48(1):105–114

Rhoades L, Eisenberger R (2002) Perceived organizational support: a review of the literature. J Appl Psychol 87(4):698–714

Rhoades L, Eisenberger R, Armeli S (2001) Affective commitment to the organization: the contribution of perceived organization support. J Appl Psychol 86(5):825–836

Ruggeri M (1994) Patients' and relatives' satisfaction with psychiatric services: the state of the art of its measurement. Soc Psychiatry Psychiatr Epidemiol 28:212–227

Schein EH (2004) Organizational culture and leadership, 3rd edn. Jossey Bass, San Francisco

Shore LM, Shore TH (1995) Perceived organizational support and organizational justice. In: Cropanzano RS, Kacmar KM (eds) Organizational politics, justice, and support: managing the social climate of the workplace. Quorum, Westport, pp 149–164

Shore LM, Tetrick LE (1991) A construct validity study of the survey of the perceived organizational support. J Appl Psychol 76:637–643

Stylianidis S (2003) Structures, institutions and psychomental approach. In: Vartzopoulos I et al (eds) Schizophrenia: phenomenological and psychoanalytical approach. Kastaniotis Publications, Athens, pp 309–330

Stylianidis S, Chondros P (2010) Mental health care in Greece today: current data and critical parameters of political health and social policy. Synchrona Themata 111:106–107

Stylianidis S, Theocharakis N, Chondros P (2007) The suspended step of psychiatric reform in Greece: a longitudinal approach featuring topical questions. Archeologia kai Technes 105:45–54

Stylianidis S, Gionakis N, Chondros P (2009) Hellenic psychiatric reform in the light of the Italian reform experience. Synapsis 15:28–44

Tsiotras N (2002) Quality improvement. Benou Publications, Athens

Tsirintani M, Giovanis A, Binioris S, Goula A (2010) A New Modelling Approach for Investigation of the Relationship between Quality of Health Care Services and Patient Satisfaction. Nosileftiki, 49(1)

Wayne SJ, Shore LM, Licen RC (1997) Perceived organizational support and leader-member exchange: a social exchange perspective. Acad Manage J 40:82–111

Xyrotyri-Koufidou S (2001) Human resources management: the challenge of the 21st century in the working environment, 3rd edn. Anikoula, Thessaloniki

Henderson C, Phelan M et al (1999) Comparison of patient's satisfaction with community-based vs. hospital psychiatric services. Acta Psychiatr Scand 99:188–195

Part IV

Empowering and Rights in Mental Health

User and Family Participation in Mental Health Services

22

Panagiotis Chondros, Stelios Stylianidis, and Michael Lavdas

Abstract

This chapter describes the different areas of user involvement (relevant interventions, type and quality of provided services, professionals and user training, research direction and criticism, supporting legal framework empowerment and implementation), the data on the extent of this involvement on European and national level and the institutional, clinical and ideological framework that determines user involvement in the issues that concern this group. The necessity of extending the debate between the involved parties (users, professionals, relatives, decision-makers at health policy level, etc.) and the terms and conditions that will make this debate equal, essential and productive are the points this chapter is focused on.

22.1 Introduction

The more we examine the different ways users are involved in mental health services and their aftermath in the process of empowerment of their voice in the improvement of issues of quality, information available and capability of choice, protection,

---

P. Chondros (✉) • M. Lavdas
Association for Regional Development and Mental Health EPAPSY, Athens, Greece
e-mail: pan_ch@otenet.gr; ml@epapsy.gr

S. Stylianidis
Department of Psychology, Panteion University, Athens, Greece
e-mail: stylianidis.st@gmail.com

rights and obligations advocacy, the more we come face to face with the resistance both among professionals and the patients to re-negotiate their roles and their relationship. So, as we look into the often difficult relationship between patients and mental health professionals and the one between patients and relatives' associations, we see two main trends in the patients' movement: one by the abolitionists, seeking to abolish psychiatry, and another seeking to reform it, the reformists (Van Hoorn 1992, p. 30). In this chapter we will describe certain matters of mostly technical nature, relevant to user participation in mental health services, such as the institutional framework dictating user involvement in the issues that concern them or the various areas of user involvement (kind and quality of provided services, professionals' and users' training, research direction and criticism, legal framework empowerment and implementation). We will, however, also refer to the framework needed for a consequent step and the establishment of a movement on which all this will be supported and solidly built. A number of the questions that arise, and we will attempt to respond to here, are the following: What is the growth process of such a movement? What will be its social role and position? What are the problems and resistances in their development? Who can guarantee their autonomy?

22.2 Conceptual and Clinical Clarifications: A Sensitive Semiology

The term (user, recipient, survivor, consumer, etc.) in each case of involvement continues to be the main problem; however this does not affect the characteristics of the social role and identity that the term carries and the interaction with society and the status quo, the professionals and the services' system. Of course, the prevailing term indicates a range of characteristics pertaining to the status quo, the social norms and the prospects. It follows that the selected terminology is not free of ethical, social and cultural origins. The user's position and role may differ to a great extent among various social groups or individuals. This is due to the representation and the degree that the specific social identity, selected or not, may causes conflict, constitute the cause for social support or, conversely, exclusion. The different roles and identities include a patient, an individual who feels inferior, a disabled person, one who is different or has special skills, a marginalised person, a dangerous person, a creative one and so on. We must note that in Greece, user and families associations have chosen the term "Receiver" (λήπτης) as opposed to user because this term, as they believe, refers in the Greek culture directly to the concept of "drug user".

The term advocacy, as well, carries enough complexity, as does any term transferred from different cultural, institutional, historical and scientific conditions. Advocacy is a way of helping an individual who believes he is victim of a prejudice or feels that his or her institutional interlocutors do not listen or respect him sufficiently and who encounters big obstacles in the exercise of his rights as a citizen to express herself or himself through the intervention of a third party.

Advocacy is a social mediation practice introducing a third party, who strengthens the request of the patient/user of the services without someone speaking in his place. Furthermore, it permits the different views to be arranged in a framework of debate that is conducted in mutual respect. As a social mediation function, the advocator covers many of the aspects of advocacy beyond the field of mental health. Supporting the Other's word, through an active process of transition from a position of disdain to a position of dignity, the individual's empowerment through his active participation comprises a conceptual framework at the opposite side of a philanthropic and welfare ideology (Stylianidis et al. 2011b).

We know that in the cases where asylum-based, closed care has primary responsibility over the individual's relations with society, the individual remains silent, is disdained, withdraws and becomes a passive recipient of services and not a citizen who is seeking his social emancipation. The term "social" includes a mosaic of levels of a reality, such as the judiciary-legal, the intersubjective, the medical, the political and the psychological. Each of these levels requires a specific response that depends on the other responses, aiming at the individual's holistic support. Accepting diversity is to open the patient's social and mental potential so he may experience what he is, without being limited within a special ghetto, in terms of his difference. This is a moral, political and social problem, not a technical one. The introduction of a third party is the necessary condition in the establishment of a place of dialogue, conversation and mutual listening: "everything is language", wrote Françoise Dolto, in 1980. One thing that is said but not heard, e.g. in the context of a therapeutic relationship of mental health team-patient, is as though it has not been said and has not been recognised as an expression of the Other.

A final term we often encounter and feel we ought to comment on is empowerment. During this process, it is the patient who rediscovers a part of his life and tries to determine "himself for himself" because the experience of mental illness is deeply debilitating and a source of self-stigmatisation for the mentally ill patient. The empowerment process describes the opposite: the recovery of the patient's negotiating power, not only with his own support but also that of the mental health professionals, volunteers, a relationship system and grid motivated by advocacy. The models to achieve something like it are different: they are related, besides the political, institutional actors, with the different cultural frameworks and the philosophy of the mental health services, but mostly with the social power of the users' movement. The medical and social axis, between which oscillates the practice of psychiatry, also shows the context in which contrasts are being managed (Stylianidis et al. 2014).

22.3 The Nature of User Involvement

The forms of participation of users and their families are manifold:

Training of other users or family members or professionals
Informing other users, family members, the general public and the mass media
Support – provision of services
Complaint
Claim
Advocacy

Programme, action and service evaluation
Research
Programme, action and services planning

In most cases, users are involved in the *provision of services* usually as persons of reference or case managers. These services differ in comparison with services that are not provided by individuals who are now or were in the past, users of the services, as to the time dedicated to supervision, individual sessions with patients or the work in the community (Simpson and House 2002). Users working in the services dedicate more time to them and less to administrative work. There are, however, cases of users working in services not as therapists, but at administrative or consultant level related to the actions being implemented. This way, they can work in the secretariat or at reception, as well as in higher positions, in steering groups or even boards of directors.

The next level where we encounter user involvement is that of *research* – given the fact that in research conducted in recent decades, 95 % of the cases pertain to objectives and methodologies that are not close to patient's preferences and priorities. The literature is therefore flooded, with the relevant resources being tied up there, by research on the effectiveness of psychotropic drugs and on the genetic factors of mental disease, while users would prefer to know more about the effectiveness of psychotherapy or methods of self-help (Hatcher et al. 2005). Unless the research agenda changes, user involvement in research increases the possibility of ensuring ethics and the participation of patients in this area. Users work in research planning, in data collection as interviewers and in results analysis.

Finally, a significant area of involvement is *training*. There is significant experience of good practice in user involvement as trainers, a characteristic example being the experience of the EMILIA project. Users can train either other users, so that they may in turn assume active roles or professionals. Having users training professionals, particularly young ones, is an emerging request in our country. Our view is that training is a privileged place for creating an important meeting place on an equal basis between professionals and users, as the relationship between the trainer and trainee may be reversed, depending on the objective and the training methodology. In training objectives, however, such as the concept of the healing and recovery process, organising and empowering the self-representation groups, there is room to extend the knowledge and experience of all, irrespective of whether they have been services users, provided there is structured and clear training philosophy and methodology (Lampaki et al. 2008).

22.4 Data Regarding Participation and Involvement

We must obtain a bigger database of studies about the effect of involvement on users and the provided services. There are still no sufficient and strong research data regarding the difference there can be at the level of symptomatology, functionality and quality of life for the user who is involved in mental health services. Other sources report an improvement in the clinical conditions and outcome on the basis of measurements related to quality of life (Thornicroft and Tansella 2005). Elsewhere (Simpson and House 2002), it is mentioned that individuals who receive services from users show the same or lower level of satisfaction from the provided services, also depending on the time period the use of the services lasts. There is also less satisfaction when patients participate in research where users are involved. According to the systematic review of relevant research, there is positive attitude with regard to training procedures, where users of the services have an active role.

In the UK, the Ministry of Health has determined an institutional framework directing all services to promote user involvement (Appleby 2000). Conversely, in the USA, the discussion differs slightly, as the relationship between users and the system is one of controversy. Here, the users' position and role came to the forefront, not for actual therapeutic reasons, but as an investigation of their position versus the services system and the insurance system in particular. This is how the terms *consumer* or *client* prevailed, as the user is the individual who receives or is entitled to the services, whether he pays or not – subsequently *survivor* for the individuals who experienced the adverse consequences of a system with tragic inequalities in dealing with patients (Andreasen 1995). As to Greece, there is a need to structure literature on the subject.

22.5 Data at European Level

The first reference to a collective movement on behalf of individuals with mental health problems was in 1845, with the Alleged Lunatics' Friend Society. The biggest growth with regard to the antipsychiatry movement occurred in the 1960s and 1970s. The oldest reference to associations in the form we currently recognise them by dates to the 1960s, in Norway and Sweden. As a result, the users' association in Sweden, Riksförbundet för Social och Mental Hälsa – Swedish National Association for Social and Mental Health (RSMH) currently numbers 8000 members. The main characteristic of the early movements was the fact that they did not stand the test of time.

The establishment and development of associations promoting participation are related to the transfer of care from asylum structures to community structures. We have to point out that historical evolution in Central and Eastern Europe was very different due to its dependence from politics.

As to the number of user associations, seven European countries (including Cyprus and Turkey) do not have any associations. Ten countries have 1 association each, 15 (with Greece among them) have 2–5, while 7 countries have 6–10 associations. Austria, Germany, Italy and Switzerland have 11–20 associations and Holland and Spain have 21–30. France and the UK have the highest number; they each have more than 30 associations. With regard to the number of family associations, the European Federation of Families of People with Mental Illness (EUFAMI) reports that its members are 37 family associations and 8 other associations from 24 countries (ENUSP).

The European Office of the World Health Organisation (WHO, 2008, 2011) provides data regarding the extent of user and family involvement and representation (on the basis of whether there is representation or guidelines):

- In committees relevant to the services (in planning, implementation, review)
- In committees relevant to actions (in stigma, prevention, promotion of mental health)

In the countries where they exist, family associations participate in the formulation and implementation of legislation in 34 % of cases on a regular basis, in 50 % on a non-regular basis and in 16 % never or rarely. For the establishment or operation of associations, there is systematic government financial support in 15 of the 42 countries. Of the EU15 countries, government support is not provided in Finland, Italy, Greece and Sweden.

Users participate in committees related to the planning of services in 20 of the 42 countries (47.6 %), as do families. In committees for the implementation of plans related to the services, we have user participation in 15 countries and family participation in 18 of the 42 (35.7 %). For review, participation in committees exists in 17 countries for users and 17 for families, out of the 42 (40.4 %).

In committees related to actions (stigma, prevention, promotion) there are 12 countries, Greece included, where there is no participation at all. Namely, users and families are not represented at any action implementation level for mental health (planning, application, review).

This WHO research for Europe does not, of course, show us the quality of involvement. However, representation may mean anything from a simple presence to participation in the decision-making. The actions and services to which we refer differ to a great extent between and within countries.

From the comparative study of the data, we arrive at a series of conclusions. The extent of representation and support is consistent with the available resources as well as each country's model of services. If there is involvement in an area, there is increased possibility of it in more areas. Users and families are represented and supported without big differences. The WHO concludes that what is missing are regulations, specific procedures, study of the involvement and relationship characteristics between associations and other involved bodies.

22.6 Data on User and Family Involvement in Greece

The law on mental health (2716/99) stipulates the participation of representatives in the Protection Committee of rights of individuals with mental disorders of the Ministry of Health. There are also family and user association representatives on the external evaluation committee established in 2013.

In March 2011, the psychiatric reform intervention implementation evaluation report for 2000–2009 says that the users' and families' views are negative with regard to the current situation. On the one hand, there has been general improvement, in the relationship between the staff and the users (which was described as "our voice is now heard") and the attitudes of society in general; on the other hand, users refer to the extensive dependence they continue to have on their families (that are often exhausted), their inability to comprehend the system and their ignorance with regard to where they should apply to receive information and help. They also noted the inhuman conditions in various hospitals (patients tied to the beds), expressed their suspicions with regard to whether the money is spent correctly, referred to the difficulties many patients experience upon entering the system (especially insofar as the housing structures) and noted the lack of respect they face (particular mention was made of the Limited Liability Social Cooperative [LLSC – KoiSPE], where patients are used as "servants").

In 2011, representatives of the Associations were included in the PSYCHARGOS Review Team. Two focus groups were conducted in the context of this team's work with the Ombudsman in April of 2012. Nineteen individuals participated in those, from seven user-family associations and from seven other bodies (e.g. Ministry of Health, committee of rights, Ombudsman, professional associations) (Stylianidis et al. 2011b).

Summarising the points recorded during these special meetings of the work group, the following were recognised as core priorities according to the participating user and family representatives (Stylianidis et al. 2011a, pp. 33–34):

- Continuing efforts to implement community psychiatry modern principles and establish psychiatric reform
- Enhancing active user and family association participation and involvement in policy planning and decision-making in mental health
- Educating psychiatric and legal community on new evaluation tools on human rights and medical ethics violations in the field of psychiatry
- Pointing out malpractice and basic human rights violations, as well as exhausting legal means to lodge complaints and seek punishment for them.
- Using evaluation tools for the level of rights and care protection, such as those advocated by the World Health Organisation
- Establishing Ombudsmen in every Healthcare District, in the context of sectorisation
- Integrating mental health service users and their families in the functioning of modern empowerment services

The result of the previous actions is the 10-year growth programme of the PSYCHARGOS C' (2011–2020) mental health units and actions, which reports in Axis 4 as a priority the "Protection of mentally ill patient rights and advocacy for their mental health, and the promotion of self-representation of mental health service users and their families".

User associations and the Federation of Families' Associations for mental health are included in the National Federation of Persons with Disabilities (ESAMEA). The latter implemented a project in 2011–2014 entitled "Empowerment of Collective Expression and Advocacy for Persons with Mental Disability". This project included organising local meetings in over 20 areas in Greece, for the purpose of informing users on the ways of organising and defending their rights and training trainers on objectives such as empowerment, advocacy, support in organising associations and, finally, user training in the corresponding subjects. The actions by ESAMEA promote the users' systematic information, in line with the Convention on the Rights of Persons with Disabilities.

22.7 The Relationship with the Mental Health Professionals: The Psychiatrist in the Forefront

In a pair such as the patient and the doctor, which is the focus of our discussion, each one is determined through their relationship with the other. There are two trends in this pair. On the one hand, the one fighting for a consensual and complementary relationship; here the doctor ideally fights to restore the patient's health and to protect him, despite the asymmetry in the relationship. According to the social norms, patients are faced with a socially deviant existence; they have to want to recover and the doctors are the ones to help. On the other hand, there is a trend describing the relationship as one of conflict. The perception is that the patient-doctor relationship, generally and particularly in the area of mental health, appears to be one of conflict and full of challenges and prevails both in the research literature and in daily institutional/clinical experience. The constant motif of both the consensual and conflicting approach is that the doctor-patient relationship is asymmetrical. The professionals obtain their power from their established authority. This in turn permits them to operate as mediators in social control (Nettleton 2002, pp. 190–1). However, the extent to which a doctor must exercise his authority remains particularly questionable. Patients have to face a double bond. On the one hand, they encounter more and more proclamations calling them to claim their rights in information and decision-making, to seek information from multiple sources and to have a say in the quality of the provided services, and on the other hand, they are required to submit to the doctor's judgement and expertise.

Let us ponder the area of psychiatry in particular. The development of psychiatry, closely following what is happening with people in society, is constantly transforming clinical-theoretical models, means of organising services and a relationship with users and their families. At the one end of the anthropographic spectrum, which is psychiatric discourse, lies biological determinism and the medicalised view of mental illness, while at the other end lie the ideas of safeguarding human rights, socially emancipating sufferers, restoring dignity and fully integrating the "patients" of medical thinking and praxis back into society.

What is the role of psychiatrists in all this? There is intense debate on how much the developments in psychiatry and its transformations as a cognitive field and as a scientific and socio-political institution have helped empower the voice of the users. Psychiatry, full of stories of oppression and abuse of authority (Johnstone 1989), appears to be evolving. We may not be too far from the times when an insane person was perceived as a form of evil, which was still true up to the start of the twentieth century, even in Europe and Greece (Stylianoudi and Chondros 2008; Stylianidis et al. 2007). There is, on the other hand, some evidence of progress: new drugs, new practices, evolved diagnostic, evaluation and monitoring methods for services and growing documentation and publications. "A key word in developments in the area of social revolution in the 20th century is post-. It was used as a prefix of numerous terms by certain generations trying to define the intellectual territory of life in the 20th century… Just like at funerals, here, these prefixes officially certified death, without involving any consent or actually certainty with regard to the nature of life after death" (Hobsbawm 1997, pp. 368–9). We are facing one of the transformations of psychiatry (Stylianidis 2006). We therefore also come to post-psychiatry. This emphasises the social and cultural context and prioritises ethics versus technology, while its purpose is to minimise medical control on interventions that include coercion (Bracken and Thomas 2001). It commands a new agreement between psychiatrists and users. It is a new trend, an alternative proposal to antipsychiatry, which, again, is attempting to place the users' voice and requests firmly in the forefront. Many fields open up under this perspective and a large number of completely new concepts and approaches, and it is to be reasonably wondered to what extent we now know more, also bearing on mind Hobsbawm's questioning.

22.8 Beyond the patient-doctor conflict: suggestions for the empowerment of users and the change in the culture of the services

The omniscience of knowledge organised opposite the ailing Other starts from this shortfall and this gap in the voice of the other. The asymmetry of the medical-healing relationship is organised around the knowledge and the know-how, around the ignorance of the individual's needs and their wishes. Thus, opinion is legalised socially and supplies the stereotype dominating relationships between the psychiatric team and patients-users, even if this is conducted in a theoretically "open" community framework and not within a total psychiatric institution (Stylianidis et al. 2008).

In this asymmetrical game, however, where one "loses" and the other "wins", each one is aware of both roles, the one stigmatising and the other being stigmatised. But in this game there are those who always loose, those who have been cast out of the game: they either choose to always loose, be marginalised in a therapeutic relationship or just leave the stage for good.

In this field, the intervention of advocacy by activating user participation plays a determining role. It redetermines the rules of the game, integrating those who have already lost or have been cast out and those who have chosen their place to be absence from the world. The traditional therapist-client relationship in this confrontation without mediation represents an entire closed totalitarian system, with its rules, rituals, language and codes, a true culture of authority in the psychiatric area.

User participation grants to those specified roles a mental, social and institutional opening, strengthening, as F. Basaglia said, the negotiating position of the weak.

Against the position-based medical-psychiatric omnipotence of the one side versus the other in a closed system, the introduction of a third party, an advocacy position, makes existing prejudice lose ground, divides and transforms the identity of the involved parties and constantly questions the narcissistic feedback of the powerful (the members of the therapeutic team), the omnipotence of knowledge, the rigidity of institutional mechanisms and the basis of the so-called (often complacently) "therapeutic alliance" with the patient.

In the therapeutic alliance, the institutional framework, transference-countertransference movements in a dual relationship, identifications, investments, anti-investments and dead-ends of the therapeutic process are no longer analysed. Everything becomes more complex to the extent that the position and audience of the Other are strengthened through the third party: patients are entered into a triangulated process where the parts of the system are obligated to converse, if they wish to exist as a system. The basis of common action and transformation of traditional psychiatric culture towards a collective democracy of health can be established from such a beginning.

In a statement regarding ethics, P. Ricoeur (1996) describes the doctor-patient relationship as an agreement of trust, *a kind of forged alliance between two people against a common enemy, disease*. However, before an agreement of trust can be established, there must be a stage of suspicion, embarrassment and reluctance. The patient expresses a request for treatment, suspicious versus the one who is in theory the expert, and the doctor who tries to reply the patient's requests, may, in turn, become suspicious of the non-compliance to the treatment prescribed by him. In order for the agreement to be established, Ricoeur (as above) tells us that both involved parties must recognise the uniqueness of this relationship, the "non-interchangeable character of one with the other". Therefore, the only possibility for this agreement to work is to consider the contracting parties as partners, which requires the active involvement of the patient in the management and development of his treatment. Medical secrecy is the legal expression of this agreement and relationship between the two sides.

We can, however, observe three paradoxes included in this agreement. The first paradox is that the subject is not an object, but the body is a part of the physical reality observed and is "objectified" by ethics, the approach and the technical arsenal of biological medicine-psychiatry. Psychiatry is often on a slippery slope, following the disconnection of body and souls in a simplistic biological reductionism, obscuring a big part of understanding and consequently the holistic care of the ailing subject.

The second paradox has to do with the fact that the individual is not a commodity, nor should medicine as a commercial product be subject to the laws of the market; however, in fact, medicine has a price and a high social cost for public health and private healthcare.

The last paradox overlaps the previous ones: anguish is private, but health is public. If all these contradictions generate conflict and if misguided psychiatrisation and the penalisation of social problems create enormous contrasts, the only possible framework where a possible solution may emerge is the consensual/conflicting process of the involved parties. On the basis of a "joint morale", we are obligated to discuss collectively and democratically the relations between disease and health and what we call personalised care, treatment and life plan to showcase a "third way" where the involved parties, namely, the social groups receiving services, the people involved in general health and mental health and local communities with their representatives, will empower their participative movement and will become involved in openly processing and evaluating a health system, where all coexist.

Through such a process, new collective responsibility, new representations of roles and relations of authority, new collective identities and new ways of social integration may emerge for those that Hanna Arendt (1961) called "useless in this world"; social practices of exclusion and neoliberal "philanthropy" may be radically challenged and a new democracy of health may be promoted. A change in the system is not at all easy. Studies show that it is usually occasional, the exception rather than the rule, while the parties involved easily return to previous, more conservative positions when they consider that the status quo is challenged or if they feel that their identity is threatened if contested. In order for change to exist, we must recognise new identity elements or even new identities for the involved parties, particularly psychiatrists and patients, so that they do not feel that change is threatening them. Up to now, we see movements gaining strength and continuity, seeking conflict as the means to change, whatever the case. Research experience, however, shows that decisiveness and will are not enough (Pérez and Mugny 1996). Validity, clear arguments and stability are also required. A strategy is needed so that there can be meaningful changes in the system and the resistance from each side can be overcome. These changes can be about specific issues. In detail:

User involvement should become national policy with a specific framework that will be structured gradually on the basis of good examples (Appleby 2000).
In cases where users offer services (care, consultancy, participation in research and research), the relationship with the service or with the action in general must be remunerated, so that obligations are met on both sides and there are no phenomena of patronising.
Training programmes must be established, structured by users for users and professionals. Programmes with specific methodology and evaluation system.

These are just some preliminary suggestions. At European level, very few users' and relatives' movements are independent and powerful in terms of funding, while most are supported by a specific few number of people and are vulnerable to crises (Rose and Lucas 2007). In order for user participation to work properly, there should be allocation of authority and recognition of user and family associations as institutional interlocutors with validity and arguments (Maza 1996), and users must be considered active citizens with rights and obligations and not faceless collateral losses of a dysfunctional system. Provided we continue to recognise the right of individuals to self-determination, besides any social dictates describing fear of the unfamiliar and the unwillingness to take on responsibility and to delete whatever is different, we can continue talking about the non-negotiable dignity inherent in any individual, irrespective and beyond social, political, financial and cultural crises or "trends" (Condylis 2003).

Bibliography

Andreasen NC (1995) Clients, consumers, providers, and products: where will it all end? Am J Psychiatry 152(8):1107–1109

Appleby L (2000) A new mental health service: high quality and user-led. Br J Psychiatry 177(4):290–291

Arendt H (1961) La condition de l'homme moderne. Calmann-Lévy, Paris, p 406

Bracken P, Thomas P (2001) Postpsychiatry: a new direction for mental health. Br Med J 322(7288):724

Condylis P (2003) On dignity. Indiktos Publications, Athens

Hatcher S, Butler R, Oakley-Brown M (2005) Evidence based mental health care. Elsevier, London

Hobsbawm E (1997) The age of extremes. The short twentieth century, 1914–1991. Themelio Publications, Athens

Johnstone L (1989) Users and abusers of psychiatry: a critical look at traditional psychiatric practice. Routledge, London

Lampaki K, Chondros P, Stylianidis S (2008) The implementation of the principles of lifelong learning for the social integration of individuals with mental disorders: the EMILIA programme. Psychiatry Workbooks 102:45–49

Maza G (1996) Structuring effective user involvement. In: Heller T, Reynolds J, Gomm R et al (eds) Mental health matters. Palgrave – Open University, Hampshire, pp 238–241

Nettleton S (2002) The sociology of health and illness. Typothito – Dardanos Publications, Athens

Pérez JA, Mugny G (1996) The conflict elaboration theory. Social influence procedures. Ulysses Publications, Athens

Ricoeur P (1996) Les trois niveaux du jugement médical. Esprit, Paris

Rose D, Lucas J (2007) The user and survivor movement in Europe. In: Knapp M, McDaid D, Mossialos E, Thornicroft G (eds) Mental health policy and practice across Europe. The future direction of mental health care. McGraw-Hill – Open University Press, Berkshire

Simpson EL, House AO (2002) Involving users in the delivery and evaluation of mental health services: systematic review. Br Med J 325(7375):1265

Stylianidis S (2006) Public health policy. In: Souliotis K (ed) Health policy and finances. Papazisis Publications, Athens, pp 537–564

Stylianidis S, Theocharakis N, Chondros P (2007) The suspended step of psychiatric reform in Greece. A timeless approach with timely questions. Archaeol Art 105:45–54

Stylianidis S, Chondros P, Lampaki K (2008) The mental health services user movement and its relation to the professionals: co-constructing a joint meaning. Psychiatry Workb 102:37–44

Stylianidis S, Lavdas M, Varvaressou X, Chondros P (2011a) Joint formulation of suggestions for the advocacy of the rights of individuals with mental disorders in the context of psychiatric reform. Ati 3:28–37

Stylianidis S, Chondros P, Varvaressou X (2011b) Improvement in the quality of rights in mental health structures: are patient rights a lost cause? Ati 3:7–8

Stylianidis S, Chondros P, Lavdas M (2014) Critical approach of an empowerment and recovery process: a case study from Greece. In: Soldatos C, Ruiz P, Dikeos D, Riba M (eds) Pluralism in psychiatry: I. Diverse approaches and converging goals. Paper presented at the 4th European Congress of the International Neuropsychiatric Association (INA) and the 1st Interdisciplinary Congress of the Hellenic Society for the Advancement of Psychiatry and Related Sciences. Nov 2012, Athens. Medimond, Bologna, pp 229–236

Stylianoudi M-G, Chondros P (2008) The representations of evil and disease in Evia, as collected from the local press from 1865 to 1940. In: Stylianidis S, Lilly Stylianoudi M-G (eds) Community and psychiatric reform: the Evia experience. Topos Publications, Athens

Thornicroft G, Tansella M (2005) Growing recognition of the importance of service user involvement in mental health service planning and evaluation. Epidemiol Psychiatr Soc 14(1):1–3

Van Hoorn E (1992) Changes? What changes? The views of the European patients' movement. Int J Soc Psychiatry 38:30–35

World Health Organization (WHO) (2011) Mental health atlas 2011. World Health Organization, Geneva

World Health Organization. Regional Office for Europe (WHO) (2008). Policies and practices for mental health in Europe: meeting the challenges. WHO Regional Office Europe

Involuntary Hospitalisation: Legislative Framework, Epidemiology and Outcome

23

Stelios Stylianidis, Lily Evangelia Peppou, Nektarios Drakonakis, and Emilia Panagou

Abstract

The involuntary hospitalisation of persons with mental health problems is a controversial issue in the provision of psychiatric care, mainly because its application is often coupled with the need to balance controversial interests: the rights of the patient, public safety and the need for treatment. Over the past few decades, the patients' movement, but also transition from asylum-type psychiatric care to community psychiatry, has shifted the focus of compulsory admission from the dangerousness and social control of the patient to his/her need for treatment. Against this background, reforms were progressively introduced into the relevant laws of most European countries, which gradually incorporated a number of texts and conventions. However, despite the similarities between such laws, there are still significant differences, which also explain to a certain extent the resulting disparities in the number of involuntary admissions in Europe and overall epidemiology of this phenomenon. Worldwide, the high rates of involuntary admissions appear to be more related with certain variables of the

S. Stylianidis (✉)
Department of Psychology, Panteion University, Athens, Greece
e-mail: stylianidis.st@gmail.com

L.E. Peppou
Association for Regional Development and Mental Health (EPAPSY), Athens, Greece
e-mail: lilly.peppou@gmail.com

N. Drakonakis • E. Panagou
Panteion University, Athens, Greece
e-mail: drnekt@gmail.com; panagou@synigoros.gr

© Springer International Publishing Switzerland 2016
S. Stylianidis (ed.), *Social and Community Psychiatry: Towards a Critical, Patient-Oriented Approach*, DOI 10.1007/978-3-319-28616-7_23

psychiatric care system than with the patients' characteristics, while the outcome appears to be satisfactory. So far, in Greece the number of involuntary hospitalisations is not recorded nationwide, systematically and reliably. The hitherto absence of systematic research into the subject of involuntary hospitalisation, as well as its determinants, also explains the absence of proposals and interventions to address the problem. However, on the basis of the first results of the Survey of Involuntary Hospitalisations in Athens and other scientific data, it appears that compulsory psychiatric treatment constitutes a first-line therapeutic solution, where the incomplete application of the law and the deficiencies of the mental health system, including its regulating culture and outlook, play a decisive role in the emergence of this issue. Therefore, the co-ordination of good practices, documented experience and ethical standards which should ensure the quality of services provided in a community framework appears to be at this stage an unrealistic endeavour for our country.

23.1 Introduction

The involuntary hospitalisation of persons with mental health problems remains a controversial issue in the provision of psychiatric care, mainly because of the restrictions imposed on the freedom and autonomy of such patients. It is set within the context of adopting coercive measures when practicing psychiatry, a fact which singularly distinguishes psychiatry from other medical disciplines. Significant issues arise in the application of such coercive measures owing to the difficulty in balancing the following controversial interests: (1) the patient's basic human rights, (2) public safety and (3) the need for treatment.

The term "compulsory admission or involuntary treatment" is understood to mean "the admission and detention for treatment of a person suffering from a mental disorder (hereinafter referred to as the "patient(s)") in a hospital, other medical establishment or appropriate place, provided this person is capable of giving his/her consent for treatment, but refuses to give such consent, or he/she is not capable of giving such consent and refuses treatment" (Council of Europe 2004).

Theoretically, compulsory admission is dictated by the principle of *parens patriae* (need for treatment) and the principle of responsibility of the state. More specifically, the principle of *parens patriae* refers to the obligation of the state to protect in a paternalistic manner its sick members who are in need of care and treatment and unable to survive without help. On the other hand, the principle of responsibility of the state places the state in the position of the protector of citizens, or society in general, from its "dangerous mentally ill members".

Since the eighteenth century, when the measure of involuntary hospitalisation was first introduced, and until the late 1960s, the predominant criterion was the principle of responsibility of the state. However, ever since and in parallel with the progressively increasing interest on human rights (patients' movement), as well as the transition from an asylum-type psychiatric care to community psychiatry, the principle of *parens patriae* gradually prevailed.

In this context, reforms were progressively introduced into the relevant legal provisions on this procedure in most European countries (Zinkler and Priebe 2002).

23.2 Legislation

Europe

National laws and policies worldwide include a broad range of rules and guarantees for the involuntary admission of persons with a mental illness. All, without exception, stipulate minimum criteria which need to be complied with in order to ensure that involuntary admission is consistent with the law. In chronological order, the most important and binding instruments are as follows:

- The European Convention for Human Rights (ECHR, 1950)
- The Recommendations of the Committee of Ministers of the Council of Europe (1983, 2004)
- The Recommendation of the Parliamentary Assembly of the Council of Europe (1994, 2004)
- The UN International Convention on the Rights of Persons with Disabilities (2006)

Specific mention is made for the first time regarding the care of the mentally ill in the European Convention for Human Right (hereinafter ECHR), which was adopted by the Council of Europe in 1950. The significance of this instrument lies in the fact that the rulings of the European Court of Human Rights (ECHR) are based on the content of this provision. The Recommendation of the Committee of Ministers of the Council of Europe of 1983 refers to the legal protection of persons suffering from mental disorders who are admitted as involuntary patients, while the Parliamentary Assembly of the Council of Europe adopted in 1994 the Recommendation on Psychiatry and Human Rights. However, the most recent Recommendation of the Committee of Ministers of the Council of Europe (2004) is the most complete and binding instrument worldwide on the protection of rights of persons with mental disorders. More specifically, it incorporates the basic principles underlying the judicial rulings of the ECHR, while taking into account the provisions of the Convention on "Human Rights and Biomedicine" of the Council of Europe, as well as the works of the European Commission for the "Prevention of Torture and Inhuman or Degrading Treatment or Punishment". This Convention includes guidelines to the Member States and calls on them to modernise and adapt their legislations along these guidelines. Finally, the UN International Convention on the Rights of Persons with Disabilities (2006) became the most recent basis for the debates regarding the current legal framework governing involuntary hospitalisation. Persons with a mental illness are specifically mentioned for the first time in a UN instrument as persons entitled to all fundamental human rights.

It is worth noting that instruments such as the Declaration of Hawaii (1977), the Resolution of the UN General Assembly (1991) and the Recommendations of the Parliamentary Assembly of the Council of Europe (1976, 1977) reflect the basic principles governing the protection of persons with a mental illness and the improvement of mental healthcare, without however binding on the Member States.

In this context, over the last decade, an attempt was made to systematically report the discrepancies between Member States regarding their current legal framework on involuntary hospitalisation. In a study funded by the EU and conducted in a time span of two years (2000–2002) with the participation of national expert representatives from every country, it was confirmed that despite the adaptation of the policies promoted by the aforementioned reports, there are still considerable differences between the national laws of EU Member States (Salize et al. 2002). The main differences are found in the criteria for involuntary hospitalisation, the opinions, the person making the decision for admission and certain aspects relating to the protection of the fundamental rights of the patients. With respect to the criteria for compulsory admission, all countries agree on the presence of mental illness, but differ with respect to the second criterion. It is worth noting that in countries where the need for treatment is specified as a criterion for involuntary admission, the relevant legislation in Ireland, Spain, Portugal, Sweden and Finland places further emphasis on the patient's lack of insight (Table 23.1).

The person rendering an opinion on the extent to which the involuntary hospitalisation criteria are met and for making the decision to admit the patient to hospital differs from country to country. As far as the former is concerned, the laws in Belgium, Denmark, Italy and Sweden allow physicians other than trained psychiatrists to make a decision, which is not the case in countries such as Austria, Greece, Ireland and Spain, where expert – and not trainee – psychiatrists are solely responsible to make a decision. As far as the decision-making for admission is concerned, the legal framework in countries such as Austria, Belgium, France, Italy and Greece authorises a state or administrative authority, such as a public prosecutor or mayor, as responsible, inter alia, for the decision. Conversely, in countries such as Denmark, Ireland and Sweden, the decision for admission is exclusively made by a medical obligation.

Finally, as far as the protection of patient rights is concerned, the patient's right to resort to appeal to court against an involuntary hospitalisation is included in every

Table 23.1 Criteria for compulsory admission in the EU

Criteria	Member states
Mental disorder + danger	Austria, Belgium, France, Germany, Luxembourg, Netherlands
Mental disorder + danger or Mental disorder + need for treatment	Denmark, Finland, Greece, Ireland, Portugal, UK
Mental disorder + need for treatment	Italy, Spain, Sweden

Replicated from Table 1.10, Salize et al. (2002)

Member State's legal framework. However, not every state's legal framework provides for the patient's right to be informed, the inclusion of a legal counsel (social worker, health professional, advocate, counsellor, etc.) and the provision of legal support free of charge.

Therefore, despite the efforts made to harmonise the laws of EU states on involuntary hospitalisation, there are significant differences between such laws.

Greece

From 1862 to 1992, two laws regulated the admission and long-term placement of patients in psychiatric hospitals in Greece: Law ΨΜΒ' of 1862 dating back to the time of King Otto and Legislative Decree 104/1973 (Bilanakis 2004).

Law ΨΜΒ' of 1862 "on the Establishment of Mental Hospitals" was the first piece of legislation of the Greek state on mental illness. In fact, this law established and developed the asylum structure in Greece, in the sense that – like all other relevant nineteenth century laws in Europe – the asylum was introduced as a place of confinement and treatment of mentally ill patients. According to this law, a mentally ill person could be admitted to a mental hospital in one of two ways: (a) admission of the patient by means of an application submitted by someone close to the patient (immediate family or relative) or (b) placement of the patient in a mental hospital by means of an order issued by a public authority (prefect, district commissioner, chief of police). In both cases, admission was based on a medical certificate which included a full description of the illness and concluded that the patient is in need for therapy and should be admitted to a mental hospital.

Law ΨΜΒ' remained in force until 1973, when Legislative Decree 104/1973 "on mental health and the treatment of the mentally ill" was introduced. According to the procedure laid down by Legislative Decree 104/1973 and the relevant ministerial decisions of the Ministry of Health adopted for the implementation thereof (Γ2β/3036/1973 και Α2β/5345/1978), a mental patient could be admitted to a mental hospital in one of three ways: (a) by voluntary admission, (b) by involuntary admission and (c) by compulsory admission of "dangerous psychiatric patients", known as "by order of the Public Prosecutor" under Article 5.

The general principle dictating this law was the complete dependency of the mental patient on the psychiatrists, since the larger framework/details and duration of the patients' treatment were determined by their opinions and decisions. The patients' admission to a mental hospital was often tantamount to a placement for an undefined period, resulting in the mental hospitals being used as custody and social care units.

The risk of arbitrariness inherent in subjecting hospitalised patients to the absolute judication of psychiatric experts, and their treatment solely as patients presumed incompetent by law and not as persons presumed competent by law, necessitated the modernisation of the relevant institutional framework on the subject of mental health in general and, more specifically, the arrangements for involuntary placement.

The current institutional framework, and the provisions of the 2071/1992 "Modernisation and Organisation of the Health Care System" law and the 2716/1999 "Development and modernisation of the Mental Health services and other provisions" law aims to protect the individual freedoms of patients. With the provisions of Law 2071/92, the legislator defines clearly the conditions and regulates in detail the procedure for involuntary placement (the content of the law is summarised in Table 23.2).

More specifically, the conditions for involuntary hospitalisation under Law 2071/92 are:

(a) The patient must suffer from a mental disorder and not be in a position to judge what is best for his/her health, and lack of hospitalisation would result in depriving him/her of the treatment for his/her condition or would lead to the deterioration of his/her condition.
(b) The patient's hospitalisation is necessary in order to prevent acts of violence against himself or others.

With respect to the procedure of admission to a mental health unit, Article 96 of Law 2071/1992 stipulates that the involuntary hospitalisation of a person who is allegedly mentally ill may be initiated by his/her spouse or close relatives by means of an application to the Public Prosecutor of the Court of First Instance of his/her place of residence or stay. If such relatives do not exist, as can happen in cases of emergency, only the Public Prosecutor can request ex officio the patient's involuntary hospitalisation. This application must be justified and describe the patients' mental illness, his/her previous and current behaviour, any past voluntary assessment interventions, his/her refusal to assessment or if such assessment is proved impossible, as precisely as possible. This application must be accompanied by two psychiatrists' reports selected from the list published every 2 years by the competent medical association. The psychiatrist should not be related to the applicant, or the patient and their opinions must be justified, i.e. they should contain the actual facts (any symptoms of illness, previous acts of violence, previous hospitalisations, where and why) and reasons why outpatient treatment is not feasible and should conclude with the diagnosis and scientific basis for such diagnosis. Provided that the Public Prosecutor determines that the legal requirements are met and that the two medical reports agree on the need for involuntary hospitalisation, the Public Prosecutor orders the patient's admission to a suitable mental health unit. There, the patient is informed by the Head of the Unit of his/her rights – particularly his/her right to appeal. A record of the proceedings is drawn up and signed by the Head of the Unit and the person accompanying the patient.

In case the patient's assessment is not feasible, because he/she has refused such assessment, the Public Prosecutor orders for the transference of the individual to a public mental clinic for assessment and for drawing up the opinions. The individual's admission is carried out under conditions ensuring the respect of the patients' personality and dignity and the patient's stay in the unit for the necessary assessment cannot exceed 48 h.

Table 23.2 Contents of Law 2071/1992

Requirements	Procedure	Result	Duration	Place/conditions of treatment	Discharge procedure
Existence of mental disorder supported by two psychiatric opinions The patient is not in a position to judge what is best for his/her health The lack of treatment would lead to the deterioration of his/her condition, or is necessary in order to prevent acts of violence against himself/herself or others	Civil court decision Possibility to attend with advocate Possibility to appoint a technical advisor as expert witness	Orders the involuntary placement of patient in a suitable mental health unit for treatment Possibility to take legal action against the decision ordering the involuntary hospitalisation	Six months with the possibility of extending hospitalisation for another 6 months upon decision of a civil court	Mental health centres, day centres, general hospital psychiatric departments, residential units, special psychiatric hospitals The conditions must first serve the therapeutic needs Possibility for leaves, outings and staying outside the mental health unit	Ex officio after a period of 6 months, unless the extension procedure is followed At any time after 6 months if the attending physician deems that the patient's condition does not impose the need for involuntary hospitalisation

Within 3 days of the patient's formal admission, the same Public Prosecutor brings the case before the Multi-member Court of First Instance. The court sits within 10 days from the Public Prosecutor's request, and where appropriate *in camera*, in order to protect the patient's private life. It should be noted that 48 h before the hearing, the patient is invited to attend and he/she has the right to appear with the aid of a lawyer and a psychiatrist as his/her technical consultant.

If the Public Prosecutor's request is not accepted, the court shall order the immediate discharge of the patient. If the Court decides that the medical reports are insufficiently convincing, the Court shall order the assessment of the patient by a third psychiatrist (preferably an assistant professor or the Chief Scientist of a public mental health unit).

If the Court rules to continue the patient's compulsory treatment, this ruling must be based on specific reasons. However, until such judgement is issued, the therapeutic responsibility for the patient lays with the Chief Scientist of the Mental Heal Unit, who continues to be scientifically and therapeutically responsible should the court order to continue his/her treatment.

Pursuant to Article 97 of Law 2071/1992, the decision of the Court of First Instance may be appealed or challenged by the patient, his/her relatives and his/her guardian in accordance with the provisions of Civil Procedure within 2 months from the publication of such decision. The appeal is heard in any event *in camera* within 15 days from lodging the appeal.

Pursuant to Article 98 of Law 2071/1992, the conditions of involuntary admission must serve the therapeutic needs. The necessary restrictive measures should not exclude the necessary therapeutic means, such as leaves, organised outings or staying in supervised spaces outside the closed institutions. In any case and throughout the placement, the patient should be treated with respect, while any restrictions imposed on his/her personal freedom are determined solely on the basis of his/her health condition and therapeutic needs.

Finally, pursuant to Article 99 of Law 2071/1992, the duration of placement may not exceed 6 months. In special cases, placement may be extended beyond the 6-month period, with the consent of three psychiatrists, one of which is the attending physician and the other two are appointed by the Public Prosecutor. Placement may, however, be terminated at any time before the end of the period of 6 months, if it is found that the conditions that led to the placement no longer apply. In this case, the Chief Scientist of the mental health unit where the patient is placed must issue a discharge certificate as well as to forward a report of the case to Public Prosecutor responsible.

A review of the provisions of Law 2071/1992 referring to the conditions, the procedure and execution of involuntary hospitalisation leads to positive conclusions as they significantly differ from the previous regime. On the positive side, the law includes the establishment of judicial guarantees to verify the legality of involuntary placement, as well as the establishment of a maximum time frame for such placement. Furthermore, the fact that the primary role of involuntary hospitalisation is shifted from the custodial to the treatment oriented highlights the explicit requirement of the legislator for respect of the personality of the patient in every case and throughout the duration of his/her placement – a requirement which, inter alia, is manifested in the latter's possibility to receive legal and psychiatric aid from a lawyer and a psychiatrist as technical consultant and to take legal action.

In addition, the enactment of Law 2716/1999 was a serious step towards improving the weaknesses of the mental healthcare system in our country. Article 1(2) ("Mental health services are structured, organised, developed and function under the provisions of this Law, in line with the principles of sectorisation and community psychiatry, the priority of primary care, outpatient care, de-institutionalisation, psychosocial rehabilitation and social re-integration, continuity of psychiatric care as well as the provision of information and voluntary assistance to the community for the purpose of promoting mental health".) was particularly significant to this positive change of direction.

The effort made to codevelop primary care coupled with post-discharge care, as well as harmonising the operation between the various units, as well as the general spirit of law, is quite clear in certain separate articles (Art. 5, 6, 7 and 8) of the law. In this respect, national legislation is brought in line (ostensibly, as detailed above) with the country's international commitments and the trends prevailing worldwide.

Since then, the law which has now been in force for more than 20 years has been subject to a number of significant changes and modifications. The competent courts' ruling on involuntary hospitalisation is no longer the Multi-member Courts of First Instance but the Single-Member Courts of First Instance. Thus, the procedure is now swifter and more flexible and, at the same time, requires fewer guarantees for the protection of the individual and the appropriateness of the decision, since one vote is now sufficient to order the involuntary admissions of a patient. At the same time, the Oviedo Convention (Convention on Human Rights and Biomedicine) led to the revocation of a second pair of conditions for involuntary hospitalisation, namely, the presence of dangerousness to self or others, a fact which the local public prosecutor authorities do not seem to be aware of. The amendment of the Civil Code, with respect to the powers of attorney, but also the introduction of a special provision according to which the involuntary hospitalisation of any person is allowed "upon the prior the authorisation of the court…", revokes the authority of the Public Prosecutor to order the involuntary placement of a patient and, as a result, defines that compulsory placement without a court decision – even if it is an interim order – is illegal (Triantafyllou and Chotamanidou 2005). On the basis of the above observations, it results that all involuntary admissions ordered by a Public Prosecutor or hospitalisations decided on the grounds of the patient dangerousness criterion are against the law. Finally, it is worth noting that the UN International Convention on the Rights of Persons with Disabilities (2006), mentioned above, has been transposed into the legislation of the Greek state (Law 4074/2012) and its provisions take precedence over any other Greek law.

However, the implementation of such legislation in Greece is found to be significantly deficient. On the international level, this is established by two decisions of the European Court of Human Rights against Greece – the Venios Case and the

Karamanof Case – while on the national level, it is reflected in the ex officio investigation of the Greek Ombudsman (2007). Specifically, with regard to the second, following the large number of complaints submitted by citizens to the Ombudsman office, an ex officio investigation was conducted to verify the extent to which the rights of involuntarily hospitalised patients are protected. The investigation was conducted in the two psychiatric hospitals in Attica – the Dromokaiteio Sanitorium and the "Dafni" Psychiatric Hospital – and included the assessment of a random sample of 89 patient records (equal representation of both sexes), who were involuntarily hospitalised in the last decade. Where the records contained information on prior involuntary hospitalisations, this information was also taken into account. This resulted in the overall analysis of 179 compulsory placements. The main deficits identified in the implementation of the law related to medical opinions, the transfer and information of the patients as well as the judicial review. Specifically, most psychiatrists did not provide a detailed explanation and the individual reasons for which the involuntary hospitalisation criteria are met. Instead, a form was used with the general preprinted statement "The conditions laid down in Law 2071/1992 are met". According to the overwhelming majority of the records (97 %), it was established that the transfer of patients was made by police and not the National Emergency Centre (EKAV), a fact which indicates that the patient is treated as potentially dangerous. At the same time, it appears that patients are not informed of their rights and, particularly, their right to take legal action. Finally, while 94 % of placements were effected in pursuance of a court order, in half of the cases a summons was not found, and in 84 % of the cases, no court decision for commitment was found. The patient did not appear in court in almost all cases, while it also appears that the procedural time frames defined by the law are not complied with. Similar findings were also observed in Thessaloniki (Kosmatos 2002). In a study conducted following the ex officio investigation conducted by the Greek Ombudsman at the "Dafni" Psychiatric Hospital, an improvement was noted as regards the content of medical opinions; however, no improvement was noted as regards issues relating to the transfer and information of patients, their appearance in court and the court decision for involuntary hospitalisation. Consequently, despite the liberal, innovative and protective nature of law 2071/1992 (Stylianidis et al. 1997), the manner in which it has been implemented in practice reminds one of both the content and perspective, of previous pieces of legislation.

The differences existing between national legislative frameworks, including Greece, are of great importance as it has been found that they are linked with the subjective perception of involuntary placed patients regarding the benefits of the treatment and of accepting its usefulness. A study carried out under the research programme EUNOMIA (European Evaluation of Coercion in Psychiatry and Harmonization of Best Clinical Practice) showed that in countries with more protective regulations, such as Slovakia and Germany, the patients' opinions regarding involuntary hospitalisation were more positive, as opposed to countries such as the UK, where regulations are less protective. At the same time, it has been suggested that the differences in legislation also explain the diversity witnessed in the epidemiological parameters of involuntary hospitalisations in Europe.

23.3 Epidemiology

Europe

Traditionally, in the epidemiology of the phenomenon, involuntary hospitalisations are expressed either as quotas of the total number of hospitalisations or as the number of hospitalisations in a population of 100,000 persons per year. With respect to these two measurement indicators, the quotas refer to the mix of patients in hospitals and, therefore, cannot be used to record the frequency of hospitalisations in the population as such (i.e. the benchmark is the clinical and not the general population). However, in most European countries, involuntary hospitalisations are recorded using both ways – if and when such information is available – although the reliability and the methods of collecting such information are often being questioned.

Over the last decade, a couple of efforts have been made in literature to catalogue findings onto the number of involuntary hospitalisations in Europe (Salize and Dressing 2004; Zinkler and Priebe 2002). More specifically, contrary to the review by Zinkler and Priebe (2002), the primary review by Salize and Dressing (2004) seems more well documented, and for this reason, it will be presented in further detail; however, the reader can refer to the other source for a more complete picture of the subject. In a study funded by the European Commission, while investigating the similarities and differences between the Member States' current legislative frameworks on involuntary hospitalisation, the method and the results of which have been discussed in the relevant subsection, an effort was made to track any changes in the number of involuntary hospitalisations over the last decade, as well as the disparities in this number between European countries. Specifically, the authors report consistent levels of involuntary hospitalisations in the last decade for Europe as a whole, although in some countries, such as the UK, Germany, France, Sweden and Finland, the numbers are rising. This result is attributed mainly to a shorter average duration of hospitalisation which, inevitably, leads to higher hospitalisation quotas. At the same time, incorporating the two involuntary hospitalisation measurement indicators mentioned above, a significant difference is noted between European countries, both in terms of the number of involuntary hospitalisations (from 6 per 100,000 in Portugal up to 218 per 100,000 in Finland) and in terms of quotas (from 3.2 % in Portugal up to 30 % in Sweden). It is worth noting that for the Mediterranean countries – Greece, Spain and Italy – the data available is incomplete, resulting in their not being taken into account in the relevant measurements.

In addition, the profile of persons who are involuntarily hospitalised has been researched by very few researchers-epidemiologists in an effort to explain the current differences between countries, although the results are often heterogeneous. In terms of socio-demographic variables, involuntarily hospitalised individuals are usually younger, single, unemployed men from ethnic minority groups, with unstable residence conditions, low socioeconomic level and low social support levels (Bindman et al. 2002; Houston and Mariotto 2001; Owens et al. 1991; Salize and Dressing 2004; Webber and Huxley 2004). In terms of clinical variables, the majority of studies indicate that they suffer from disorders of the schizophrenic spectrum; their symptomatology is quite severe and has more previous hospitalisations and in particular involuntary (Houston and Mariotto 2001; Owens et al. 1991; Salize and Dressing 2004). However, the studies focusing on the socio-demographic and clinical characteristics of patients place the burden of involuntary hospitalisation on the patient. While personal variables were found to be linked to a large extent with involuntary hospitalisation, other parameters – more systemic – seem to play a more significant role.

At the opposite end of studies exploring the correlations between involuntary hospitalisation and the patients' particulars, other studies focus on characteristics associated with the mental health services. Specifically, a higher incidence of involuntary hospitalisations is observed in areas with limited access to such services (Hansson et al. 1999) or poor networking between such services (Durbin et al. 2006; Weirdsma and Mulder 2009). At the same time, it has been found that the number of involuntary hospitalisations is higher in areas with low standards of living, insufficient resources and poorly organised services (Huxley and Kerfoot 1993). Furthermore, a study by Bindman and his associates in the UK showed that the levels of compulsory placements in 34 geographical are linked, on a statistically significant level, to the quality of service indicators: delays in finding beds in hospital departments or residential units for acute cases and absence of home visits after a specific time to patients who are in an acute phase, as well as the standard of living in the relevant area (Bindman et al. 2002). It is worth noting that in addition to service networking, areas with improved community networks, i.e. networks which include welfare services, accommodation organisations and local police, demonstrate lower levels of involuntary admissions (Weirdsma et al. 2007).

Greece

In Greece, the number of studies on the epidemiology of involuntary hospitalisation is very limited. The percentage of involuntary hospitalisations in 1979, and before the enactment of law 2071/1992, amounted to 97 %. However, the corresponding percentages after the introduction of this law are not recorded nationwide, although they are believed to range between 4-% and 50-% (Liakos 2004; Greek Ombudsman 2007) or higher (Livaditis 2010).

In a prospective study conducted by Bozikas and his associates in the 1st Psychiatric Clinic of the Aristotle University of Thessaloniki, data was obtained from 204 consecutive admissions (Bozikas et al. 2003). Of these, 54,9 % were found to be involuntary, while the patients who presented a higher likelihood of being admitted against their will were single, diagnosed with a psychotic disorder or bipolar disorder, self-employed and skilled or unskilled workers and had a higher number of previous involuntary admissions. Variables relating to social support or mental health services were not examined.

In a more recent prospective study, the court order documents which included the records kept by police stations nationwide together with special forms created for the purposes of the study and completed by the chief of each police station were examined (Douzenis et al. 2012). The study covered the conditions of involuntary assessment of patients, following the initiation of the relevant procedure by a relative or ex officio, as well as the characteristics of patients whose involuntary assessment led to an involuntary admission. Of the 2,038 files examined, involuntary assessment led to an involuntary admission in the vast majority of cases (87.5 %). A cause for apprehension and concern was the finding that in 58.1 % of the cases, police officers were present, presented a concerning factor, although most patients did not oppose the procedure in any way. A comparison between patients whose involuntary assessment led to involuntary admission to those who ultimately were not admitted did not identify any statistically significant differences in terms of gender, age or nationality.

In light of the above, Greece appears to have high involuntary hospitalisation rates; nevertheless, no adequate scientific explanation could be extracted for the reasons behind this.

23.4 Outcome

The issue of outcome is closely related to the criterion of need for therapy, but also with the moral justification of involuntary hospitalisation. In other words, persons suffering from mental illness are deprived of their fundamental freedoms, because of the expected positive outcome of their placement, which could not have occurred in any other manner than by their involuntary hospitalisation. This is why the investigation of the outcome/effectiveness of involuntary admission has drawn such strong scientific interest over the past years.

International literature on the subject differs methodologically in terms of the outcome indicators used to assess, readmission, symptomatology, insight, functionality, adherence to treatment and medication and treatment satisfaction, but also the time of assessment of the outcome. Discharge and/or follow up assessment may be unavailable, make it relatively difficult to reconcile the results and draw conclusions. In this context, two systematic efforts were made by two teams from the UK (Katsakou and Priebe 2006) and Germany (Kallert et al. 2008) to review the relevant literature.

The first review attempted to examine the outcome of involuntary hospitalisation both in terms of clinical indicators as well as in terms of subjective perception of the patients (Katsakou and Priebe 2006). Subsequently, it attempted to determine the socio-demographic and clinical characteristics associated with more positive and more negative outcomes. The primary studies were assessed on the basis of specific methodological criteria relating to the size of the sample, the cross-sectional or longitudinal nature of research planning, response rates and the presence of a bias error, prior to being included in the review. Of the 521 articles identified, only 23 satisfied such criteria and corresponded to 18 international studies. The result of the review substantiated the clinical effectiveness of involuntary hospitalisation, while at a later stage most patients were mainly favourably disposed towards hospitalisation. However, a significant proportion of patients did not feel that their hospitalisation was justified or beneficial. Patients showing a significant clinical improvement were found to express more positive outlook on involuntary hospitalisation (Katsakou and Priebe 2006).

The second review was focused on the outcome of the treatment of involuntarily hospitalised patients compared to those voluntarily hospitalised (Kallert et al. 2008). The primary works included in the review were previously evaluated on the basis of methodological parameters, such as those described above. The analysis of these 17 studies showed that involuntarily hospitalised patients were either highly likely to be readmitted in the years following their discharge (the reassessment time frames vary considerably between studies, from 30 days after discharge to 17 years), especially involuntarily. Concerning the clinical indicators, no differences between the two teams were identified as far as the degree of general psychopathology and commitment to therapy are concerned, during measurements following discharge. In terms of social functionality, involuntarily hospitalised patients show lower levels both at the time of admission and at the time of discharge. However, improvement with regard to this specific indicator is in the same range and magnitude as that of voluntarily hospitalised patients. Finally, as far as the subjective indicators used to evaluate the treatment are concerned, involuntarily hospitalised patients were found more likely to consider their hospitalisation unjustified and less satisfied with their treatment.

The low to average quality of most studies on this specific subject and their heterogeneity as regards the various methodological aspects highlight and stress the need to conduct methodologically sound studies under daily clinical routine conditions. The use of weighted outcome tools, enlistment of a sufficient number of patients and clarity in determining follow-up measurements are key to a good methodological approach in accordance with current literature.

No studies have been conducted in Greece on the outcome of the treatment of persons with mental disorders.

23.5 Study on Involuntary Hospitalisations in Athens (MANA)

Against this background and on the basis of the limited number of studies on the epidemiology of involuntary hospitalisation in Greece, the Association for Regional Development and Mental Health (EPAPSY), in cooperation with the Panteion University, has, since 2011, developed a research programme investigating compulsory admissions in Athens area and exploring different facets of the issue in depth. Through different research questions and by adopting different methodologies, the programme attempts to give a full picture of involuntary commitment in the "Dafni" Attica Psychiatric Hospital. The following questions represent some of the main themes under examination:

- What is the proportion of involuntary hospitalisations in "Dafni" APH and which socio-demographic and clinical characteristics are associated with the involuntary nature of admission?
- What is the cohort outcome of involuntarily hospitalised patients?

- What is the subjective opinion of involuntarily hospitalised patients on their treatment?
- What is the subjective opinion of voluntarily hospitalised patients on their treatment?
- What is the perspective of relatives of patients who are involuntarily hospitalised?
- To what extent are the legal requirements concerning the content of medical opinions complied with?
- To what extent do involuntarily hospitalised patients believe they have benefited from their hospitalisation and that it was justified? Which factors contribute to such favourable opinions.
- What proportion of the sample meets the "revolving door" criteria? What are the characteristics of such patients and what is the outcome of their hospitalisation?
- What are the views of mental health professionals in community structures as well as the staff working at the "Dafni" APH on mental health and involuntary hospitalisation?
- Which patients are more likely to become mechanically restrained and what is the outcome of their hospitalisation?
- What are the views of mental health professionals, patients and their relatives on mechanical restrain?

A mixed methodology (quantitative and qualitative) is adopted to investigate all the above questions, depending on the nature of the question and the availability of current literature on the subject. All the sub-studies are carried out with the help of undergraduate Psychology students, while the authors of this chapter are the ones responsible for the overall co-ordination and supervision of the project.

The first results of the study reveal that a large proportion of involuntary hospitalisations in the "Dafni" APH is explained by the shortcomings of the mental health services as a whole. For instance, it is noted that the only forecasting indicator for involuntary hospitalisation is the previous number of involuntary hospitalisations, while a large proportion of patients was found to meet the "revolving door" criteria (36.4 %). On the same note, a large proportion of patients hospitalised in "Dafni" (about 85–89 %), were referred to the hospital's outpatient clinic instead of community settings after hospitalisation to the hospital's outpatient clinic and not to community structures, while focus groups of the hospital's mental health professionals stress the obstacles and difficulties in communication between hospital and community structures. It is worth noting that, based on the sub-question concerning the view of mental health professionals working in community structures on mental illness and involuntary hospitalisation, it appears that elements of the "asylum" culture, especially as to the dangerousness of mentally ill patients and need for social control, are also found in community structures.

The aggregation of the findings of this specific programme is expected to result in an in-depth understanding of the mechanisms promoting the establishment of involuntary hospitalisation as a routine practice in the mental health system. At a later stage, the programme aims to link these results to the design and implementation of tailored interventions for the effective management of the problem.

Conclusions

In modern psychiatry, the questions concerning restrictive measures during the psychiatric hospitalisation of patients remain pressing. This is because the association of mental illness to antisocial behaviour and dangerousness is still dominant. A direct outcome of this standpoint is the tendency to exclude, isolate and marginalise individuals suffering from mental illnesses, "penalise" mental illness and, ultimately, stigmatise it, as a solution for preventing possible risks (Gravier and Eytan 2011). Respectively, mentally ill patients facing social exclusion, and all the more so assert their self-evident rights.

The involuntary assessment and hospitalisation process is an exceptional – in the sense of departing from the norm – experience in people's lives (in modern societies), in which they undergo the restrictions of their freedoms and are being, without consenting to either of the two aforementioned procedures. The infrequency of this experience, supported by the weight of the resulting threat to their personal freedom and dignity, calls for the establishment of a very clear legal framework outlining all authorised or unauthorised implementation procedures, as well as the operation of a reliable system to record and control the above procedures (Fytrakis 2007).

The need to comply with the law could be said to be a preoccupation for some legal practitioners ignoring the reality as well as the individuals being in need of help. In this respect, psychiatrists working in hospitals often argue that "a person in crisis cannot be helped with legislative articles but with appropriate therapy". Even the Code of Medical Conduct [Law 3418/2005, Art. 28(8)] requires involuntary hospitalisation "to comply with the terms and conditions laid down by the laws in force". Nevertheless, psychiatrists' knowledge of involuntarily commitment as well as on the rights of the people suffering from mental illness is in need of improvement.

Of course, the experience of the members of the prosecution or the judiciary on the specific subject is rather negligible, since their training and briefing on the procedure is non-existent, and whatever experience they have is gained in the field. Thus, Thomas Szasz's aphorism regarding the threat posed to individual freedoms from a conspiracy between state authority and psychiatry no longer sounds threatening but a tangible reality (Szasz and Kraus 2007). In Greece, the poor implementation of the law on involuntary hospitalisation in practice frequently finds health professionals and the judiciary directly involved in a "silent complicity" against mentally ill persons. At the same time, the absence of reliable national data on the number of involuntary hospitalisations in Greece is an additional aspect of this silent complicity, as the magnitude of the problem is not exposed, the reasons for its existence are not scientifically substantiated and there are no recognised fields and ways of intervention to deal with it.

Scientific data on involuntary hospitalisations from studies in Greece, as well as the evaluation of psychiatric reforms, highlight the many and multilevel shortcomings of the mental health system – which cannot even be classified as a system and which, basically, is also accountable for the country's high involuntary hospitalisation levels. Social welfare shortcomings, the relief of the family, the fatigue and evasion of responsibility of mental health professionals, the indifference of judicial authorities and fragmented nature of treating the mental disease result in transforming involuntary hospitalisation from a measure of last resort to social automatism.

It appears that the current structure of the mental health services "system" defines both the procedure and the outcome of the therapy for persons with a serious mental illness. In this context, social automatism reproduces on all three levels – structure, procedure, outcome – the aforementioned deficiency and malfunction of the system, as well as its accompanying ethical deadlocks (Stylianidis et al. 2014). Therefore, the co-ordination of good practices, documented experience and ethical standards which should ensure the quality of service in a community framework seems at this stage unrealistic.

Bibliography

Bindman J, Tighe J, Thornicroft G, Leese M (2002) Poverty, poor services and compulsory psychiatric admission in England. Soc Psychiatry Psychiatr Epidemiol 37:341–345

Bilanakis N (2004) Psychiatric care and human rights in Greece. Athens: Odysseas

Bozikas V, Tsipropoulou V, Desseri C, Kosmidou M, Bogiatzi M, Pitsavas S, Karabatos T (2003) Study of factors affecting involuntary hospitalisation of patients in mental clinic. Psychiatriki 14:110–120

Council of Europe (2004) Recommendation of the committee of ministers to member states concerning the protection of the human rights and dignity of persons with mental disorder. Available at http://www.coe.int/t/dg3/healthbioethic/texts_and_documents/Rec(2004)10_e.pdf

Douzenis A, Michopoulos I, Economou M, Rizos E, Christodoulou C, Lykouras L (2012) Involuntary admission in Greece: a prospective national study of police involvement and client characteristics affecting emergency assessment. Int J Soc Psychiatry 58:172–177

Durbin J, Goering P, Streiner DL, Pink G (2006) Does systems integration affect continuity of mental health care? Adm Policy Ment Health 33:705–717

Fytrakis E (2007) Involuntary hospitalisation today: a black hole in the rule of law. Tetradia Psychiatrikis 100:109–120

Gravier B, Eytan A (2011) Enjeux ethiques de la psychiatrie sous contrainte. Rev Med Suisse 7:1806–1811

Hansson L, Muus S, Saarento O, Vinding HR, Gostas G, Sandlund M et al (1999) The Nordic comparative study on sectorized psychiatry: rates of compulsory care and use of compulsory admissions during a 1-year follow-up. Soc Psychiatry Psychiatr Epidemiol 34:99–104

Houston KG, Mariotto M (2001) Outcomes for psychiatric patients following first admission: relationships with voluntary and involuntary treatment and ethnicity. Psychol Rep 88:1012–1014

Huxley P, Kerfoot M (1993) Variation in requests to social services departments for assessment for compulsory psychiatric admission. Soc Psychiatry Psychiatr Epidemiol 28:71–76

Kallert TW, Glockner M, Schutzwohl M (2008) Involuntary vs. voluntary hospital admission: a systematic literature on outcome diversity. Eur Arch Psychiatry Clin Neurosci 258:185–209

Katsakou C, Priebe S (2006) Outcomes of involuntary hospital admission: a review. Acta Psychiatr Scand 114:232–241

Kosmatos K (2002) Involuntary hospitalisation in Mental Health Unit. Experiences, findings and prospects from the implementation of Law 2071/1992. Criminal Law Series, 22. A. Sakkoula Publications, Athens-Komotini

Liakos A (2004) Contribution in the proceedings of the first meeting for compulsory hospitalization by the president of the Greek committee for the protection and care of the mentally ill. University Mental Health Research Institute, Athens

Livaditis M (2010) Involuntary psychiatric treatment in modern Greece. Psychiatriki 21:15–16

Owens D, Harrison G, Boot D (1991) Ethnic factors in voluntary and compulsory admissions. Psychol Med 21:185–196

Salize HJ, Dressing H (2004) Epidemiology of involuntary placement of mentally ill people across the European Union. Br J Psychiatry 184:163–168

Salize HJ, Dressing H, Peitz M (2002) Compulsory admission and involuntary treatment of mentally ill patients – legislation and practice in EU-member states/final report. Central Institute of Mental Health, Manheim

Stylianidis S, Mitrosouli M, Ploumbidis D (1997) On the implementation of the new Greek law in psychiatry. Tetradia Psychiatrikis 60:152–155

Stylianidis S, Peppou S, Drakonakis N (2014) Moral and ethical issues relating to compulsory psychiatric hospitalisation. In: Douzenis A, Lykoura L (eds) Moral and ethics in mental health. VITA Medical Publications, Athens

Szasz T, Kraus K (2007) Aphorisms on psychiatry and psychoanalysis. Ekdotiki Thessalonikis, Thessaloniki

The Greek Ombudsman (2007) Ex officio study of the independent Greek Ombudsman authority on the involuntary hospitalisation of mentally ill patients. Special report. Access from http://www.synigoros.gr/reports/Eidiki_Ekthesi_Akousia_Nosileia_17_5_07.pdf

Triantafyllou G, Chotamanidou P (2005) The court order for involuntary admission of persons with mental disorders in MHUs following the amendment of the Civil Code (Law 2447/1996). *Armenopoulos*: J Thessaloniki Bar Assoc

Webber M, Huxley P (2004) Social exclusion and risk of emergency compulsory admission: a case-control study. Soc Psychiatry Psychiatr Epidemiol 39:1000–1009

Weirdsma AI, Mulder C (2009) Does mental health service integration affect compulsory admissions? Int J Integ Care 9:1–8

Weirdsma AI, Poodt HD, Mulder C (2007) Effects of community-care networks on psychiatric emergency contacts, hospitalization and involuntary admission. J Epidemiol Community Health 61:613–618

Zinkler M, Priebe S (2002) Detention of the mentally ill in Europe: a review. Acta Psychiatr Scand 106:3–8

The Impact of the Economic Crisis in Greece: Epidemiological Perspective and Community Implications

24

Marina Economou, Lily Evangelia Peppou, Kyriakos Souliotis, and Stelios Stylianidis

Abstract

The global financial crisis has triggered a sustained recession in Greece with wide-ranging socioeconomic consequences. Throughout the 5 years of economic turmoil in the country, unemployment rates have rocketed, while financial strain has become omnipresent. As a corollary of these, the population health has declined, while substantial increases in suicide mortality have been recorded. A series of repeated nationwide cross-sectional studies by the University Mental Health Research Institute has corroborated a gradual but steady increment in 1-month prevalence of major depression, while 1-month prevalence of suicidality was found to be on the rise until 2011. Nonetheless, in spite of the growing

---

M. Economou (✉)
First Department of Psychiatry, Medical School, Eginition Hospital,
National & Kapodistrian University, Athens, Greece

University Mental Health Research Institute (UMHRI), Athens, Greece
e-mail: meconomu@otenet.gr

L.E. Peppou
Association for Regional Development and Mental Health (EPAPSY), Athens, Greece
e-mail: lilly.peppou@gmail.com

K. Souliotis
Faculty of Social and Political Sciences, University of Peloponnese, Corinth, Greece

Department of Hygiene, Epidemiology and Medical Statistics,
Centre for Health Services Research, Medical School, National & Kapodistrian University,
Athens, Greece
e-mail: soulioti@hol.gr

S. Stylianidis
Department of Psychology, Panteion University, Athens, Greece
e-mail: stylianidis.st@gmail.com

mental health needs of the population, the mental healthcare system seems incapable of fulfilling them, as the economic downturn has also impinged on healthcare. Different types of interventions have been recommended for offsetting the dire impact of the crisis in Greece, including restructuring of mental health services, enhancing the social capital of the community and implementing active labour market and debt relief programmes; however, any action along these lines relies heavily on local initiatives taken by specific service providers. Concerted efforts for ameliorating the mental health effects of the recession in Greece are urgently needed, in order to prevent further exacerbation of psychiatric morbidity in the foreseeable future and to avoid a potential outbreak of suicides.

24.1 Introduction

The global financial crisis is considered to be the worst economic downturn since the Great Depression in the 1930s. It started off in the US banking sector, when a rise in interest rates resulted in borrower defaults, which in turn led to bank defaults and eventually to a crash in the housing and stock markets (Financial Crisis Inquiry Commission 2011). The turmoil was soon diffused to European banks causing the vast majority of European countries to fall into deep recessions. In Europe, it was Ireland and the Mediterranean countries – the so-called PIGS – that were more strongly hit by the crisis.

In the wake of the crisis, the Greek economy was regarded as the 27th largest economy in the world by nominal gross domestic product (GDP) with 32,100 USD GDP per capita (Eurostat 2010). Nonetheless, as a corollary of the global recession and the local unrelenting spending, the country entered a prolonged and sustained economic downturn since early 2009.

The GDP in Greece started displaying negligible growth rate since the last months of 2007 and negative growth rate until 2014, when it reached a positive 0.8 % (World Bank 2015). Concomitantly, the national debt rose from 105.4 % of GDP in 2007 to 175 % in 2013 and 177.1 % in 2014 (Eurostat 2015). To tackle the grave financial situation and in an attempt to avoid a potential default that would further endanger the stability of the global economy, the international community and the Greek government agreed on two bailout packages – the so-called Memoranda of Economic and Financial Policies, one amounting to 110 billion euros in 2010 and another one amounting to 158 billion euros in 2011. In return, the Greek government was expected to implement large-scale structural reforms and austerity measures under the close supervision of the European Commission, the European Central Bank and the International Monetary Fund – collectively known as "Troika" – while it proceeded to curbing public spending.

The wide-ranging social and health-related consequences of the enduring recession have now begun to unfold. The present chapter will elaborate on the mental health effects of the financial crisis in Greece, arguing for a substantial negative impact in the form of elevated rates of suicides as well as of major depression. However, in spite of the growing mental health needs of the population, there has been no policy framework for offsetting the mental health impact of the recession.

24.2 Socioeconomic Consequences

The hallmark of the social landscape in Greece during the ongoing financial crisis has been the sharp rises in unemployment rates. Unemployment figures had clustered around the 10 % mark in the first half of the previous decade, while before May 2008, they were at their lowest level for over a decade, reaching 6.6 % of the labour force (i.e. 325,000 people). Nonetheless, since then, they started displaying an upward course, with the number of employed individuals being reduced by 20 % (i.e. 930,000 people) during the time period 2010–2013. In particular, as a corollary of the implemented measures that disrupted and dismantled the labour market, unemployment rates rocketed amid the economic downturn with germane figures being 7.7 % in 2008, 9.5 % in 2009, 12.6 % in 2010, 17.7 % in 2011, 24.3 % in 2012, 27.5 % in 2013 and 26.5 % in 2014 (Eurostat 2015). It merits noting that in year 2015, 25.6 % of citizens were found to be unemployed, the highest figure recorded in the Eurozone (Eurostat 2015). Data emanating from monthly reports of Manpower Employment Organization provide additional information about the predicament of unemployment in the country. In the July 2015 report, the number of registered people seeking for work was found to be 817,787 (Manpower Employment Organization 2015). Among them, 463,595 individuals (i.e. 56.69 %) were looking for work for more than a year, underscoring the long duration of unemployment in Greece. Furthermore, during the particular month only 101,257 citizens (i.e. 12.38 %) received benefits for their status.

According to a report elaborating on the social impact of the Greek crisis, labour market institutions and norms in Greece protected male breadwinners at the expense of their wives and grown-up children prior to the outset of the recession (Matsaganis 2013) The rationale for this had been to ensure that unemployment was not translated into poverty. In other words, unemployed and poor people seemed to correspond to two different population subgroups, with the former category entailing predominantly wives of employed men and young people living with their parents, whereas the latter included the elderly and those residing in rural regions (Matsaganis 2013). Nonetheless – in accord to the same report – primary earners were gravely hit by the crisis. A decrease in employment rate was more pronounced among male workers aged between 30 and 44 years: from 93.8 % in 2008 to 74.1 % in 2013, a substantial drop of 21 % in less than 5 years. It is therefore clear that population subgroups that were protected against the pernicious effects of unemployment during the previous decades were also at stake amid the recession with vast implications for themselves and their families.

The second defining feature of the social landscape in Greece amid the economic contraction has been the rising rates of poverty. In accordance to data provided by the Hellenic Statistical Authority, the population who is at risk of poverty or social exclusion was found to rise from 28.1 % in 2008 to 35.7 % in 2013 and 36 % in 2014 (Hellenic Statistical Authority 2015). Moreover, a survey by the Hellenic Confederation of Professionals, Craftsmen and Merchants (GSEVEE) documented substantial income loss for 93.7 % of households since the beginning of the crisis with ensuing reductions in expenses for basic goods and food (GSEEVE 2014). Furthermore, one out of three households reported being in arrears, while 42.5 % of respondents were pessimistic about the adequacy of their income to meet upcoming financial obligations. The negative impact of the financial crisis on Greek households is also substantiated by reports on the child population. According to data emanating from UNICEF, a stark increase in child poverty rate from 23 % in 2008 to 40.5 % in 2012 has been recorded (UNICEF 2014). Apart from poverty and income loss, it merits noting that throughout the recession income inequality has also widened in Greece and in fact to a larger extent than the one observed in other European countries (Matsaganis and Leventi 2014).

Therefore, the economic crisis has yielded adverse consequences on the social landscape in Greece, which in turn have impinged on the health of the population.

24.3 Health Consequences

Reviews on the health effects of the financial crisis in Greece have suggested a gradual deterioration of public health (Kentikelenis et al. 2014; Simou and Koutsogeorgou 2014). In a single-country analysis and by employing a difference-to-difference approach, Vandoros and colleagues have substantiated a negative impact of the financial crisis on self-rated health in Greece (Vandoros et al. 2013). In a further study, a difference-to-difference analysis was performed in order to examine trends in self-rated health in Greece and Ireland as compared to a control country – Poland (Hessel et al. 2014). Evidence from the particular study suggests that the financial crisis has resulted in higher prevalence of poor health in Greece but not in Ireland.

Apart from self-report health indicators, it has been reported that during the time period 2009–2011, Greece has experienced unevenly high morbidity and mortality burden of certain large-scale epidemics, including an outbreak of West Nile virus infections and malaria and a major outbreak of HIV among injected drug users (Bonovas and Nikolopoulos 2012). Arguably, while most of these outbreaks have been attributed to environmental triggers, the preventive public health measures that would have contained the spread of these epidemics were not properly implemented, most likely due to dismantling of pertinent services (Kondilis et al. 2013).

In a recent article questioning the claim of a "major health tragedy" in Greece amid the recession, potential changes in 30 mortality-based health indicators during the financial crisis were investigated in three countries: Finland, Iceland and Greece (Tapia Granados and Rodriguez 2015). Findings indicate that only five indicators displayed significant deterioration in Greece: HIV incidence, maternal mortality, ill-defined conditions, infant mortality and suicide. Consistent with this, it seems that the impact of the crisis on the health of the Greek population is not across the board and it has influenced the incidence of particular diseases. Similarly, a recent study investigating trends in cardiovascular risk factors during the recession by analysing three waves of the "Hellas Health" survey in years 2006, 2008 and 2011 revealed that while fruit and vegetable consumption decreased to an alarming degree during the crisis, trends in smoking prevalence and physical activity were favourable (Filippidis et al. 2014). Additionally, socioeconomic disparities in fruit and vegetable consumption, physical activity and tobacco use were documented, rendering certain people – especially those of lower socioeconomic level – particularly vulnerable to cardiovascular disease.

In line with the aforementioned, the impact of the recession on health is not uniform in Greece, as it has particularly affected the onset of specific diseases and it has afflicted different population subgroups unevenly.

24.4 Mental Health Consequences: Suicide

The effect of the financial crisis on suicides has engendered a lively debate in Greece (Economou et al. 2011; Fountoulakis et al. 2012; Kentikelenis et al. 2011; Kontaxakis et al. 2013; Liaropoulos 2012; Stuckler et al. 2011). Recently, a 30-year interrupted time series analysis exploring the influence of austerity- and prosperity-related events on the occurrence of suicide during the time period 1983–2012, based on data provided by the Hellenic Statistical Authority, corroborated a significant, abrupt and sustained increase in total suicides (by 35.7 %) after the passage of new austerity measures in June 2011 (Branas et al. 2015). Similarly, another ecological study performed a joint point analysis to identify discontinuities in suicide trends between the time periods 2003–2010 and 2011–2012 as well as it sought to explore their association with GDP and unemployment throughout the entire period (Rachiotis et al. 2015). Results from this study confirmed a rise in total suicide rate by 35 % between 2010 and 2012. Moreover, a significant correlation between suicide mortality and unemployment, especially among working-age men, was also demonstrated. The strong correlation between suicide mortality and unemployment has also been supported by another study, which has advanced existing knowledge about the correlates of suicide mortality in Greece by providing evidence for its substantial association with public debt, HIV incidence and homicides (Madianos et al. 2014).

Congruent with these, the recession and the pertinent austerity measures have gravely impinged on the health of the population by triggering an increase in suicide mortality. The steep rises in unemployment rates seem to be playing a prominent role in driving this phenomenon.

24.5 Mental Health Consequences: Common Mental Disorders

On the grounds of the socioeconomic turmoil in the country and based on international evidence suggesting an increase in the prevalence of affective disorders as a corollary to the global recession (Lee et al. 2010; Wang et al. 2010; WHO 2011), the

University Mental Health Research Institute (UMHRI) designed and implemented a series of repeated nationwide cross-sectional surveys on the prevalence of major depression and suicidality in years 2008, 2009, 2011 and 2013. All telephone surveys had a similar methodology and drew different samples from the base population. The sampling frame was the national phone-number databank, which provides coverage for the vast majority of households in the country. A random sample of telephone numbers belonging to individuals were selected from the directory, and within each household, the person who had their birthday last was selected for the interview. Response rates were high and all samples were comparable and representative of the Greek population. For the detection of major depression and suicidality, the germane modules of the Structured Clinical Interview (SCID-I) were employed (First et al. 1996). Respondents, who reported experiencing one or both of the two core symptoms of major depression for at least 2 weeks in the month preceding the interview, were asked about experiencing seven additional symptoms most of the time throughout the same time period. Participants recounting at least five symptoms overall were further enquired about the extent to which the symptoms interfered with their level of functioning at work and at home and with their interpersonal relationships. Moreover, they were asked four additional questions in an attempt to disentangle the presence of major depression from symptoms explained by a general medical condition, the direct physiological effect of a substance (medication and/or street drugs) and bereavement. The diagnosis was found to have good psychometric properties.

For assessing participants' degree of financial strain, the Index of Personal Economic Distress, an original, self-constructed scale, was used (Madianos et al. 2011). The particular scale encompasses eight items tapping respondents' difficulty in fulfilling daily financial demands of a household during 6 months preceding the interview. Responses were made on a three-point scale, reflecting a frequency dimension, (1) never, (2) sometimes and (3) often, while the overall scale score can range from 8 (no economic hardship) to 24 (serious economic hardship). In the 2013 survey, an item was added in the Index enquiring about participants' difficulty in meeting financial obligations related to paying taxes and health/pension contributions. The persistent nature of the recession in Greece has engendered different sources of financial strain throughout the years necessitating therefore the revision of the scale.

All interviews were conducted by well-trained interviewers, graduates of social sciences.

The findings of all four surveys indicate a gradual but steady increase in 1-month prevalence of major depression. In particular, in 2008, when the crisis had not begun in Greece, 1-month prevalence of major depression was 3.3 % (Madianos et al. 2011). Since then, an upward course has been recorded: 6.8 % in 2009, 8.2 % in 2011 and 12.3 % in 2013 (Madianos et al. 2011; Economou et al. 2013b, 2015). On the contrary, 1-month prevalence of suicidality had increased during the time period 2008–2011; however it declined thereafter. Specifically, pertinent figures for suicidal ideation were found to be 2.4 % in 2008, 5.2 % in 2009, 6.7 % in 2011 and 2.6 % in 2013, while for suicidal attempt, they were 0.6 % in 2008, 1.1 % in 2009, 1.5 % in

2011 and 0.9 % in 2013 (Economou et al. 2016). This different pattern of results has also been observed in South Korea as a result of the Asian economic crisis (Organization for Economic Cooperation & Development 2007), and it can be explained in line with evidence suggesting that while depression involves a prolonged course of symptoms prior to reaching the threshold of a clinical diagnosis, suicidal acts may constitute an acute response to the onset of a crisis (Hong et al. 2011).

Regarding the risk factors for major depression, throughout the 5-year period of the recession in Greece, different variables have appeared to be heightening the odds of suffering from the disorder. The only variable that has consistently constituted a risk factor for major depression in all four surveys is financial distress. It merits noting that the strong association between economic hardship and major depression has been recorded in other studies as well (Ahnquist and Wamala 2011; Meltzer et al. 2012). Surprisingly, the strong influence of unemployment on major depression has predominantly emerged in the 2013 survey (Economou et al. 2016), perhaps due to the steep rises in unemployment rates after 2011 and the growing realisation of its long duration.

Interestingly, when the impact of unemployment and financial hardship on suicidality is explored, their effects are retained, even after controlling for the presence of major depression (Economou et al. 2015). In this rationale, during the economic crisis in Greece, there are suicidality symptoms related to the presence of major depression as well as symptoms independent of the disorder and pertinent to the socioeconomic turmoil in the country. This is congruent with the view that apart from the clinical manifestations of affective disorders in certain individuals in Greece, there is a widespread "social sorrow" which should not be overlooked or underestimated (Stylianidis 2011) – for an elaboration on the concept of "social sorrow", the reader is encouraged to refer to the germane chapter of the present book. Moreover, evidence from the UK suggests that in 2010 and 2011 issues pertaining to financial hardship and employment contributed substantially to 13 % of suicides, while they were the key contributing factor in 4 % of them (Coope et al. 2015). It is therefore clear that the occurrence of major depression and suicidality is greatly influenced by the socioeconomic hallmarks of the recession in Greece: unemployment and economic hardship.

In sharp contrast to the findings related to major depression, the prevalence of generalised anxiety disorder (GAD) was found to be impervious to the influence of the financial crisis. Similarly to major depression, its presence was assessed through incorporating the corresponding module of the SCID-I in all three surveys (First et al. 1996). In 2008, 1-year prevalence of GAD was 3.7 %, in 2009 it was 3.8 %, and in 2011 it was 4 %. In a publication delineating changes in 1-year prevalence of GAD between 2009 and 2011, it was shown that the most substantial increases were observed in men, people of working age, married individuals, respondents who had completed undergraduate studies, employed participants and citizens of Athens (Economou et al. 2013a). These results are possibly explained by the adverse working conditions in the country. The fast-paced increases in unemployment as well as the popularity of part-time employment regimes seem to have created an omnipresent fear of job loss and job insecurity, which in turn has given rise to the development of GAD.

Interestingly, when a potential protective influence of cognitive social capital on the presence of major depression and GAD was investigated, the findings were contrary to expectations (Economou et al. 2014b). Specifically, interpersonal and institutional trust, the two indices of cognitive social capital employed, were found to be inversely related to the presence of major depression but not to GAD. It is highly likely that trust may alleviate the anxiety triggered by certain environmental stimuli but cannot cover the full range of events eliciting worry in people who suffer from the disorder, hence the non-significant impact. Nonetheless, the particular findings were recorded for people reporting low economic distress. On the other hand, in people experiencing high financial distress, trust was no longer a protective factor for neither major depression nor GAD, indicating in this way a moderating influence of financial strain. The particular finding resembles to some extent research on high-poverty areas in the USA, where social capital has been linked to elevated rates of mental distress (Mitchell and LaGory 2002). The authors of the aforementioned study have argued that community connections in these areas can engender a number of obligations, leading people to tackle converging difficulties, stemming from both their personal life and the community. In this reasoning, close interpersonal relationships, which are founded on trust, can result in additional emotional burden through social contagion pathways. In line with this, the findings of the epidemiological surveys in Greece echo the conclusions drawn by other researchers that promoting social capital alone, i.e. without addressing socioeconomic indicators, may be ineffective means for promoting mental health and preventing the onset of mental disorders (Ahnquist et al. 2012; Phongsavan et al. 2006).

Apart from the surveys conducted by the UMHRI, complementary evidence for the mental health effects of the financial crisis in Greece are yielded from the 2009 to 2010 Psychiatric Morbidity Survey and from data gleaned in the context of the UMHRI Depression Helpline. The Psychiatric Morbidity Survey was conducted by the University of Ioannina on a nationally representative sample of the adult population in Greece (Skapinakis et al. 2013). It was a household survey and data were collected between September 2009 and February 2010 (i.e. amid financial crisis). For assessing participants' psychiatric morbidity, the Revised Clinical Interview Schedule (CIS-R) was employed for tapping common mental disorders as well as the Alcohol Use Disorders Identification Test (AUDIT) for alcohol use. The response rate of the survey was 54 % and it estimated 1-week prevalence of common mental disorders. The results of the survey showed that 14 % of the population suffered from clinical significant psychiatric morbidity. Generalised anxiety disorder was the preponderant disorder (prevalence, 4.1 %), followed by depression (2.9 %), phobias (2.79 %), mixed anxiety-depression (2.67 %), panic disorder (1.88 %) and obsessive-compulsive disorder (1.69 %). Harmful alcohol use was recorded for 12.69 % of the population. Regarding the risk factors for mental disorders, female gender, divorced or widowed marital status, low educational attainment and unemployment were positively associated with clinical significant psychiatric morbidity. Differences in the prevalence of major depression between the UMHRI surveys and the 2009–2010 Psychiatric Morbidity Survey can be accounted for by the different methodologies adopted: household survey vs. telephone survey (Crete was excluded from the 2009 to 2010 Psychiatric Morbidity Survey), 1-week prevalence vs. 1-month prevalence and CIS-R vs. SCID-I.

With regard to the UMHRI Depression Helpline, a nationwide telephone helpline providing information on mental health issues and brief counselling services from 2008 to 2014, a steep increase is documented in calls with direct or indirect reference to the economic decline during the first half of 2010 and onwards (Economou et al. 2012). The callers who referred to the recession manifested depressive symptomatology of clinical significance to a greater extent than callers who made no such reference. In addition, a higher frequency of depressive symptoms was discerned among unemployed individuals, whereas employed people were found to experience anxiety symptoms to a higher degree. It merits noting that anxiety and depression symptoms were assessed with the pertinent Goldberg scales (Goldberg et al. 1988).

Concerning self-reported indicators of mental health, the findings are similar to the ones derived by the use of clinical instruments, employed in the aforementioned studies (SCID, CIS-R, Goldberg Depression and Anxiety Scales). Data emanating from two cross-sectional nationwide surveys in years 2006 and 2011 were compared with regard to depressive symptoms, assessed with the question: "During the last 4 weeks, how often did you feel sad/depressed and that nothing could improve your mood?" (Mylona et al. 2014). Findings from this study support that in 2011 there was greater likelihood of respondents reporting feeling sad or depressed as compared to 2006. Additionally, income, education and unemployment were found to constitute decisive determinants of depressive symptomatology.

It is therefore conspicuous that the sustained recession in Greece has resulted in increasing prevalence rates of major depression for the population as a whole. Rises in unemployment and financial hardship emerge as the most plausible accounts for this impact.

24.6   Healthcare Consequences

In spite of the growing mental health needs of the population, the ongoing financial crisis has impinged on the healthcare system as well (Economou et al. 2014a). In the wake of the economic crisis in Greece, the National Health System (NHS) had already been in a state of crisis, as demonstrated by substantial problems in efficiency, healthcare provision, organisation, structure and management as well as a fragmented administrative framework, an extensive private sector, a dearth of primary healthcare services and insufficient hospitals and workforce (Emmanouilidou and Burke 2013). Moreover, the absence of a functioning referral system between primary- and higher-level care in tandem with problematic pricing and provider reimbursement mechanisms resulted in poor coordination of care, large informal payments and a sizable black economy, hindering further the system's ability to deliver equitable financing and access to services (Liaropoulos et al. 2008).

Congruent with these, the recession has brought the country's healthcare system in the throes of collapse (McKee et al. 2012). According to a systematic literature review on the topic, the economic downturn has incurred deleterious consequences on healthcare, including curbing of public health expenditures, reductions in the number of health professionals and their salaries, cuts in pensions, decreases in the procurement of medical supplies, rapid reforms in the pharmaceutical and social insurance sectors as well as inadequate primary healthcare services (Simou and Koutsogeorgou 2014). Furthermore, access to and provision of healthcare services are hampered, out-of-pocket contributions have persisted and monitoring and efficiency issues have been discerned. It is noteworthy that while there is a growing unwillingness on the part of citizens to pay informally for healthcare services, an increasing demand for these payments, either as a prerequisite for access to services or to redeem services provided, has been recently demonstrated (Souliotis et al. 2016).

Similar problems have been documented in the mental healthcare system. Mental health services have downsized their operations and personnel, while public funding for mental health was reduced by 20 % between 2010 and 2011 and by additional 55 % between 2011 and 2012 (Anagnostopoulos and Soumaki 2013). The psychiatric and neurology departments of the Eginition Hospital are on the verge of collapse, psychiatric inpatient departments of general hospitals have to tackle an enormous workload as they are operating at 120 % of their capacity and mental health professionals suffer from burnout and impaired morale (Hyphantis 2013).

Therefore, in spite of the growing mental health needs of the population during the recession in Greece, the mental healthcare system appears incapable of addressing them.

24.7 Alleviating the Mental Health Effects of the Crisis

Various papers have been published in order to provide a comprehensive framework for mitigating the mental health effects of the economic crisis (Christodoulou and Christodoulou 2013; Wahlbeck and McDaid 2012; World Health Organization 2011); however, not all of their recommendations fit neatly to the Greek reality. Restructuring of mental health services should become a top priority, accompanied by active labour market programmes, debt relief programmes and enhancement of social capital. In particular, to meet the growing mental health needs of the economic crisis, emphasis should be given on buttressing community-based mental health services, which have been shown to prevent against suicide mortality (Pirkola et al. 2009; While et al. 2012). An integrated care approach promoting service provision in primary care will facilitate access to mental healthcare and shift the focus to prevention and early detection of mental health problems. Concomitantly, the mental healthcare system must cultivate resilience-strengthening elements in the community, to create a comprehensive and accessible network while targeting the stigma attached to mental disorders in order to make services both accessible and acceptable.

Active labour market programmes usually endeavour to improve changes of people finding gainful employment and usually encompass public employment services, labour market training, special programmes for young people in transition from school to work and programmes to provide or promote employment for people with disabilities. In light of the alarmingly high rates of unemployment in the country, there is an urgent need for the implementation of this type of interventions.

Regarding debt relief programmes, reforms of bankruptcy laws and establishment of debt management advisors may be helpful in protecting mental health. Generally, there is a need for national initiatives to encourage cooperation and communication between health services and debt management agencies. Debt management advisers should be trained to refer clients to mental healthcare when needed, and conversely, mental health providers should acknowledge the role of financial strain and refer people with mental health problems to debt advice bureaus (Fitch et al. 2009).

For enhancing social capital, participation in community activities should be encouraged, in line with evidence suggesting that social networks, such as trade unions, religious congregations and sport clubs, seem to constitute a safety net against the adverse repercussions of rapid macroeconomic changes (Stuckler et al. 2009).

To the authors' knowledge, no policy framework specific to offset the mental health impact of the recession in Greece has been designed nor implemented.

The only intervention to tackle with the increasing prevalence of major depression in a cost-effective and empowering manner, while promoting the social capital of the community amid the recession in Greece, is the joint initiative "Citizens Against Depression". In particular, the Regional Development and Mental Health Association (EPAPSY), the Greek Association for Mood Disorders (MAZI), the Charity Office of the Archdiocese of Athens and the Association of Families and Friends of Mental Health of Northern Attica collaborate in order to promote self-help groups for fighting depression in the community. In March 2014, in the context of "We Are All Citizens" programme funded by EEA Grants for Greece, the Regional Development and Mental Health Association and the Salten Psychiatric Centre in Bodo, Norway, developed a bilateral partnership for sharing their knowledge and experiences of self-help groups. Their programme includes the following:

(i) Development of a training module
(ii) Development of an e-learning platform, after adjusting training material to an e-learning format
(iii) Training of professionals who will be involved in ten key areas of Greece
(iv) Group therapy for depression and suicide prevention
(v) Training of users in organising and coordinating self-help groups
(vi) Facilitating self-help groups through establishing local meeting points in four target areas
(vii) Evaluation
(viii) Dissemination

The Maison Blanche Hospital in Paris has joined this effort by designing the evaluation of the initiative.

The programme is expected to empower individuals suffering from depressive symptoms, to reduce their perceived isolation and to reinforce their social networks, therefore fostering resilience. This is a currently ongoing effort and results are anticipated in the ensuing months.

Conclusion

The persistent recession in Greece has triggered a cascade of dire socioeconomic consequences, which in turn have impinged on the mental health of the population. While mounting evidence corroborates the growing mental health needs of the population, existing mental health services are incapable of addressing them. However, there has been no systematic effort on the part of national policy to design and implement interventions geared towards mitigating the mental health effects of the crisis. Echoing the conclusions drawn by the ex post evaluation of the implementation of psychiatric reform in the country (Loukidou et al. 2013), any plan to counteract the untoward effects of the financial crisis on mental health in the country relies on local initiatives by particular service providers. Congruent with this, the contention that the economic downturn may provide a window of opportunity for restructuring mental healthcare in Greece (Karamanoli 2011; Liaropoulos 2012) seems overoptimistic, if not futile. Concerted efforts – from policymakers, epidemiologists, health economists, clinicians, patients and their families – for ameliorating the mental health impact of the recession in Greece are urgently needed, in order to militate against exacerbation of psychiatric morbidity in the foreseeable future and to avoid a potential outbreak of suicides.

References

Ahnquist J, Wamala S, Lindstrom M (2012) Social determinants of health – a question of social or economic capital? Interaction effects of socioeconomic factors on health outcomes. Soc Sci Med 74:930–939

Ahnquist J, Wamala SP (2011) Economic hardships in adulthood and mental health in Sweden. The Swedish National Public Health Survey 2009. BMC Public Health 11:788–798

Anagnostopoulos DC, Soumaki E (2013) The state of child and adolescent psychiatry in Greece during the international financial crisis: a brief report. Eur Adolesc Child Psychiatry 22: 131–134

Bonovas S, Nikolopoulos G (2012) High- burden epidemics in Greece in the era of economic crisis. Early signs of a public health tragedy. J Prev Med Hyg 53:169–171

Branas C, Kastanaki A, Michalodimitrakis M, Tzougas J, Kranioti E, Theodorakis P et al (2015) The impact of economic austerity and prosperity events on suicide in Greece: a 30-year interrupted time-series analysis. BMJ Open 5(1):e005619–e005619

Christodoulou N, Christodoulou G (2013) Financial crises: impact on mental health and suggested responses. Psychother Psychosom 82(5):279–284

Coope C, Donovan J, Wilson C, Barnes M, Metcalfe C, Hollingworth W et al (2015) Characteristics of people dying by suicide after job loss, financial difficulties and other economic stressors during a period of recession (2010–2011): a review of coroners' records. J Affect Disord 183:98–105

Economou M, Madianos M, Theleritis C, Peppou L, Stefanis C (2011) Increased suicidality amid economic crisis in Greece. Lancet 378:1459

Economou M, Peppou L, Komporozos A, Mellou A, Stefanis C (2012) Depression telephone helpline: help seeking during the financial crisis. Psychiatriki 23:17–28

Economou M, Peppou L, Fousketaki S, Theleritis C, Patelakis A, Alexiou T et al (2013a) Economic crisis and mental health: effects on the prevalence of common mental disorders. Psychiatriki 24:247–261

Economou M, Madianos M, Peppou L, Patelakis A, Stefanis C (2013b) Major depression in the Era of economic crisis: a replication of a cross-sectional study across Greece. J Affect Disord 145(3):308–314

Economou C, Kaitelidou D, Kentikelenis A, Sissouras A, Maresso A (2014a) The impact of the financial crisis on health and the health system in Greece – case study. WHO/European Observatory on Health Systems and Policies, Copenhagen

Economou M, Madianos M, Peppou L, Souliotis K, Patelakis A, Stefanis C (2014b) Cognitive social capital and mental illness during economic crisis: a nationwide population-based study in Greece. Soc Sci Med 100:141–147

Economou M, Peppou L, Souliotis K (2015) Recent epidemiological data on the mental health effects of the economic crisis. Presentation, presented at the 19th congress of the Italian Society of Psychopathology, Milan

Economou M, Angelopoulos E, Peppou LE, Souliotis K, Stefanis C (2016) Suicidal ideation and suicide attempts in Greece during the economic crisis: an update. World Psychiatry, 15:83–84

Emmanouilidou M, Burke M (2013) A thematic review and a policy-analysis agenda of Electronic Health Records in the Greek National Health System. Health Policy 109(1):31–37

Eurostat (2010) Report of the revision of the Greek Government Deficit and Debt Figures. Available at: http://epp.eurostat.e.c.europa.eu/cache/ITY

Eurostat (2015) Eurostat statistics database 2015. Retrieved from http://epp.eurostat.ec.europa.eu

Filippidis F, Schoretsaniti S, Dimitrakaki C, Vardavas C, Behrakis P, Connolly G, Tountas Y (2014) Trends in cardiovascular risk factors in Greece before and during the financial crisis: the impact of social disparities. Eur J Public Health 24(6):974–979

Financial Crisis Inquiry Commission (2011) The financial crisis inquiry report. US Government Printing Office, Washington, DC

First M, Spitzer R, Gibbon M (1996) Structured clinical interview for DSM-IV axis I disorders, clinical version (SCID-CV). American Psychiatric Press, Washington, DC

Fitch C, Hamilton S, Bassett P, Davey R (2009) Debt and mental health: what do we know? What should we do? Royal College of Psychiatrists and Rethink, London

Fountoulakis K, Grammatikopoulos I, Koupidis S, Siamouli M, Theodorakis P (2012) Health and the financial crisis in Greece. Lancet 379:1001–1002

Goldberg D, Bridges K, Duncan-Jones P, Grayson D (1988) Detecting anxiety and depression in general medical settings. BMJ 297:897–899

Hellenic Confederation of Professionals, Craftsmen and Merchants (2014) Research on household income and expenses. GSEEVE, Athens

Hellenic Statistical Authority (2015) Risk of poverty. Research on income and living conditions of households 2014. HSA, Piraeus

Hessel P, Vandoros S, Avendano M (2014) The differential impact of the financial crisis on health in Ireland and Greece: a quasi-experimental approach. Public Health 128:911–919

Hong J, Knapp M, McGuire A (2011) Income-related inequalities in the prevalence of depression and suicidal behaviour: a 10-year trend following economic crisis. World Psychiatry 10:40–44

Hyphantis T (2013) The "depression" of mental health care in general hospitals in Greece in the era of recession. J Psychosom Res 74:530–532

Karamanoli E (2011) Debt crisis strains Greece's ailing health system. Lancet 378:303–304

Kentikelenis A, Karanikolos M, Papanicolas I, Basu S, McKee M, Stuckler D (2011) Health effects of financial crisis: omens of a Greek tragedy. Lancet 378(9801):1457–1458

Kentikelenis A, Karanikolos M, Reeves A, McKee M, Stuckler D (2014) Greece's health crisis: from austerity to denialism. Lancet 383:748–753

Kondilis E, Giannakopoulos S, Gavana M, Ierodiakonou I, Waitzkin H, Benos A (2013) Economic crisis, restrictive policies, and the population's health and health care: the Greek case. Am J Public Health 103:973–979

Kontaxakis V, Papaslanis C, Havaki-Kontaxaki B, Tsouvelas G, Giotakos O, Papadimitriou G (2013) Suicide in Greece: 2001–2011. Psychiatriki 24:170–174

Lee S, Guo W, Tsang A, Mak A, Wu J, Ng K, Kwok K (2010) Evidence for the 2008 economic crisis exacerbating depression in Hong Kong. J Affect Disord 126(1–2):125–133

Liaropoulos L (2012) Economic crisis and health in Greece, 2009–2012. BMJ 345:e7988

Liaropoulos L, Siskou O, Kaitelidou D, Theodorou M, Katostaras T (2008) Informal payments in public hospitals in Greece. Health Policy 87:72–81

Loukidou E, Mastroyannakis A, Power T, Craig T, Thornicroft G, Bouras N (2013) Greek mental health reform: views and perceptions of professionals and service users. Psychiatriki 24: 37–44

Madianos M, Economou M, Alexiou T, Stefanis C (2011) Depression and economic hardship across Greece in 2008 and 2009: two cross-sectional surveys nationwide. Soc Psychiatry Psychiatr Epidemiol 46:943–952

Madianos M, Alexiou T, Patelakis A, Economou M (2014) Suicide, unemployment and other socioeconomic factors: evidence from the economic crisis in Greece. Eur J Psychiatry 28(1):39–49

Manpower Employment Organization (2015) Brief report: registry of Manpower Employment Organization-July 2015. Manpower Employment Organization, Athens

Matsaganis M (2013) The Greek crisis: social impact and policy responses. Friedrich Ebert Stiftung, Berlin

Matsaganis M, Leventi C (2014) Poverty and inequality during the great recession in Greece. Polit Stud Rev 12(2):209–223

McKee M, Karanikolos M, Belcher P, Stuckler D (2012) Austerity: a failed experiment on the people of Europe. Clin Med 12:346–350

Meltzer H, Bebbington P, Brugha T, Farrell M, Jenkins R (2012) The relationship between personal debt and specific common mental disorders. Eur J Public Health 23:108–113

Mitchell C, LaGory M (2002) Social capital and mental distress in an impoverished community. City Community 1(2):199–222

Mylona K, Tsiantou V, Zavras D, Pavi E, Kyriopoulos J (2014) Determinants of self-reported frequency of depressive symptoms in Greece during economic crisis. Public Health 128:752–754

Organization for Economic Cooperation and Development (2007) OECD health report. Organization for Economic Cooperation and Development, Paris

Phongsavan P, Chey T, Bauman A, Brooks R, Silove D (2006) Social capital, socio-economic status and psychological distress among Australian adults. Soc Sci Med 63(10):2546–2561

Pirkola S, Sund R, Sailas E, Wahlbeck K (2009) Community mental-health services and suicide rate in Finland: a nationwide small-area analysis. Lancet 373:147–153

Rachiotis G, Stuckler D, McKee M, Hadjichristodoulou C (2015) What has happened to suicides during the Greek economic crisis? Findings from an ecological study of suicides and their determinants (2003–2012). BMJ Open 5(3):e007295

Simou E, Koutsogeorgou E (2014) Effects of the economic crisis on health and healthcare in Greece in the literature from 2009 to 2013: a systematic review. Health Policy 115:111–119

Skapinakis P, Bellos S, Koupidis S, Grammatikopoulos I, Theodorakis P, Mavreas V (2013) Prevalence and sociodemographic associations of common mental disorders in a nationally representative sample of the general population of Greece. BMC Psychiatry 13:163

Souliotis K, Golna C, Tountas Y, Siskou O, Kaitelidoy D, Liaropoulos L (2016) Informal payments in the Greek health sector amid the financial crisis: old habits die last. Eur J Health Econ, 17:159–170

Stuckler D, King L, McKee M (2009) Mass privatisation and the postcommunist mortality crisis: a cross-national analysis. Lancet 373:399–407

Stuckler D, Basu S, Suhrcke M, Coutts A, McKee M (2011) Effects of the 2008 recession on health: a first look at European data. Lancet 378(9786):124–125

Stylianidis S (2011) The clinical perspective on what is temporary – aspects of individual and social sorrow: clinical and social questions from a psychoanalytic standpoint. Oedipus 5:229–249

Tapia Granados J, Rodriguez J (2015) Health, economic crisis, and austerity: a comparison of Greece, Finland and Iceland. Health Policy 119:941–953

United Nation's Children's Fund (2014) Children of the recession: the impact of the economic crisis on child well-being in rich countries. UNICEF, Florence

Vandoros S, Hessel P, Leone T, Avendano M (2013) Have health trends worsened in Greece as a result of the financial crisis? A quasi-experimental approach. Eur J Public Health 23:727–731

Wahlbeck K, McDaid D (2012) Actions to alleviate the mental health impact of the economic crisis. World Psychiatry 11:139–145

Wang J, Smailes E, Sareen J, Fick G, Schmitz N, Patten S (2010) The prevalence of mental disorders in the working population over the period of global economic crisis. Can J Psychiatry 55:598–605

While D, Bickley H, Roscoe A, Windfuhr K, Rahman S, Shaw J et al (2012) Implementation of mental health service recommendations in England and Wales and suicide rates, 1997–2006: a cross-sectional and before-and-after observational study. Lancet 379:1005–1012

World Bank (2015) GDP growth (% annual), 2015. Retrieved from http://data.worldbank.org/indicator/NY.GDP.MKTP.KD.ZG

World Health Organization (2011) Impact of economic crises on mental health. WHO, Geneva

Afterword: The Economic Crisis and Mental Health

25

Stelios Stylianidis, Panagiotis Chondros, and Michael Lavdas

Abstract

In this chapter, we provide a brief description of the European and Greek political and social context of the economic crisis, in order to gain a better understanding of the effects of these circumstances on public health and particularly on mental health. Then, we refer to the impact of the economic crisis on mental and general public health. Finally, we present certain proposals and innovative initiatives in the mental health field. Unlike the recurrent distorted ideas and paralysing inward-looking approach so common in modern Greek psychiatric institutions, we choose to present specific examples of *interventions* which are in keeping with the spirit of critical rationality and reflection which pervades this book.

25.1 Introduction

The economic crisis produced a number of significant changes on a microeconomic level, such as loss of jobs and social insecurity about the future, increase in household debts and rapidly increasing social inequality which threaten social cohesion and resilience of every person as well as of social links and networks.

S. Stylianidis
Department of Psychology, Panteion University, Athens, Greece
e-mail: stylianidis.st@gmail.com

P. Chondros • M. Lavdas (✉)
Association for Regional Development and Mental Health (EPAPSY), Athens, Greece
e-mail: pan_ch@otenet.gr; ml@epapsy.gr

Such changes – dramatic both in terms of intensity and quality – are decisive for the life and survival of citizens, as well as the ability to invest in a better future, insofar as this ability is closely linked to the economic, mental and family resources of rapidly growing and expanding excluded social groups.

It is generally acknowledged, based on research data from the public health and public mental health field, that unemployment, poverty, homelessness, breakdown of family and social bonds and the difficulty and/or lack of access to health services have a negative impact on the mental health indicators of the general population (Saraceno et al. 2007; Saraceno and Barbui 1997; Mezzich and Saraceno 2007; Drew et al. 2005). All available literature demonstrates that social inequalities have the most negative impact on the outcome of the mental health of individuals, along with unemployment, part-time employment, job insecurity, low educational and social level (Marmot 2005, 2013; Patel et al. 2010; Bambra 2010). A degraded urban environment and low quality of life lead to an increase in the prevalence of mental disorders.

The impact of the economic crisis on southern European countries has led, inter alia, to budget cuts for health, mental health, social services and programmes, as well as to significant cuts in the social benefits and disability pensions.

In Greece, the multilevel crisis and protracted recession have had a decisive effect on the rise in prevalence of mental disorders in the general population and, in particular, the increase in cases of depression and attempted suicide, as well the increase in applications for psychiatric and psychological help and treatment, while at the same time, the dismantlement of public mental health service system, due to underfunding, is under way (Stylianidis 2012).

Consequently, the major challenges faced by the partners in the field mental health and the suspended psychiatric reforms should be "preventive" in nature and are as follows:

To prevent the exclusion or degradation of mental health due to social policy priorities and health policies in general
To prevent the further fragmentation and weakening of the network of mental health structures and to reduce staff burnout
To stimulate the resourcefulness of therapeutic teams and public health policymakers and to provide innovative responses to a range of new social suffering, social exclusion and psychopathology issues
To develop new innovative actions and cooperations and to substantiate their effectiveness under the current conditions and opportunities arising from the protracted crisis

It goes without saying that the management of and response to these challenges exceed the limits of the psychiatric community and the wider field of mental health in general. For this reason, we are setting out below a broad introduction to the sociological framework of the crisis at European level. In an overall systemic crisis, such as the current crisis, there is an urgent need for the active participation of professionals, the movements of families and users of mental health services in the development of political interventions and proposals which operate effectively on the local level and to plan interventions on the national and European level.

25.2 The Deficit of Democracy in Europe, Social Insecurity and Vulnerable Social Ties

The European project was initially based by its fathers on a political and cultural vision and the desire to unify the old continent after two destructive wars, which had begun in Europe. The original core Member States of the former EEC had a sound basis of common financial interests as well as the political will to develop a rule of law and a strong social protection net for its most vulnerable social groups. Free access of European citizens to quality health, social welfare and education services, as well as the declared aim of reducing social inequalities and social exclusion formed part of the European identity, a non-negotiable axiological system.

According to Castel (2003), there are two main types of protection:

(a) *Constitutional protection*, which guarantees the basic freedoms and safety of goods and persons in a framework based on the rule of law
(b) *Social protection*, which covers the basic risks that could lead a person to a deterioration of his/her situation, such as illness, accidents, old age, social exclusion situations and "transience" of existence

These two keystones are the basis of the European project under the shared vision for a post-war Europe. These principles of protection came close to such an axiological, ethical, legal and institutional level that Western Europe was characterised a "secure" society, in the sense that it was capable of providing security and protection to its members. The position we advocate here is that the manner in which democracy operates in the European region in these times of systemic crisis has a dark side to it, an increasing deficit which creates insecurity, instability and threat against citizens, people previously protected by the rule of law.

In a very sketchy way, we can describe three main deficits of democracy:

(a) A *policy deficit* in relation to the dominant narrative of market overinvestment without regulatory measures consistent with a globalised economy, the protection of banks and stock exchanges – a deficit which, inter alia, results in the marginalisation of the traditional policy role. Today, policy, and, moreover, the composition of governments, is imposed by the markets and not by the political institutions.

   For instance, the increasing accumulation of capital is not invested in the establishment of new innovative enterprises and the creation of new jobs and, consequently, to curb the phenomenon of unemployment and its numerous implications. This stagnation reproduces the vicious cycle of increasing social inequalities and social exclusion, the vulnerability of new social groups and also wars or threats of war.
(b) A *deficit of democracy* in the functioning of European institutions and, notably, the European Commission. If we consider the matter from a purely formal perspective, there is no deficit in the EU, insofar as its leaders are elected by the

national and European elective bodies. However, the decision-making process and crisis management of both economic and international conflicts, lack of procedural transparency and lobbying in various areas (foreign policy, financing, targeted controls, criteria governing the selection of programmes, etc.) indicate this is a "nondemocratic" democracy. Prime ministers are elected by the citizens of the Member States. However, they are just pawns in a geopolitical chess game determined by the International Monetary Fund (IMF), the European Central Bank (ECT) and European Commission bureaucrats. The real influence of the European Parliament is in fact insignificant in this complicated jigsaw puzzle of interests, just as marginal as the influence of civic society and the Council of Europe.

Daily, we are seeing a crisis of confidence which defines the relationship between the EU and its citizens. The citizens' lukewarm participation in European elections confirms this claim. In fact, European institutions cannot claim any real legitimacy without a minimum level of economic, social and cultural cohesion. By way of illustration, we refer to a recent article by Jäcklein (2014), "10 threats to Europeans", published in the respected *Monde Diplomatique* where the above information can be found in one place:

Disregard of basic worker's rights
Reduction of workers' rights to collective representation
Relaxation of technical norms and standards
Restrictions on the free movement of people
Absence of sanctions against abuse
The progressive disappearance of public services
Increased unemployment
Loss of confidentiality of personal data
Subordination of people to intellectual property rights
Subordination of states to laws tailor made for multinationals

Unable to react in the face of these "threats", national governments – as also witnessed in Greece – are experiencing a dramatic weakening of their role. There are two basic reasons for this: First, because every decision taken by a Member State government comes up against a faceless bureaucratic mechanism of the European Commission which requires compliance with the rules and previous agreements, aimed at the so-called European harmonisation of the partners. Second, because traditional political parties can no longer perform the role of representing their social base, insofar as they are confronted with insurmountable difficulties in effectively fulfilling the citizens' agenda in the face of the above-mentioned "grey area" of how European institutions operate.

We find ourselves between an illusion and a tragedy: this Europe does not interest its citizens-electors enough to mobilise them in order to radically change this hopeless situation. Conversely, the rise of Eurosceptics, populists and extreme right-wing parties with their divisive rhetoric in the last elections makes this change a far more complex and difficult task.

A fundamental antithesis which allows us to gain a better understanding of the current crisis is that a process of alliance aimed at creating a common currency was brought forward. However, this "Euro agreement" was not supported by a relevant process to ensure the political union of the Member States. As a direct result, "economic stabilisation" rather than the political management of the crisis was imposed, under German leadership, through the imposition of extreme austerity measures. Unemployment was the key weapon in reducing the southern European country competitiveness deficit, resulting, inter alia, in a lack of growth, drop in family income, worsening of budgetary deficits, a huge social cost and a dramatic increase in social inequalities (Lapavitsas 2014). In short, neoliberal policy imposed stabilisation through the destruction on the European South.

25.3 Social Insecurity and Uncertainty About the Future

These dramatic changes, both political and economic, have many implications on the cohesion of every social structure. The last decade for most European countries was marked by a rather latent and less clear move towards individualism, growing insecurity and weakening of collectivism. Everyone is fighting for themselves, their individual survival or the strengthening of their own group's narrow special interests. Systemic media present such profound transformations of society, financial disaster and breakdown of interpersonal and social relations as a "matter of course" and as a current requirement for mobility, adaptation, temporary redundancy of workers and "flexicurity", as the institutionalization of job insecurity has been shamelessly defined in EU "jargon". Everything is fluid and mobile; without fixed points of reference, everything is ephemeral, both labour relations and emotional relationships and human relationships (Bauman 2013a, b).

When the implementation of the rules of "deregulation" of labour relations meets with serious resistance, when the model of "precarious growth" is not established (Beck 1992), then a tough austerity policy is imposed to remove the obstacles arising from budgetary deficits. Austerity policies which are promoted with dogmatic fanaticism in Europe by the mechanisms of German hegemony – with a protestant flavour to them – should be imposed exclusively since "There Is No Alternative" (TINA).

Within the framework of such dominance of the neoliberal model of economic and social governance, every social solidarity concept and tradition is degraded and discredited as resistance to market liberalisation, competitiveness and self-regulation of free trade. Every coherent social protection programme which, of course, differs from the various humanitarian actions promoted by the Media is considered a relic of the past, part of a costly and ineffective welfare state, which stands in the way of "unlocking" creativity and autonomy in the area of "entrepreneurship" of every free individual. Hereat, we note a full distortion of reality by the mandarins of the markets, which is based on certain actual problems and failures of the welfare state, in Greece and in Europe: instead of improving and evaluating the services and benefits, we close down services and cancel social protection (Sakellis 2012).

However, new vulnerable social groups are emerging as a result of the crisis: the poor, the disabled, the homeless and the elderly, children without protection, unprotected mothers, single-parent families, migrating populations due to wars and disasters, economic migrants and political refugees and the long-term unemployed. All these people are living in a vicious cycle of poverty, social exclusion and physical and mental vulnerability, which in turn leads to their greater marginalization (see also conclusions in the Chap. 4). It is self-evident that the way to deal with and care for all these "outcasts" of a system which produces increasing inequalities cannot be to classify them into diagnostic categories and create – in a setting of shortage of resources – specialised services for each separate category. As aptly put by Castel (2000, 2013), addressing the complex needs of such populations is not just about securing material resources, but primarily about redesigning a social policy which takes seriously into account the growing process of social disaffiliation.

The conclusions of the researchers participating in the study of the social phenomena of globalisation and the systemic features of the economic crisis are largely in agreement (Giddens 2004; Beck 1992, 2006).

25.4 Greece's Special Situation

There is an immense volume of literature about the special features of the Greek crisis in the wider European context, too much in fact to be presented in the context of this chapter. Unavoidably, we shall limit ourselves to making our observations on certain aspects of the crisis which are directly or indirectly related to the failure of the reforms in our country and, consequently, the suspended step of Greek psychiatric reform and the enormous challenges facing the fragmented system of mental health services in our country under extreme crisis conditions.

The need for bold reforms in Greece was already clear since the birth of the Greek state in the face of the "ineffective, irrational and/or morally unacceptable mode of operation of its institutions" (Veremis et al. 2011).

For several years, various clandestine processes have been underway which have brought the country to the brink of the abyss, namely, the autistic political system, the gradual weakening and unbridled partisanship of institutions, widespread corruption, lawlessness and impunity, distorting of incentives and national introversion (Veremis, Tsoukas op. cit.: 12).

As Pantazopoulos (2013) characteristically points out regarding the common logic after the transition from dictatorship to democracy: "The people's proactive creativity was blocked, social responsibility was undermined and political elitists were 'coerced' in becoming a component of society because of the way in which the social bond was symbolically represented within a self-victimising but, at the same time, resistant society. The problem, therefore, is political and cultural. Political in that the political order is not independent of social interests, therefore, the first is high-jacked by the latter. Cultural in that meaning-generating structures remained intact (political nationalist-populism)".

Greece became, once again, Europe's utopia, but which Europe and what kind of utopia? Tsoukalas (2012) wrote that the European Union is not characterised by a deficit of democracy as claimed so far. It has developed into a mechanism detached from European societies, which operates as the battering ram of the general interests of the financial system. It is forcibly trying to make European societies adapt to a new bare market capitalism model, devoid of any pre-capitalism remnants and also devoid of social compensation mechanisms which date from the historical compromises dictated, inter alia, by post-war social-democratic politics. It is the triumph of market ethics and principles, which is expressed via a punitive speech code and a possessive morality. Greece represents the utopia of implementing such a policy. That is why everyone is aware that the challenge is not to write off the debt but to change the country based on the European new neoliberal model.

25.5 Economic Crisis and Mental Health

From 2009 and onwards, a number of articles were published, at both European and national level, in scientific and other publications about the effects of the economic crisis on health (Karanikolos et al. 2013; Marmot and Bell 2009). The World Health Organisation already since 2001 makes it perfectly clear that the correlation between socioeconomic factors, such as unemployment, the uncertain work environment, the move down the social ladder, housing and other specific health indicators, is undisputable and substantiated by solid research facts (WHO 2003, 2009). The depletion and lack of resources, at the personal and state level, appear to be affecting the quality of life, access to adequate and appropriate care and the population's level of health (Tsiantou and Kyriopoulos 2010).

As far as Greece is concerned, there is a division of opinion as to whether specific indicators, such as, for instance, suicides, have worsened and whether this is a result of the crisis (Kentikelenis et al. 2011, 2012, 2014; Madianos et al. 2011; Fountoulakis and Theodorakis 2014; Fountoulakis et al. 2012). In the 1990s, while researching the role of various factors which could help us interpret this data, such as dietary habits or informal care networks, we frequently encountered the term "paradox of health" (Philalithis 2001) which described the fact that health indicators, e.g. life expectancy, cardiovascular diseases, etc., in Greece – despite its fewer health resources – were better. According to the OECD's data (2014a), the paradox, on a first reading of "hard" indicators, seems to have persisted. Health expenditure as a percentage of GDP increased from 8 % in 2000 to 9.3 % in 2012 and was even up to 10 % in 2010. However, per capita spending on health fell from 3,000 USD to 2,100 USD compared to an average of 3,100 and 3,200, respectively (OECD 2014b). The number of available doctors increased from 4.3 per 1,000 persons to 6.2 in 2011 (highest rate in OECD countries) and the number of nurses from 2.7 per 1,000 persons to 3.3 in 2009 (one of the lowest rankings, 32nd out of 34 countries). Life expectancy at birth increased from 78.2 years in 2000 to 80.7 in 2012 and mortality due to cancer and cardiovascular disease fell at a rate matching the average of OECD countries.

On the other hand, however, there is a long list of data showing the existence of considerable problems, a wide disparity in access to adequate care and low levels of meeting needs. When the patients' personal opinion is required and the evaluation is based on self-reference (which, methodologically, is particularly important in the field of social psychiatry), the findings are highly unfavourable.

In relation to the use of health service, studies show that (Kyriopoulos 2014; National School of Public Health 2013):

- One out of three Greeks is forced to modify his/her therapy, by reducing their medication dosage because of financial difficulties.
- Sixty percent of chronically ill patients have no access to health services or are on a long waiting list.
- Chronically ill patients have reduced by 30 % their visits to primary health services in the period 2011–2013.
- Chronically ill patients have reduced by 50 % their primary healthcare spending in the period 2011–2013.
- Hospitalisations for major depression owing to the economic crisis have increased by 50 %.
- Life expectancy is expected to decrease by 3 years as a result of the deterioration in the quality of life.
- Since 2008, infant mortality has increased from 3.31 to 4.28 in 2009, 4.36 in 2010 and 4.01 in 2011.
- The annual public per capita pharmaceutical expenditure will amount approximately to €170, which is the lowest figure in OECD countries.
- Eight out of ten Greeks are forced to reduce spending for daily necessities in order to afford their medication.
- Four out of ten Greeks have reduced spending for food to save money for their medication.

According to a survey conducted on behalf of the Athens Medical Association (2014) on doctors-members of the AMA (ISA), insured persons of the EOPYY (National Organisation for Healthcare Services Provision) and patient associations, the data on patient access to health were unfavourable (sample: 200 AMA members, 800 persons >29 years old and 10 patient associations). Patients quit their treatment because they cannot afford their contribution towards the cost of it. One out of three patients reported that they were unable to find an associated doctor. Sixty-six percent of doctors believe that health services have deteriorated. The most important problem put forward by patients is that they did not find an EOPYY associated doctor, while a considerable percentage stated that they were forced to discontinue their treatment or omit a dose because they could not afford to pay their contribution. Specifically, 18 % of respondents stated that they could not afford to pay for their medication, whereas 11 % were unable to find their medication easily.

And although the specific data were obtained from a sample pertaining to Athens, a study by the Hellenic Open University and the Centre for Health Studies of the University of Athens Faculty of Medicine, conducted on a representative sample of

1,000 people in October 2010 (Pappa et al. 2013), showed that 99 people, 10 % of the total sample, reported that their healthcare needs were not being met and that the two basic reasons for this were cost and lack of time.

More specific data show that the possibility of not receiving essential health services is increased where children are concerned, in the case of women and in the case of individuals with mental disorders or individuals with secondary education only. Therefore, the findings suggest that the socio-demographic characteristics and level of health are important factors which explain why healthcare needs are not being met. Researchers report that such needs will continue to grow, a fact which will exacerbate inequalities in health and access to healthcare services. Another study has shown a significant 15 % increase in the level of non-satisfaction of health needs in a period of 2 years (Kentikelenis et al. 2011).

The data correlated from two studies conducted nationwide by the Department of Health Economics of the National School of Public Health in 2006 and 2011 provide information on 10,572 individuals (Zavras et al. 2013). The results showed that poor health levels by self-reference are more often found in the elderly, the unemployed, pensioners, housewives and individuals suffering from chronic diseases. By contrast, men, individuals with a higher educational level and those with higher benefits, are more likely to report a better level of health for themselves. Also, the likelihood of poor health level reports increases during an economic crisis.

The Hellenic National Committee for UNICEF, in its annual Report "The Situation of Children in Greece 2014 – The Effects of the Economic Crisis on Children", which was prepared in cooperation with the University of Athens and outlines the situation of children in our country, states that the number of children exposed to the risk of poverty in Greece in 2012 was over half a million and actually stood at 521,000, a number which corresponds to 26.9 % of all children, compared to 23.7 % in 2011. The number children exposed to the risk to poverty or social exclusion amount to 686,000 in 2012, compared to 30.5 % in 2011. 52 % of poor households with children in 2012, compared to 44.3 % in 2011, reported being unable to afford a diet which includes the consumption of chicken, meat, fish or vegetables of equal nutritional value every second day.

Social protection benefits for 2011 amounted to 28.0 % of GDP or €60.1 billion and decreased by 4.9 % compared to 2009, a year where they amounted to €63.2 billion. Specifically, family-children social protection benefits to meet family-children-related needs remain unchanged compared to the GDP rate, standing at 1.8 % for 2011, below the EU average (2.2 %), and amount to €3.7 billion, down by 513 million or 12.1 % from 2009 (€4.2 billion). It is estimated that a considerable number of children in Greece have no medical and hospital care as a result of their parents losing social security rights, while other alternative forms of delivery of medical and hospital care do not cover the entire population.

Generally, children's living conditions have deteriorated, as 74.1 % of poor households with children and 29.5 % of nonpoor households reported being unable to meet their extraordinary but also daily living costs. The inability to meet such needs, particularly where children are concerned, lowers their living standards, can expose them to serious health risks, limit their growth potential and push them to the fringes of society (UNICEF 2014, page 35).

Finally, the economic crisis has affected health and healthcare in Greece. It is obvious that apart from the question of how such data should be methodologically defined and measured, there is also the question of how such data should be interpreted in political terms and used and, subsequently, to respond to the crisis. It should be noted that when Sir Douglas Black produced the first reports on inequalities in health based on socioeconomic criteria in the late 1970s (Black Report 1982), the conservative government in the UK prevented their publication. Nevertheless, they prompted large the scale studies later conducted by the WHO and other international organisations. Furthermore, in 2010, Sir M. Marmot, former president of the International Institute for Society and Health and Chairman of the WHO Commission on Social Determinants in Health, expressed his concern at the way in which reports on inequalities in health and cuts in resources are being accepted. Finally, in 2012, in a system such as the British system, where control and monitoring, fulfilment of indicators and criteria and systematic reporting prevails, the disclosure that 43 persons in hospital wards died of reasons which was unrelated to their pathology caused quite an uproar. This disclosure caused Prime Minister Cameron to intervene, and it was considered a national disgrace by the British people. The report on the Mid Staffordshire NHS Foundation Trust Public Inquiry by Sir R. Francis, which followed after the scandal, is a landmark in the history of the difficulties arising in any thorough assessment and surveillance of a health system, calling attention to the need to take in account not just numeric indicators but also the opinions of patients and employees.

It is still too early to provide a clear answer as to the precise extent and manner in which the economic crisis will impair the health of the citizens and healthcare. Although various structures and actions seem to be absorbing a large part of this social and economic strain, all actions to address inequalities, the protection of vulnerable groups and the restructuring of health resources must be immediate.

25.6 Economic Crisis, Social Protection System and Mental Health

It has been established (WHO 2003) that individuals who are at the lower end of the social ladder are two times more likely to suffer from a mental disorder. The effects of the economic crisis on the mental health of adults are particularly evident in the higher rates of mental disorders and, specifically, depression running at 8.2 % in 2011 as opposed to 3.3 % in 2008 (Economou et al. 2013). Furthermore, suicidal ideation among individuals who already receive medication has increased to 22.7 % (2011) compared to 4.5 % in 2009 (Economou et al. 2013), while the use of antidepressants has increased by 34.8 % (2006–2011) (Kyriopoulos 2014). Mental disorder rates have increased considerably; however, only one out of four patients suffering from a mental disorder is receiving treatment.

In children and adolescents, the cases of psychosocial problems have increased by 40 %. Specifically, behavioural disorders rose by 28 %, suicide attempts by 20 % and school dropout by 25 %. Cases of domestic tension have increased by 51 % (due to a parent's unemployment, serious financial problems and debts) (Anagnostopoulos and Soumaki 2013). A study by Stylianidis et al. (2014) is currently underway and already demonstrates high involuntary hospitalisation rates (60 % in the "Dafni" Psychiatric Hospital and 50 % in the Sismanogleio General Hospital), while one of its most important findings includes the fragmentation of mental healthcare where the rates of the "revolving door" phenomena are high.

The fragmentation characterising the provision of mental health services, as demonstrated by the "ex-post evaluation" (MHSS 2010, 2012), is a structural weakness of the public system which has a direct impact on the particularly high therapeutic gap in Greece, standing at 75 % (Skapinakis et al. 2013).

The current socioeconomic conditions and their effect on mental health can be interpreted using the "social determinants" model, as more and more studies substantiate the development of mental disorders caused by the coexistence of one or more aggravating factors. For example, the development of depression has been associated with people of low social and economic status, people whose social position has been undermined or who have experienced violence and the stigma which is becoming a characteristic of persons who are in such a position. Panoussis (2012) classifies the homeless, the working poor, the unemployed and the temporarily employed as an "other people" category and not just poorer and continues saying that "Income poverty and the lack of resources lead to human poverty which is understood to mean the denial of common values. […] A poor person feels entitled and automatically justified in his/her final rejection of the constant ultimate value of life and the values of the society in which he/she lives. On the other hand, poverty is often defined as weakness, poor people are blamed for their failure, solidarity and compassion are continuously disparaged, the enrichment of one person is dramatic for another person and, ultimately, excluded persons are doomed to share between them only the public ills". This gives us an idea of the connection with depression as we are not referring to a loss and a consequent bereavement but a process which includes blame and shame, factors which significantly add to the likelihood of associating the loss with the development of a depressive symptomatology (Kendler et al. 2008). On the basis of the social determinants already mentioned, it is apparent that social and economic inequality has a significant impact on mental health, perhaps greater than poverty in the strict sense of the limited financial resources. In the current crisis, people in vulnerable groups are faced with the "freedom of no choice" (Panoussis 2012), and therefore, they not only have to face their limited financial resources but also uncertainty, limited access to health and mental health services, a low sense of self-esteem, shame and guilt which create a "poverty culture". The current phenomena of psychiatric symptomatology constitute, according to

Stylianidis (2011), "the transient clinic". In his own words: "The clinical signs of the psychotic function which could easily create confusion with a mass of people who live (survive better) in a state of extreme social exclusion and lack of symbolic, imagined and actual inclusion in and integration into a social group" and goes on to define the "transient clinic" as the psychopathology of the "street", through which emerges the same symptomatology found in a prepsychotic or antecedent schizophrenic syndrome. This symptomatology is found "in many social groups, such as the 'healthy' poor and destitute, the homeless, drug addicts without shelter, alcoholics, immigrants looking for work, the long-term unemployed, political refugees seeking asylum, mental patients wondering about expressing – often in a loud manner – their delirious activities" (Stylianidis 2011).

The "Gini" index, where values from 0 (absolute equality) to 1 (absolute inequality) are assigned, is used in an attempt to "measure" economic inequality. In Greece, the specific index (0.3448 in 2009 to 0.3678 in 2012) has increased significantly from 2009 to 2012 (0.3448 in 2009 to 0.3678 in 2012). Thus, as noted by Matsaganis and Leventi (2013), although the austerity measures theoretically targeted the rich, in practice they led to a dramatic loss of income for population groups at the bottom of the income ladder, adversely affecting their already difficult financial situation. They specifically note that persons at the bottom of the income ladder lost 24.2 % of their precrisis income between 2009 and 2012. And if we adjust this percentage on the basis of income distribution in 2012, then the poorer 10 % of the population has lost 56.5 % of its income, and these percentages are clearly lower as we climb up the income ladder.

We realise even more that the conditions of the socioeconomic crisis call for the development of good practices to achieve the best possible result with few resources (cost effective) to support and protect vulnerable social groups.

25.7 Actions to Counter and Overcome the Crisis

In light of the considerations set out in the introduction from a sociological perspective, it is clear that such actions must be specifically designed to address the complex needs arising and must also be innovative. For this reason, we should first examine the macro-level importance of innovative actions in the formulation of mental health policies. Unavoidably, the question of whether individual experiences of innovative actions can provide answers to the questions of a mental health system is raised. According to Bachrach (1980), the differences between a mental health system and a "model programme" are significant and substantial leading to the failure of the latter to provide comprehensive answers to the general problems facing a mental health system. The differences lie in the objectives set, the groups targeted, the techniques used to identify "cases", the allocation of resources and funds and the evaluation procedures applied. In conclusion, it could be argued that innovative actions contribute little to the problems of a mental health system. However, the importance of innovative actions lies in their experimental and pioneering orientation and the principles they are attempting to apply. What are the characteristics of an innovative action?

Innovative Actions

Implement new and original ideas to a limited extent, i.e. an idea or a series of ideas is put into practice for the first time on a small scale. Such new actions challenge established practices and all that they signify (attitudes, perceptions and mentalities) or modify them creatively by setting, for the most part, improvement as their main objective (in both cases).

They are experimental oriented: a change is introduced which also includes an assumption about their outcome.

They try new approaches and practices in order to test their effectiveness. Actually, they are an assumption which is under examination aiming to improve understanding of the phenomena currently being studied or to provide better answers to the hoped-for result of such actions.

They are subject to internal and/or external evaluation. The evaluation of innovative actions is deemed necessary in order to validate or otherwise the effectiveness of the new actions being tested. Usually, such evaluations concern comparative procedures, i.e. the products of such innovative actions by comparing them to the respective products resulting from existing, established practices.

They comprise a cluster of numerous and specific attributes – e.g. combined use of dissimilar resources, specialised or highly trained staff and more favourable funding, which renders them unique events frozen in the specific time period in which they are taking place.

Despite the unique character of innovative actions, they aspire to be disseminated, reproduced and generalized on a greater scale. This, however, depends on a number of factor which usually include the characteristics of the framework in which such innovative action takes place, the degree and extent of its specific characteristics and the contents of the evaluation in relation to the effects triggered by its implementation (as also described above, an innovative action is more of an assumption than a definitive answer to a hoped-for result).

The admissibility of an innovative action by those to which it is addressed or involves is differentiated depending on the time it takes place. Its experimental and/or sometimes radical orientation might cause some form of resistance which subsequently subsides.

The substantiation of an innovative action as such needs to be validated principally by those who are affected by such planned changes or expected effects.

The innovation may involve a new idea, approach and/or mode of implementation.

25.8 Innovative Actions: Implementation Examples

Mobile Mental Health Units

The organisation of mobile units (for a detailed description, see relevant Chapter) involves some elements of innovation and is a community type of care which provides answers to the needs of the community.

Self-Help, Networking and Therapeutic Support in Treating Depression

To counter the effects of the economic crisis, actions are needed to enhance social sustainability. The objective of the WHO-EC Partnership Project on User Empowerment in Mental Health (2008–2011) was to support Member States improve user and carer empowerment strategies and actions. The basic qualities of empowerment according to the WHO and the EU are:

Self-reliance
Dignity and respect
Power – ability to decide
Access to information and resources
Sense of belonging and contributing to a wider community

At the community level, the above is achieved according to the experts and the good practice examples reported by:

State funding for the establishment and operation of local user and carer associations
Self-help groups and other user and carer community networks
Training provided to social partners, such as employers, police officers and the Media, on combating stigma (WHO, Regional Office for Europe 2011)

Therefore, according to these principles, any action promoting the concept and practices of self-help promotes social sustainability. Depression and suicidal tendency are directly linked to social exclusion and the wider social conditions and, as a result, also include population groups mentioned in the above matters of horizontal interest. The action is based on the concept of empowerment of mental health service users and persons with a psychiatric disability. Empowerment aims to change the degree of choices, influence and control of a person in his/her life. The key to empowerment is the removal of barriers preventing access to training, care and representation actions and the transformation of power relationships, such as the patient-specialist relationship (WHO 2011).

The action aims to create a support model for depression which can be disseminated at no great cost. The main purpose is to train mental health service users, people with depressive symptomatology in organising self-help groups for depression. An intervention will be implemented in stages as follows: (a) design of the intervention (training material for the therapeutic intervention and training in self-help), (b) development of an online platform and systemisation of training material in electronic format for e-learning, (c) training of trainers to intervene in ten action areas, (d) therapeutic groups for depression and suicidal tendency, (e) user training on the organisation of self-help groups, (f) development and support of self-help groups, (g) evaluation and (h) dissemination of results.

This action could increase the provision of social welfare services to vulnerable social groups. Depression often leads people to isolation and has a significant impact on their quality of life. It also leads to the disruption of social ties. It affects groups of people living both in urban as well as in remote areas. This action aims to create a support model which can be disseminated at no great cost, even in areas where mental health services are not available or limited. It combines therapeutic treatment, the training of people suffering from depression to cope with the disease and the organisation of self-help groups using the self-organisation methodology. The WHO and EU guidelines stress the importance of user empowerment actions and self-help actions. Therefore, the purpose of this project is to provide social welfare services to people suffering from depression and to train user groups to set up self-help groups. The distance learning method through the online platform will enable users throughout Greece to receive training on the methodology of self-help.

Implementation of the WHO mhGAP Package to Train Non-specialists in Identifying and Dealing with Mental Health Problems

Mental health services cover only a small fraction of the general population's psychiatric morbidity. In countries with a developed primary healthcare (PHC) system, most mental disorders, primarily those known as "common mental disorders", such as anxiety disorders, depression, etc., are covered by the PHC services, which are key contributors to the follow-up of serious mental disorders, always in cooperation with the mental health services in each area (Üstün and Sartorius 1995). The causes vary, from the stigmatisation of the mental disorder and the subsequent unwillingness of patients to receive treatment, the difficulty in accessing mental health services, the absence of education of PHC personnel to the identification and management of mental disorders, etc. This action includes educational interventions as well as the monitoring and evaluation of the function of PHC services and mental health services in mental health regions where it is implemented.

Therefore, as already mentioned in detail above, the implementation of such action is appropriate for the Greek health system which is facing tremendous challenges in the provision of care services and the protection of human rights of people with mental, neurological and substance use disorders. At the same time, mental, neurological and substance use disorders interfere, in substantial ways, with the ability of children to learn and the ability of adults to function in families, at work, and in society at large. Also, there is a widely shared but mistaken idea that improvements in mental health require sophisticated and expensive technologies and highly specialised staff. However, what is required is increasing the capacity of the primary healthcare system for delivery of an integrated package of care by training, support and supervision. That is why, in October 2010, the WHO launched the Mental Health Gap Action Programme (mhGAP), to address the lack of care, especially in low- and middle-income countries, for people suffering from mental, neurological and substance use disorders. Against this background, the WHO designed the "mhGAP Intervention Guide for Mental, Neurological and Substance Use Disorders in Non-Specialized Health Settings", a technical tool for implementation of the mhGAP Programme. It provides the full range of recommendations to facilitate high-quality care services provided at first and second level facilities by non-specialist healthcare providers in resource-poor settings.

Direct and Indirect Beneficiaries
Patients in the field and their families
PHC services
Mental health services

Expected Results
Increase in treated psychiatric morbidity in the field and consequent reduction of "covert" psychiatric morbidity
Improvement of the skills of PHC professionals in identifying and managing mental disorders
Improvement of cooperation between mental health services and PHC
Improvement of follow-up of patients with serious mental disorders and reduction of losses in follow-up

Potential Obstacles to Implementation
Indifference of local mental health entities or PHC.
Doctors' lack of time.
General practitioners believe they are already trained.
Reactions of local stakeholders.

Employment Support to Persons with a Mental Disorder: The Example of Social Cooperatives

It would be ironic, in a period of high long-term unemployment rates – youth unemployment and social exclusion – to set the objective of occupational integration and rehabilitation of persons with a mental disorder. However, good practices in the field of social economy in Greece and abroad show that it is possible to identify innovative actions and synergies with other alternative social economy fields which can widen the possibilities for the users' social reintegration by creating new jobs. Gainful employment is a crucial issue for the mental health of every person. Unemployment rates for persons with mental disorders are higher compared to those with any other disability. The current socioeconomic conditions also make the employment of persons with mental disorders more difficult. Social cooperatives (Koi.SPE) are an innovative legal form of social enterprise in the European area introduced in 1999 by Article 12 of Law 2716/1999 "Development and modernisation of mental health services and other provisions". It is designed for "the socio-economic and occupational integration of persons with serious psychosocial problems and contributes to their treatment and greatest possible financial independence". As mentioned by Mitrouli and as provided by the instruments of incorporation of the social cooperative, "A Social Cooperative is both a therapeutic unit and a cooperative social enterprise. It is a commercial law legal entity whose members have limited liability. It may engage in any economic activity and may, at the same time, produce, supply, consume and, generally, provide services and goods. It is established in a Municipality and the idea is that one Social Cooperative should be set up in each Mental Health Region". So far, 23 social cooperatives have been created and operate throughout Greece, while, at the same time, a second level Panhellenic body was set up in 2011 to represent social cooperatives, the Panhellenic Social Cooperative Association to enhance their representation and interconnection with public and international organisations [Additional information is available on the POKOISPE website].

Development of a Consultation Stations Network to Promote Dementia Prevention and Intervention Actions in Urban Areas and Remote Islands

Services and structures for dementia in Greek are mainly initiatives by non-profit organisations, Alzheimer Societies, and are found principally in the two larger urban centres, Athens and Thessaloniki. There are at present 23 memory clinics, 16 day centres for dementia patients and 3 care at home programmes for dementia patients in Greece, while the recorded number of families with persons suffering from dementia amounts to 200,000. The needs are ever increasing, and the supply of services is limited and often irregular due to underfunding problems (Efthymiou et al. 2012).

The aim of the Athens Association for Alzheimer's Disease and Related Disorders initiative in cooperation with the Regional Development and Mental Health Association (EPAPSY) and CMT Prooptiki is the development of dementia services, to be provided in spaces and structures that the target population are able to visit on a daily basis. In addition, the development of an online distance learning platform will support the training of health professionals within the areas where consultation stations operate as well as every interested health professional in general, by providing access to educational material on dementia and other interactive services as well.

This action covers the operation of 17 consultation stations for dementia prevention and intervention for the general population in Athens and the Cyclades. The project will be implemented in stages as follows: (a) development of standards and scientific planning by a group of experts, (b) set-up and training of an implementation team consisting of 11 health professionals, (c) operation of dementia consultation stations which will provide the population dementia prevention programmes (assessment of mental functions/screening, mental empowerment groups for healthy elderly people, informational speeches in the community) and dementia intervention programmes (operation of memory clinics, non-pharmaceutical interventions for dementia patients and their carers), (d) distance learning for health and care professionals from all over Greece to enable the widest possible implementation of the programme to as many areas as possible, (e) publicity measures and measures for dissemination of results and (f) assessment of the programme.

Host Families: Case Example of Implementation by the Patras SOPSY (Association of Families for Mental Health)

Tomaras et al. (2005) report that, at the national level, Law 2716/1999 on the "Development and modernisation of mental health services and other provisions" (Government Gazette 96/A/17.5.1999) counts "host families" among psychosocial units or programmes. Ministerial Decisions No. 19353 (Government Gazette 1433/B/22.10.2001) and 35724 (Government Gazette 485/B/19.4.2002) work out the details of the provisions of the law. Finally, Ministerial Decision No. 39321 (Government Gazette 453/B/16.4.2010) allows the development of "organised foster and host families" (among several other "complementary actions") by mental health units which, according to Law 2716/1999, belong to non-profit private law entities.

The Patras SOPSY foster family programme, in cooperation with the General Hospital of Arta Psychiatry Department, fulfils all the conditions to become an example of good practice because of the substantial involvement of families, users and citizens and an innovative programme linked to the entire range of sectorised mental health and social welfare services with specific actions at local and national level.

Indications regarding the use of foster families as a psychosocial rehabilitation tool are more focused on the patient's personal history and a competently prepared individual care plan than on diagnostic criteria. The persons put forward for placement in foster families have a disadvantage (temporary or lasting) in managing their daily lives which is associated with their mental disorder. Therefore, the framework of foster families is situated midway between a *care* and *psychosocial rehabilitation* space and a *life place*.

The interdisciplinary team responsible for the final selection of such patients needs to take seriously into account the foster family's resilience, ability and potential psychopathology (Stylianidis et al. 2013). As Stylianidis et al. (2013) go on to say, based on a review of literature and good practices, although no strong empirical basis exists to support their validity and effectiveness, two conclusions can be drawn:

- The main objective set for the first therapeutic foster family type model is the *continuity of psychosocial rehabilitation*, housing and social integration in the shift from the hospital to independent living in the community.
- The second type focuses on the main objective of *stabilising* the course of the serious mental disorder and reduces relapses and readmissions with the least possible economic cost.

It is self-evident that the *first type*, that of the continuous dynamic rehabilitation-recovery-cure and independent living process, has to be the *strategic choice* of this programme, with the following specific objectives:

Improvement of initial symptomatology of patients
Prevention of relapses
Prevention of readmissions
Social inclusion and independent living
Improvement of quality of life of patients
Increase of patient satisfaction compared to traditional psychosocial rehabilitation housing structures
Savings
Improved networking and synergies between foster families and various services within the framework of sectorisation
Promotion of patient empowerment and participation throughout the social inclusion process

Assertive Community Treatment (ACT) and Community Care

Home intervention – (Assertive Community Treatment) – is an intensive intervention programme in the community for people with serious mental conditions (usually schizophrenia or psychotic disorders). The programme may prove to be particularly effective in preventing repeated hospitalisations, by reducing not only costs but also the mental and emotional effect of hospitalisations, particularly after a court order for involuntary psychiatric assessment. The ACT model is already implemented at the EPAPSY Day Centre, Fifth Psychiatric Region (for more information, please see the Chap. 13).

Telepsychiatry

The use of technologies to provide remote mental health services in areas with limited access to health services for geographic or socioeconomic reasons is particularly important. Online consultation and teleconferencing in a telepsychiatry setting may prove particularly useful practices in crisis intervention (e.g. in supervising professionals), the consultation, prevention and rehabilitation of a person (for more information, please see the Chap. 16).

25.9 Conclusions: Comments

As mental health professionals, it is important to overcome our paralysing introversion, the result of numerous frustrations and accumulated disappointment on the suspended step of so-called reform. In addition, we must look at European reality and its institutions not just as a source of financing and a substitute for the crumbling Greek state but also as an area of challenges, exchanges and know-how.

We must create a shared vision of change in a European social solidarity and cohesion setting. It is also important not to consider the problem of public mental health from one dimension only, demanding things from an untrustworthy state but also blaming it, but also to promote new types of synergies, innovations and networking with stakeholders and persons who do not belong to the narrow field of mental health.

Such types of synergies which provide a stable framework for advanced psychiatric reform practices are (a) the empowerment and involvement of the families, friends and users of mental health services at all mental health service levels, assessment and participation in the decision-making process to enable the operation of the system and (b) the systematic synergy and integration of mental health actions (psychiatric care, prevention, etc.), particularly under crisis and dramatic lack of resources conditions, to more comprehensive social and healthcare structures so as to fully meet the people's basic needs.

We must develop what we refer to as the routine of clinical practice, repetition and burnout of staff in mental health units and, by utilising new ideas and knowledge, transform it to what the great art critic, Arthur Danto, defined as "transfiguration of the commonplace". We can move towards collective demands together with other social and political forces, to achieve a new social state which creates a framework for the development of equal possibilities and opportunities for all citizens; towards the rationalisation, reorganisation and qualitative improvement of existing services; and towards the development of a new structure for the social state through education, assessment, targeted operation, economic growth, as well as the necessary changes in policy and institutional processes (Stylianidis 2014).

Bibliography

Anagnostopoulos D, Soumaki E (2013) The status of mental health of children and adolescents in Greece during the crisis. Synapsis 9:11–26 [in Greek]

Athens Medical Association (2014) Presentation of the results for surveys conducted for the Athens Medical Association. Retrieved on 12/07/2014 from http://www.isathens.gr/images/eggrafa/PRESENTATION_ISA_PRESS.pdf

Bachrach LL (1980) Overview: model programs for chronic mental patients. Am J Psychiatry 137(9):1023–1031

Bambra C (2010) Yesterday once more? Unemployment and health in the 21st century. J Epidemiol Community Health 64(3):213–215

Bauman Z (2013a) Liquid love: on the frailty of human bonds. Wiley, New York

Bauman Z (2013b) Liquid modernity. Wiley, New York

Beck U (1992) Risk society: towards a new modernity. Sage, London

Beck U (2006) Living in the world risk society: a hobhouse memorial public lecture given on wednesday 15 February 2006 at the London School of Economics. Econ Soc 35(3):329–345

Black Report (1982) Inequalities in health: black report pelican series. Penguin Books, New York

Castel R (2000) The roads to disaffiliation: insecure work and vulnerable relationships. Int J Urban Reg Res 24(3):519–535

Castel R (2003) From manual workers to wage laborers: transformation of the social question. TransAction Publishers, New Jersey

Castel R (2013) L'insécurité sociale: Qu'est-ce qu'être protégé? Seuil, Paris

Drew N, Funk M, Pathare S, Swartz L (2005) Mental health and human rights. In: Promoting mental health. WHO Press, Geneva

Economou M, Madianos M, Peppou LE, Patelakis A, Stefanis CN (2013) Major depression in the era of economic crisis: a replication of a cross-sectional study across Greece. J Affect Disord 145:308–314

Efthymiou A, Margiotis E, Nikolaou K, Sakka P (2012) Low cost good practices in dementia in Greece. In: Stylianidis S, Ploumpidis D (eds) Minutes of the panhellenic conference for psychosocial rehabilitation: what changes for which new needs. EPAPSY, Athens, pp 111–112

Fountoulakis KN, Theodorakis PN (2014) Austerity and health in Greece. Lancet 383(9928):1543

Fountoulakis KN, Grammatikopoulos IA, Koupidis SA, Siamouli M, Theodorakis PN (2012) Health and the financial crisis in Greece. Lancet 379(9820):1001–1002

Giddens A (2004) The welfare state in a modern European society. Lecture at IX Jornada d'Economia. El future de l'estat del benestar. Retrieved at 8.8.2014 from http://www.uoc.edu/symposia/caixamanresa/jornadaeconomia/eng/giddens.pdf

Jäcklein W (2014) … et dix menaces pour les peuples européens. Le Monde diplomatique, Retrieved at 8.8.2014 from http://www.monde-diplomatique.fr/2014/06/JACKLEIN/50485

Karanikolos M, Mladovsky P, Cylus J, Thomson S, Basu S, Stuckler D, … McKee M (2013) Financial crisis, austerity, and health in Europe. Lancet 381(9874):1323–1331

Kendler K, Myers J, Zisook S (2008) Does bereavement-related major depression differ from major depression associated with other stressful life events? Am J Psychiatry 165(11): 1449–1455

Kentikelenis A, Karanikolos M, Papanicolas I, Basu S, McKee M, Stuckler D (2011) Health effects of financial crisis: omens of a Greek tragedy. Lancet 378(9801):1457–1458

Kentikelenis A, Karanikolos M, Papanicolas I, Basu S, McKee M, Stuckler D (2012) Health and the financial crisis in Greece–authors' reply. Lancet 379(9820):1002

Kentikelenis A, Karanikolos M, Reeves A, McKee M, Stuckler D (2014) Greece's health crisis: from austerity to denialism. Lancet 383(9918):748–753

Kyriopoulos G (26 Jan 2014) National Health System: 30 years later, I Efimerida ton Syntakton. Retrieved on 08/08/2014 from http://www.efsyn.gr/?p=169087

Lapavitsas K (Feb 2014) Impact of financial crisis on economy and society. Lecture at the 6th International Congress on Brain & Behaviour of the International Society on Brain and Behaviour & 19th Thessaloniki Conference of the South-East European Society for Neurology and Psychiatry, Thessaloniki

Madianos M, Economou M, Alexiou T, Stefanis C (2011) Depression and economic hardship across Greece in 2008 and 2009: two cross-sectional surveys nationwide. Soc Psychiatry Psychiatr Epidemiol 46(10):943–952

Marmot M (2005) Social determinants of health inequalities. Lancet 365(9464):1099–1104

Marmot M (2013) Fair society, healthy lives. Inequalities in health: concepts, measures, and ethics. 282

Marmot MG, Bell R (2009) How the financial crisis affect health? Br Med J 338:1314

Matsaganis M, Leventi C (2013) The distributional impact of the Greek crisis in 2010*. Fisc Stud 34(1):83–108

Mezzich JE, Saraceno B (2007) The WPA-WHO joint statement on the role of psychiatrists in disasters response. World Psychiatry 6(1):1

Ministry of Health and Social Solidarity (YYKA) (2010) Report on the assessment of the implementing interventions of Psychiatric Reform for the period 2000–2009. http://www.psychargos.gov.gr/Documents2/Ypostirixi%20Forewn/Ypostirixi%20EPISTHMONIKH/Ex%20Post%20%CE%A0%CE%91%CE%A1%CE%91%CE%94%CE%9F%CE%A4%CE%95%CE%9F%202%20Teliko.pdf. Accessed on: 20 Jul 2014

Ministry of Health and Social Solidarity (YYKA) (2012) Report of the Task Force for the Review of the PSYCHARGOS Programme – National Action Plan PSYCHARGOS C' (2011–2020). MHSS, Athens. Available at: http://www.psychargos.gov.gr/Documents2/%CE%9D%CE%95%CE%91/%CE%A8%CE%A5%CE%A7%CE%91%CE%A1%CE%93%CE%A9%CE%A3%20%CE%93'%20(2011–2020).pdf. Accessed on 31 Jul 2014

National School of Public Health (2013) 30% of Greeks cut back on their medication for financial reasons. Survey conducted by ΚΑΠΑ Research under the supervision of National School of Public Health Department of Epidemiology and Biostatistics. Retrieved on 08/08/2014 from http://www.onmed.gr/ygeia-politiki/item/301209-to-30-ton-ellinon-meionei-ta-farmaka-tou-gia-oikonomikous-logous#ixzz39oeMmoO3

OECD (2014a) Health Statistics 2014. How does Greece compare? Retrieved on 15/07/2014 από http://www.oecd.org/els/health-systems/Briefing-Note-GREECE-2014.pdf

OECD (2014b) Society at a Glance 2014 highlights: Greece The crisis and its aftermath

Panoussis J (Mar 2012) Economic collapse and mental health. In: Stylianidis S, Ploumpidis D (eds) Minutes of the panhellenic conference for psychosocial rehabilitation. Main presentation at the Panhellenic Conference for Psychosocial Rehabilitation: what changes for Which new needs. EPAPSY, Athens, pp 47–49

Pantazopoulos AO (2013) Left-wing nationalism-populism 2008–2013. Epikendro Publications, Thessaloniki

Pappa E, Kontodimopoulos N, Papadopoulos A, Tountas Y, Niakas D (2013) Investigating unmet health needs in primary healthcare services in a representative sample of the Greek population. Int J Environ Res Public Health 10(5):2017–2027

Patel V, Lund C, Hatherill S, Plagerson S, Corrigall J, Funk M, Flisher AJ (2010) Mental disorders: equity and social determinants. In: Equity, social determinants and public health programmes, p 115

Philalithis AE (2001) If I were minister of health: the Greek Health Paradox and the Health Policy Conundrum. In: Towards unity for Health Geneva. Geneva, World Health Organization, 4, pp 13–15

Sakellis G (Mar 2012) Welfare state in crisis. In: Stylianidis S, Ploumpidis D (eds) Minutes of the Panhellenic conference for psychosocial rehabilitation. Main presentation at the Panhellenic conference for psychosocial rehabilitation: what changes for which new needs. EPAPSY, Athens, pp 30–39

Saraceno B, Barbui C (1997) Poverty and mental illness. Can J Psychiatry 42(3):285–290

Saraceno B, van Ommeren M, Batniji R, Cohen A, Gureje O, Mahoney J, … Underhill C (2007) Barriers to improvement of mental health services in low-income and middle-income countries. Lancet 370(9593):1164–1174

Skapinakis P, Bellos S, Koupidis S, Grammatikopoulos I, Theodorakis PN, Mavreas V (2013) Prevalence and sociodemographic associations of common mental disorders in a nationally representative sample of the general population. BMC Psychiatry 13:163–176

Stylianidis S (2011) The transient clinic. Aspects of a personal and social anguish. Clinical and social questions from a psychoanalytical perspective. Oedipus 5:229–249

Stylianidis S (Mar 2012) Psychosocial rehabilitation under economic crisis conditions: what changes for which new needs. Introduction A'. In: Stylianidis S, Ploumpidis D (eds) Minutes of the Panhellenic conference for psychosocial rehabilitation. Main presentation at the Panhellenic conference for psychosocial rehabilitation: what changes for which new needs. EPAPSY, Athens, pp 6–14

Stylianidis S (Aug 2014) Psychiatric reform in cain and titanic Greece. TVXS. Retrieved on 08/08/2014 from http://tvxs.gr/news/egrapsan-eipan/psyxiatriki-metarrythmisi-stin-ellada-toy-kain-kai-toy-titanikoy

Stylianidis S, Peppou L, Mentis E (2013) Therapeutic foster placement of a family of adults with a mental illness: Patras SOPSY. Patras SOPSY, Patras

Stylianidis S, Peppou L, Drakonakis N (2014) Moral and ethical issues on involuntary psychiatric hospitalisation. In: Douzeni A, Lykoura L (eds) Integrity and ethics in mental health. VITA Medical Publications, Athens

Tomaras V, Papageorgiou A, Soldatou M, Gournellis P, Christodoulou GN (2005) Towards the rehabilitation of a chronic mental patient: a pilot foster placement programme. Psychiatriki 16:217–225

Tsiantou V, Kyriopoulos G (2010) The economic crisis and its effect on health and healthcare. Hell Med Arch 27(834):840–21

Tsoukalas K (2012) Greece in limbo and reality. Themelio Publications, Athens

UNICEF (2014) Report: the situation of children in Greece 2014 – the effects of the economic crisis on children. Hellenic National Committee for UNICEF, Athens, Retrieved on 17/07/2014 from: http://www.unicef.gr/uploads/filemanager/PDF/2014/children-in-greece-2014.pdf

Üstün TB, Sartorius N (eds) (1995) Mental illness in general health care: an international study. Wiley, Chichester

Veremis T, Kalyvas S, Kouloumpis T, Pagoulatos G, Tsoukalis L, Tsoukas C (2011) The anatomy of the crisis. Skai Publications, Athens

World Health Organization (WHO) (2003) The solid fActs: social determinants of health, 2nd edn. WHO Europe, Copenhagen

World Health Organization (WHO) (2009) The financial crisis and global health. Report of a High-Level Consultation. World Health Organization, Geneva. Ανασύρθηκε στις 5.7.2014 από: http://www.who.int/mediacentre/events/meetings/2009_financial_crisis_report_en_.pdf

World Health Organization (WHO) (2011) mhGAP intervention guide. WHO Press, Geneva

Zavras D, Tsiantou V, Pavi E, Mylona K, Kyriopoulos J (2013) Impact of economic crisis and other demographic and socio-economic factors on self-rated health in Greece. Eur J Publ Health 23(2):206–210

Index

A

Abstraction, 29
Abuse, child, 345
Alcohol Use Disorders Identification Test (AUDIT), 464
American Nervousness (Beard), 7
Anglo-Saxon movement, 22
Animal magnetism, 7
Antipsychiatry, 12–13, 22, 23, 26, 32, 33, 98
Assertive community treatment (ACT), 491
   abnormality, 250
   accommodation facilities, 269
   and AOT teams, UK
      daycare structures, 255
      housing structures, 256
      inpatient services, 255
   Association for Regional Development, 263–264
   characteristics, 252
   clinical orientation, 251, 270–271
   by CMHT, UK (*see* Community Mental Health Teams (CMHT))
   "coercion", concept of, 250
   commitment, 269, 272
   daily life skills activities, 268, 271
   Franco Basaglia Daycare Centre, 238
   frequency of visits, 268, 271
   Global Assessment of Functioning, 265
   in Greece, 262–263
   interventions, 271
   medication regimen, 268, 271
   methodological tools, 265
   patient self-empowerment system, 250
   psychopathological illnesses, 251
   psychosocial history, 266–267, 270
   quality of life, 251
   rehabilitation and accommodation, 272
   social welfare benefits and financial aid, 272
   team intervention, 267–268
   in USA, 252–253

Asylums. *See also* Madness; Mental health
   in eighteenth century, 6
   first, in Valencia, 5
   Hôpital Général, 5
   locking, 5, 7
   in mid-seventeenth century, 5

B

Being and Time (Heidegger), 31
The Birth of the Clinic (Foucault), 22
Brief psychotherapy
   cognitive-behavioural treatment, 291
   conventional evaluation methods, 292
   EPAPSY Day Centre, 296–298
   Gestalt experiential techniques, 292
   historical overview
      "cathartic" method, 278
      clinical approaches, 280
      "corrective emotional experience", concept of, 281
      early psychoanalytical attitude, 279
      early therapeutic approaches and techniques, 278
      Freud's theory, 279
      patient's regression, 279
      Rank's theory, 280
      therapeutic interventions, 280
   initial assessment, 282–284
   and interpersonal psychotherapy (IPT), 291
   longer-term benefits, 290
   methodological limitations, 292
   "open" psychotherapy treatments, 278
   patient's transference, 287
   psychodynamic approach
      interpersonal existence and interpretation, 287
      Malan's technique, 289

Brief psychotherapy (*cont.*)
   personality and mental health development, 288
   psychic representations, 288
   randomised control trials (RCTs), 289
   self, concept of, 287
   triangle of conflict, 288
   socioeconomic crisis conditions, 278
   socioeconomic framework, 281–282
   supplementary sessions, 286
   theoretical approaches and technical intervention, 290
   therapeutic alliance, 284–285, 292–293
   therapist's attitude, 285–286, 293–295
   training and supervision, 295–296

C

Causality relations
   confidence interval, 43
   confounding, 46–47
   direction of causality, 47
   information bias, 44
   investigator bias, 45
   misclassification error, 44
   non-participation, 46
   randomised controlled test, 43
   recall bias, 44
   selection bias, 44, 45
   significance testing, 43
   testing methods, 44
   types, 44
Child psychiatry
   definition, 195–196
   mobile mental health units, NE and Western Cyclades
   ACT, 198
   assessment and recording, 206–208
   child abuse, 209
   Children's Health Fund, 198
   demographic variables, 201
   diagnosis, 201, 202
   economic crisis, 210
   emotional disorders and behavioural problems, 205
   historical background, 196–197
   international conventions and declarations, 194
   mental disorders prevalence, 194
   mental health prevention and promotion actions, 208–209
   parental involvement, 199
   parental stress, 205
   physical and psychological effects, 195
   primary healthcare doctors, 199
   psychological and social functionality, 193
   resources and consistency, lack of, 209
   rights of children, 194
   schools and teachers, 199
   social integration and participation, 195
   socioeconomic and cultural crisis, 197, 200, 204
   sources of referrals, 203–204
   supervision, role of, 206
Chiswick Women's Aid, 346
Citizens and Madness (Dorner), 12
Clinical governance (CG), 410
Clinical psychology, 10
Community care, 491
Community Mental Health Teams (CMHT)
   assessment and brief treatment/referral teams, 260
   care co-ordinator/case manager, 258
   characteristics, 256–257
   crisis resolution and home treatment teams, 261
   early intervention psychosis teams, 261
   emergency duty teams/out of hours teams, 261
   fixated threat assessment teams, 261
   forensic mental health teams, 261–262
   homeless outreach teams, 262
   recovery and rehabilitation teams, 260–261
   staff, 259
Community psychiatry
   Daycare Centres for Autistic Children, 99–100
   effects on mental health, 128
   ethnopsychiatric approach, 107–108
   Halfway Houses, 100–104
   institutional framework, 376
   Kulturarbeit, 105, 106
   mental pathologies, 107
   neurotic inhibitions and symptoms, 105
   postmodernism, 106, 107
   psychiatric reform, 98–99
   psychoanalytical institutes, 97–98
   psychosocial rehabilitation and recovery, 382
   TT dynamics, 377
The Construction of the Psychoanalytical Space, 372
Continuing day treatment (CDT) programmes, 216
Continuous quality improvement (CQI) framework, 410
Critical psychiatry, 12, 18–21, 146, 317

D

Daseinsanalyse. *See* Psychiatric phenomenology
Daycare units/hospitals
  admission, 217
  for Alzheimer's disease, 218
  for autism spectrum disorders, 218
  case management
    care system, 229
    community ties, 230
    day-to-day skills, 230
    medication, 229
    patient's environment, 229
    professional integration, 230
    replases, prevention of, 230
    support and supervision, 230
    theoretical model and principles, 227–229
  CDT programs, 216
  complementary service, 217
  costs and care, 242–243
  definition, 217
  factors and parameters, 243
  Franco Basaglia Daycare Centre
    ACT, 238
    diagnoses of attendees, 232
    money management, 236
    psychiatric diagnosis and follow-up, 236
    psychosocial rehabilitation unit, 233–236
    psychotherapy service, 237
    self-care and health promotion groups, 236
    social club, 237
    social skills training, 236
  historical development, 218–219
  infrastructure, 224
  mental health services, 217
  multidisciplinary team, 224–226
  neo-institutionalism and asylum's functions, 242
  networking
    and mental health promotion, 238–239
    PSCYHARGOS III Programme, 240
    social cohesion, 239
    social cooperatives, 239
  psychosocial rehabilitation, 216, 218
  recovery model, 216
  research, evaluation and documentation, 240–241
  services, 226–227
  social clubs, 218
  social integration and recovery, 217
  staff, 224
  theoretical model
    Bion's containment and concepts, 221
    cognitive-behavioural therapy (CBT), 223
    cognitive model, 223
    milieu therapy, 220
    negative beliefs, 223
    preconscious, 222
    psychoanalytical theoretical approach, 221, 222
    psychocognition, 222
    quality of life, 223
    schizophrenia, 223
    social skills models, 224
    therapeutic community, 220, 221
  transitional day hospitals, 217
  WARP Declaration, 216
Deficit of democracy and European Union
  constitutional protection, 475
  "Euro agreement", 477
  European harmonisation, 476
  policy deficit, 475
  social protection, 475
Deinstitutionalisation movement, 12–13
Disability-adjusted life years (DALY), 63
Doctor–patient relationship
  biological determinism, 432
  collective democracy of health, 434
  daily institutional/clinical experience, 432
  psychiatric culture, 434
  self-determination, 435
  training programmes, 435
  user involvement, 433
Dolhuysjes, 5
Domestic violence
  anger and stress management skills, 356–357
  child abuse, 345
  communication development, 356–357
  counselling women, 353–355
  criminal mediation, 346
  cultural admixtures and migration, 344
  definitions, 344–345
  family idealisation, 343–344, 348
  feminist theory, 346
  financial resources, 344
  fluid circumstances, 344
  Greek financial crisis, 347
  group therapy, 356
  health sciences, 344
  identification and assessment (*see* Risk assessment)

Domestic violence (*cont.*)
  male victims, 349
  management
    with adult victims, 351–353
    with minor victims, 357–358
  mental health community service, child abuse, 358–360
  Panhellenic study, 347
  primary victims, 347
  self-determination and human dignity, 346
  social exclusion and mental disorders, 344
Double alienation, 22
Dysfunction of the mental health system, 37, 180, 223, 235

E
Economic and social crisis
  British system, 482
  children's living conditions, 481
  deficit of democracy in Europe, 475–477
  Greece
    GDP, 458
    healthcare consequences, 460–461, 465–466
    health-related consequences, 458, 466–468
    mental disorders, 461–465
    socioeconomic consequences, 459–460
    suicide, 461
    Troika, 458
  innovative actions
    ACT, 491
    consultation stations network, 489–490
    dementia prevention and intervention actions, 489–490
    employment support, 488–489
    mobile units, 485
    networking and therapeutic support, 486–487
    patient-specialist relationship, 486
    Patras SOPSY, 490–491
    self-help, 486
    state funding, 486
    telepsychiatry, 491
    WHO mhGAP package, 487–488
  insecurity and ties, 477–478
  multilevel crisis, 474
  protracted recession, 474
  psychiatric and psychological help and treatment, 474
  reflection, 462
  social inequality, 473
  and social protection system, 482–484
  socio-demographic characteristics, 481
  sociological perspective, 484
Electroconvulsive therapy (ECT), 11
E-mental health
  counselling, 333
  "difficult" calls, 335
  information, 333
  online psychological support
    benefits, 338
    counselling via live chat, 337
    determination, 337
    e-mails, 337
    ethical considerations, 338–340
    online self-help/support groups, 338
    video conferencing, 337–338
  psychological support helpline, 332–333
  support, 333
  telepsychiatry
    clarification, issues, 334
    closure, 334
    content exploration, 334
    defintion, 336
    relationship establishment, 334
    service, 336–337
EPAPSY-Association for Regional Development and Mental Health
  chi-square statistical verification, 412–413
  management, 410–411
  mental health promotion, 409
  PROJECT method, 410
  PSYCHARGOS, 409
  psychosocial rehabilitation, 409
  sample rated performance, 414
  sound impact indicators, 410
Epidemiology
  Europe, 449–450
  Greece, 450–451
  investigative design (*see* Investigative design)
Ethical and moral issues, 159
Ethnopsychiatry, 107–108, 315–317
Europe
  compulsory admission criteria, 442
  ECHR, 441
  epidemiology, 449–450
  legal support provision, 443
  mental illness, 442
  national laws and policies, 441
  user involvement, 429–430
European Court of Human Rights (ECHR), 441
European Federation of Families of People with Mental Illness (EUFAMI), 429
Evaluation, social psychiatry services
  administrative procedures and outcomes, 390
  assessment indices, 393
  clinical-therapeutic programmes, 390
  cost/effectiveness analysis, 395

Index

decision-making process, 390
efficacy and effectiveness, 392
extended health system, 390
financial quality, 392
high-quality services, 391
and human rights, 401, 402
interpersonal component, 391
matrix model, 393
medical quality, 392
mental health services, 393–395
pubic health system, 399–401
service quality, 391
social quality, 392
structure-process-outcome, 391
treatment protocols, 393
Evidence-based medicine, 53–54
Existentialism
Anglo-Saxon movement, 22
and asylums, 21–23
biomedical model, 24
Burton's and Basaglia's notion, 22
critical psychiatry, 19–20
double alienation, 22
existence, 19
and Foucault, 21–26
institutional neurosis, 22
moral treatment, 21
pathology of madness, 23
Pinel, 21–24, 26
Renaissance, 25

F
Feminist theory, 346
Freudian theory, 10

G
Generalised anxiety disorder (GAD), 463
Global Burden of Disease (GBD), 63
Global mental health
accessibility, 60, 61, 65, 66, 71
DALY, 63
definition, 59
depression and suicidality, 73
economic burden of mental disorders, 64
estimate cost types, 64
GBD, 63
human rights, 61
life expectancy, 65
local services, 65
in low-, middle-and high-income settings, 60, 61
material conditions, 65
MGMH, 61–62
national level, 65
and online databases and platforms, 66–67
parental behaviour, 65
personal and social level, 61
psychotropic drugs, 62
resource availability
DALYs, 67–68
high conditions, 69–70
low conditions, 67, 69
middle conditions, 69
rights to mental health, 59
self-directed psychological treatment exercises., 62
social determinants, 64, 67, 72, 73
social support, 65
treatment gap, 60–63
trust and security, 65
World Health Report, 2008, 64
Governing the Soul (Rose), 33
Great confinement, 5, 17, 23, 25
Greece
epidemiology, 450–451
EUNOMIA, 448
financial crisis, 347
involuntary hospitalisation, 444, 446
National Emergency Centre (EKAV), 448
patient's assessment, 444
psychiatric epidemiology, 54–55, 57
therapy, 443
user involvement, 430–432
Greece's special situation, 478–479
Greek mental health system, 78, 399
Group therapy, 12

H
Halfway Houses
deinstitutionalisation, 102
in institutions, 101
mental health institution, 102–104
residential units and sheltered accommodation, 100–101
Hard biomedical model, 18, 19
Health. *See also* Mental health
aspects of, 119
functional definition, 118
historic definition of, 118
illness prevention, 121
interdependence, mental and physical, 118
promotion, 120–121
WHO definition, 118
Health promotion, 120–121
The History of Madness (Foucault), 12, 21, 23
Hôpital Général, 5
Human superorganism, 128
Husserlian phenomenology, 29–32
Hypnotism, 8

I

Illness prevention, 121
Individual and social pain
   ethnopsychiatric approach, 107–108
   Kulturarbeit, 105, 106
   mental pathologies, 107
   neurotic inhibitions and symptoms, 105
   postmodernism, 106, 107
Individualised socialisation, 35
In-patient services and out-patient–social mental health centres, 99
Institutional neurosis, 22
Insulin comas, 11
International Association for Child and Adolescent Psychiatry, 123
International Convention on the Rights of Persons with Disabilities (CRPD), 61
Interpersonal cognitive problem-solving programme (ICPS), 122
Interpersonal psychotherapy (IPT), 291
Investigative design
   advantages and disadvantages, 48, 49
   case-control studies, 51
   classic cohort studies, 51–52
   ecological studies, 48, 50
   and evidence-based medicine, 53–54
   experimental studies, 48
   involuntary hospitalisation, 47–48
   observational studies, 48
   randomised controlled tests, 52–53
   synchronic/cross-sectional studies, 50–51
   systematic review of abstracts, 48
Involuntary hospitalisation
   in Athens, 452–453
   clinical indicators, 451
   compulsory admission/involuntary treatment, 440
   epidemiology (*see* Epidemiology)
   human rights (patients' movement), 440–441
   psychiatric care, 440
   public safety, 440
   study of outcomes, 451–452
   treatment, 452
Italian deinstitutionalisation movement, 12

L

Legislative framework
   Europe (*see* Europe)
   Greece (*see* Greece)
Lived experiences, 26–32

M

Madness. *See also* Asylums; Mental health
   as alienation, 22–25
   cause of, 6
   ethics and hermeneutics of, 18
   Foucault's theory on, 25–26
   partial/occasional, 21
   pathology of, 23
   traitement moral, 4–7
Manu militari, 14
Matrix model, 240, 392–393
Mental disorders
   AUDIT, 464
   GAD, 463, 464
   Index of Personal Economic Distress, 462
   psychometric properties., 462
   SCID-I, 462
   UMHRI, 461–462, 464
   unemployment and financial hardship, 463
Mental health. *See also* Asylums; Health; Madness; Promotion, mental health
   antiquity, 4
   biomedical model, 13
   Byzantine Empire, 4–5
   development of, 4
   DSM-III, 13
   hypnotism, 8
   Italian deinstitutionalisation movement, 12
   managed care, 13
   Mental Health Declaration for Europe, 118
   nervous disorders, 7
   neurasthenias, 7–8
   neuroses, 8
   nineteenth century, end of, 7
   Ottoman Empire, 5
   prevalence, mental disorder, 119–120
   prevention, 8–9
   promotion (*see* Promotion, mental health)
   psychiatric revolution, 14
   psychotherapists, in USA, 4
   Victorian era illnesses, 7–8
   WHO definition, 119
Mental health community service, child abuse, 358–360
Mental health movement
   clinical psychology, 10
   Freudian theory, 10
   military activities, 9–10
   prefrontal lobotomies, 11
   shell shock, 10
   shock treatments, 11
   WWI, 9–10
   WWII, 10

Mental health structures
  classification system, 396
  clinical information, 397–398
  epidemiological research, 396
  ethical and deontological basis, 86
  political support, 85
  psychiatric reform, 393–395
  psychiatric treatments, 87
  quality assurance, 393
Mental institution, 370, 375, 377, 419
Mental states, 28
Mesmerism, 7
Metropolitan Athens
  classes and ethnic minorities, 135
  data analysis, 137
  discrimination and sense of insecurity, 142
  feasibility sampling, 136
  interview tool, 137
  mental illnesses, 140
  migrants and homeless population, 135
  physical illnesses, 139
  poverty, 136
  self-image, 138
  socio-demographic profile, 137–138
  stress and depression, 136
  substance dependence, 140–141
Micro-social crises, 22
Migrants' mental healthcare
  access to rights, 324
  Babel Day Centre, in Athens
    client-centred network, 319
    communication, 320
    community links, 322
    daily routine, 322
    education, 325–326
    external circumstances, 321
    family constellation, 321
    legal position, 322
    media campaign, 318
    mental resilience, 319
    networking, 325
    nostalgic disorientation, 320
    Papadopoulos' theoretical approach, 320, 321
    physical health, 321
    psychological/psychiatric state, 322
    reception process, 322
    volunteering, 326
  chronic pain, 311
  cultural competence, 313–314
  cultural mediation, 315
  definition, 310
  ethnopsychiatry, 315–317
  identity, 323
  inadequacy of resources, 324
  personal characteristics, 311
  political and socioeconomic framework, 311
  post-migration stress and weight, 312
  prevalence, 311
  PTSD, 311
  risk of victimisation, 325
  social interaction characteristics, 311
  therapeutic alliance, 323–324
Military neuroses, 10
Modern psychiatry, transformation
  "agentic" subjectivities, 34
  contemporary approaches, 33–35
  globalised capitalism, 34
  Miller's approach, 33
  narratives, 34
  new therapeutic techniques, 34
  psychotherapeutic drugs, 34
  subjective-existential experience, 33
Moral treatment, 21
The Myth of Mental Illness (Szasz), 12

N
Neoliberalism
  exile of the paternal figure, 35
  "hedonist" ideal, 35
  internal exile, 35
  mass media and advertising, 35–36
  passive attitude, 35
  professional life, 36
  social bond, 36, 37
  social disaffiliation, 37
  social insecurity, 36
Neo-liberal model, 36, 477, 479
Nervous system diseases, 7–9
Neurasthenias, 7–8
Neuroleptics, 11
Neutral introspection, 27
The New Psychology and Its Relation to Life (Tansley), 10
The Normal and the Pathological (Canguilhem), 24
Not Made of Wood (Foudraine), 12

O
Observational neutrality, 28
Online counselling
  counselling via live chat, 337
  exchange of e-mails, 337
  video conferencing, 337–338

Online psychotherapy
  benefits, 338
  counselling via live chat, 337
  determination, 337
  e-mails, 337
  ethical considerations, 338–340
  online self-help/support groups, 338
  video conferencing, 337–338
Operation procedures, mental health system, 390, 393–395
Organisational culture
  assessment scale, 406
  behavioural norms, 407
  EPAPSY (*see* EPAPSY-Association for Regional Development and Mental Health)
  factorial analysis, 414
  graphic rating scale, 406
  health sector, quality and performance, 409
  intervention limitations, 418
  macro-culture theory, 407
  microculture theory, 407
  qualitative analysis, 416–417
  rating of structures, 415

P
Patras SOPSY (Association of Families for Mental Health), 490–491
Phenomenology. *See* Subject and phenomenology
Philosophical foundations. *See* Subject and phenomenology
Positive and Negative Syndrome Scale (PANSS), 265
Postmodern individualism, 33
Post-traumatic stress disorder (PTSD), 311
The Power of Psychiatry (Miller and Rose), 33
Prefrontal lobotomies, 11
Promoting Alternative Thinking Strategies (PATHS) programme, 122
Promotion, mental health
  in Cyclades, 2, 12
  in Greece
    assertive learning, 124–125
    awareness-raising groups, 125
    disadvantage, 128
    experiential learning, 125
    intellectual and emotional processes, 125
    planning interventions, 124–125
    primary protection, children and adolescents, 123–124
    programme evaluation, 126–127
    web of life, 128
  ICPS, 122
  importance of, 121–122
  International Association for Child and Adolescent Psychiatry, 123
  intervention programme, for adolescents, 122, 123
  parents and teachers, primary school, 123
  PATHS programme, 122
  RIPP programme, 122
  school environment, 122, 123
Psychiatric epidemiology
  causality relations
    bias, 44–46
    confounding, 46–47
    direction of causality, 47
  definition, 42
  documentation, 42, 50, 53
  and evidence-based medicine, 53–54
  in Greece, 54–55
  homogenisation, 57
  methodology, 42, 52
  prevalence of disorders, 42, 43
Psychiatric institutions, 376, 380, 381, 383
Psychiatric phenomenology, 29–32. *See also* Subject and phenomenology
Psychiatric reform
  in Greece
    cost-benefit, 87
    education system, 77
    epidemiological data, 83, 88
    ethical and deontological basis, 86
    evidence-based best practices, 89
    health system, 79
    mental disorder, 83
    mental health and care services, legal framework, 80
    objections, 87–88
    political support, 85
    primary healthcare, 77
    PSYCHARGOS programme, 81
    psychiatric treatments, 87
    public health perspective, 88
    resource availability, 79, 87
    social principles, 78
    welfare network, 85
  of mental health system, 393–395
  quality assurance, 393
Psychiatrists
  madness and neurasthenia, 8
  military, 9–10
  schizophrenia, 11
  social work, 8

Index	517

Psychiatry and Anti-psychiatry (Cooper), 12
Psychiatry and psychocognition, 222, 242
Psychoanalytical structures in the community
   in hospital services and in community, 97–104
   individual and community pain, 104–108
   mental health structures, 108
   processuality, 109
   subjectivity and mental pain (*see* Subject of mental pain)
Psychoses
   adolescence, 369
   chronic psychotic pathology, 369
   healthcare institutions, 369
   mental life, 368
   schizophrenia, 368
   sexuality, 367
   subjectification process, 370
Psychotherapists, 4, 8, 11
Pubic mental health system evaluation, 399–401

Q
Quality assurance, 392, 393, 395

R
Radicalism, 11–13
Rationalism, 13–14
Reactivity, 374
Reductionism, 11, 17, 18, 21, 434
Reflexive knowledge, 27
Renaissance, 22, 25, 26
Responding in Peaceful and Positive Ways (RIPP) programme, 122
Revised Clinical Interview Schedule (CIS-R), 464
Risk assessment
   medical care, 351
   physical injuries, 350
   psychological symptoms, 350
   psychosomatic symptoms, 350

S
Safety plan, 351–353
Sexuality of patients
   acute psychotic episode, 380–381
   countertransference particularities, 372–375
   deinstitutionalisation, 366
   institutional psychotherapy, 366

patient's sexual impulses, 366
psychoanalytical development, 366
psychosocial rehabilitation and recovery, 382
and psychotic disorders (*see* Psychoses)
psychotic pathology, 366
recovery process, 382
supervision process, 383
TT (*see* Therapeutic team (TT))
Shell shock, 10
Social disaffiliation, 37
Socio-economic inequality, 194–195, 483
Sociological foundations
   community psychiatry, 18
   critical psychiatry, 18
   great confinement, 17
   hard biomedical model, 18, 19
   reductionism, 17, 18
   social psychiatry, 18
   soft biomedical model, 18, 19
   traditional psychiatry, 18
Soft biomedical model, 18, 19
Staff assessment, mental health *see* Organisational culture
Stavros Niarchos Foundation, 123–124
Structured Clinical Interview (SCID-I), 462
Subject and phenomenology
   abstraction, 29
   analogic and symbolic components, 31
   analysis of existence, 31
   Cartesian approach, 28–29
   conscious experience, 27
   epokhe, Husserl, 29, 30, 32
   Heidegger phenomenology, 31–32
   Husserlian phenomenology, 29–32
   introspective approach, 28
   Jackson's thesis, 28
   jealousy, 28
   mental states, defined, 28
   nonrepresentation, 30–31
   observational neutrality, 28
   pain and anger, 27
   phenomenology, defined, 26–27, 29
   preconceptions, 29
   reflexive knowledge, 27
Subject of mental pain
   atheoretical classification system, 96
   clinical approach, 96
   diagnostic and therapeutic value, 95
   subject-based psychiatry, 97
   traitement moral, 95
Systemic family psychotherapy, 12
System structural elements, 269

T

Telepsychiatry, 491
   clarification, issues, 334
   closure, 334
   content exploration, 334
   defintion, 336
   relationship establishment, 334
   service, 336–337
Therapeutic team (TT)
   collective illusion, 370
   connection and transformation processes, 370
   "counterfeit", 371
   group matrix, 370
   group mental instrument, 370
   human communication, 371
   mental institution, 370
   psychoanalysis, 371
   psychotic psychopathology, 370
   recovery-healing, mental disease, 371
   "relational grid", 372
Transference-counter-transference (CT)
   autoerotic/aloerotic function of release, 374
   collateral CT, 374, 375
   Freudian concept, 373
   personal analysis, 372
   projective identification, 374
   psychoanalytical theory, 375
   psychotic patient's disease, 376
   saviour syndrome, 373
   transmutation, 374
Treaties of Madness (1758), 6

U

University Mental Health Research Institute (UMHRI), 461–462
User and family participation
   advocacy, 426–427
   asylum-based, closed care, 427
   EMILIA project, 428
   empowerment process, 425–426
   at European Level, 429–430
   functionality, 428–429
   in Greece, 430–432
   mental health professional relationship, 432–435
   quality of life, 428–429
   social role and position, 426
   symptomatology, 428–429

V

Victorian era illnesses, 7–8

W

Web of life, 128

Y

Years lived with disability (YLD), 62

Printed by Printforce, the Netherlands